The Vulva

EDITED BY

Constance Marjorie Ridley
MA BM FRCP

Consultant Dermatologist, Elizabeth Garrett Anderson, Royal Northern and Whittington Hospitals, London

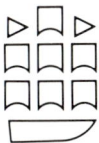

CHURCHILL LIVINGSTONE
EDINBURGH LONDON MELBOURNE AND NEW YORK 1988

CHURCHILL LIVINGSTONE
Medical Division of Longman Group UK Limited

Distributed in the United States of America by Churchill
Livingstone Inc., 1560 Broadway, New York, N.Y. 10036, and
by associated companies, branches and representatives
throughout the world.

First published 1988

ISBN 0 443 03265 3

British Library Cataloguing in Publication Data

The Vulva.
  1. Vulva—Diseases
  I. Ridley, Constance Marjorie
  618.1′6   RG261

Library of Congress Cataloging in Publication Data

The Vulva.

  Rev. ed. of: The vulva/Constance Marjorie Ridley.
1975.
  Includes index.
  1. Vulva—Diseases.   I. Ridley, Constance Marjorie.
[DNLM: 1. Vulvar Diseases.   WP 200 V991]
RG261.V85   1988   618.1′6   87-13837

Produced by Longman Group (FE) Ltd
Printed in Hong Kong

Preface

The reason thought to justify publication of The Vulva in 1975 is that for the compilation of this larger volume now; the need, that is, for a comprehensive survey of conditions affecting the vulval area.

These conditions may be infective, neoplastic, or neither. To unravel their causation and to institute effective treatment may call for the skills of several types of specialist, clinical and non-clinical. Publications on relevant matters are scattered in the literature of the various specialities and it is hoped that to collate them will be of value in management of patients. Furthermore, juxtaposition of such diverse material will perhaps at once prompt useful discussion between specialists and provide a basis for it.

The sheer amount of material available, the recondite nature of some of it and sometimes the need for it to be transmuted into terms intelligible to the clinician has led me to call upon several authors.

Multi-author works however are vulnerable to problems of overlap and even of disagreement. While trying to minimise these trends, I have not been Draconian in eliminating them since confrontation of different views is valuable, and to cut out all overlap would curtail the natural development and continuity of thought by the individual author.

It is inevitable in a book of this sort that some chapters will be of little direct relevance to any particular reader and that some will contain much more detail than that reader may require. This consideration applies in particular to the detailed accounts of the embryology and anatomy of the lower genital tract, and of techniques for virological diagnosis. To have ample accounts of topics not to be easily found discussed as a whole elsewhere is however one of the aims of this volume.

London, 1988

C.M.R.

Acknowledgements

I should like to thank all my contributors for their involvement. My thanks also go to many colleagues who have supplied photographs and have enabled me to see many interesting patients. My colleagues in the departments of histopathology and photography at the Whittington Hospital have been most helpful. I am indebted to Professor K Dover and to Mr L Payne for some historical information.

I am grateful to those who have coped with the laborious typing of this work. The staff of Churchill Livingstone have been very helpful and supportive and I should like to thank especially Mrs Sylvia Hull, Miss Georgina Bentliff, Miss Yvonne O'Leary and Mr James Dale. My thanks are also extended to the compiler of the index.

Professor Fox and Dr Buckley wish to thank Mrs Linda Chawner for her invaluable assistance in the preparation of the photomicrographs of chapters 8, 9 and 10.

Contributors

John J Bradley MB FRCP FRCPsych
Consultant Psychiatrist, Whittington Hospital.
Hon Senior Lecturer, Royal Free Hospital School
of Medicine, London

C Hilary Buckley MD FRCPath
Senior Lecturer in Gynaecological Pathology,
University of Manchester. Honorary Consultant
Histopathologist, St Mary's Hospital for Women
and Children, Manchester

Michael J Campion BSc MB BS DRCOG
Fellow in Gynaecological Oncology, Royal
Northern Hospital, London

H Fox MD FRCPath FRCOG
Professor of Reproductive Pathology, University of
Manchester. Honorary Consultant Pathologist,
St Mary's Hospital, Manchester

Dennis J McCance BSc PhD
Senior Lecturer in Microbiology, Guys Hospital
Medical School, London

J M McLean MB BS BSc MD
Senior Lecturer in Anatomy, University of
Manchester

J D Oriel MD
Consultant Physician in Genitourinary Medicine,
University College Hospital, London

C Marjorie Ridley MA BM FRCP
Consultant Dermatologist, Elizabeth Garrett
Anderson, Royal Northern and Whittington
Hospitals, London

A Singer PhD FRCOG
Consultant Gynaecologist, Royal Northern and
Whittington Hospitals, London

EN ceſte figure ſont demonſtrez les Membres eſtant en la femme, quant a la ſituatiõ, liaiſon, & entremeſlurc. A. demõſtre la partie de la veine du foye, autremẽt dicte, caué. BB. les veines ſeminales, elles ſont de coleur blanchaſtre: par ces vaines eſt icíte la ſemence. CC. ſont les veines, les q̃lles embraſſent l'amarri, ou matrice. DD. les couillõs de la femme. F. l'amarri, matrice. la portiere. GG. les cornes de la matrice. H. lentree deans la matrice, ou l'oriſice interieux. I. le col de la matrice, aultremẽt, la partie honteuſe. KK. le tronc de la vei ne du foye, caué. plante par les cuiſſes au bas du genou. LL. ceſt le tronc de la plus grãde ar tere dicte aorte, a cauſe qu'elle eſt la ſource de toutes les aultres Arteres. M. monſtre la veſ ſie. QQ. petiz conduictz par ou paſſe l'ourine en la veſſie, dictz en grec vriteres. PP. Les reins, ou roignõs. OO. les veines   deſcendãt aux roignõs de couleur blãchatre.

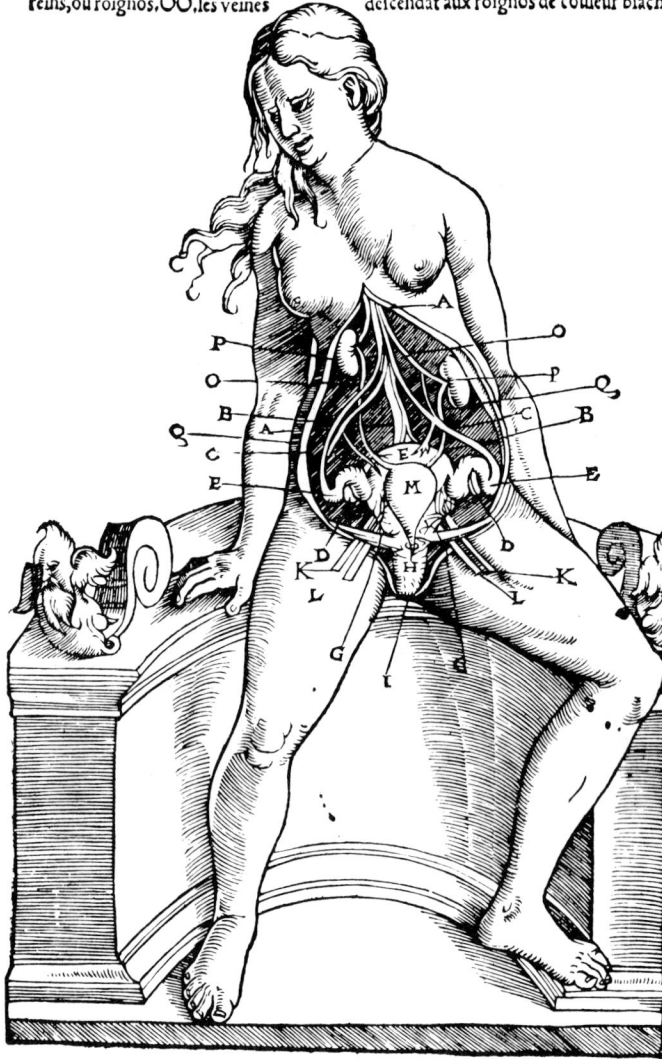

IN HAC FIGVRA GENERATIONIS MEMBRA IN muliebri ſexu quo ad ſitum & colligantiam demonſtrantur. A. pars venæ cauæ eſt. BB. venæ ſeminales candidæ. CC. venæ vterum amplexantes. EE. inuolucrum ex ſeminarijs venis & arterijs conſtans. DD. mulieris teſticuli. F. matrix ſiue vterus. GG. cornua matricis. H. orificium matricis interius. I. collum matricis, pudibunda. KK. venæ cauæ truncus in crura implantatus. LL. arteriæ aortæ truncus eſt. M. ve ſica. QQ. vreteres. PP. renes. OO. venæ albæ renales.

Seated female showing viscera. Walter Hermann Ryff (fl. 1539). From the original in the Wellcome Library by courtesy of the Trustees.

Contents

Embryology and congenital anomalies of the vulval area
J M McLean

Initially the embryonic pelvis or tail fold contains only the hindgut, which terminates at the cloacal membrane. Subsequently the urorectal septum divides the hindgut and cloacal membrane into the ventral or anterior urogenital sinus and genital membrane and the dorsal or posterior terminal gastrointestinal tract and anal membrane. At a later stage the female reproductive tract develops within the urorectal septum and in doing so incorporates part of the urogenital sinus and body wall elements associated with the genital membrane. Thus the pelvis eventually accommodates parts of the urinary, reproductive and gastrointestinal systems, all of which communicate with the exterior at the pelvic outlet. That part of the pelvic outlet caudal to the pelvic floor is the anatomical perineum, which is divided by a line joining the ischial tuberosities into an anterior urogenital triangle and a posterior anal triangle. The anal triangle, bounded by the sacrotuberous ligaments, contains the anal canal and ischiorectal fossae. The urogenital triangle, contained within the subpubic arch, is occupied by the vulva.

Although the critical events in the embryogenesis and organogenesis of the female reproductive tract are genetically determined the subsequent processes of differentiation are also crucial to the development of the urinary system and terminal part of the gastrointestinal system. Thus congenital abnormalities of the female reproductive tract, including the vulva, may occur in isolation or in association with urinary or gastrointestinal abnormalities. Some of the aetiological factors responsible for abnormal or ambiguous human sexual development have now been established. This information has helped to rationalise the medical management of affected individuals. In addition these 'experiments of nature' have provided much information concerning the biological mechanisms underlying normal sexual development.

EMBRYOLOGY

Because development is a continuous process various means have been used to identify and tabulate the progression of events during normal human embryogenesis. The founder of the Department of Embryology at the Carnegie Institution in Washington, Franklin Mall, was the first to introduce staging into human embryology. His observations and those of Streeter, his successor at the Carnegie Institution, form the basis upon which the first 8 weeks of human development, which constitute the embryonic period, are described in 23 Carnegie stages. Alternatively, embryonic length or age may be used as a means of identifying the developmental stage and in this account the reference point will be the postovulatory age, that is, the length of time since the last ovulation, related, when appropriate, to the Carnegie stage. Since ovulation and fertilisation are closely related in time the postovulatory interval is an adequate measure of embryonic age. Embryonic age, length and stage are all interrelated. Age, however, conveys an immediate meaning since it is a familar yardstick, but it must be recognised that prenatal ages are only as useful as postnatal ages, since they are reference points for the usual pattern or range of developmental events.

Fertilisation

Human life and development begin at fertilisation when the spermatozoon and ovum fuse to form the zygote or conceptus. The normal haploid set of 23 chromosomes in each human gamete yields a zygote with the diploid set of 46 chromosomes. Each female gamete begins its first meiotic division during intra-uterine life and completes it at ovulation, while its second meiotic division is completed during the process of fertilisation (Uebele-Kallhardt 1978). This protracted reduction division delivers 22+ X chromosomes to the newly formed zygote, which also receives 22+ X or 22+ Y chromosomes from the male gamete. The resulting chromosomal complement of the zygote is 44+ XX or 44+ XY and thus its genetic or chromosomal sex is established.

Sex chromosomes

While studying spermatogenesis in the insect *Pyrrochoris apterus* the German cytologist Henking (1891) observed that one of the chromosomes remained undivided. This chromosome was therefore present in only half of the spermatozoa produced by the adult male insect. When it was later suggested (McClung 1902) that this chromosome might have a sex-determining role, it had already been designated the X chromosome (McClung 1899) and so it has remained. Thus the male *P. apterus* with only one sex chromosome is XO and the female with two sex chromosomes is XX. Stevens (1905) subsequently noted a variant of the two types of spermatozoa. In the common mealworm beetle *Tenebrio molitor* she observed that spermatozoa had either ten large chromosomes or nine large chromosomes and a single small chromosome. Since adult female cells possessed 20 large chromosomes and adult male cells one small and 19 large chromosomes, she suggested that the character of the spermatozoon determined the sex of the progeny. About the same time Wilson (1906) made identical observations and referred to the small chromosome as the Y chromosome. Thus in *Drosophila melanogaster*, so beloved of geneticists, males are XY and females XX. The Y chromosome, however, was not considered to have any male-determining function since, in *Drosophila*, flies with XXY chromosomes are normal fertile females while those with XO chromosomes are sterile males (Bridges 1916). Indeed the chromosomal constitution of the human male was thought to be XO (von Winiwarter 1912, Oguma & Kihara 1923) until the Y chromosome was demonstrated in man (Painter 1924).

Before the introduction of modern cytological techniques observations on human chromosomes were not wholly reliable. With the use of dividing cells in tissue culture, however, Tjio and Levan (1956) established the human diploid number of chromosomes as 46. This was confirmed by Ford & Hamerton (1956) who also provided unequivocal evidence of the presence of an X and a Y chromosome in human male cells. These new techniques not only established the normal male and female sex chromosome constitutions, they also revealed a number of sex chromosome abnormalities associated with familiar clinical syndromes. The XXY sex chromosome pattern in Klinefelter's syndrome (Jacobs & Strong 1959) and the XO pattern in Turner's syndrome (Ford et al 1959) suggested that, contrary to the situation in *Drosophila*, the human Y chromosome was male determining and the number of X chromosomes had no major effect on the process of sex determination.

Sexual differentiation and determination

Procreation by sexual means allows an infinite range of genetic variation, the opportunity of its unique expression and its subsequent conservation for future generations. Gonochorism, whereby males and females develop as separate individuals, may arise by the operation of environmental factors such as temperature in reptiles or host size in nematodes (Bull 1981). It is generally, although not unanimously, accepted that environmental sex determination was the first and most primitive mechanism for producing two sexes and that this was later replaced by the XX/XY genotypic mechanism (Witschi 1929, Ohno 1967, Mittwoch 1971, 1975). The majority of mammalian species conform to the XY/XX system with the Y chromosome being male determining (Vorontsov 1973). The variety and diversity of sex-determining mechanisms occurring in animals and plants and their evolution has been authoritatively reviewed by Bull (1983).

Reference to sex-determining chromosomes draws attention to the problems of distinguishing between determination and differentiation during embryogenesis. Determination describes events which irrevocably commit cells to a certain course of development and differentiation describes the processes whereby these cells achieve this development. Since the sex of the human individual is established at fertilisation this may be regarded as the definitive act of determination with all that follows being processes of embryonic differentiation. This is a sequential process whereby the genetic or chromosomal sex of the zygote determines the gonadal sex of the embryo, which itself regulates the differentiation of the internal and external genital apparatus and hence the sexual phenotype of the individual. At puberty the development of secondary sexual characteristics reinforces the phenotypic manifestations of the sexual dimorphism, which achieves its biological fulfilment in successful procreation. Both male and female embryos possess the same indifferent gonadal and genital primordia which have an inherent tendency to feminise unless specifically prevented from doing so by masculinising factors. The indifferent gonads differentiate into ovaries in the absence of the testis-organising factor regulated by the Y chromo-

some. Thereafter female differentiation of the internal and external sexual organs continues in the absence of specific masculinising factors which are normally secreted only by the developing testes. This process of female differentiation is not dependent on the presence of ovaries and will occur in the agonadal embryo. The sexual dimorphism that results from sexual differentiation in placental mammals is therefore mediated by the testis and its secretions. Furthermore this male differentiation takes place in an environment of high oestrogen and progestagen concentrations.

In humans these differentiating processes are regulated by at least 30 specific genes located in sex chromosomes or autosomes that act through a variety of mechanisms, including organising factors, sex steroid and peptide secretions and specific tissue receptors (Grumbach & Conte 1981)

Early embryogenesis

Progress in assisted human reproduction and the publication of the Warnock Report (1984) has focused attention on the early stages of human

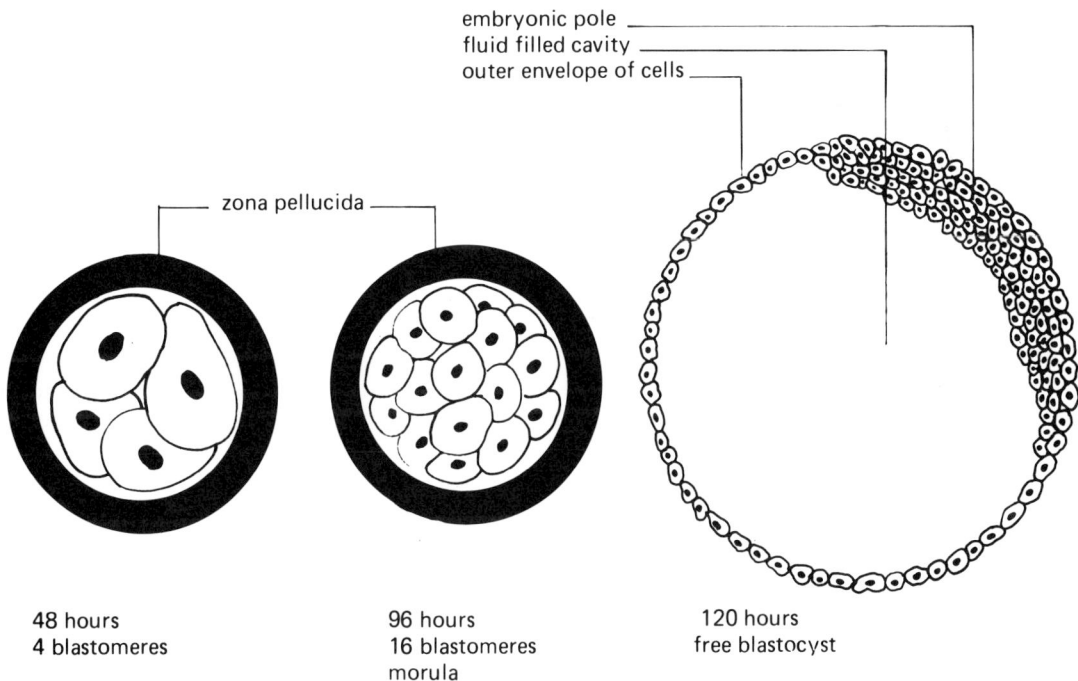

Fig. 1.1 The conceptus, as the morula, is enclosed within an acellular envelope, the zona pellucida. Dissolution of the zona pellucida allows formation of the blastocyst with an embryonic pole or inner cell mass, and a characteristic fluid-filled cavity.

embryogenesis. The events of this period are critically important for the subsequent development of all organ systems including the genitourinary and terminal gastrointestinal systems.

Carnegie stage 1 embraces the process of fertilisation in which the human zygote, with its XX or XY sex chromosome constitution, is conceived in the distal third of the uterine tube (Croxatto & Ortiz 1975). Carnegie stage 2 extends from the two-cell embryo through the dissolution of the zona pellucida to the appearance of the fluid-filled segmentation cavity which identifies the blastocyst and enables embryonic and trophoblastic cells to be specifically identified. Carnegie stage 3 is the period of development during which the blastocyst (Fig. 1.1) normally lies free within the female reproductive tract. The embryo subsequently adheres to,

penetrates and is eventually buried within the endometrium during the process of implantation which extends from the 6th to the 12th postovulatory day and embraces Carnegie stages 4 and 5 (O'Rahilly 1973).

The primitive amniotic cavity develops some 7½ days after fertilisation (Blechschmidt 1968, Luckett 1973) and its floor forms the primary ectoderm. The primary endoderm is probably formed from ectoderm by cells which migrate around the blastocoelic cavity (Hauser & Streeter 1941) and enclose the yolk sac. The opposed layers of ectoderm and endoderm form the bilaminar embryonic disc (Fig. 1.2).

During the 13th, 14th and 15th postovulatory days (Carnegie stage 6) several significant events occur within the conceptus, one of which is the

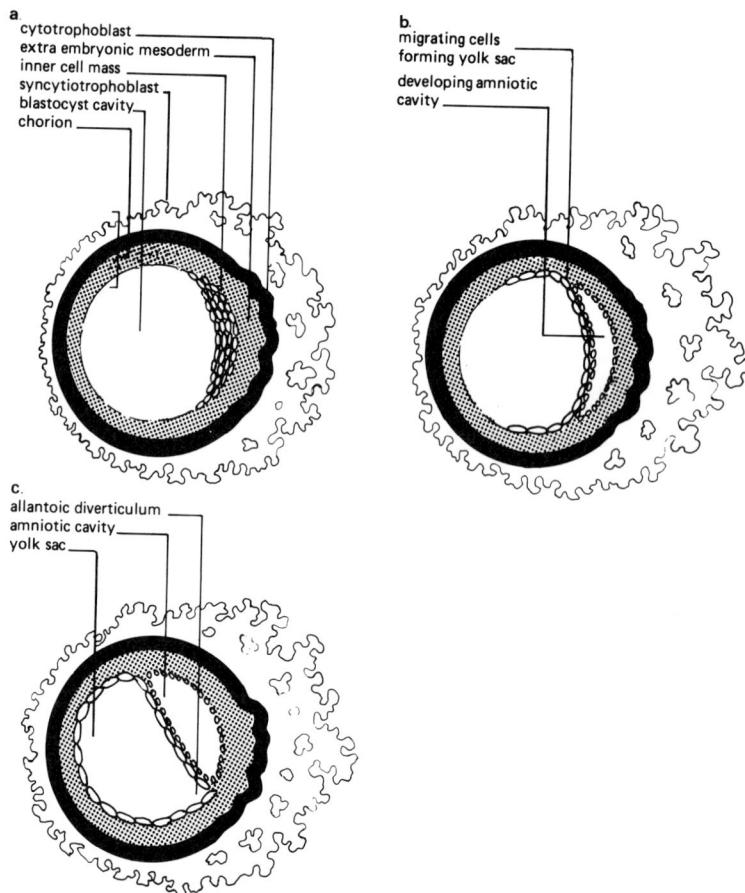

a.
cytotrophoblast
extra embryonic mesoderm
inner cell mass
syncytiotrophoblast
blastocyst cavity
chorion

b.
migrating cells
forming yolk sac
developing amniotic
cavity

c.
allantoic diverticulum
amniotic cavity
yolk sac

Fig. 1.2 The conceptus continues to differentiate forming (**a**) the chorion, (**b**) the amniotic cavity and (**c**) the yolk sac. The area of contact between amniotic cavity and yolk sac is the bilaminar embryonic disc.

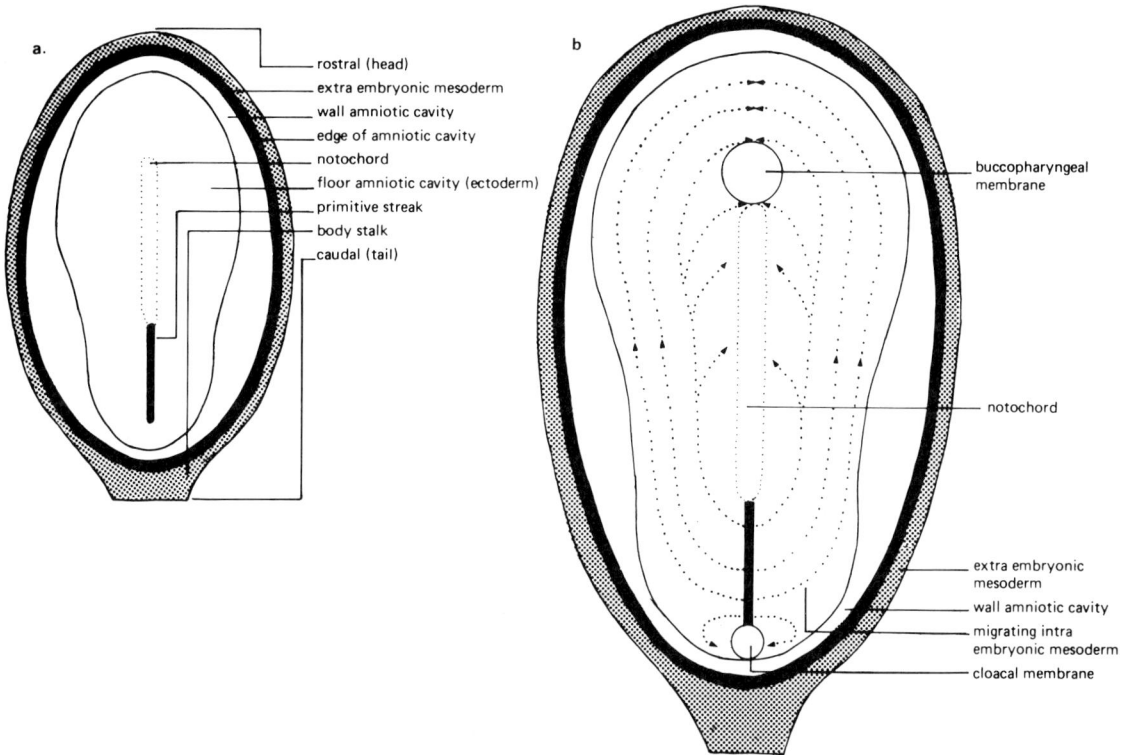

Fig. 1.3 (**a**) A diagrammatic view of the floor of the amniotic cavity, the dorsal surface of the bilaminar embryonic disc, revealing the primitive streak and notochord. (**b**) Intra-embryonic mesoderm, generated by the primitive streak and interposed between the floor of the amniotic cavity and roof of the yolk sac, converts the bilaminar embryonic disc into a trilaminar disc. The bucco-pharyngeal and cloacal membrane remain bilaminar.

formation of the primitive streak (Fig. 1.3) lying caudally in the midline of the embryonic disc (Hauser & Streeter 1941). The primitive streak generates intra-embryonic mesoderm, which migrates through the embryonic disc, in the plane between ectoderm and endoderm (Fig. 1.3), and converts the bilaminar embryonic disc into a trilaminar disc. Two areas of ectoderm:endoderm apposition remain, the cloacal membrane immediately caudal to the primitive streak (Fig. 1.3), and the buccopharygneal membrane. At the same time the intra-embryonic coelom, the forerunner of the pericardial, pleural and peritoneal cavities, is being formed within the intra-embryonic mesoderm (Fig. 1.4).

Carnegie stage 9, from the 19th to the 21st day, heralds the onset of that phase of embryogenesis dominated by the formation of the neural folds and subsequently the neural tube (Fig. 1.5 and 1.6). During the next 5 days the neural ridges fuse and the primitive neural tube is buried in the underlying mesoderm.

The growth of the nervous system initially produces a simple dorsal convexity and ventral concavity (Fig. 1.7a). Eventually the portion of the embryo which accommodates the neural tube attains maximum dorsal convexity (Fig. 1.7b) and the once rostral and caudal portions of the embryo are so displaced ventrally that the neural tube is freed from their constraining influences. Unimpeded the neural tube extends rostrally and caudally, overriding the now ventrally displaced original rostral and caudal regions of the embryonic disc which are therefore inverted and reversed in the formation of the head and tail folds (Fig. 1.7c). Neural tube closure and growth has also effected significant folding in the transverse plane, producing the lateral folds (Fig. 1.6d). This process of flexion re-orientates the primitive embryonic tissues and structures and establishes new

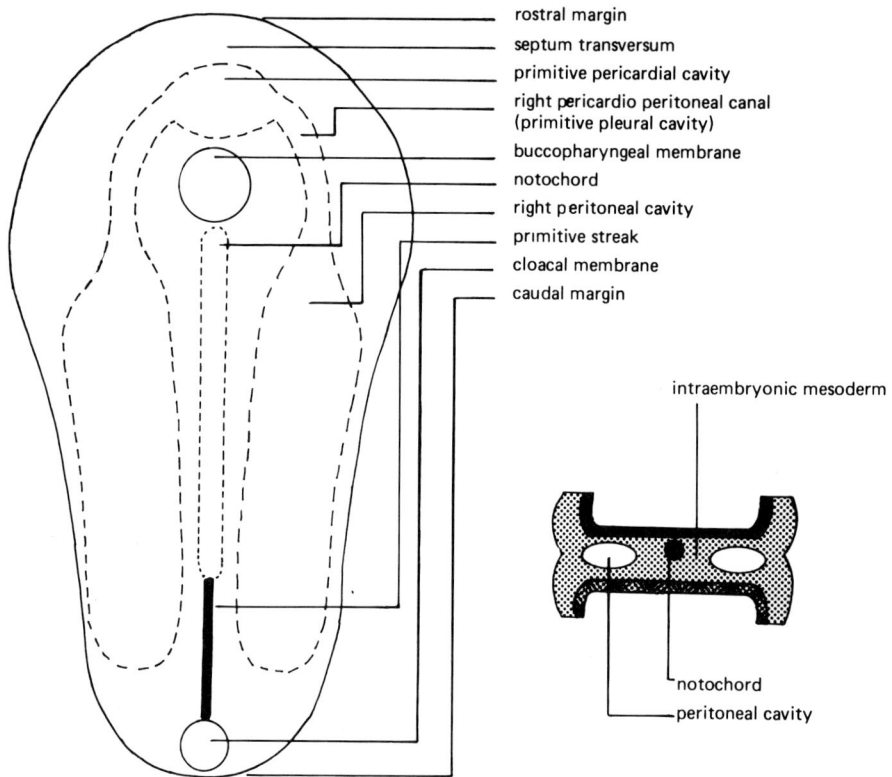

rostral margin
septum transversum
primitive pericardial cavity
right pericardio peritoneal canal
(primitive pleural cavity)
buccopharyngeal membrane
notochord
right peritoneal cavity
primitive streak
cloacal membrane
caudal margin

intraembryonic mesoderm

notochord
peritoneal cavity

Fig. 1.4 The intra-embryonic coelom forms within the intra-embryonic mesoderm of the trilaminar embryonic disc.

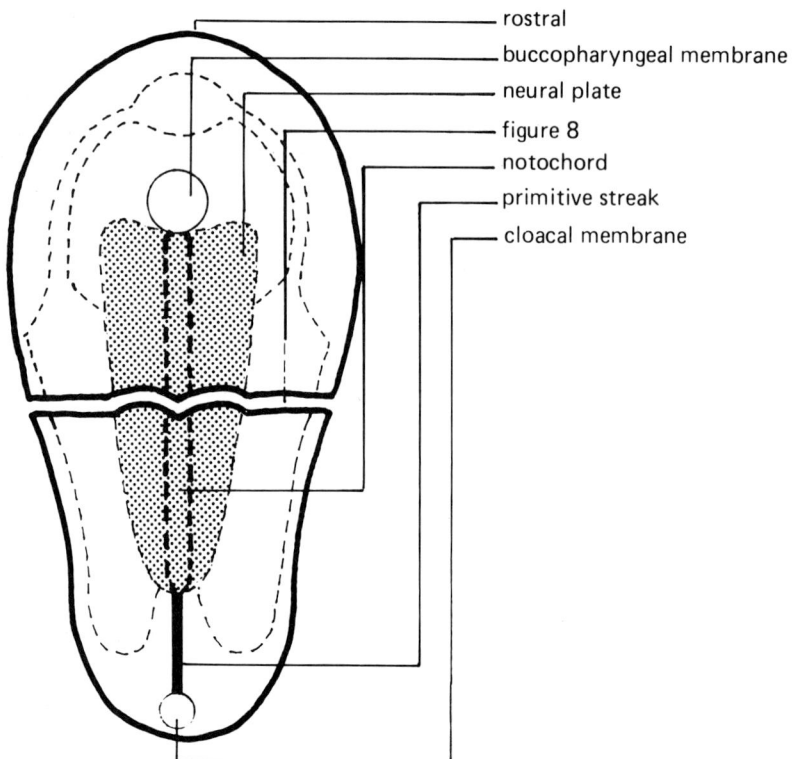

rostral
buccopharyngeal membrane
neural plate
figure 8
notochord
primitive streak
cloacal membrane

Fig. 1.5 The ectoderm on the dorsal surface of the trilaminar embryonic disc overlying the notochord forms the neural plate.

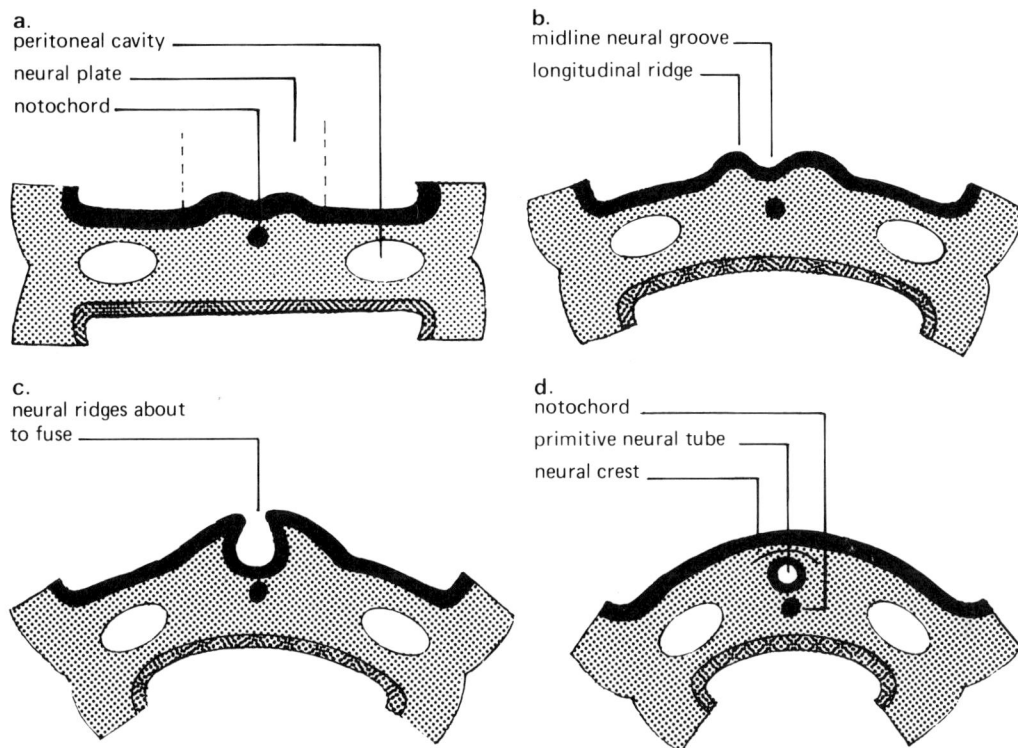

Fig. 1.6 (a) A midline longitudinal groove appears in the neural plate ectoderm. (b) The neural groove deepens with elevation of the neural ridges. (c) The neural ridges approximate and fuse to form the neural tube. (d) As the neural tube is enclosed by the intra-embryonic mesoderm the trilaminar embryo folds in the transverse plane displaying a dorsal convexity and ventral concavity.

relationships between them which are essential to subsequent development. The endoderm of the dorsal part of the yolk sac is drawn into the ventral concavity of the embryo and is subdivided into foregut, midgut and hindgut. The hindgut is caudal to the rostral limit of the allantoic diverticulum and also dorsal and rostral to the cloacal membrane (Fig. 1.8a). The intra-embryonic mesoderm in the midembryo region (Fig. 1.8b) is subdivided into paraxial mesoderm, lateral mesoderm and intermediate mesoderm. The paraxial mesoderm surrounds the neural tube and is the site of somite formation. The lateral mesoderm, so named because of its location in the flat trilaminar embryo, is carried ventrally by the formation of the lateral folds. The lateral mesoderm accommodates the primitive peritoneal cavity which divides it into splanchnopleuric mesoderm, associated with endoderm and destined to form the visceral muscle of the gut derivates, and somatopleuric mesoderm associated with ectoderm and destined to partici-

pate in the formation of the body wall. The intermediate mesoderm lies between the paraxial and lateral mesoderm. It is within the intermediate mesoderm that important elements of the genitourinary system develop.

The indifferent embryo

The intermediate mesoderm extends the length of the body cavity. It is lateral and ventral to the paraxial mesoderm and adjacent to the midline dorsal mesentry of the gut tube which is itself being formed at this time (Keith, 1948). At the caudal limit of the intra-embryonic coelom or primitive peritoneal cavity the intermediate mesoderm is in continuity with the mesoderm investing the terminal or cloacal portion of the hindgut (Fig. 1.9). Change and differentiation are continuous during organogenesis and several events are taking place during the same period of time which are relevant to more than one system. In particular, some of the

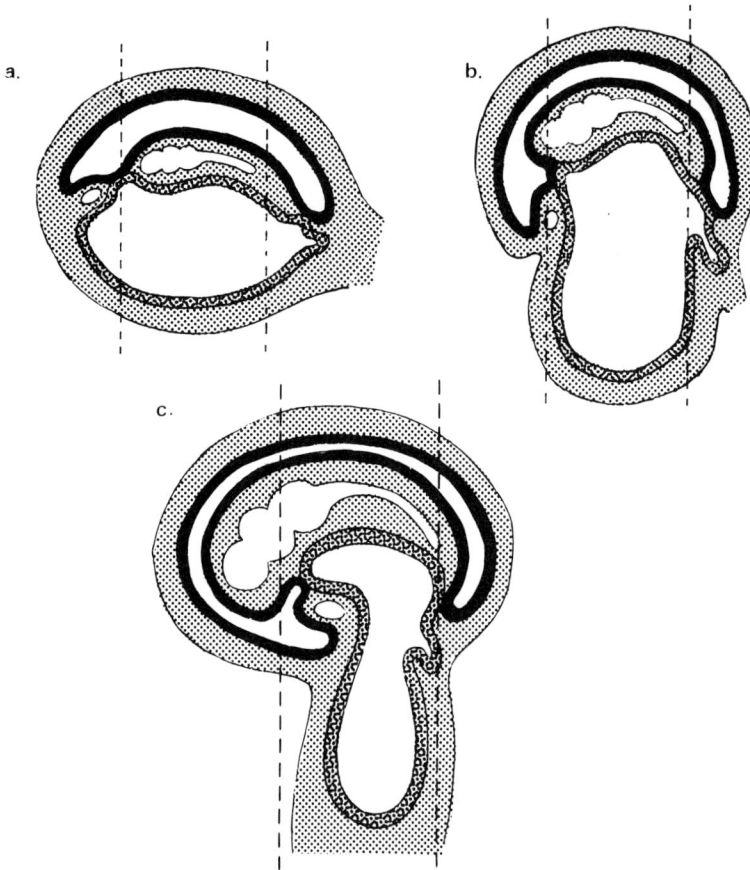

Fig. 1.7 (a) As the neural tube is enclosed within the intra-embryonic mesoderm it lengthens and expands rostrally, causing a dorsal convexity and ventral concavity. (b) Further growth of the neural tube increases this curvature in the longitudinal plane, (c) with the eventual formation of the head and tail folds.

events involved in the development of the urinary system, reproductive system and terminal part of the digestive system are interrelated and interdependent.

The urorectal septum

The hindgut appears about the 20th postovulatory day, during Carnegie stage 9 (O'Rahilly 1973) and is established during the process of flexion as that part of the primitive yolk sac enclosed within the tail fold of the embryo. In this situation the hindgut lies caudal to the rostral limit of the allantoic diverticulum and dorsal and rostral to the cloacal membrane (Fig. 1.10a). The mesoderm at the rostral limit of the allantoic diverticulum extends dorsally then caudally, in line with the curvature of the tail

fold, dividing the hindgut into ventral and dorsal parts. As the division proceeds the two parts of the hindgut remain in continuity with each other caudal to the advancing mesoderm of the urorectal septum (Fig. 1.10b). The mesoderm reaches the cloacal membrane at 30–32 days (O'Rahilly 1977) as the Carnegie stage moves from 13 to 14 (O'Rahilly 1973). As the urorectal septum fuses with the cloacal membrane the embryonic hindgut is completely divided into the ventral (anterior) urogenital sinus and dorsal (posterior) rectum (Fig. 1.10c). The formation of the urorectal septum transforms the caudal part of the embryo. In the future pelvis the block of mesoderm, interposed between the dorsal gut tube and the ventral urogenital sinus, is in direct continuity across the side wall of the gut tube with the intermediate mesoderm. Indeed the caua.

ectoderm of dorsal surface
of body
neural tube
intra embryonic mesoderm
foregut
midgut
hindgut
pericardial cavity
allantoic diverticulum
vitello intestinal duct
ventral yolk sac
body stalk or ventral surface
of body

b. paraxial mesoderm
somite
intermediate mesoderm
somatopleuric mesoderm
peritoneal cavity
splanchnopleuric mesoderm
intra embryonic coelom
continous with extra
embryonic coelom
body stalk

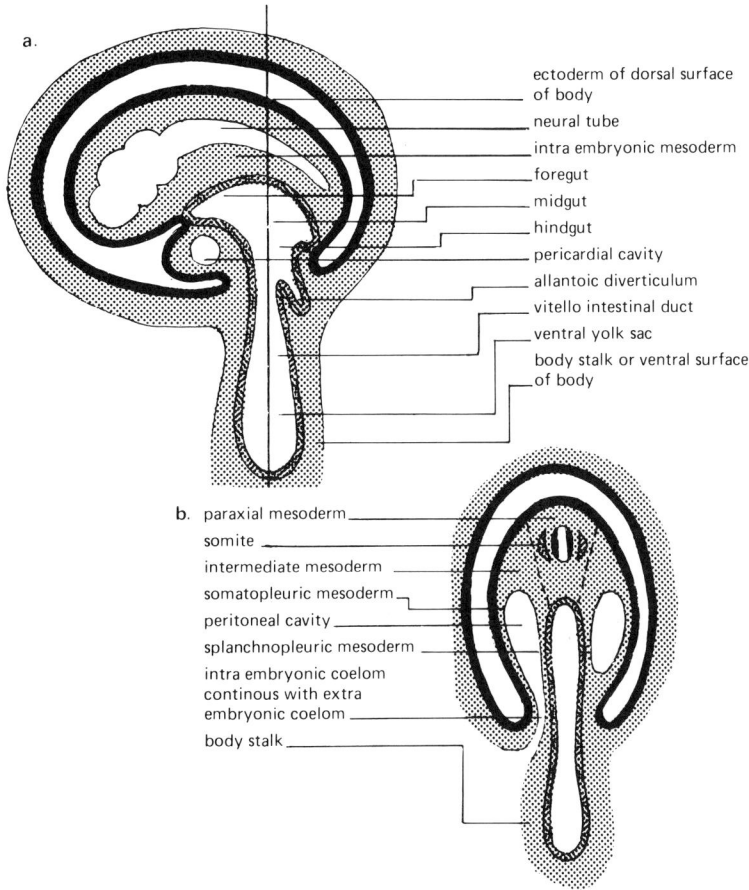

Fig. 1.8 (a) A midline section of the embryo after formation of the head and tail folds.
(b) A transverse section of the mid-embryo region after formation of the lateral folds.

dal limit of the intermediate mesoderm 'runs into' the urorectal septum (Fig. 1.11).

The mesonephric ducts

The first indication of the urinary system in the human embryo appears at 21 days when mesonephric vesicles develop within the intermediate mesoderm (O'Rahilly and Muecke 1972). Medially these vesicles are immediately associated with branches of the dorsal aorta. Laterally they are associated with a solid rod of cells which develops within the lateral part of the intermediate mesoderm at 24 days. This solid rod of cells acquires a lumen at 26 days and forms the mesonephric duct. The mesonephric vesicles open into the mesonephric duct as it extends caudally through the intermediate meso-

derm. Skirting the gastrointestinal hindgut the bilateral mesonephric ducts enter the developing urorectal septum to reach the posterior (dorsal) surface of the urogenital sinus, still incompletely divided from the rectum. The mesonephric ducts open into the urogenital sinus at 28 days during Carnegie stage 13 (O'Rahilly 1977). Thereafter the urorectal septum completes the separation of the urogenital sinus from the rectum. The functioning mesonephros produces an increase in pressure in the closed urogenital sinus which ruptures the ventral part of the cloacal membrane and allows the urogenital sinus to communicate with the amniotic cavity (Ludwig 1965).

In 1759, Caspar Friedrich Wolff, in a publication concerned with the embryology of the chick, described a symmetrical pair of paravertebral

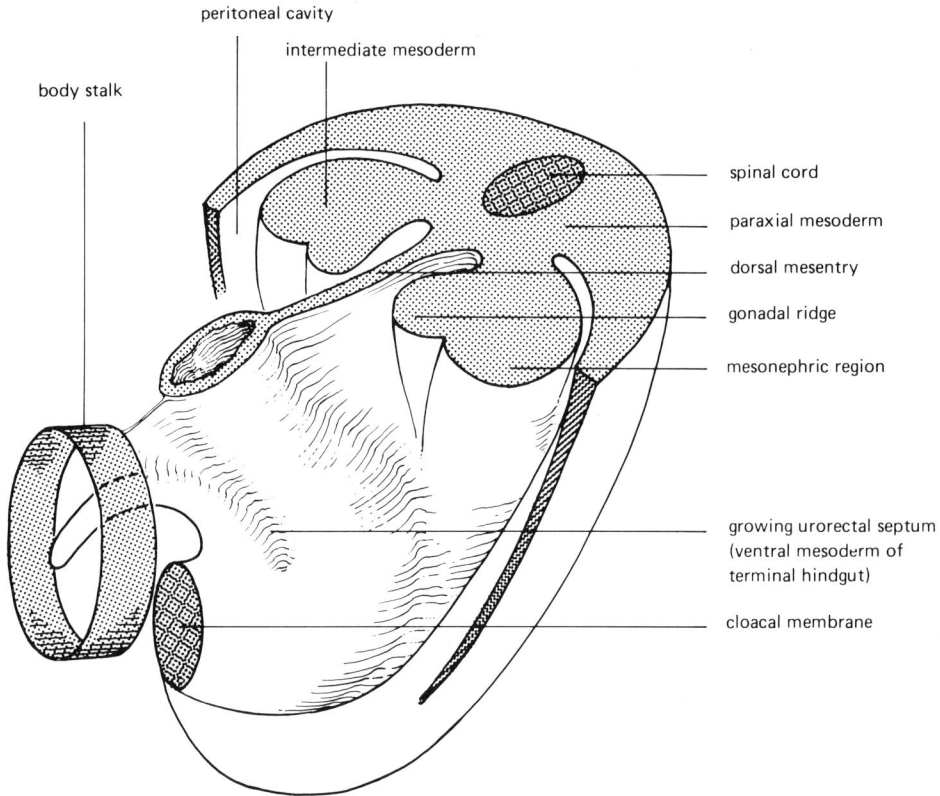

Fig. 1.9 The caudal half of the embryo showing the gonadal ridge and mesonephric region of the intermediate mesoderm which, at its caudal limit, is continuous with the mesoderm investing hindgut.

swellings as being the precursors of the kidneys. Later Rathke (1825) referred to these areas in which the mesonephros was developing as 'Wolffian bodies after Wolff'. The term Wolffian was subsequently used by other investigators to describe the duct and vesicles of the mesonephros (Stephens 1982). The mesonephros has only a transient renal function in the human embryo but its excretory duct is crucial to the subsequent development of the metanephros. As the urorectal septum reaches the cloacal membrane at 30 to 32 days, the caudal end of each mesonephric duct, having already opened into the urogenital sinus, gives origin to a ureteric bud and begins to be incorporated into the posterior wall of the urogenital sinus (Keith 1948). The portion of each duct incorporated into the urogenital sinus subsequently forms the trigone of the bladder and the posterior wall of the urethra (Fig. 1.12). The ureteric bud arising from the mesonephric duct ascends the duct's path of

descent and, acquiring a lumen, eventually forms the collecting system and ureter of the ipsilateral kidney. As the ureteric bud appears intermediate mesoderm condenses at its growing end to form the metanephric cap within which nephrons develop. The mesonephros achieves its maximum size and maximum excretory function in the human embryo at 42 days (Potter & Osathanondh 1966). At the same stage of development nephrons appear in the metanephric cap (Kissane 1974) and begin to function at 50 days (Potter & Osathanondh 1966). Thereafter the metanephros begins to take over the excretory function of the mesonephros and the mesonephric vesicles begin to degenerate.

The paramesonephric ducts

Johannes Müller (1830), in a publication concerned with genital development, described a cord (of cells) on the outer aspect of the Wolffian body

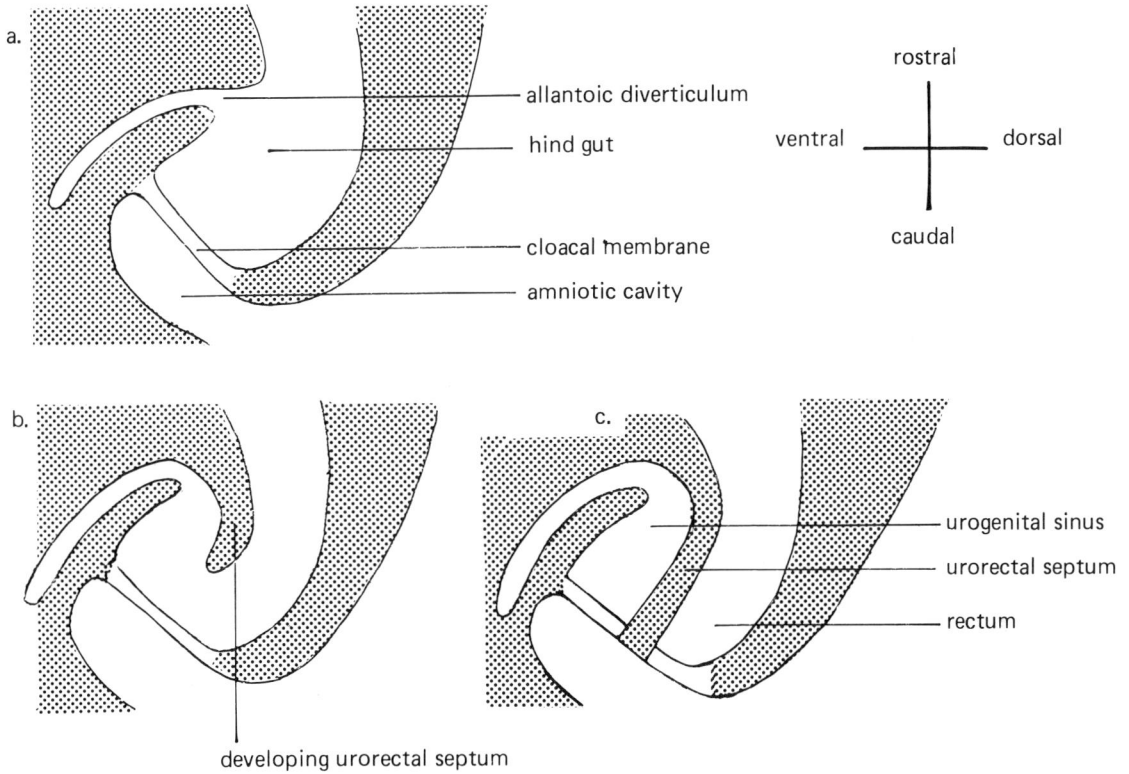

Fig. 1.10 (**a**) The primitive hindgut is enclosed within the embryonic tailfold. (**b**) The developing urorectal septum grows dorsally and caudally from the rostral limit of the allantoic diverticulum. (**c**) The fusion of the urorectal septum with the cloacal membrane divides the hindgut into urogenital sinus and rectum.

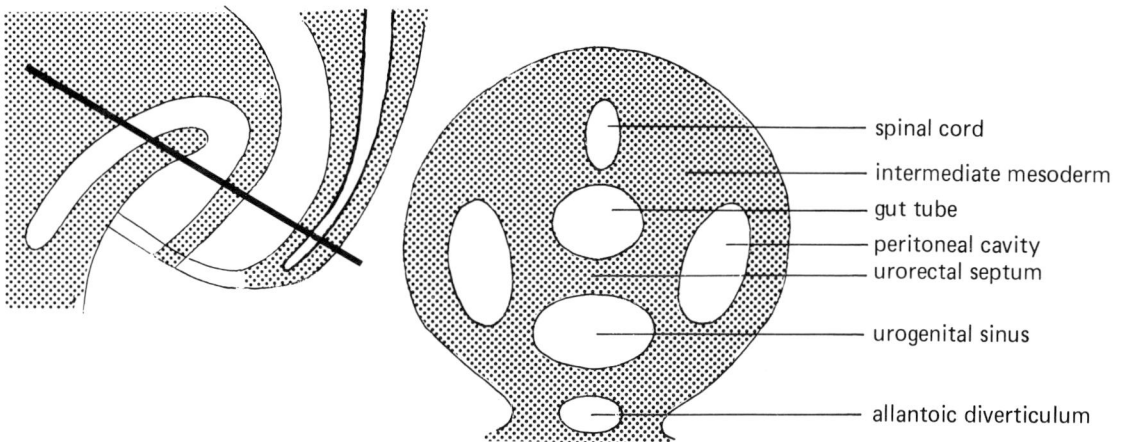

Fig. 1.11 A transverse section through the embryonic pelvis demonstrates the continuity of the intermediate mesoderm with the mesoderm of the urorectal septum.

a.

allantoic diverticulum

urogenital sinus

mesonephric duct

ventral cloacal
membrane

b.

mesonephric duct

ureteric bud

c.

metanephric cap
ureteric duct
mesonephric duct

ventral cloacal
membrane absent

d.

ureter

future trigone of bladder

future urethra

mesonephric duct

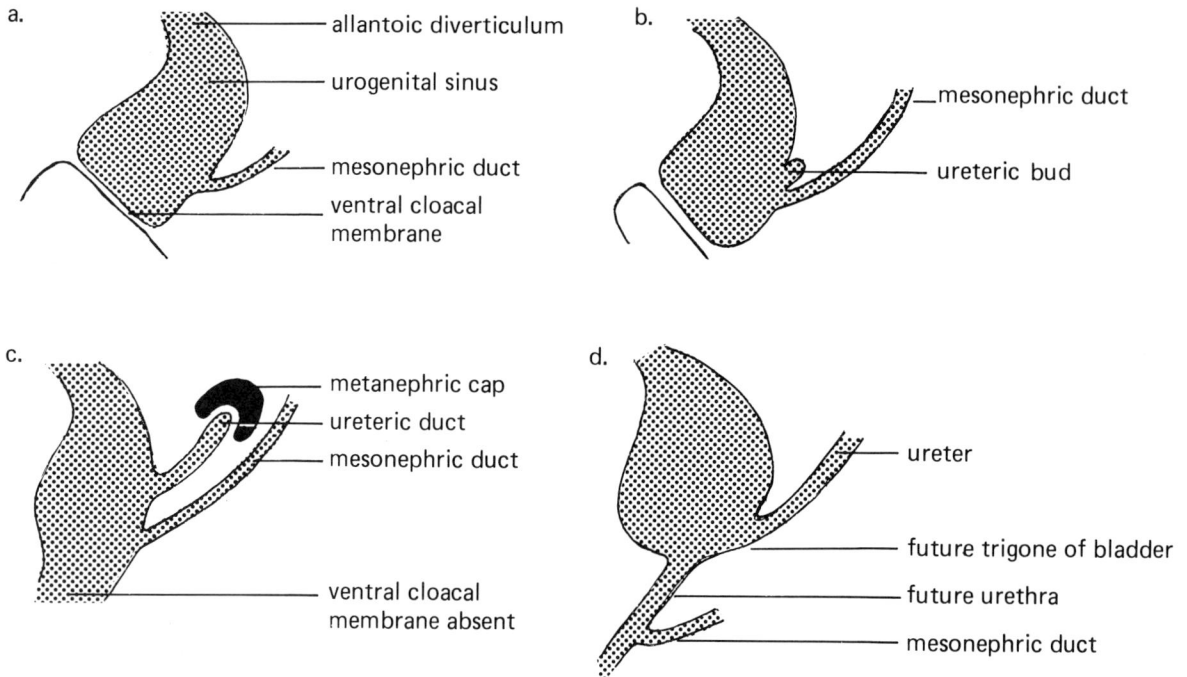

Fig. 1.12 (**a**) The mesonephric duct, within the urorectal septum, opens into the urogenital sinus. (**b**) The caudal limit of the mesonephric duct gives origin to the ureteric bud. (**c**) The metanephric cap forms at the growing end of the ureteric bud or duct. (**d**) The mesonephric duct forms the ureter, trigone of the bladder and posterior wall of the urethra.

which was much thinner than the Wolffian cord. He concluded that although the two cords were either attached or adjacent to each other they were 'two quite different things'. These Müllerian ducts are now referred to as the paramesonephric ducts and they appear in the human embryo at about 40 days. Each duct is initially observed as a thickening and invagination of the coelomic epithelium on the lateral aspect of the intermediate mesoderm at the cephalic end of the mesonephros (Felix 1912, Faulconer 1951). The site of the invagination later becomes the abdominal ostium of the uterine tube with its associated fimbriae. The precursor of each paramesonephric duct extends caudally as a solid rod of cells in the intermediate mesoderm, in close association with and initially lateral to the mesonephric duct. The mesonephric duct has been shown experimentally both to induce the paramesonephric duct (Didier 1973a, b) and to guide its descent (Gruenwald 1941); indeed the growing caudal tip of the paramesonephric duct lies within the basement membrane of the mesonephric duct (Frutiger 1969). As the paramesonephric cord of

cells continues its descent a lumen appears in its cranial portion which is in continuity with the intra-embryonic coelom. This lumen extends caudally behind the growing tip of the paramesonephric cord converting it into a duct. During descent the paramesonephric ducts pass ventral to the mesonephric ducts and, coming into close association with one another, reach the posterior aspect of the urogenital sinus within the urorectal septum (Fig. 1.13). Indeed as soon as the two paramesonephric ducts come into contact they begin to fuse even before their growing ends reach the urogenital sinus (Koff 1933). The external surface of their medial walls, initially in apposition, begin to fuse and eventually the duct lumina are separated only by a median septum (O'Rahilly 1977). At 49 days before the paramesonephric ducts reach the urogenital sinus a tubercle appears on the internal aspect of its posterior wall between the openings of the mesonephric ducts. This tubercle is not formed by the paramesonephric ducts but identifies the site at which the common paramesonephric duct fuses with the posterior wall of the

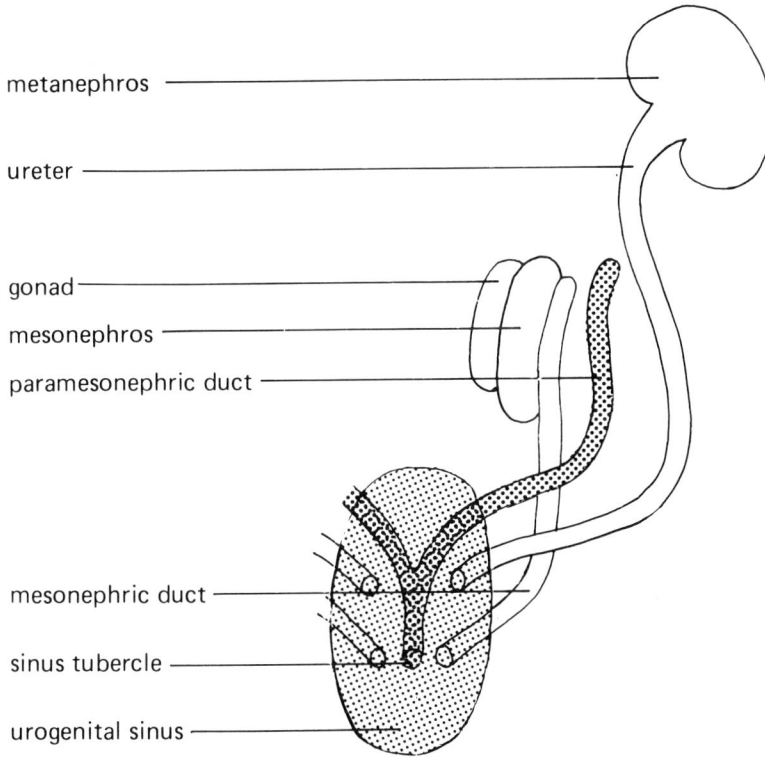

Fig. 1.13 The indifferent human embryo possesses mesonephric and paramesonephric ducts. The terminal paramesonephric ducts fuse within the urorectal septum and reach the urogenital sinus at the sinus tubercle situated between the openings of the two mesonephric ducts.

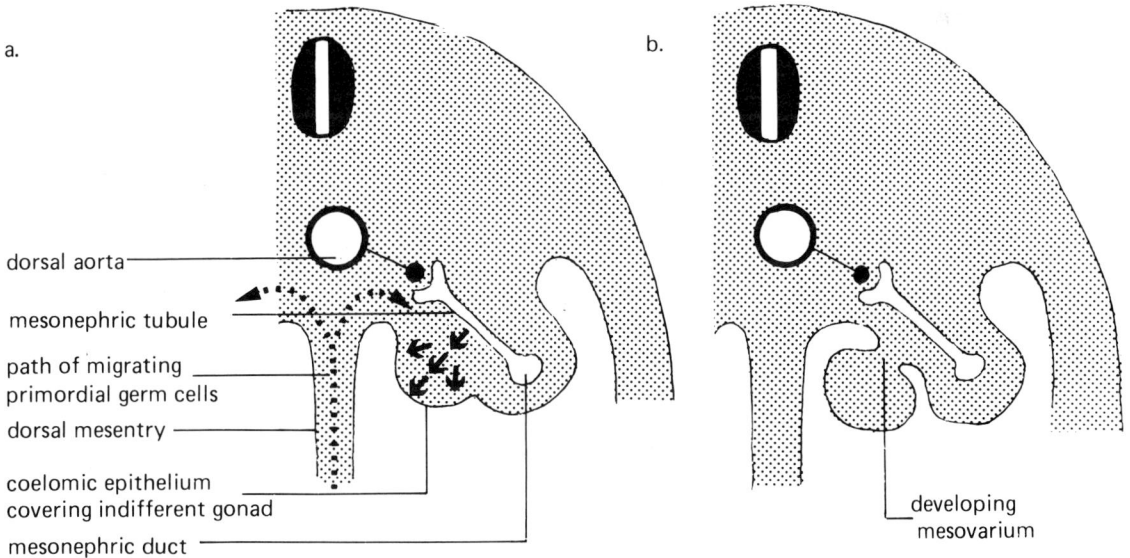

Fig. 1.14 A transverse section showing (**a**) the invasion of the indifferent gonad by mesonephric cells and primordial germ cells and (**b**) the developing mesovarium.

urogenital sinus at 56 days (Glenister 1962, Josso 1981).

Primordial germ cells

Perhaps the most significant event of early embryogenesis is the separation of a clone of gonia or primordial germ cells, subsequently capable of meiosis, from the pool of somatic cells capable only of mitosis. In the female mammal these gonia also retain two functional X chromosomes, in contrast to the somatic cells which possess only one functional X chromosome (Lyon 1974). Primordial germ cells are unquestionably present in the allantoic diverticulum and adjacent parts of the yolk sac in 17–20-day embryos (Jirasek 1977). From this location the primordial germ cells migrate (Figs. 1.9 and 1.14a) through the mesoderm surrounding the hindgut and into the dorsal mesentery (Hardisty 1978). The destination of these migrating cells is the medial aspect of the intermediate mesoderm adjacent to the mesonephros and they begin to reach this area in the human embryo at 35 days (Jirasek 1971). The mechanisms that initiate and direct the migration of the gonia to the future gonad are unknown.

The indifferent gonad

Although the concept of an indifferent gonad has recently been challenged by the demonstration of sex-specific proteins in the gonadal blastema of rat embryos during the morphologically indifferent state (Müller et al 1984), the area to which the primordial germ cells migrate is referred to as the indifferent gonad until gonadal sex is established. At 35 days the indifferent gonad begins to be formed on the medial aspect of the mesonephros by the invasion of that area of the intermediate mesoderm by three other cell types: the primordial germ cells, cells from overlying coelomic epithelium and cells from the adjacent mesonephros. In normal circumstances the primordial germ cells, having entered the mesoderm of the indifferent gonad, undergo rapid mitotic proliferation. Before the gonads are established as testes or ovaries the pattern of germ cell proliferation is similar in both sexes.

The basal lamina of the somatic coelomic epithe-lium overlying the medial aspect of the intermediate mesoderm in the region of the mesonephros is incomplete, and dividing epithelial cells readily invade the underlying mesoderm. The proliferating coelomic epithelial cells at the cranial end of the mesonephros condense to form the primordium of the suprarenal cortex (Crowder 1957). Just caudal to this suprarenal area is the gonadal mesoderm. The epithelial cells link up with other cells originating from the mesonephros to establish the urogenital connection (Brambell 1956). These events occur between day 35 and day 42 (Jirasek 1977) and establish the main features of the indifferent gonad.

Emergent gonadal sex

Until approximately 42 days of gestation male and female embryos are indistinguishable morphologically (Fig. 1.15). At this stage there are 300–1300 primordial germ cells within the indifferent gonads destined to become either spermatogonia or oogonia. The close association between gonad and adrenal at this early stage of development can result in adrenal cells being sequestered in the gonad to retain their function in the mature ovary or testes (Grumbach & Conte 1981).

The transformation of the indifferent gonad into an embryonic testis occurs in 43- to 49-day-old embryos during Carnegie stage 18 (Jirasek 1977). After differentiation of the testes, Leydig cells become evident at 56 days. Their numbers increase, are maximal between 90 and 120 days, decline thereafter and disappear shortly after birth (Mancini et al 1963). Testosterone production, which is directly related to the number of Leydig cells in the testes (Zondek & Zondek 1979), begins at 56 days and reaches a peak towards midgestation (Siiteri & Wilson 1974). In addition to testosterone the developing testes secrete another hormone, as predicted by Jost (1947). Anti-Müllerian hormone (AMH) is synthesised by Sertoli cells (Blanchard & Josso 1974), present in the differentiating testes at 60 days (Jirasek 1977). Secretion of AMH begins shortly after testicular differentiation and continues into the perinatal period. It is functional, however, for only a short critical period during early gestation (Josso et al 1977).

The transformation of the indifferent gonad into an embryonic ovary occurs gradually in 45- to 55-

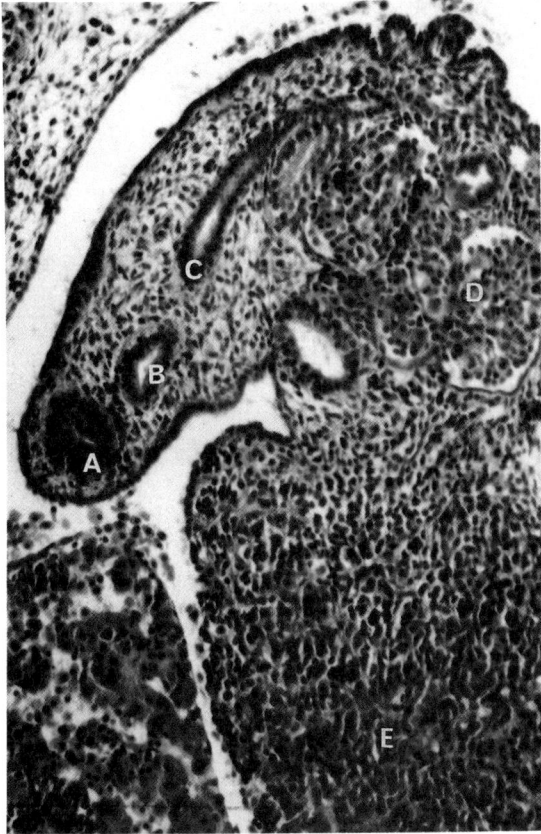

Fig. 1.15 A transverse section of the right side of the upper abdomen of a 42-day embryo showing: (**a**) the paramesonephric duct with a barely discernible lumen; (**b**) the mesonephric duct; (**c**) a mesonephric tubule; (**d**) the mesonephros; (**e**) the gonad (H & E, × 210).

day-old embryos during Carnegie stages 18 to 22 (Jirasek 1977). An indifferent gonad with germ cells in meiosis is an ovary (Peters 1970) since meiotic division does not occur in the testes until puberty. The stage of ovarian develpment at which meiosis begins varies between species (Grinsted & Aagesen 1984). In the human embryo germ cells are distributed evenly throughout the gonad and their entry into meiosis follows the early stages of ovarian differentiation. The onset of meiosis begins at the centre of the ovary (Waldeyer 1870, Winiwarter & Sainmont 1908) and is said to occur in the human embryo at 56 to 60 days (Jirasek 1977) although other investigators maintain that meiosis does not occur until 70 to 84 days (Baker 1963). This discrepancy probably results from difficulty in identifying the earliest stage of the first meiotic division. In the human ovary follicles begin to form sometime between 12 weeks (Gondos & Hobel 1973) and 16 weeks (Jirasek 1977) of gestation.

Mechanisms of gonadal differentiation

As indicated earlier investigation of patients with numerical abnormalities of the sex chromosomes has shown the Y chromosome to be extremely potent in inducing testicular differentiation (Ford et al 1959, Jacobs & Strong 1959).

The H-Y transplantation antigen

Using a highly inbred mouse strain, Eichwald and Silmser (1955) observed that skin grafts from male donors to male recipients and those from female donors to either female or male recipients survived, while grafts from male donors to virgin female recipients were rejected. This rejection was attributed to a male specific transplantation antigen determined by a gene on the Y chromosome. Since the genes governing expression of histocompatibility antigens in mice were already designated H-1, H-2, H-3, etc. (Snell 1948), the new gene was called H-Y and its product the H-Y antigen. The H-Y antigen, initially demonstrated in skin, has now been shown to be present on all male tissues studied (Gasser & Silvers 1972).

Following the identification of antibodies to H-Y antigen in the sera of female mice after rejection of male skin grafts (Goldberg et al 1971), anti-H-Y serum was generated in female mice or rats by repeated injections of male spleen cells. Such antisera can be used to assay H-Y antigen expression on target cells (Wachtel & Koo 1981). The methodology of H-Y antigen assays is still developing and undoubtedly problems of specificity and reproducibility exist in the various tests applicable to humans (Grumbach & Conte 1981). There are also uncertainties about the relationship, if any, which exists between the immunologically active and biologically active sites of the H-Y antigen.

H-Y antigen is invariably associated with the heterogametic sex in a wide variety of species. This widespread phylogenetic conservation of H-Y antigen, together with its early appearance in eight cell mouse embryos (Krco & Goldberg 1976), has led to the suggestions that: (a) it is the factor responsible for inducing differentiation of the heterogametic gonad, and (b) it is the product of the testes-organising gene (Wachtel et al 1975).

Action of the H-Y antigen

The undifferentiated embryonic mammalian gonad is induced to become a testis in the presence of a Y chromosome and an ovary in its absence. Subsequent male differentiation is induced by hormones secreted by the newly formed testes. If the testis fails to secrete these hormones or if some defect blocks their action the embryo differentiates as a female. The sex-determining role of the Y chromosome and its associated H-Y antigen is thus limited to the induction of the testis. Testicular differentiation therefore should always be associated with the expression of H-Y antigen regardless of sexual phenotype or apparent karyotype (Wachtel & Koo 1981).

The biologically active H-Y antigen is a protein composed of hydrophobic peptide subunits linked by disulphide bonds (Ohno et al 1979). It has been detected on all cell membranes from normal XY males except immature germ cells, but the only gonadal cell which secretes the H-Y antigen is the primitive Sertoli cell (Ohno 1979). Two types of cell membrane receptor for H-Y antigens have been identified (Ohno 1979, Ohno et al 1979, Wachtel & Ohno 1979). One, associated with β_2-microglobulin, is non-specific and represents the stable anchorage site on all male cells. The second receptor site is only on gonadal cells, both male and female, and it binds the H-Y antigen with much higher affinity than the non-specific receptor site.

The role of H-Y antigen in testicular differentiation is still emerging. Dissociated rodent testicular cells from XY neonates have been shown to reorganise as ovarian follicles after application of H-Y antibody (Ohno et al 1978, Zenzes et al 1978a) while indifferent gonads from XX rodent embryos form testes after exposure to H-Y antigen (Zenzes et al 1978b). These experiments provide direct evidence that H-Y antigen is indeed responsible for testicular organisation. It is suggested (Wachtel & Ohno 1979) that the Y chromosome contains a locus or loci which either codes for the cell membrane H-Y antigen or regulates its expression. The

H-Y antigen is disseminated by the primitive Sertoli cells in the indifferent gonad, it binds to the gonad-specific H-Y receptors and induces differentiation of the testes. The indifferent gonad has an inherent tendency to form an ovary in the absence of H-Y antigen or its specific gonad receptor.

Regulation of H-Y antigen expression

Recently several groups of workers have reported positive expression of H-Y antigen in unexpected circumstances; in patients with XO gonadal dysgenesis and in phenotypic females with primary hypogonadism or gonadal dysgenesis, associated with either autosomal translocations or structural abnormalities of the X chromosomes (Grumbach & Conte 1981). These patients had neither testicular tissue nor a detectable Y chromosome.

The major problem therefore is the location of the structural gene which codes for the H-Y antigen. Initially it was thought to be located on the Y chromosome, possibly as multiple copies. Subsequent studies of H-Y antigen positive familial forms of XX males in several species suggest a more complex genetic control of H-Y antigen expression (Wachtel & Ohno 1979, Wachtel 1979). In recent reviews of the genetic control of H-Y antigen synthesis (Polani & Adinolfi 1983) it has been suggested that several forms of H-Y antigen may be produced, only one of which is biologically active in testicular differentiation. To account for the presence of serologically detectable H-Y antigen in the absence of testicular differentiation, it has been posited that H-Y antigen is initially produced as a biologically inactive precursor substance under the control of an autosomal structural gene. This precursor substance H-Yp is converted into the testes-differentiating antigen H-Ya under the influence of a gene located on the Y chromosome and designated H-Y^a. It is further suggested that anti H-Y sera will cross-react with H-Yp and H-Ya. Another gene designated H-Y^r is present on the pairing segment of the distal part of the short arm of the X chromosome which escapes inactivation. This gene, expressed in double dose by normal females, converts the precursor substance H-Yp into an H-Y product which is serologically undetectable and biologically inactive in terms of testicular differentiation. The gene H-Y^r is expressed in single dose by XO individuals in whom its effect is insufficient to render the precursor substance H-Yp wholly undetectable although it remains biologically inactive. The single dose expression of H-Y^r in normal males is overriden by the effect of H-Y^a on the Y chromosome. Furthermore an exchange of H-Y^r and H-Y^a genes between the X and Y chromosomes during XY crossover could subsequently result in XX zygotes expressing both H-Y^r products and H-Y^a products, and XY zygotes expressing only H-Y^r products. Individuals developing from such zygotes will appear to have inappropriate gonads for their chromosomal constitution as well as possible aberrant H-Y antigen expression.

Ovarian differentiation

The observations concerning the expression and action of H-Y antigen presented in the previous section suggest that ovarian differentiation is a passive event which occurs in the absence of a testis inducer. It has, however, been known for some time that two functional X chromosomes are required for normal ovarian differentiation in the human embryo (Ford et al 1959). In XO individuals the germ cells do not survive meiosis, follicular formation fails and the resulting streak gonad is sterile and devoid of endocrine activity (Carr et al 1968). In contrast an XO chromosomal constitution in the mouse does not prevent the development of fertile functioning ovaries (Cattanach 1962). The occurrence of familial XX gonadal dysgenesis, transmitted as an autosomal recessive trait, also suggests that autosomal genes are essential for ovarian organogenesis in humans (Grumbach & Conte 1981). It is possible that a counterpart to the H-Y antigen exists in the female and that it determines ovarian differentiation. The supernatant from fetal ovarian tissue does inhibit testicular organogenesis in cell suspensions, which would otherwise organise as testes (Wachtel & Hall 1979), but this supernatant factor may not be an ovarian organiser.

X chromosome inactivation

The X chromosome is large and genetically active whereas the Y chromosome is small and almost inert. Many of the genes on the X chromosomes are not involved in sexual differentiation. Any dosage difference between the sexes for this chromosome, that is, XX, XY, suggests a compensating mechanism to avoid the effects of aneuploidy. This phenomenon was studied in *Drosophila* and the term 'dosage compensation' was introduced to describe the mechanism which allows normal development (Müller et al 1931). In mammals dosage compensation is achieved by X chromsome inactivation (Lyon 1961). At some stage in the early development of the female embryo one of the X chromosomes in each cell is inactivated so that the effective dosage of X-linked genes is equivalent in males and females. In placental mammals inactivation is random and fixed from cell to cell so that the female becomes a cell mosaic of paternally and maternally active X chromosomes. It is possible to detect this mosaicism if the female is heterozygous for certain X-linked markers. A number of studies on mosaicism have demonstrated that X inactivation does not occur until the blastocyst stage in the mouse (Nesbitt 1971) and in many other species including humans (Park 1957). The sex chromatin body is found in the interphase nuclei of female cells and is a heterochromatic structure formed by the inactive X chromosome. Cytological studies of sex chromatin confirm the absence of X inactivation during early cleavage of the embryo (Park 1957, Melander 1962). The absence of any dosage compensation during this early phase of embryogenesis must be of some functional significance in view of the potentially lethal effect of aneuploidy in mammals.

When the primordial germ cells reach the indifferent gonad in human, rat and rabbit embryos there is no longer any cytological evidence of X inactivation (Ohno et al 1961, Teplitz & Ohno 1963, Ohno 1964). These results suggest, and it is generally accepted, that inactivation does occur in primordial germ cells but that reactivation follows when the oogonia reach the gonadal mesoderm. Both X chromosomes appear isopycnotic and several studies of X-linked gene expression in human and mouse oocytes are consistent in demonstrating activity of both X chromosomes in each oocyte (Gartler & Cole 1981).

In somatic cells X inactivation does not involve the entire X chromosome, otherwise XO and XXY individuals would not demonstrate any somatic defects. It has been argued that a group of genes on the Y chromosome are homologous with a group of genes on the X chromosome. These genes therefore function in double dose in the somatic cells of XX and XY individuals. In XO individuals the presence of these genes in only a single dose contributes to their somatic defects (Burgoyne 1981). Partial synapsis of the X and Y chromosomes, with the formation of a synaptonemal complex, has been clearly demonstrated, at the zygotene stage of meiotic prophase, in a number of mammalian species including humans (Solari 1974).* Since it is now widely accepted that pairing of autosomes during cell division is confined to homologous associations, it is reasonable to assume that the pairing of the X and Y chromosome is a consequence of homology. In the human pairing occurs between the short arms of the X and Y chromosomes (Pearson & Bobrow 1970) and, when maximal, involves most of the distal third of the X short arm and extends almost to the Y centromere (Moses et al 1975, Solari 1980). Using these facts to present his case Burgoyne (1982) suggests that the segment of the X chromosome which pairs with the Y chromosome escapes inactivation.

Ovarian development

One of the distinguishing features of the developing gonads is the rapid proliferation of primordial germ cells by mitosis, followed in the ovary by their entry into meiosis. Meiosis is essential to gametogenesis and consists of two cell divisions. The first, a specialised reduction division, is followed by the second, which is a modified mitotic division. During reduction division, meiosis I, genetic material is exchanged between the original maternal and paternal chromosomes of each homologous pair. This exchange enables meiosis, at its completion, to generate genetically unique gametes. Meiosis I begins during intra-uterine life and is completed at ovulation, some 15 to 45 years later. Meiosis II occurs only at fertilisation.

---

*Synapsis: The pairing of homologous chromosomes during meiosis.
Synaptonemal complex: A ribbon-like structure spanning the space between paired chromosomes during meiosis.

Gonadal induction

The transformation of the indifferent gonad into an embryonic ovary occurs gradually in 45- to 55-day-old embryos during Carnegie stages 18 to 22 (Jirasek 1977). The early fetal stage is defined by Jirasek (1977) as extending from the end of the embryonic period until the completion of the 16th week of gestation. During the first week of this early fetal period oogonia at the centre of the gonad enter meiosis. The onset of meiosis rapidly extends peripherally to reach oogonia at the surface of the ovary. No differences have been observed in the structure of the early fetal ovaries from 45X and 46XX individuals. Normal meiotic oocytes in the early fetal ovaries of 45X individuals suggest that the presence of two X chromosomes is not necessary for the beginning of meiosis (Jirasek 1977).

The late fetal stage begins at the completion of the 16th week of gestation (Jirasek 1977). Primary follicles, which begin to form in the fetal ovary after the 16th week, are characterised by an oocyte, completely surrounded by a single layer of follicular cells and separated from the follicular cells of adjacent primary follicles by connective tissue. Oocytes which are incompletely surrounded by follicular cells degenerate. The formation of primary follicles requires the presence of two normal X chromosomes, since all the oocytes in 45X individuals degenerate because the envelope of follicular cells is incomplete (Jirasek 1977).

The fetus achieves legal viability at 28 weeks of gestation. At this stage some of the ovarian follicles consist of growing oocytes surrounded by several layers of cuboidal granulosa cells. The stroma surrounding these growing follicles becomes organised into a cellular theca interna and a fibrous theca externa. Towards the end of gestation some of these compact multilayered growing follicles become vesicular and cells of the associated theca interna demonstrate a well-developed smooth endoplasmic reticulum and contain 3β-hydroxysteroid dehydrogenase. These growing vesicular follicles degenerate and disappear from the ovary within 6 months of birth and are not normally present again until the onset of puberty (Jirasek 1977).

During the early fetal stage the ovaries contain five million primordial germ cells, oogonia and oocytes (Witschi 1962) and some seven million at 20 weeks of gestation (Baker 1963). Their numbers decline thereafter and about five million germ cells degenerate before, or at, the primary follicle stage during the remainder of gestation. This process continues after birth and it has been estimated that only 400 000 oocytes remain in the ovaries at the onset of puberty. Since no more than 400 of these will be ovulated during a woman's reproductive life, 99.9% degenerate and disappear in follicular atresia (Jirasek 1977).

Genital duct differentiation

At the end of the embryonic period the fetus has gonads which are recognisable as either testes or ovaries, but possesses both mesonephric and paramesonephric duct systems (Fig. 1.13). Subsequent sexual differentiation of these ducts is governed by fetal testicular hormones (Jost 1947) which cause regression of the paramesonephric ducts and further development of the mesonephric ducts. In the female fetus the absence of testicular hormones allows regression of the mesonephric ducts and development of the paramesonephric ducts.

Male differentiation

Paramesonephric duct. In the human male fetus paramesonephric duct regression begins in that part of the duct adjacent to the caudal pole of the testis at 56 to 60 days (Jirasek 1977). Once initiated regression extends caudally and cranially and is complete at 70 days (Jirasek 1971). The inhibitory effect of the fetal testes on paramesonephric duct development is not caused by testosterone, since high testosterone levels have no effect on paramesonephric ducts in the castrated male rabbit fetus (Jost 1947). The inhibitory substance, a glycoprotein termed anti-Müllerian hormone (AMH), is produced by fetal and neonatal Sertoli cells (Blanchard and Josso 1974, Price 1979) which are first identified in the human testes at 60 days (Jirasek 1977). AMH is capable of causing paramesonephric duct regression for only a very limited time during intra-uterine life. Unless its action is initiated at the end of the embryonic period and

rapidly completed the paramesonephric ducts become resistant to any inhibitory effect of AMH (Josso et al 1977). The mechanism of AMH's action on the paramesonephric ducts has not yet been elucidated (Josso 1981). The fetal and neonatal testis continues to produce AMH and it has been detected in male infants up to 2 years of age (Donahoe et al 1977). Although its role during this period is unknown, it may be involved in the process of testicular descent (Hutson 1985). Persistence of paramesonephric ducts has been observed in otherwise normal human males and in some animals (Jost 1965, Josso 1979). This abnormality is X linked (Sloan & Walsh 1976) and may be due to a defect in AMH production or a block to its action.

Mesonephric duct. The second aspect of male differentiation is the integration of the mesonephric duct into the genital system after it has completed its excretory function with the mesonephric kidney. The persistence of the mesonephric duct and its incorporation into the genital system of the male fetus is referred to as stabilisation of the duct and is testosterone dependent. Mesonephric ducts removed from testicular influence by castration or explantation regress unless testosterone is administered exogenously or added to the culture medium (Jost 1947, Price & Pannabecker 1959). Testosterone production by the Leydig cells of the human testis begins at 56 days (Siiteri and Wilson 1974) and stabilisation of the mesonephric ducts occurs between 56 and 70 days in synchrony with the degeneration of the paramesonephric ducts (Price et al 1975). Testosterone secretion by the fetal testis is controlled by maternal chorionic gonadotrophin, which binds to fetal testicular cells (Hudson & Burger 1979). Stabilisation of the mesonephric ducts is brought about by testosterone, not by dihydrotestosterone (DHT) since the undifferentiated mesonephric ducts lack 5α-reductase, the enzyme necessary to generate dihydrotestosterone (Siiteri & Wilson 1974).

Mesonephric ducts in young female embryos can be stabilised by exposure to testosterone before the end of the 'critical period' for sex differentiation. In humans this critical period embraces the end of embryogenesis and the beginning of early fetal life, after which exposure of the female fetus to testosterone does not prevent the degeneration of the mesonephric ducts (Josso 1981).

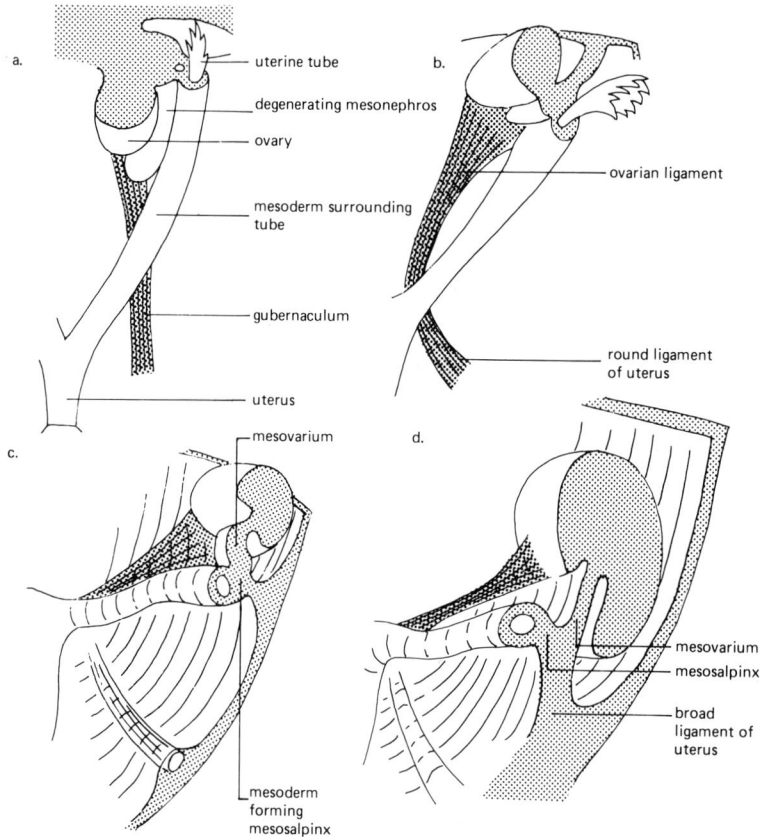

Fig. 1.16 Sequential stages in the descent of the ovary into the pelvis.

Female differentiation

At the time of apparent male differentiation in the XY fetus the comparable undifferentiated structures in the XX fetus are already irreversibly committed to female organogenesis. When the male paramesonephric ducts begin to degenerate at 56 days in the human fetus the female paramesonephric ducts no longer respond to AMH (Josso et al 1977). Female organogenesis involves stabilisation of the paramesonephric ducts and regression of the mesonephric ducts.

Paramesonephric duct. At the end of the embryonic period the caudal segments of the two paramesonephric ducts have fused within the urorectal septum (O'Rahilly 1977).

Uterine tube. The upper segment of each paramesonephric duct develops fimbria at its cephalic end and subsequently forms the uterine tube. The tube is lined by ciliated columnar epithelium which

is thrown into deep folds in the ampullary region. The transverse lie of the uterine tubes is established by the descent of the ovary (Fig. 1.16). As descent occurs the ipsilateral uterine tube and ovary are juxtaposed and cellular exchange takes place between them (O'Rahilly 1977). The utero-tubal junction is demarcated by an abrupt increase in the diameter of the uterine segment. These changes occur progressively during the first half of intra-uterine life and at term the uterine tube in the human infant is very well developed (Josso 1981).

Uterus. In the female embryo as soon as the paramesonephric ducts come into apposition within the urorectal septum and begin to fuse the uterus is being formed. At 63 days Hunter (1930) refers to the fused paramesonephric ducts as the uterus and identifies the body and the cervix by the presence of a constriction between them. The genital canal is established at 80 days when resorption of the median septum completes the fusion of the paramesonephric ducts (Koff 1933). The genital canal continues to lengthen by further fusion of the paired paramesonephric ducts at its cephalic end, by interstitial growth and by continued growth of its caudal end (O'Rahilly 1977). This growing caudal end, at its point of contact with the posterior wall of the urogenital sinus, is involved in additional cellular proliferation, which is essential to the development of the vagina.

The cervix, which forms the caudal two-thirds of the fetal uterus (Pryse-Davies & Dewhurst 1971), is generally believed to be of paramesonephric origin (Koff 1933, Forsberg 1965, Witschi 1970). It has, however, been claimed that its mucous membrane is derived from the urogenital sinus (Fluhmann 1960) but the exact contribution of paramesonephric and sinus tissue to the cervix remains uncertain (Davies & Kusama 1962). About the 17th week cervical glands appear (Koff 1933) and the future os is identifiable (Bulmer 1957). It has been variously reported that at 22 weeks the cervical canal is lined with stratified squamous epithelium with an entropion present (Eida 1961), while from 22 weeks to term the squamocolumnar junction is said to be situated some distance external to the os producing the congenital ectropion (Davies & Kusama 1962). The cervical epithelium of the newborn is described as stratified or pseudostratified columnar epithelium (Davies & Kusama 1962). Around the 19th week the corpus begins to differentiate into layers of mucosa, muscle and serosa (Hunter 1930, Witschi 1970) and approximately a week later glands begin to form in the simple columnar epithelium (Koff 1933). A well-marked fundus is apparent at 26 weeks and 'the change in the form of the upper limit of the uterus from a V-shaped notch to a convex curve . . . is due to the general thickening of its walls, brought about by the growth and development of muscle tissue' (Hunter 1930). At birth the endometrium is lined by a low columnar or cuboidal epithelium (Fluhmann 1960) and the endometrium itself may resemble either the proliferative or the secretory mucosa of the adult (Song 1964).

Vagina. For many years the conflicting opinions expressed concerning the development of the vagina were of little more than academic interest. Since the early 1970s, however, many publications have associated the occurrence of cervical and vaginal ridges, vaginal adenosis, ectropion and clear-cell carcinoma of the vagina in young adult females with prenatal exposure to diethylstilboestrol (Greenwald et al 1971, Herbst et al 1971, Fetherston et al 1972, Herbst et al 1972, Hill 1973, Pomerance 1973, Barber & Sommers 1974, Herbst et al 1974). The drug was considered to have had a teratogenic effect on the developing lower genital tract. Uterine synechiae and hypoplasia in 60% of exposed females indicates that the teratogen also affects the upper genital tract (Kaufman et al 1977). In addition some 20% of exposed males demonstrate some abnormality of their reproductive tracts such as epididymal cysts, hypoplastic testes, cryptorchidism and spermatozoal deficiencies (Gill et al 1976). It has been variously suggested that the vagina develops solely from the paramesonephric ducts (Felix 1912), the mesonephric ducts (Forsberg 1973), the urogenital sinus (Bulmer 1957, Fluhmann 1960), or from a combination of paramesonephric and mesonephric tissue (Witschi 1970), paramesonephric and sinus tissue (Koff, 1933, Agogué 1965), or mesonephric and sinus tissue (Forsberg 1973) with the relative contributions of each tissue an additional matter for controversy (O'Rahilly 1977). The following account of the development of the vagina is derived largely from O'Rahilly (1977).

At 49 days, before the paramesonephric ducts reach the urogenital sinus, a tubercle appears on the internal aspect of its posterior wall between the openings of the two mesonephric ducts. This is the sinus tubercle which identifies the site at which the fused paramesonephric ducts make contact (Fig. 1.17a) with the posterior wall of the urogenital sinus at 56 days (Glenister 1962, Josso 1981). The fusion of the paramesonephric ducts is complete at 80 days with the formation of the genital canal. The growing caudal end of the canal impinges on the posterior wall of the urogenital sinus and induces additional cellular proliferation. At 87 days three dorsal projections of the posterior wall of the urogenital sinus are identified, one in the midline and one on either side (Fig. 1.17b). These projections, or sinuvaginal bulbs, are probably of sinus origin (Koff 1933, Bulmer 1957), although other authors dispute this. Proliferation of the lining epithelium of these sinuvaginal bulbs converts them into solid tissue projections at 95 days.

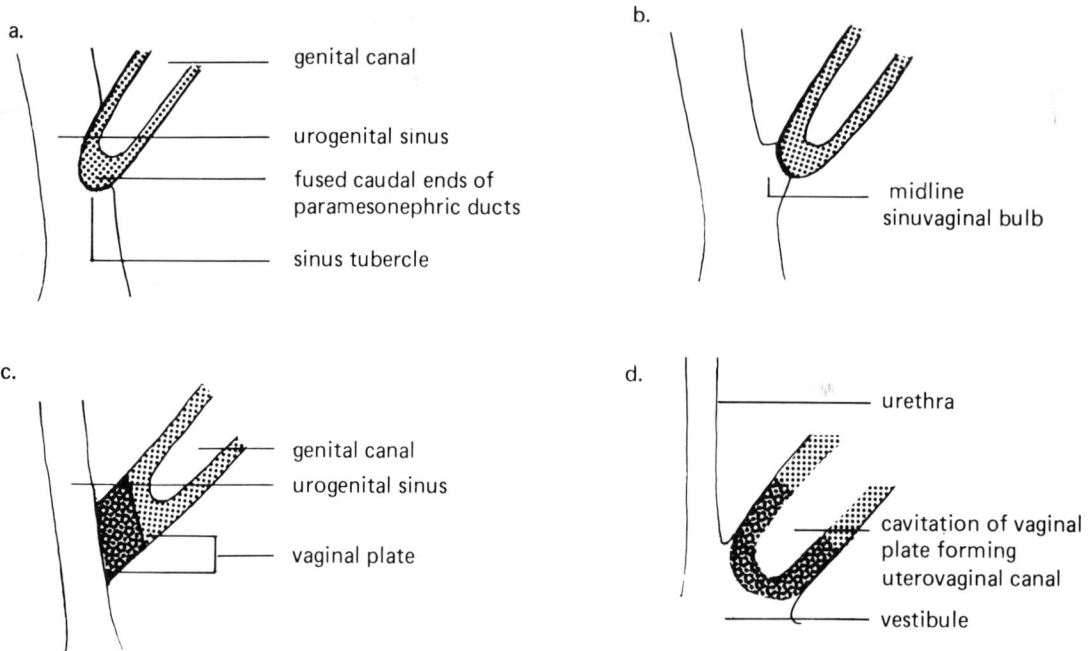

Fig. 1.17 (a) The fused paramesonephric ducts form the genital canal, the solid caudal end of which abuts on the posterior wall of the urogenital sinus at the sinus tubercle. (b) Cellular proliferation of the sinus epithelium generates the sinuvaginal bulbs which displace the genital canal dorsally. (c) Further cellular proliferation converts the sinuvaginal bulbs into solid tissue projections which participate in the formation of the vaginal plate. (d) Extensive caudal growth of the vaginal plate brings its lower surface into the primitive vestibule.

Together these projections displace the original genital canal in a dorsal direction (Fig. 1.17b). The solid sinuvaginal outgrowth and the solid caudal end of the genital canal together form the vaginal plate (Fig. 1.17c). The vaginal plate is recognisable between 87 and 95 days and its formation is complete at 19 weeks. Desquamation of cells from the vaginal plate precedes the formation of the vaginal lumen (O'Rahilly 1977).

The establishment of the vaginal plate is followed immediately by extensive growth caudally (Figs. 1.17d and 1.18) so that by the 16th week the vaginal rudiment approaches the cloacal vestibule (Witschi 1970). It has long been assumed that lengthening of the uterovaginal canal was achieved by cephalic extension, whereas Witschi (1970) maintains that 'the lower end of the vagina is sliding down the urethra to its separate opening'. At this stage the sinus element and the paramesonephric element are equally represented in the uterovaginal canal. At approximately 14 weeks the uterovaginal canal has a cephalic dilatation representing the corpus and a cervical dilatation which marks the region of the vaginal fornices (Koff 1933). The transition from pseudostratified columnar to stratified squamous epithelium observed at 17 weeks is considered to identify the cervicovaginal junction (Bulmer 1957, Davies & Kusama 1962).

The cervix is generally considered to be of paramesonephric origin (Koff 1933, Forsberg 1965, Witschi 1970) but Fluhmann (1960) claimed its mucous membrane to be of sinus origin and this indeed may be so. It has been suggested that the cervix and the upper segment of the vagina are initially lined by paramesonephric tissue which subsequently degenerates to be replaced by sinus tissue. In explanation of the teratogenic effect of diethylstilboestrol it has been further suggested that the drug prevents this degeneration and replacement and adversely affects the persisting paramesonephric tissue (Ulfedder & Robboy 1976). Certainly the occurrence of upper genital tract abnormalities associated with prenatal exposure to diethylstilboestrol (Kaufman et al 1977) supports these suggestions.

Cavitation of the vaginal plate, according to the

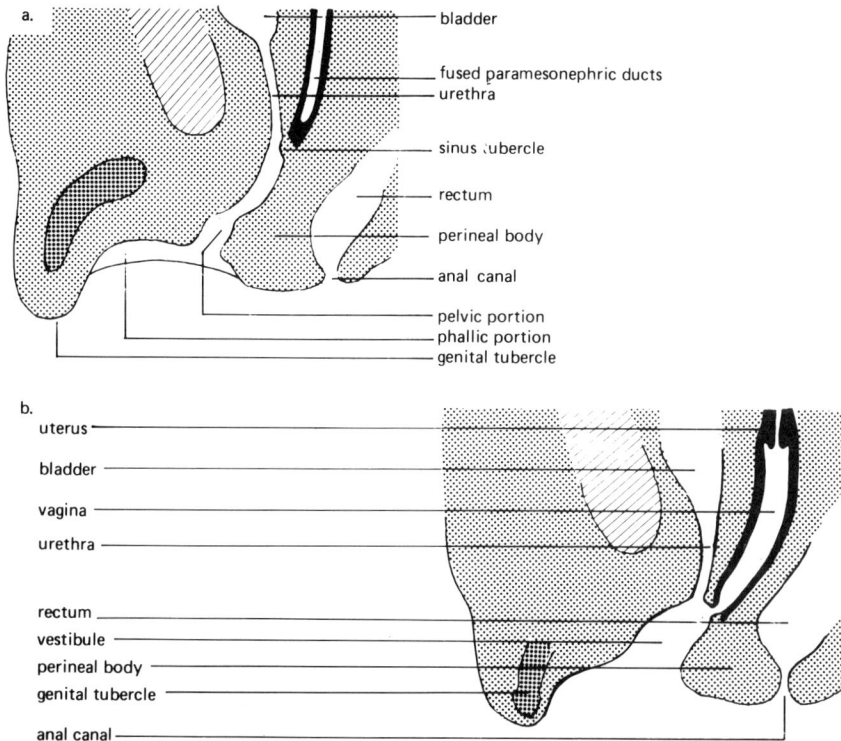

Fig. 1.18 (**a**) The fused paramesonephric ducts abut on the posterior surface of the urogenital sinus at the sinus tubercle. Above the sinus tubercle the urogenital sinus forms the bladder and urethra while below the tubercle it is divided into pelvic and phallic portions. (**b**) After the formation of the vaginal plate its extensive caudal growth transfers the vaginal opening into the vestbule.

various authorities cited by O'Rahilly (1977) is complete at about the midpoint of gestation, with the uterovaginal canal then having access to the exterior. More recently, however, it has been shown that at 14 weeks the vagina, uterus and uterine tubes have a continuous lumen accessible by intravaginal injection of a rapidly setting silicon liquid (Terruhn 1980). At approximately 17 weeks the high oestrogen levels in the maternal circulation begin to influence the fetal vagina although there is no evidence of an oestrogen response in the uterine corpus (Witschi 1970). In the newborn the stratified squamous epithelium of the vagina shows evidence of a marked oestrogen response. The site of the junction between the cervical and vaginal epithelia is variable and there is a range of normal appearance.

Oestrogens appear to have no role in the normal development of the paramesonephric ducts in the female since castration (Jost 1947), or explantation to steroid-free culture media (Picon 1969), is fol-

lowed by normal differentiation. However, in some experimental animals oestrogen has been shown to modify paramesonephric organogenesis and oestrogen receptors have been demonstrated in the paramesonephric ducts of late fetal rats (Somjen et al 1976) and guinea pigs (Pasqualini et al 1976).

Mesonephric duct. As the urorectal septum reaches the cloacal membrane at 30–32 days the caudal end of the mesonephric duct, having already opened into the urogenital sinus, gives origin to the ureteric bud and begins to be incorporated into the posterior wall of the urogenital sinus (Keith 1948). The portion of each duct incorporated into the urogenital sinus subsequently forms the trigone of the bladder and the posterior wall of the urethra (Fig. 1.12). At 30–32 days cells from cephalic mesonephric vesicles invade the coelomic epithelium on the medial aspect of the adjacent intermediate mesoderm (Fig. 1.14a) to induce the formation of the indifferent gonad (Wartenberg 1982). Meanwhile the mesonephric vesicles and ducts provide a functional excretory system for the developing embryo. This role begins to be taken over by the metanephric kidney before the end of embryogenesis and in the female fetus the mesonephric system then becomes redundant. It has, however, been suggested that the mesonephric ducts contribute to the formation of the uterine wall (Witschi 1970) and that their caudal ends are involved in vaginal organogenesis (Forsberg 1965).

Towards the end of embryogenesis the mesonephric vesicles begin to degenerate together with the mesonephric ducts. The lumen of the mesonephric duct is obliterated at 75 days and only remnants persist at 105 days (Josso 1981). A number of mesonephric derivatives may be located in the adult female. A constant finding is the epoophoron associated with the ovary and derived from the cephalic mesonephric duct and adjacent vesicles (Duthie 1925). A more caudal portion of the mesonephros may be encountered in the broad ligament as the paroophoron, while remnants of the terminal mesonephric duct may persist lateral to the uterus and vagina or incorporated into the cervix (O'Rahilly 1977, Buntine 1979). Adjacent to the lower genital tract such remnants are referred to as Gartner's ducts.

Development of the external genitalia

Urogenital sinus

The urorectal septum divides the hindgut into the urogenital sinus anteriorly and the terminal portion of the gastrointestinal tract posteriorly. This subdivision is completed at 30–32 days, but at 28 days the growing ends of the mesonephric ducts, within the urorectal septum, open into the posterior aspect of the developing urogenital sinus. Immediately the terminal mesonephric ducts give origin to the ureteric buds and are themselves incorporated into the urogenital sinus. This incorporation separates the mesonephric ducts and ureters, and at 49 days the mesonephric ducts terminate in the urogenital sinus on either side of the sinus tubercle. Cranial to the sinus tubercle the urogenital sinus is referred to as the vesico-urethral canal, and from it arise the bladder, the whole of the female urethra and the intramural and prostatic parts of the male urethra (Jirasek 1977). The por-

tion of the urogenital sinus caudal to the sinus tubercle continues to be referred to as the urogenital sinus and is subdivided into pelvic and phallic portions (Fig. 1.18).

Perineum

At the completion of flexion, about day 24, the anterior limit of the extensive cloacal membrane abuts on the base of the umbilical cord. On either side of the cloacal membrane just below the umbilical cord are the paired primordia of the genital tubercle. During the next few days retraction of the anterior end of the cloacal membrane from the base of the umbilical cord allows formation of an anterior body wall caudal to the umbilicus. The paired primordia of the genital tubercle fuse. Extending posteriorly from the base of the tubercle on either side of the cloacal membrane are the cloacal folds, lateral to which are the genital swellings. At 30–32 days the urorectal septum reaches the cloacal membrane and divides it into an anterior genital membrane and a posterior anal membrane. The anterior component of each cloacal fold becomes the genital fold and the posterior component the anal fold. The genital membrane ruptures soon afterwards, due to the increasing pressure associated with the functional mesonephric kidney (Ludwig 1965), as also does the anal membrane (Jirasek 1977). After the rupture of the genital membrane the phallic portion of the urogenital sinus is limited anteriorly by the underside of the genital tubercle. The genital tubercle elongates and is referred to as a phallus. This indifferent state, when phenotypic sex cannot be determined from the appearance of the external genitalia, lasts until day 63 (Jirasek 1977).

Masculinisation of the external genitalia

In the normal male fetus masculinisation begins between 63 and 70 days with the lengthening of both the phallus and the anogenital distance (Jirasek et al 1968). The genital folds fuse carrying the opening of the phallic portion of the urogenital sinus to the base of the phallus. Thereafter the cavernous urethra, enveloped in its spongy tissue, is completely closed and its opening is carried to the distal end of the phallus. These changes are completed by 84 to 98 days and during the same period the genital swellings fuse in the midline to form the scrotum (Jirasek 1977).

Feminisation of the external genitalia

In the normal female fetus feminisation begins between 63 and 77 days when the phallus, without lengthening, bends caudally (Jirasek 1977). During this period the anogenital distance remains unchanged, there is no fusion of the genital folds and the phallic portion or the urogenital sinus remains open. Some time between 14 weeks (Terruhn 1980) and 20 weeks (O'Rahilly 1977) the vagina opens into the pelvic portion of the urogenital sinus converting it into the vaginal vestibule. During the second half of gestation the urethral and vaginal openings separate. As they do so the phallus becomes the clitoris, being incorporated within the fused anterior ends of the genital folds, which become the labia minora. The genital swellings, lateral to the labia minora, become the labia majora and are continuous with the future mons pubis, anterior to the clitoris.

Mechanism of differentiation

Testosterone is the only steroid hormone produced by the fetal gonad at the time of sexual differentiation (Wilson & Siiteri 1973, Siiteri & Wilson 1974) and it enters its target cells by diffusion. In cells possessing the enzyme 5α-reductase testosterone is converted to dihydrotestosterone (DHT), otherwise it remains as testosterone. Within the cell the androgen, as either testosterone or DHT, is bound by a specific high affinity cytosol protein receptor. The androgen receptor complex is activated and translocated to the nucleus where it initiates gene transcription. After transcription and processing of the messenger RNA, the specific RNA within the cytoplasm is involved in the synthesis of new androgen-induced proteins (Liao 1978).

The synthesis of the androgen cytosol protein receptor is regulated by genes at the X-linked Tfm locus (Ohno 1977). Therefore both sexes possess the cellular apparatus for androgen action with the limiting factor being the plasma concentration of testosterone. Male differentiation of the mesonephric ducts is testosterone dependent since the undifferentiated ducts lack the enzyme 5α-

reductase (Wilson & Lasnitzki 1971, Siiteri & Wilson 1974). In contrast male differentiation of the urogenital sinus and external genitalia is DHT dependent and 5α-reductase is present in these tissues, in both sexes, before sexual differentiation begins (Wilson & Lasnitzki 1971, Wilson 1973).

In the female fetus the absence of testosterone allows the mesonephric ducts to degenerate and enables the urogenital sinus and external genitalia to follow their inherent tendency and differentiate according to the female phenotype. In the male fetus any defect which prevents the effective action of androgen will impair masculinisation of the internal and/or external organs of reproduction. Failure to synthesise the cytosol protein receptor prevents the action of testosterone on the mesonephric ducts and of DHT on the urogenital sinus and the external genitalia. This receptor defect causes complete or incomplete androgen insensitivity, as observed in the testicular feminisation syndromes (Morris 1953). Failure to synthesise 5α-reductase prevents the conversion of testosterone to its intracellular metabolite DHT, which is necessary for the virilisation of the urogenital sinus and external genitalia (Imperato-McGinley et al 1974). This enzyme defect, transmitted as an autosomal recessive (Simpson et al 1971, Peterson et al 1979), causes the clinical syndrome first described by Novakowski & Lenz (1961) in which patients have female external genitalia in association with normal testes and male internal reproductive organs.

The external genitalia of the human male fetus are completely masculinised by 84 to 98 days (Jirasek 1977). If a female fetus is exposed to significant androgen levels before the end of this period of development complete external virilisation will occur (Grumbach & Ducharme 1960), while lower levels or later exposure will produce various forms of incomplete virilisation.

CONGENITAL ANOMALIES

The sex of the newborn is established from the appearance of the external genitalia. Occasionally this may not be possible because of the ambiguous nature of the external genitalia. In such circumstances, despite parental anxiety, sex should not be assigned on the basis of approximation to male or female phenotype. Such assignment must await careful examination of the pudenda, karyotyping to establish chromosomal complement and if necessary full endocrine and cytogenetic investigations. These latter procedures may be necessary since the genital appearances of an undermasculinised male, a masculinised female and an hermaphrodite are essentially similar (Dewhurst 1980). Some of these abnormalities are known to be caused by genetic defects while others are caused by endogenous or exogenous factors which influence development at certain critical periods of embryogenesis. There are certain conditions of abnormal sexual differentiation in which the apparent sex of the infant, assigned on the basis of pudendal phenotype, will not accord with the chromosomal, gonadal or genital duct sex of the child. In such cases the associated problems will not present until adolescence or later. In addition there are a number of readily recognisable structural defects involving the lower female genital tract and external genitalia in which the cause is unknown.

A. Ambiguous external genitalia

In infants, children or adults in whom the external genitalia are not characteristic of male or female phenotype there are a number of possible presentations. Almost all such individuals, however, possess a phallus enlarged to a varying degree with a small opening on its ventral surface, at its base or on the perineum through which urine is voided. A second opening or depression may be identified more posteriorly, while on either side of the midline virilisation, ranging from rugose labia-majora-like structures to scrotal sacs, may be seen (Dewhurst 1980). A structural classification of such conditions is possible since comparable anatomical findings occur in a variety of clinical syndromes. However, the following classification, derived from Grumbach & Conte (1981) and Simpson (1982), is preferred. It is based upon aetiological mechanisms and clinical syndromes and comprises three main groups:

1. Disorders of gonadal differentiation.
2. Female pseudohermaphroditism.
3. Male pseudohermaphroditism.

1. Disorders of gonadal differentiation

(a) Ovarian dysgenesis. Approximately 50% of all patients with ovarian dysgenesis have a chromosomal complement of 45X; a further 25% have sex chromosomal mosaicism without a structural chromosomal abnormality (45X/46XX; 45X/46XY) while the remainder have either a structurally abnormal X or Y chromosome or no detectable chromosomal abnormality (Simpson 1982).

(i) 45X Turner's syndrome. Only a small number of 45X embryos survive intra-uterine life (Boué et al 1975). At birth the genital ducts and external genitalia are entirely female although clitoral enlargement may occasionally be present (Grumbach & Conte 1981). The ovaries are associated with the broad ligaments. They consist of fibrous stroma and are termed streak gonads. Secondary sexual development does not usually occur but some 45X individuals do menstruate and very occasionally bear children (King et al 1978, Kohn et al 1980). Patients with Turner's syndrome are of short stature and exhibit a range of somatic abnormalities including webbing of the neck, coarctation of the aorta and renal anomalies. Also associated with the condition is a predisposition to develop diabetes mellitus (Engel & Forbes 1965).

(ii) 45X/46XX mosaicism and X chromosome abnormality. In these conditions the phenotype is invariably female. Some of the affected individuals will be indistinguishable from those with 45X. Others, who exhibit no somatic defects, will nevertheless have streak gonads, will not undergo secondary sexual development and will fail to menstruate.

(iii) 45X/46XY mosaicism and Y chromosome abnormality. A highly diverse phenotype is encountered in 45X/46XY mosaicism since the presence of a Y-bearing cell line may induce some testicular differentiation. Such individuals may appear typically male or female or may possess ambiguous external genitalia with varied genital duct development. In a series of 111 patients with 45X/46XY mosaicism, two-thirds were reared as females (Zah et al 1975). Several cases of structural abnormality of the Y chromosome have been reported (Davis 1981). The affected individuals are phenotypic females with bilateral streak gonads who remain sexually immature.

(iv) 46XX, 46XY. Gonadal dysgenesis may occur in association with apparently normal 46XX or 46XY karyotypes. These individuals are phenotypically female but have streak gonads and remain sexually immature. The 46XX form of gonadal dysgenesis appears to be inherited as an autosomal recessive condition (Simpson et al 1971). The genetic heterogeneity of this form of gonadal dysgenesis is evidenced by its occurrence in some families in association with neurosensory deafness, which may also afflict otherwise normal male siblings (Pallister & Opitz 1979). The 46XY form of gonadal dysgenesis occurs in both H-Y positive and H-Y negative forms. Clitoral enlargement is not uncommon but the most important aspect of this condition is the increased incidence of gonadal neoplasms, which are more likely to occur in the H-Y positive form (Simpson 1982). Bilateral gonadectomy is therefore indicated as a prophylactic measure (Dewhurst 1980, Grumbach & Conte 1981).

In all forms of ovarian dysgenesis oestrogen replacement therapy is recommended at 12–13 years of age eventually to be cycled monthly with progesterone (Grumbach & Conte 1981).

(b) True hermaphroditism. True hermaphrodites possess both ovarian and testicular tissue, with an ovary on one side and a testis on the other or, more commonly, with ovotestes situated bilaterally or unilaterally (Grumbach & Conte 1981). The differentiation of the genital tract, the appearance of the external genitalia and the development of secondary sexual characteristics are variable. Although the external genitalia are often ambiguous (Fig. 1.19) three-quarters of reported cases have been reared as males because of the size of the phallus (van Niekerk 1976). Despite the tendency to rear these patients as males the majority of their gonads exhibit oocytes but not spermatozoa, a uterus is almost invariably present and 60% of them have a 46XX karyotype; indeed four 46XX true hermaphrodites have become pregnant (Tegenkamp et al 1979). The remaining 40% of true hermaphrodites in van Niekerk's 1976 review were equally distributed between 46XY karyotypes, 46XX/46XY chimeras and sex chromosome mosaics.

(c) Seminiferous tubular dysgenesis. Two forms of seminiferous tubular dysgenesis have been identified. In both the external genitalia are typical-

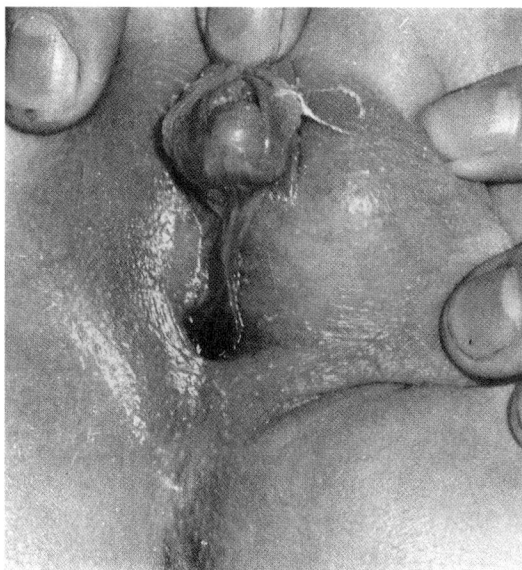

Fig. 1.19 External genitalia of a true hermaphrodite. (From Dewhurst 1980 with permission)

ly male but show no maturation with approaching adulthood. Within the testes the seminiferous tubules remain undeveloped, Leydig cells are functionally inadequate and spermatogonia are rarely seen.

(i) Klinefelter's syndrome. Males with at least one Y chromosome and at least two X chromosomes have Klinefelter's syndrome. About 1 per 800 liveborn males has a 47XXY karyotype which is characterised by seminiferous tubule dysgenesis and androgen deficiency. This phenotype may also be associated with 46XY/47XXY, 48XXYY, or 49XXXXY karyotypes (Simpson 1982).

(ii) 46XX males. These individuals are sex-reversed phenotypic males. Since they are H-Y positive the presumptive aetiology must involve either an X-Y or Y-autosome translocation (de la Chapelle 1981).

(d) Gonadal agenesis. In this condition abnormal external genitalia are associated with hypoplastic Müllerian and Wolffian derivatives. A small phallus, ill-developed labia majora and fusion of the labioscrotal folds are features of the external genital appearance (Sarto & Opitz 1973). Such individuals have a 46XY karyotype and are H-Y positive (Schulte 1979). The frequent association of somatic anomalies suggests a possible teratogen.

2. Female pseudohermaphroditism

Female pseudohermaphrodites are 46XX individuals with normal ovaries, normal Müllerian duct derivatives and atypical female external genitalia. The clitoris is enlarged, labial fusion produces a variable vaginal orifice and the urethral opening may not be distinct from the vagina. The external genitalia of the male fetus are completely masculinised by 84 to 98 days (Jirasek 1977). If a female fetus is exposed to significant androgen levels in the presence of 5α-reductase before the end of this period of development complete virilisation will occur (Grumbach & Ducharme 1960), while lower levels or later exposure will produce various forms of incomplete virilisation. The source of the virilising influence may be fetal, maternal or exogenous.

(a) Fetal. Congenital adrenal hyperplasia accounts for most of the cases of female pseudohermaphroditism and approximately half of all patients with ambiguous external genitalia. There are several types of congenital adrenal hyperplasia and all are transmitted as an autosomal recessive trait (Grumbach & Conte 1981). The common denominator in all types is impaired cortisol formation due to an enzyme defect on the steroid biosynthetic pathway. Depressed cortisol synthesis produces hypersecretion of adrenocorticotrophic hormone (ACTH) through the negative feedback mechanism and consequent hyperplasia of the adrenal cortex. There are essentially two types of enzyme defect. The first, caused by 21-hydroxylase deficiency or 11β-hydroxylase deficiency, limits cortisol production and diverts the synthetic pathway towards overproduction of adrenal androgens and androgen precursors. The second, caused by 3βol-dehydrogenase deficiency or 17α-hydroxylase deficiency, limits cortisol production and also impairs the synthesis of sex steroids by the gonads and adrenals.

(i) 21-hydroxylase deficiency. Since the adrenal begins to function during the third month of intra-uterine life excessive production of adrenal androgens will virilise the fetal female external genitalia (Fig. 1.20). Several forms of 21-hydroxylase deficiency exist, some of which are associated with sodium depletion and are therefore life threatening in the neonatal period. All deficiency states result from a mutant autosomal recessive gene, located on

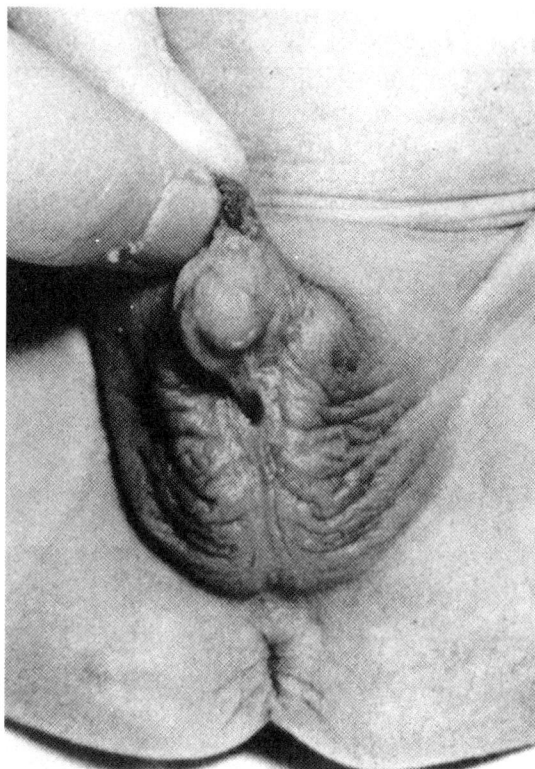

Fig. 1.20 External genitalia of a female child with congenital adrenal hyperplasia. (From Dewhurst 1980 with permission)

chromosome 6, which is closely linked to the HLA locus (Du Pont et al 1977). Linkage to the HLA locus permits antenatal diagnosis (Simpson 1982) and the possibility of pharmacological suppression of the fetal adrenal gland in utero. Such intervention, beginning at the tenth week of gestation, with dexamethasone administration to the mother, is not harmful to the fetus (Evans et al 1985). In affected individuals adrenal hormone supplementation is required postnatally.

(ii) 11β-hydroxylase deficiency. This enzyme deficiency, also inherited in an autosomal recessive fashion, is less common than 21-hydroxylase deficiency. Sodium depletion does not occur in association with this defect.

(iii) 3βol-dehydrogenase deficiency. With this enzyme defect the only androgen synthesised is dehydroepiandrosterone (DHEA), which is relatively weak. Females with this deficiency are less virilised than females with 21- or 11β-hydroxylase deficiencies. In fact DHEA is such a weak androgen that males with 3βol-dehydrogenase deficiency may fail to masculinise (Simpson 1982).

(iv) 17α-hydroxylase deficiency. Females with this enzyme defect have normal female external genitalia at birth but show no secondary sexual development at puberty (Simpson 1982).

(b) Maternal. In rare instances, virilisation of the female fetus may occur if the mother is suffering from certain ovarian or adrenal tumours or has unrecognised congenital adrenal hyperplasia. The absence of virilisation in the mother does not exclude a maternal source since the level of androgen required to virilise the external genitalia of the early female fetus is much less than would be required to have a virilising effect on the adult female (Grumbach & Ducharme 1960).

(c) Exogenous. Virilisation of the external genitalia of female infants has been frequently observed following maternal ingestion of testosterone or synthetic progestational agents during the first trimester of pregnancy (Grumbach & Ducharme 1960, Wilkins 1960, Dewhurst & Gordon 1984, Reschini et al 1985). Administration of such agents between the 8th and 12th week of gestation causes marked virilisation (Fig. 1.21), while later in pregnancy their use causes clitoral enlargement (Fig. 1.22). These agents, as well as stilboestrol, were often prescribed in the past for women with habitual or threatened abortion. Although exposure to stilboestrol during intra-uterine life is known to cause malformations in the reproductive tracts of both sexes and an increased incidence of cervical and vaginal neoplasia (Herbst et al 1972, 1974), it has also been shown to cause female pseudo-hermaphroditism (Bongiovani et al 1959). More recently intra-uterine exposure to danazol (Danocrine®, Chronogyn®), a carbon-17-alkylated derivative of ethinyltestosterone used in the treatment

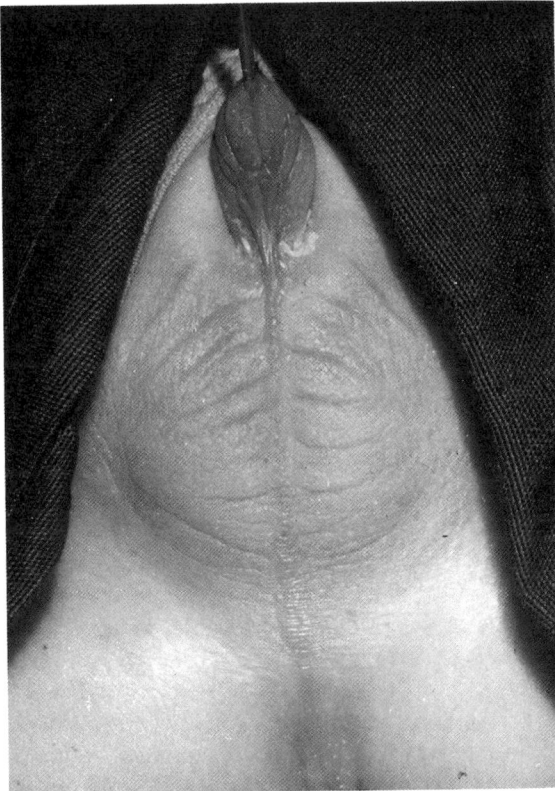

Fig. 1.21 Marked virilisation of a female child caused by maternal androgen therapy during early pregnancy. (From Dewhurst 1980 with permission)

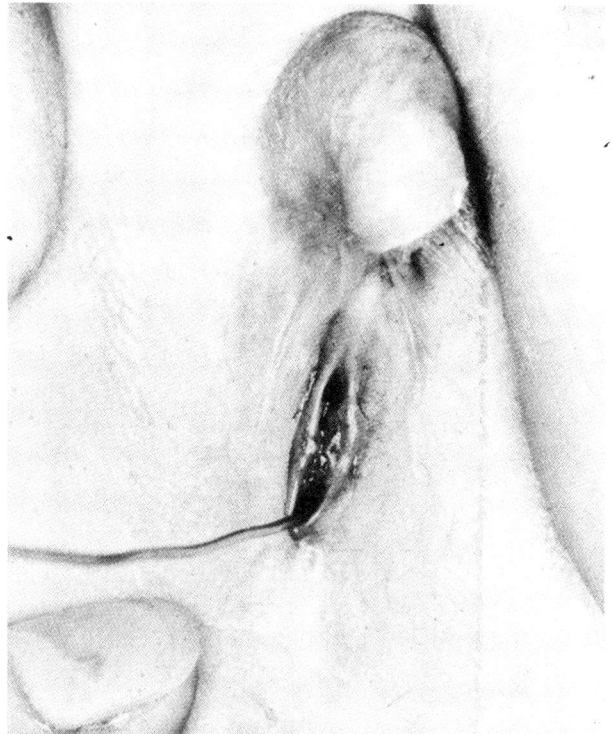

Fig. 1.22 Partial virilisation of a female child caused by maternal androgen therapy during pregnancy. (From Dewhurst 1980 with permission)

of endometriosis and of hereditary angio-oedema, has been associated with the occurrence of female pseudohermaphroditism (Rosa 1984, Shaw & Farquhar 1984).

3. Male pseudohermaphroditism

In male pseudohermaphroditism the testes, which are always present, are unable to effect complete masculinisation of the genital ducts and external genitalia (Fig. 1.23). This functional defect can occur at any of several stages in the masculinisation process and will therefore produce varying degrees of the female phenotype.

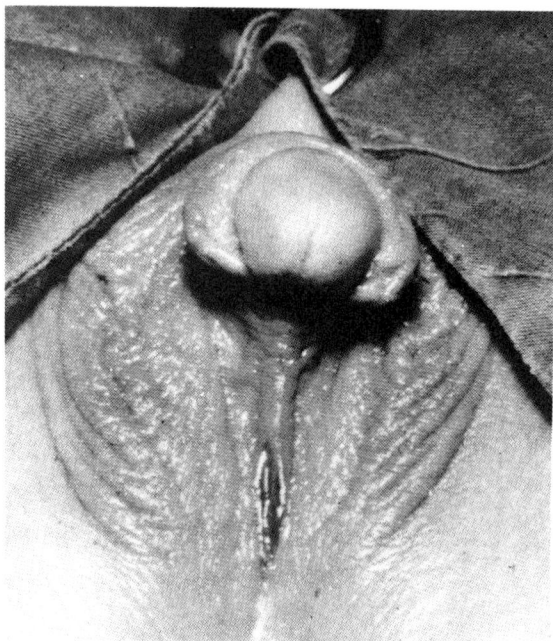

Fig. 1.23 External genitalia of an incompletely masculinised male child in whom there was partial testicular failure. (From Dewhurst 1980 with permission)

(a) *Lack of testicular response to gonadotrophin.* Production of testosterone by the Leydig cells of the fetal testes is essential for Wolffian duct stabilisation and masculinisation of the external genitalia. An individual with Leydig cell agenesis or a receptor abnormality, resulting in their unresponsiveness to gonadotrophins, has female external genitalia, no Wolffian reproductive tract derivatives and, because of AMH production by Sertoli cells, absent Müllerian derivatives (Berth-

ezene et al 1976, Brown et al 1978). Such individuals have ectopic testes and exhibit no secondary sexual characteristics with the approach of adulthood.

Any defect in Sertoli cell response to gonadotrophins, or a lack of responsiveness by the Mullerian ducts to AMH, results in the presence of internal female organs of reproduction in otherwise normal males.

(b) *Enzyme defects in testosterone biosynthesis.* Five familial enzymatic defects in testosterone biosynthesis have been identified, one at each of the enzymatic steps required for the coversion of cholesterol to testosterone (Grumbach & Conte 1981). Three of these defects involve enzymes affecting both glucocorticoid and sex steroid biosynthesis while the remaining two involve enzymes principally concerned with testosterone biosynthesis in the testes. The first group of patients will therefore require adrenal hormone therapy throughout life and all will require appropriate sex steroid therapy at puberty depending on the degree of surgical intervention and the sex of rearing.

Each of these enzyme defects is inherited as an autosomal or X-linked recessive trait. In general their effect is to produce external genitalia ranging from the normal female appearance to that of an hypospadic male. Müllerian duct derivatives are invariably absent but a blind-ending vaginal pouch is common in affected individuals. The Wolffian duct derivatives may be normal or hypoplastic while the testes are usually ectopically situated. Pubertal masculinisation may be pronounced in some of these conditions when the child, because of the appearance of the external genitalia, has been raised as a girl (Fig. 1.24).

(c) *Defects in androgen dependent target tissue.* Effective biosynthesis of testosterone is essential, but not sufficient, for full masculinisation of the 46XY fetus. Male differentiation of the external genitalia is effected by DHT, produced from testosterone by the enzyme 5α-reductase. The action of testosterone on the Wolffian ducts and of DHT on the external genitalia is dependent on a specific intracellular cytosol protein receptor which, after binding the androgen, is activated to initiate gene transcription which achieves the masculinising effect (Liao 1978).

(i) *Androgen receptor and postreceptor defects.* The

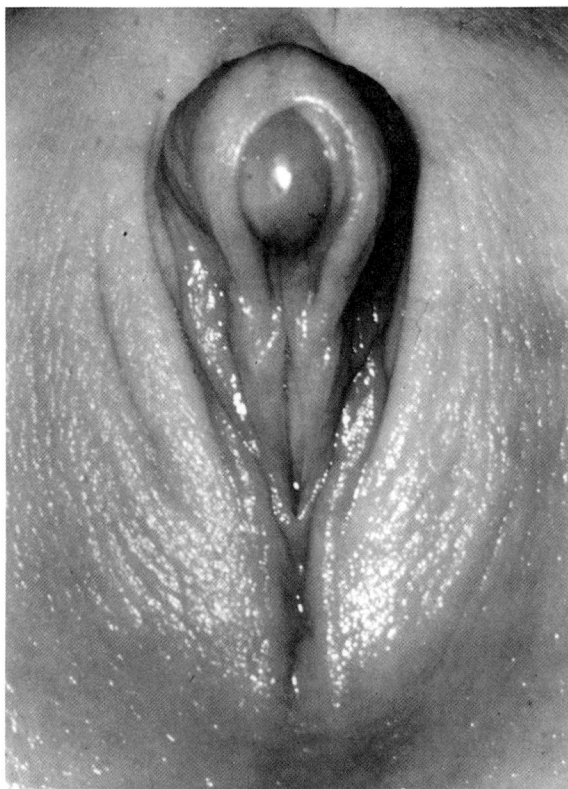

Fig. 1.24 External genitalia of an XY child reared as a girl. (From Dewhurst with permission)

synthesis of the androgen cytosol protein receptor is regulated by genes at the Tfm locus on the X chromosome (Ohno 1977). Failure to synthesise the receptor or activate the receptor–androgen complex effectively blocks the androgen's masculinising role. Such receptor defects cause complete or incomplete androgen insensitivity, typical of the testicular feminisation syndrome (Morris 1953).

In the complete androgen insensitivity syndrome H-Y positive males are phenotypically female and possess a blind vaginal pouch. They develop female secondary sexual characteristics at puberty but fail to menstruate since Müllerian duct derivatives are absent. The Wolffian duct derivatives are also absent or vestigial while the testes are intra-abdominal or situated in the labial or inguinal regions (Grumbach & Conte 1981). The incomplete syndrome presents in a variety of forms due to decreased numbers of cytosol androgen receptors in the target tissues (Griffin et al 1976).

(ii) 5α-reductase deficiency. This familial type of male pseudohermaphroditism was first reported by Novakowski & Lenz (1961) who described it as 'pseudovaginal perineoscrotal hypospadias'. Affected individuals at birth have a clitoris-like hypospadic phallus, a bifid scrotum and a urogenital sinus opening on the perineum. Further investigation shows a 46XY karyotype, normally differentiated ectopic testes, male internal ducts and no Müllerian derivatives. This abnormality of sexual development, transmitted as an autosomal recessive trait (Simpson et al 1971, Peterson et al 1979) was later shown to be due to an absence of 5α-reductase from the external genital tissue. Failure to synthesise 5α-reductase prevents the conversion of testosterone to DHT, which is now known to be necessary for masculinisation of the external genitalia (Imperato-McGinley et al 1974). Perhaps the most striking but as yet unexplained phenomenon associated with this condition is the masculinisation occurring at puberty: the voice deepens, muscle mass increases, the phallus enlarges, the bifid scrotum becomes rugose and pigmented while the enlarging testes descend into the labioscrotal folds (Grumbach & Conte 1981).

B. Structural defects

Various abnormalities may arise in the genital system, as in other systems, due to inherent defects of development, migration, canalisation and fusion. The interdependence during development of the reproductive, urinary and terminal gastrointestinal systems causes some genital defects to be associated with renal, rectal or anal anomalies. In this account brief reference will be made to abnormalities of the upper reproductive tract in so far as they affect the lower reproductive tract. It is evident from the notifications of congenital malformations of the external genitalia in England and Wales over the period 1964 to 1983 that their incidence is falling in females but rising in males (Matlai and Beral 1985).

Upper reproductive tract

Absence of the uterine tubes without associated uterine abnormalities is very rare (Warkany 1971). Partial absence or atresia of a tube, with or without the presence of tubal diverticula, has been reported, the latter form of isolated abnormality being associated with tubal pregnancy (McNalley 1926). Absence of the uterus is common in some disorders of gonadal differentiation and in male pseudohermaphroditism but it may occur in otherwise normal females in whom the Müllerian ducts have failed to develop. More often, however, there is unilateral Müllerian duct development and this type of anomaly is associated with renal agenesis (Frost 1958). Fusion defects of the Müllerian ducts can cause abnormalities ranging from a bicornuate uterus with various degrees of cervical and vaginal septation to the formation of two uteri and two vaginae. In some of these latter cases there has been duplication of the vulva, urethra and bladder (Warkany 1971).

Congenital or later prolapse of the uterus is not uncommon in the female spina bifida infant, when the protrusion between the labia minora exhibits a cervical opening. The cause of this condition is thought to be paralysis of the pelvic floor musculature arising as a consequence of the neural tube defect (Torpin 1942).

Lower reproductive tract

(a) **Vaginal agenesis.** The absence of a vagina forms part of the presenting clinical picture in some patients with male or female pseudohermaphroditism. Agenesis of the vagina may, however, occur in 46XX females who are not pseudohermaphrodites. Total vaginal agenesis is usually found in association with tubal and uterine agenesis presumably as a consequence of complete Müllerian aplasia. Occasionally the upper reproductive tract is normal and functional and the vaginal agenesis has resulted from a partial Müllerian defect or because the vaginal plate has failed to form or cavitate. In a survey of 167 women with total vaginal agenesis one-third of them had associated renal tract defects while others had skeletal abnormalities (Evans et al 1981). The authors of this study suggest familial transmission, the variable expression of an underlying recessive trait or the action of a teratogen as the most likely cause of this condition, in which the average age at presentation was 16 years. In some patients with vaginal agenesis a very shallow vaginal opening may be present; when this is associated with a rudimentary upper reproduc-

tive tract it is referred to as the Rokitansky–Kuster–Hauser syndrome (Simpson 1982).

(b) **Vaginal atresia.** In this condition the urogenital sinus fails to form the inferior portion of the vagina. The lower vagina is replaced by fibrous tissue above which there is a normal reproductive tract (Simpson 1976).

(c) **Vaginal septa.** Transverse vaginal septa are said to be located at the junction of the upper third and lower two-thirds of the vagina (Simpson 1976). The probable cause of transverse vaginal septa formation is the failure of either the Müllerian or urogenital sinus contributions to the vagina to cavitate completely. This aetiology would therefore cause transverse septa to form at any level in the vagina. In the Amish community this abnormality is inherited as an autosomal recessive trait (McKusick et al 1964). Patients with transverse vaginal septa may present at puberty with retained menstrual products or alternatively with a continuous vaginal discharge.

A longitudinal vaginal septum may present in the midline as the result of a fusion defect in the Müllerian system and will be associated with abnormalities of the upper reproductive tract. More usually longitudinal septa are formed by aberrant cellular proliferation, which can occur in any plane and are rarely associated with clinical problems.

(d) **Imperforate hymen.** This is commonly caused by the failure of the central epithelial cells of the hymenal membrane to degenerate. However this condition may arise as the result of an inflammatory reaction in the hymen after birth. The majority of cases are identified with the onset of puberty.

(e) **Vaginal cysts.** In the neonatal period vaginal cysts may be found posterior to the urethral meatus. These cysts arise from the anterior or lateral walls of the vagina at the introitus and usually rupture spontaneously (Warkany 1971). Occasionally one or more of these cysts may enlarge and obstruct the urethra. These cysts are thought to be inclusions from the urogenital sinus epithelium and may persist asymptomatically into adulthood (Robboy et al 1978). Certainly mucous cysts were found in the same location, interior to the labia minora and external to the hymen, in about 3% of adults attending a vulval clinic (Friedrich & Wilkinson 1973). In addition the Wolffian ducts, which degenerate in the female, leave caudal remnants in the lateral walls of the vagina and at the vulva. These remnants may undergo cystic degeneration, when they are termed Gärtner's cysts.

External genitalia

Various abnormalities of the vulva are caused by disturbances of sexual differentiation which lead to an ambiguous appearance of the external genitalia. Other vulvar defects, such as duplication, occur in association with abnormalities of the upper reproductive tract and urinary system. Congenital anomalies of the vulva that occur in isolation involve the clitoris and the labia.

(a) Clitoris. The clitoris may be absent (Falk & Hyman 1971), probably as a result of the genital tubercles remaining hypoplastic or failing to fuse. It is, however, more likely that failure of the genital tubercles to fuse will be interpreted as duplication of the clitoris.

(b) Labia minora. Hypertrophy and/or an asymmetry of the labia minora may occur without demonstrable aetiology. True hypoplasia of the labia minora occurs infrequently, and may be a sign of defective steroidogenesis.

Fusion of the labia minora may occur in association with defective sexual differentiation but it may also be observed in the postnatal period as a result of inflammatory adhesion (see also p. 194).

Vulval and urinary system abnormalities

(a) Kidney. Bilateral renal agenesis is a lethal congenital malformation (Potter 1946) and in the female is frequently associated with deformation of the external genitalia, absence of the uterus and vagina and abnormalities of other systems (Potter 1965).

Unilateral renal agenesis, which is compatible with a long and active life, is also associated with malformation of the external genitalia. The incidence of genital anomalies in unilateral renal agenesis is about 40% in females and 12% in males (Warkany 1971).

(b) Ureter. The ureteric bud arises from the Wolffian (mesonephric) duct. It is eventually separated from the Wolffian duct as the latter structure is incorporated into the urogenital sinus to form the trigone of the bladder and urethra. Failure of dissociation between the ureteric bud and Wolffian duct in the female will allow the ureteric orifice to be located at any site along the caudal remnant of the Wolffian duct (Gärtner's duct). Vaginal drainage of the ectopic ureter occurs because of secondary rupture of Gärtner's duct into the vagina (Weiss et al 1984).

(c) Bladder. Exstrophy of the bladder is caused by a failure of the subumbilical portion of the anterior abdominal wall to meet in the midline above the genital tubercles. The genital tubercles remain as paired primordia and the anterior wall of the bladder is either partially or totally absent. This condition may therefore exist as incomplete or complete bladder exstrophy and is always associated with epispadias and other abnormalities of the external genitalia. A more severe form of this structural defect is cloacal exstrophy in which the urorectal septum fails to divide the hindgut and the abdominal wall deficit gives access not only to the bladder but also to the terminal gastrointestinal tract (Diamond and Jeffs 1985). In comparison with the urinary and/or intestinal abnormalities those of the external genitalia may seem minor. However, these conditions are now capable of surgical repair and it is important to refashion the external genitalia in accordance with the chromosomal and gonadal sex of the infant in so far as this is possible (Dewhurst 1980).

(d) Urethra. Congenital abnormalities of the urethra occur predominantly in the male. Those that occur in females have a lower incidence than in males. In duplication of the urethra, a cause of urinary incontinence in the female, the accessory urethra usually arises from the trigone and opens on to the anterior wall of the vagina (Williams 1958). Mild forms of epispadias may occur in the female giving rise to disturbance of bladder control and urinary incontinence. In this condition the urethral opening lies deep to the mons veneris between two clitoral elements (Williams 1958). Hypospadias, when it occurs in the female, does so in association with female pseudohermaphroditism. In both epispadias and hypospadias, the female urethra is congenitally short (Burbige & Hensle 1985). Meatal stenosis is uncommon in the female but may simulate bladder neck obstruction (Warkany 1971). Prolapse of urethral mucosa

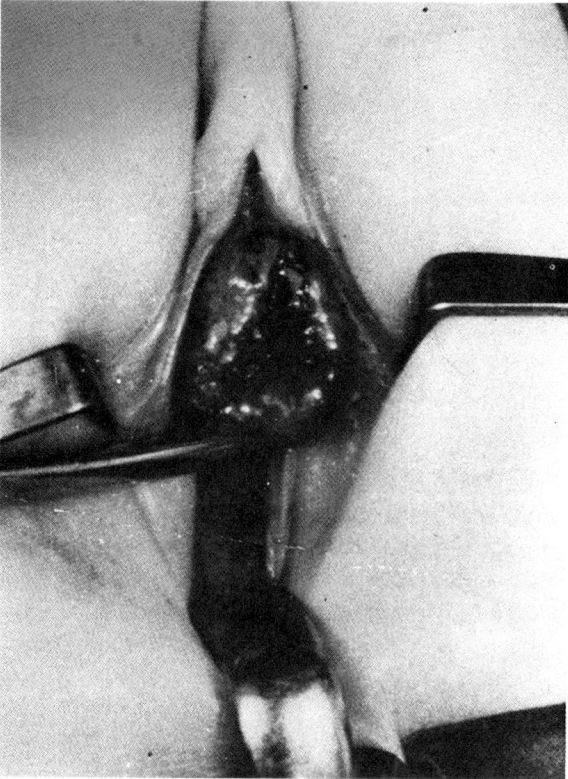

Fig. 1.25 Prolapse of urethral mucosa in a child. (By courtesy of Ridley, C M 1975 The Vulva. Major Problems in Dermatology 5. Lloyd Luke).

(Fig. 1.25) occurs only in the female (Capraro et al 1970). Urethral cysts may develop in Skene's glands which open at the termination of the urethra. Inadequate drainage or infection will cause recurrent urinary symptoms. Finally, an ectopic ureter may open into the urethra.

These various urethral abnormalities may present as urinary incontinence although lesser degrees of incontinence may cause constant vulval wetness and skin irritation. They are all amenable to surgical repair.

Vulval and intestinal abnormalities

In the female an imperforate anus or anal stenosis may be associated with a variety of abnormalities of the genital tract and vulva (Hall et al 1985). An ectopic bowel opening may be found in the vagina or elsewhere in the perineum. When a rectovaginal fistula is formed there are often urinary tract abnormalities present also.

Vulval mammary tissue

The number of mammary glands is determined by the average number of young delivered with each pregnancy. During embryogenesis paired thickenings of ectoderm descend the ventral body wall, on either side of the midline, from the base of the fore limb bud to the medial aspect of the hind limb bud. The caudal two-thirds of these 'milk-lines' disappear in the human and the breast primordia are restricted to the thoracic region. Persistence of the most caudal elements of the milk-lines in the human will therefore involve the labia majora of the vulva; hence ectopic vulval breast tissue (p. 228).

REFERENCES

Agogué 1965 Dualité embryologique du vagin humain et origine histologique de sa muqueuse. Gynécologie et Obstetriques 64: 407–414

Baker T G 1963 A quantitative and cytological study of germ cells in human ovaries. Proceedings of the Royal Society of London Series B 158: 417–433

Barber H R K, Sommers S C 1974 Vaginal adenosis, dysplasia and clear-cell adenocarcinoma after diethylstilboestrol treatment in pregnancy. Obstetrics and Gynecology 43: 645–682

Bérthezene F, Forest M G, Grimaud J A, Clanstrat B, Mornex R 1976 Leydig cell agenesis; a cause of male pseudohermaphroditism. New England Journal of Medicine 295: 969–972

Blanchard M G, Josso N 1974 Source of the anti-Müllerian hormone synthesized by the fetal testes. Paediatric Research 8: 968–971

Blechschmidt E 1968 Vom Ei zum Embryo. Deutsche Verlags-Austalt, Stuttgart

Bongiovani A M, DiGeorge C, Grumbach M M 1959 Masculinization of the female infant associated with estrogen therapy alone during gestation. Journal of Clinical Endocrinology and Metabolism 19: 1004–1010

Boue J, Boue A, Lazar P 1975 Retrospective and prospective epidemiological studies of 1500 karyotyped spontaneous human abortions. Teratology 12: 11–16

Brambell F W R 1956 Ovarian changes. In: Parkes A S (ed) Marshall's physiology of reproduction. Vol. 1. Longmans Green, London pp 397–544

Bridges C B 1916 Non-disjunction as proof of the chromosome theory of heredity. Genetics 1, 1–52

Brown D M, Markland C, Dehner L P 1978 Leydig cell hypoplasia: a cause of male pseudohermaphroditism. Journal of

Clinical Endocrinology and Metabolism 46: 1–7

Bull J J 1981 Evolution of environmental sex determination from genotypic sex determination. Heredity 47: 173–184

Bull J J 1983 Evolution of sex determining mechanisms. Benjamin/Cummings, Menlo Park

Bulmer D 1957 The development of the human vagina. Journal of Anatomy 91: 490–509

Buntine D W 1979 Adenocarcinoma of the uterine cervix of probable Wolffian origin. Pathology 11: 713–718

Burbige K A, Hensle T W 1985 Surgical management of urinary incontinence in girls with congenitally short urethra. Journal of Urology 133: 67–71

Burgoyne P S 1981 The genetics of sex in development. In: Hamilton D, Naftolin F (eds) Basic reproductive medicine Vol 1. Basis and development of reproduction. MIT Press, Cambridge, p 1–31

Burgoyne P S 1982 Genetic homology and crossing over in the X & Y chromosomes of mammals. Human Genetics 61: 85–90

Capraro V J, Bayonet-Rivera N P, Magoss I 1970 Vulvar tumors in children due to prolapse of urethral mucosa. American Journal of Obstetrics and Gynecology 108: 572–575

Carr D H, Haggar R A, Hart A G 1968 Germ cells in the ovaries of XO female infants. American Journal of Clinical Pathology 49: 521–526

Cattanach B M 1962 XO mice. Genetic Research 3: 487–490

Crowder R E 1957 Development of the adrenal gland in man, with special reference to origin and ultimate location of cell types and evidence in favour of the 'cell migration' theory. Contributions to Embryology 36: 195–210

Croxatto H B, Ortiz M E S 1975 Egg transport in the Fallopian tube. Gynecologic Investigation 6: 215–225

Davies J, Kusama H 1962 Developmental aspects of the human cervix. Annals of the New York Academy of Science 97: 534–550

Davis R M 1981 Localization of male determining factors in men. Journal of Medical Genetics 18: 161–195

de la Chapelle A 1981 The etiology of maleness in XX-man. Human Genetics 58: 105–116

Dewhurst J 1980 Practical pediatric and adolescent gynecology. Marcel Dekker, New York, Basel

Dewhurst J, Gordon R R 1984 Fertility following change of sex: a follow up. Lancet ii: 1461–1462

Diamond D A, Jeffs R D 1985 Cloacal exstrophy: a 22 year experience. Journal of Urology 133: 779–782

Didier E 1973a Recherches sur la morphogenèse du canal de Müller chez les oiseaux. I Étude descriptive Wilhelm Roux Archives 172: 271–286

Didier E 1973b Recherches sur la morphogenèse du canal de Müller chez les oiseaux. II Étude experimentale Wilhelm Roux Archives 172: 287–302

Donahoe P K, Ito Y, Morikawa Y, Hendren W H 1977 Müllerian inhibiting substance in human testes after birth. Journal of Paediatrics 12: 323–330

Du Pont B, Oberfield S E, Smithwick E M, Lee T D, Levine L S 1977 Close genetic linkage between HLA and congenital hyperplasia 21-hydroxylase deficiency. Lancet ii, 1309–1312

Duthie G M 1925 An investigation of the occurrence, distribution and histological structure of the embryonic remains in the human broad ligament. Journal of Anatomy 59: 410–431

Eichwald E J, Silmser C R 1955 Untitled communication. Transplantation Bulletin 2: 148–149

Eida T 1961 Entwicklungsgeschichtliche Studien über der Verschiebung der Epithelgrenze an der Portio vaginalis cervicis. Yokohama Medical Bulletin Supplement 12: 54–63

Engel E, Forbes A P 1965 Cytogenic and clinical findings in 48 patients with congenitally defective or absent ovaries. Medicine 44: 135–164

Evans M I, Chrousos G P, Mann D W, Larsen J W, Green I, McClusky J, Loriaux D L, Fletcher J C, Koons G, Overpeck J, Schulman T D 1985 Pharmacological suppression of the fetal adrenal gland in utero. Journal of the American Medical Association 253: 1015–1020

Evans T N, Poland M L, Boving R L 1981 Vaginal malformations. American Journal of Obstetrics and Gynecology 141: 910–920

Falk H C, Hyman A B 1971 Congenital absence of clitoris: a case report. Obstetrics and Gynecology 38: 269–271

Faulconer R J 1951 Observations on the origin of the Müllerian groove in human embryos. Contributions to Embryology 34: 159–164

Felix W 1912 The development of the urogenital organs. In: Keibel F, Mall F P (eds) Manual of human embryology. Lippincott, Philadelphia, p 752–979

Fetherston W C, Meyers A, Speckhard M E 1972 Adenocarcinoma of the vagina in young women. Wisconsin Medical Journal 71: 87–93

Fluhmann C F 1960 The developmental anatomy of the cervix uteri. Obstetrics and Gynecology 15: 62–69

Ford C E, Hammerton J L 1956 The chromosomes of man. Nature 178: 1020–1023

Ford C E, Jones K W, Polani P E, de Almeida J C, Briggs J H 1959 A sex chromosome anomaly in a case of gonadal dysgenesis (Turner's syndrome). Lancet i: 711–713

Forsberg J G 1965 Origin of vaginal epithelium. Obstetrics and Gynecology 25: 787–791

Forsberg J G 1973 Cervicovaginal epithelium: its origin and development. American Journal of Obstetrics and Gynecology 115, 1025–1043

Friedrich E G, Wilkinson E J 1973 Mucous cysts of the vulvar vestibule. Obstetrics and Gynecology 42: 407–414

Frost I F 1958 Case report of a patient with a true unicornuate uterus with unilateral renal agenesis. American Journal of Obstetrics and Gynecology 75: 210–212

Frutiger P 1969 Zur Frühentwicklung der Ductus paramesenephrici und des Müllerschen Hügels beim Memschen. Acta Anatomica 72: 233–245

Gartler S M, Cole R E 1981 Mammalian X-chromosome inactivation. In: Austin C R, Edwards R G (eds) Mechanisms of sex differentiation in animals and man. Academic Press, London, ch 3, p 113–143

Gasser D L, Silvers W K 1972 Genetics and immunology of sex linked antigens. Advances in Immunology 15: 215–247

Gill W B, Schumacher G F B, Bibbo M 1976 Structural and functional abnormalities in the sex organs of male offspring of mothers treated with diethylstilboestrol. Journal of Reproductive Medicine 16: 147–152

Glenister T W 1962 The development of the utricle and of the so called 'middle' or 'median' lobe of the human prostate. Journal of Anatomy 96: 443–455

Goldberg E H, Boyse E A, Bennett D, Scheid M, Carswell E A 1971 Serological demonstration of H-Y (male) antigen on mouse sperm. Nature 232: 478–480

Gondos B, Hobel C J 1973 Interstitial cells in the human fetal ovary. Endocrinology 93: 736–739

Greenwald P, Barlow J J, Nasca P C, Burnett W S 1971 Vaginal cancer after maternal treatment with synthetic estrogens. New England Journal of Medicine 285: 390–392

Griffin J E, Punyashthiti K, Wilson J D 1976 Dihydrotestosterone binding by cultured human fibroblasts. Journal of Clinical Investigation 57: 1342–1351

Grinsted J, Aagesen L 1984 Mesonephric excretory function related to its influence on differentiation of fetal gonads. Anatomical Record 210, 551–556

Gruenwald P 1941 The relation of the growing Müllerian duct to the Wolffian duct and its importance for the genesis of malformations. Anatomical Record 81: 1–19

Grumbach M M, Conte F A 1981 Disorders of sex differentiation. In: Williams R H (ed) Textbook of endocrinology, 6th edn. Saunders, Philadelphia, ch 9, p 423–514

Grumbach M M, Ducharme J R 1960 The effects of androgens on fetal sexual development, androgen-induced female pseudo-hermaphroditism. Fertility and Sterility 11: 157–180

Hall R, Fleming S, Gysler M, McLorie G 1985 The genital tract in female children with imperforate anus. American Journal of Obstetrics and Gynecology 151: 169–171

Hardisty M W 1978 Primordial germ cells and the vertebrate germ line. In: Jones R E (ed) The vertebrate ovary. Plenum Press, New York, p 1–45

Henking H 1891 quoted by Emery A E H 1974 Elements of medical genetics, 3rd edn. Churchill Livingstone, Edinburgh

Herbst A L, Ulfelder H, Pozkanzer D C 1971 Adenocarcinoma of the vagina: association of maternal stilboestrol therapy with tumor appearance in young women. New England Journal of Medicine 284: 878–881

Herbst A L, Kurman R J, Scully R E 1972 Vaginal and cervical abnormalities after exposure to stilboestrol in utero. Obstetrics and Gynecology 40: 287–298

Herbst A L, Robboy S J, Scully R E, Poskanzer D C 1974 Clear-cell adenocarcinoma of the vagina and cervix in girls: analysis of 170 registry cases. American Journal of Obstetrics and Gynecology 119: 713–724

Hertig A T 1935 Angiogenesis in the early human chorion and in the primary placenta of the macaque monkey. Carnegie Institution of Washington Publication 459 Contributions to Embryology 25: 37–81

Hertig A T 1968 Human trophoblast. Thomas, Springfield Illinois

Heuser C H 1932 A presomite human embryo with a definite chorda canal. Carnegie Institution of Washington Publication 433 Contributions to Embryology 23: 251–267

Heuser C H, Streeter G L 1941 Development of the macaque embryo. Carnegie Institution of Washington Publication 525 Contributions to Embryology 29: 15–55

Hill E C 1973 Clear cell carcinoma of the cervix and vagina in young women. A report of six cases with association of maternal stilboestrol therapy and adenosis of the vagina. American Journal of Obstetrics and Gynecology 116: 470–484

Hudson B, Burger H G 1979 Physiology and function of the testes. In: Shearman R P (ed) Human reproduction physiology, 2nd edn. Blackwell Scientific Publications, Oxford

Hunter R H 1930 Observations on the development of the human fetal genital tract. Contributions to Embryology 22: 91–108

Hutson J M 1985 A biphasic model for the hormonal control of testicular descent. Lancet ii: 419–421

Imperato-McGinley J, Guerrero L, Gauther T, Peterson R E 1974 Steroid 5α-reductase deficiency in man; an inherited form of male pseudohermaphroditism. Science 186: 1213–1215

Jacobs P A, Strong J A 1959 A case of human intersexuality having a possible XXY sex determining mechanism. Nature 183: 302–303

Jenkinson S D, Mackinnon A E 1984 Spontaneous separation of fused labia minora in prepubertal girls. British Medical Journal 289: 160–161

Jirasek J E 1971 Development of the genital system in human embryos and fetuses. In: Cohen MM (ed) Development of the genital system and male pseudohermaphroditism. Johns Hopkins Press, Baltimore

Jirasek J E 1977 Morphogenesis of the genital system in the human. In: Blandau R J, Bergsma D (eds) Morphogenesis and malformation of the genital system. Liss, New York

Jirasek J E, Rabock V, Uher J 1968 The relationship between the development of gonads and external genitalia in human fetuses. American Journal of Obstetrics and Gynecology 101, 830

Josso N 1979 Development and descent of the fetal testes. In: Bierich J R, Giarolo A (eds) Cryptorchidism. Academic Press, London

Josso N 1981 Differentiation of the genital tract: stimulators and inhibitors. In: Austin C R, Edwards R G (eds) Mechanisms of sex differentiation in animals and man. Academic Press, London.

Josso N, Picard J Y, Tran D 1977 The anti-Müllerian hormone. In: Blandau R J, Bersma D (eds) Morphogenesis and malformations of the genital system. Liss, New York

Jost A 1947 Recherches sur la differenciation sexuelle de l'embryon de Lapin. Archives d'Anatomie Microscopic et Morphologue Experimental 36: 271–315

Jost A 1965 Gonadal hormones in the sex differentiation of the mammalian fetus. In: de Haan R L, Ursprung H (eds) Organogenesis. Holt, Rinehart & Winston, New York

Kaufman R H, Binder G L, Grav P M Jr, Adam E 1977 Upper genital tract changes associated with exposure in utero to diethylstilboestrol. American Journal of Obstetrics and Gynecology 128: 51–56

Keith A 1948 Human embryology and morphology, 6th edn. Arnold, London

King C R, Magenis E, Bennett S 1978 Pregnancy and the Turner Syndrome. Obstetrics and Gynaecology 52: 617–624

Kissane J M 1974 Development of the kidney In: Hepinstall R H (ed) Pathology of the kidney, 2nd edn. Little Brown, Boston, ch 2, p 51–68

Koff A K 1933 Development of the vagina in the human fetus. Contributions to Embryology 24: 59–90

Kohn G, Yarkonis S, Cohen M M 1980 Two conceptions in a 45X woman. American Journal of Medical Genetics 5: 339–343

Krco C J, Goldberg E H 1976 H-Y (male) antigen: detection on 8-cell embryos. Science 193: 1134–1135

Liao S 1978 Molecular actions of androgens. In: Litwack G (ed) Biochemical actions of hormones, Vol. 4. Academic Press, New York

Luckett W P 1973 Amniogenesis in the early human and rhesus monkey embryos. Anatomical Record 175: 375 abstract

Ludwig E 1965 Über die Beziehungen der kloakenmembran zum septum urorectale beimenschlichen embryonen von 9 bis 33 mm SSL 2. Anatomische Entwicklung 124: 401–413

Lyon M F 1961 Gene action in the X chromosome of the mouse (Mus musculus L). Nature 190: 372–373

Lyon M F 1974 Mechanisms and evolutionary origins of variable X chromosome activity in mammals. Proceedings of the Royal Society of London Series B 187: 243–268

McClung C E 1899 A peculiar nuclear element in the male reproductive cells of insects. Zoology Bulletin 2: 187–197

McClung C E 1902 The accessory chromosome—sex determinant? Biology Bulletin 3: 43–84

McKusick V A, Bauer R L, Koop C E, Scott R B 1964 Hydrometrocolpos as a simply inherited malformation. Journal of the American Medical Association 159: 813–816

McNally F P 1926 The association of congenital diverticula of the Fallopian tube with tubal pregnancy. American Journal of Obstetrics and Gynecology 12: 303–318

Mancini R E, Vilar O, Lavieri J C, Andrada J A, Heinrich J J 1963 Development of the Leydig cells in the normal human testis. American Journal of Anatomy 112: 203–210

Matlai P, Beral J 1985 Trends in congenital malformations of external genitalia. Lancet i: 108

Melander Y 1962 Chromosomal behaviour during the origin of sex chromatin in the rabbit. Hereditas 48: 645–661

Mittwoch U 1971 Sex determination in birds and mammals. Nature 231: 432–434

Mittwoch U 1975 Chromosomes and sex differentiation. In: Reinboth R (ed) Intersexuality in the animal kingdom. Springer-Verlag, Berlin

Morris J M 1953 The syndrome of testicular feminization in male pseudohermaphrodites. American Journal of Obstetrics and Gynecology 65: 1192–1211

Moses M J, Counce S J, Paulson D F 1975 Synaptoneural complex of man in spreads of spermatocytes, with details of the sex chromosome pair. Science 187: 363–365

Müller H J, League B B, Offerman C A 1931 Effects of dosage changes of sex-linked genes and the compensatory effects of other gene differences between male and female. Anatomical Record (Suppl.) 51: 110 abstract

Müller J 1830 Bildungsgeschichte der Genitalien aus anatomischen Untersuchangen en Embryonen des menschen und der Thiere. Arnz, Düsseldorf

Müller U, Schindler H, Schemp W, Schott K, Neuhoff V 1984 Gene expression during gonadal differentiation in the rat. Developmental Genetics 5: 27–42

Nesbitt M N 1971 X-chromosome inactivation mosaicism in the mouse. Developmental Biology 26: 252–263

Novakowski H, Lenz W 1961 Genetic aspects in male hypogonadism. Recent Progress in Hormone Research 17: 53–95

Oguma K, Kihara H 1923 Etudes des chromosomes chez l'homme. Archives de Biologie (Paris) 33: 493–516

Ohno S 1964 Life history of female germ cells in mammals. Proceedings of the Second International Conference of Congenital Malformations 36–40

Ohno S 1967 Sex chromosomes and sex linked genes. Springer-Verlag, Berlin

Ohno S 1977 Testosterone and cellular response. In: Blandau R J, Bergsma D (eds) Morphogenesis and malformation of the genital system. Alan R Liss New York, p 99–106

Ohno S 1979 Major sex determining genes. Springer-Verlag, Berlin

Ohno S, Kaplan W D, Kinosita R 1961 X chromosome behaviour in germ and somatic cells of Rattus norvegicus. Experimental Cell Research 22: 535–544

Ohno S, Nagai Y, Ciccarese S 1978 Testicular cells lysostripped of H-Y antigen organic ovarian follicle-like aggregates. Cytogenetic Cell Genetics 20: 351–364

Ohno S, Nagai Y, Ciccarese S, Smith R 1979 Testes organizing H-Y antigens and the primary sex determining mechanism of mammals. Recent Progress in Hormone Research 35: 449–470

O'Rahilly R 1977 The development of the vagina in the human. In: Blandau R J, Bergsma D (eds) Morphogenesis and malformation of the genital system. Liss, New York, p 123–136

O'Rahilly R, Muecke E C 1972 The timing and sequence of events in the development of the human urinary system during the embryonic period proper. Zeitschrift Anatomische Entwicklung 138: 99–109

O'Rahilly R 1973 Developmental stages in human embryos.

Part A: Embryos of the first three weeks. Carnegie Institution of Washington

Painter T S 1924 The sex chromosomes of man. American Naturalist 58: 506–524

Pallister P D, Opitz J M 1979 The Perrault syndrome; autosomal recessive ovarian dysgenesis with faculative, non-sex-linked sensorineural deafness. American Journal of Medical Genetics 4: 239–246

Park W W 1957 The occurrence of sex chromatin in early human or macaque embryos. Journal of Anatomy 91: 369–373

Pasqualini J R, Sumida C, Gelly C, Nguyen B L 1976 Specific ^{3}H-estradiol binding in the fetal uterus and testes of guinea pig. Journal of Steroid Biochemistry 7: 1031–1038

Pearson P L, Bobrow M 1970 Definitive evidence for the short arm of the Y chromosome associating with the X during meiosis in the human male. Nature 226: 959–961

Peters H 1970 Migration of genocytes into the mammalian gonad and their differentiation. Philosophical Transactions of the Royal Society of London 259: 91–101

Peterson R E, Imperato-McGinley J, Gautier T, Sturla E 1979 Hereditary steroid 5α-reductase deficiency. In: Vallet H L, Porter I H (eds) Genetic mechanisms of sexual development. Academic Press, New York, p 149–174

Picon R 1969 Action du testicule foetal sur le developpement in vitro des canaux de Müller chez le rat. Archives de Anatomie et Microscopie 58: 1–19

Polani P E, Adinolfi M 1983 The H-Y antigen and its functions: a review and a hypothesis. Journal of Immunogenetics 10: 85–102

Pomerance W 1973 Post-stilbestrol secondary syndrome. Obstetrics and Gynecology 42: 12–18

Potter E L 1946 Bilateral renal agenesis. Journal of Pediatrics 29: 68–76

Potter E L 1965 Bilateral absence of ureters and kidneys. A report of 50 cases. Obstetrics and Gynecology 25: 3–12

Potter E L, Osathanondh V 1966 Normal and abnormal development of the kidney. In: Mostofi F Km, Smith D E (eds) The kidney. Williams & Wilkins, Baltimore, ch 1, p 1–16

Price D, Pannabecker R 1959 Comparative responsiveness of homologous sex ducts and accessory glands of fetal rats in culture. Archives of Anatomy and Microscopy 48: 223–244

Price D, Zaaijer J J D, Oriz E, Brinkmann A O 1975 Current views on embryonic sex differentiation in reptiles, birds and mammals. American Zoology 15: 173–195

Price J M 1979 The secretions of Müllerian inhibiting substance by cultured isolated Sertoli cells of the neonatal calf. American Journal of Anatomy 156: 147–158

Pryse-Davies J, Dewhurst C J 1971 The development of the ovary and uterus in the foetus, newborn and infant, a morphological and enzyme histological study. Journal of Pathology and Bacteriology 103: 5–25

Rathke M H 1825 quoted by Stephens 1982

Reschini E. Giustina G, D'Alberton A, Candiani G B 1985. Female pseudohermaphroditism due to maternal androgen administration: 25 year follow up. Lancet i: 1226

Robboy S J, Ross J S, Prat J, Keh P C, Welch W R 1978 Urogenital sinus origin of mucinous and ciliated cysts of the vulva. Clinical Obstetrics and Gynecology 51: 347–351

Rosa F W 1984 Virilization of the female fetus with maternal danazol exposure. American Journal of Obstetrics and Gynecology 149: 99–100

Sarto G E, Opitz J M 1973 The XY gonadal agenesis syndrome. Journal of Medical Genetics 10: 288–293

Schulte M J 1979 Positive H-Y antigen testing in a case of XY gonadal absence syndrome. Clinical Genetics 16: 438–440

Shaw R W, Farquhar J N 1984 Female pseudohermaphroditism associated with danazol exposure in utero. British Journal of Obstetrics and Gynaecology 91: 386–389

Siiteri O K, Wilson J D 1974 Testosterone formation and metabolism during male sexual differentiation in the human embryo. Journal of Clinical Endocrinology and Metabolism 38: 113–125

Simpson J L 1976 Disorders of sexual differentiation. Academic Press, New York

Simpson J L 1982 Abnormal sexual differentiation in humans. Annual Review of Genetics 16: 193–224

Simpson J L, Christakos A C, Horwith M, Silverman F S 1971a Gonadal dysgenesis in individuals with apparently normal chromosomal complements. Birth Defects 7: 215–228

Simpson J L, New M, Peterson R E, German J 1971b Pseudo-vaginal periscrotal hypospadias in sibs. Birth Defects 7: 196–200

Sloan W R, Walsh P C 1976 Familial persistent Müllerian duct syndrome. Journal of Urology 115: 459–461

Snell G D 1948 Methods for the study of histocompatibility genes. Journal of Genetics 49: 87–108

Solari A J 1974 The behaviour of the XY pair in mammals. International Review of Cytology 38: 273–317

Solari A J 1980 Synaponemal complexes and associated structures in microspread human spermatocytes. Chromosoma 81: 315–337

Somjen G J, Kaye A M, Linder H R 1976 Demonstration of 8-S-cytoplasmic oestrogen receptor in rat Müllerian duct. Acta Biochemica and Byophysics 428: 787–791

Song J 1964 The human uterus: morphogenesis and embryological bases for cancer. Thomas Springfield, Illinois

Stephens T D 1982 The Wolffian ridge: history of a misconception. Isis 73: 254–259

Stevens N M 1905 Studies in spermatogenesis with special reference to the accessory chromosome. Carnegie Institution Washington Publication 36: 1–32

Tegenkamp T R, Brazzell J W, Tegenkamp I, Labidi F 1979. Pregnancy without benefit of reconstructive surgery in a bisexually active true hermaphrodite. American Journal of Obstetrics and Gynecology 135: 427–428

Teplitz R, Ohno S 1963 Postnatal induction of oogenesis in the rabbit. Experimental Cell Research 31: 183–189

Terruhn V 1980 A study of impression moulds of the genital tract of female fetuses. Archives of Gynecology 229: 207–217

Tjio J H, Levan A 1956 The chromosome number of man. Hereditas 42: 1–6

Torpin R 1942 Prolapsus uteri associated with spina bifida and club feet in newborn infants. American Journal of Obstetrics and Gynecology 43: 892–894

Uebele-Kallhardt 1978 Human oocytes and their chromosomes. Springer-Verlag, Berlin

Ulfedder H, Robboy S J 1976 Embryologic development of human vagina. American Journal of Obstetrics and Gynecology 126: 769–776

Van Niekerk W A 1976 True hermaphroditism. An analytic review with a report of 3 new cases. American Journal of Obstetrics and Gynecology 126: 890–907

Vorontsov N N 1973 The evolution of sex chromosomes. In: Chiarelli A B, Capanno E (eds) Cytotaxonomy and vertebrate evolution. Academic Press, London, p 619–657

Wachtel S S 1979 Immunogenetic aspects of abnormal sexual differentiation. Cell 16: 691–695

Wachtel S S, Hall J L 1979 H-Y binding in the gonad, inhibition by a supernatant of the fetal ovary. Cell 17: 327–329

Wachtel S S, Koo G C 1981 H-Y antigen in gonadal differentia-

tion. In: Austin C R, Edwards R G (eds) Mechanisms of sex differentiation in animals and man. Academic Press, London, ch 7, p 255–299

Wachtel S S, Ohno S 1979 The immunogenetics of sexual development. Progress in Medical Genetics 3: 109–142

Wachtel S S, Ohno S, Koo G C, Boyse E A 1975 Possible role for H-Y antigen in the primary determination of sex. Nature 257: 235–236.

Waldeyer W 1870 Eierstock und Ei. Enzelmann, Leipzig

Warkany J 1971 Congenital malformations. Year Book Medical Publishers, Chicago

Warnock M 1984 Report of The Committee of Inquiry Into Human Fertilisation and Embryology. Her Majesty's Stationery Office, London, Cmnd 9314

Wartenberg H 1982 Development of the early human ovary and role of the mesonephros in the differentiation of the cortex. Anatomy and Embryology 165: 253–280

Weiss J P, Duckett J W, Snyder H M 1984 Single unilateral vaginal ectopic ureter: is it really a rarity? Journal of Urology 132: 1177–1179

Wilkins L 1960 Masculinization of female fetus due to use of orally given progestins. Journal of the American Medical Association 172: 1028–1032

Williams D L 1958 Urology in childhood. In: Encyclopedia of Urology, Vol. XV. Springer-Verlag, Berlin

Wilson E B 1906 Studies on chromosomes III The sexual differences of the chromosome groups, with some considerations on the determination and inheritance of sex. Journal of Experimental Zoology 3: 1–40

Wilson J D 1973 Testosterone uptake by the urogenital tract of the rabbit embryo. Endocrinology 92: 1192–1199

Wilson J D, Lasnitzki I 1971 Dihydrotestosterone formation in fetal tissues of the rabbit and rat. Endocrinology 89: 659–668

Wilson J D, Siiteri P K 1973 Development pattern of testosterone synthesis in the fetal gonad of the rabbit. Endocrinology 92: 1182–1191

Winiwarter H von 1912 Études sur la spermatogenèse humaine. Archives de Biologie 27: 91–188

Winiwarter H von, Sainmont G 1908 Nouvelles recherches sur l'ovogenèse et l'organogenèse de l'ovaire des mammiferes (chat). Archives de Biologie 24: 373–431

Witschi E 1929 Studies on sex differentiation and sex determination in amphibians. Journal of Experimental Zoology 54: 157–223

Witschi E 1962 Embryology of the ovary. In: Gray H G, Smidt D E (eds) The ovary. Williams & Wilkins, Baltimore, p 1–10

Witschi E 1970 Development and differentiation of the uterus. In: Mack H C (ed) Prenatal life. Wayne State University Press Detroit p 11–35

Wolff C F 1759 Theoria generationis quoted by Adelman H B 1966 Marcello Malphigi and the evolution of embryology. Cornell University Press, New York

Zah W, Kalderon A E, Tucci J R 1975 Mixed gonadal dysgenesis. Acta Endocrinologica (Suppl.) 197: 1–39

Zenzes M T, Wolf U, Engel W 1978b Organization in vitro of ovarian cells into testicular structures. Human Genetics 44: 333–338

Zenzes M T, Wolf U, Güunther E, Engel W 1978a Studies on the functions of H-Y antigen: dissociation and reorganization experiments on rat gonadal tissue. Cytogenetic Cell Genetics 20: 365–372

Zondek L H, Zondek T 1979 Observations on the determination of foetal sex in early pregnancy. Contributions to Gynaecology and Obstetrics 5: 91–108

2

Anatomy and physiology of the vulval area
J M McLean

The perineum is that part of the pelvic outlet caudal to the pelvic diaphragm. It is divided into an anterior urogenital triangle and a posterior anal triangle. The vulva lies principally within the urogenital triangle but extends beyond it to overlie the pubic symphysis and adjacent parts of the pubic bones while the anal canal and ischiorectal fossae are wholly accommodated within the anal triangle. Embryologically the perineum is a junctional zone being derived from body wall ectoderm, hindgut endoderm and the intervening mesoderm surrounding the original cloacal membrane. The perineum is therefore not simply an area of skin, but forms an essential part of the female genital tract, urinary tract and gastrointestinal tract. Although the elements of the genital, urinary and gastrointestinal tracts within the perineum are distinct and separate structures, the anatomical location of the perineum determines their functional interrelationship and shared vulnerability to certain pathological conditions. Indeed, changing patterns of sexual behaviour indicate that the female anal canal has assumed a sexual function. A recent paper on the treatment of perianal condylomata acuminata states that 33% of the female patients regularly acquiesced in anal penetration (Jensen 1985).

THE PELVIC FLOOR

The pelvic floor, or pelvic diaphragm, is a sheet of muscle slung around the midline urethra, vagina and anal canal. The muscles of the pelvic floor are coccygeus and levator ani but Last (1959) suggests they be regarded as one morphological entity; ischiococcygeus, iliococcygeus and pubococcygeus. These three named muscles have a linear origin,

the white line, which extends from the ischial spine across the side wall of the pelvis, overlying the obturator fascia, to the body of the pubis. They are inserted into the sacrum, coccyx, anococcygeal raphe and perineal body (Fig. 2.1). From this linear origin on either side, the muscle fibres slope downwards and backwards to their midline insertion forming a gutter shaped pelvic floor which slopes downwards and forwards.

The ischiococcygeus muscle arises from the ischial spine and is inserted into the side of the fifth sacral vertebra and the coccyx. The other two muscles, iliococcygeus and pubococcygeus, are often separated from each other by a triangular gap despite the fact that their fibres arise in linear continuity from the ischial spine to the body of the pubis. The iliococcygeus arises from the posterior half of the fibrous linear origin and, overlying the pelvic surface of ischiococcygeus, it is inserted into the coccyx and anococcygeal raphe. This raphe is the interdigitation of muscle fibres from the right and left sides and it extends from the tip of the coccyx to the anorectal junction.

The pubococcygeus arises from the anterior half of the fibrous linear origin and from the posterior surface of the body of the pubis. The muscle fibres arising from the fibrous linear origin sweep backwards on the pelvic surface of iliococcygeus to be inserted into the anococcygeal raphe. Those fibres arising from the pubic bone form a muscle sling around the anorectal junction which produces a forward angulation of the junction. This part of pubococcygeus is referred to as pubo-rectalis and it lies beneath the anococcygeal raphe and intermingles with the deep part of the external anal sphincter. The most medial fibres arising from the pubis form a muscle sling around the vagina. This part of

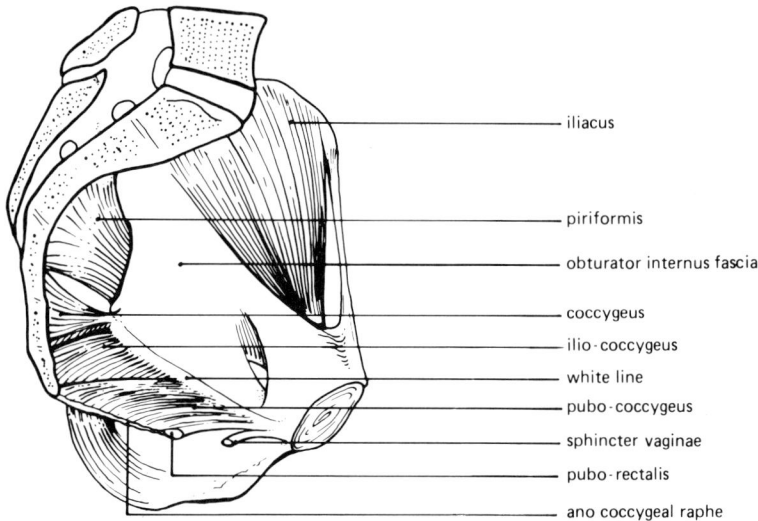

Fig. 2.1 The muscles of the pelvic walls and pelvic floor.

pubococcygeus is the sphincter vaginae and behind the vagina its fibres intermingle with the fibromuscular tissue of the perineal body. The midline gap between the medial edges of the sphincter vaginae is occupied by the pubovesical ligaments and the deep dorsal vein of the clitoris.

The nerve supply of the pelvic diaphragm is from the lumbosacral plexus (S.2,3,4) and its principal function is to assist in the maintenance of continence when intra-abdominal pressure is raised during episodes of coughing, sneezing and muscular effort. The posterior midline portion of the pelvic diaphragm is an important component of the postanal plate (Wendell-Smith & Wilson 1977) upon which the terminal rectum rests.

THE ANAL TRIANGLE

The anal canal

The anorectal junction, lying at the level of the pelvic floor, is angled forward by the puborectalis muscle. The anal canal is about 4 cm long and extends from the anorectal junction downwards and backwards to the anal orifice. Posteriorly the fibromuscular anococcygeal raphe tethers the anal canal to the coccyx. Anteriorly it is separated from the lower vagina by another fibromuscular mass, the perineal body (Fig. 2.2), while laterally it is related to the ischiorectal fossae. The whole length of the

anal canal however is enclosed in sphincter muscles which normally keep it closed.

The lining of the anal canal is said to reflect its dual embryological origin from the hindgut and body wall ectoderm. Certainly in the upper two-thirds, or hindgut portion, the mucosa is thrown into several longitudinal folds termed anal columns. Each column contains a terminal radical of the superior rectal artery and vein; the largest ones being in the left lateral, right posterior and right anterior quadrants. These are the principal sites of internal haemorrhoid formation. The lower ends of the anal columns are linked by short crescentic folds of mucosa, the anal valves. An anal valve may be torn during defaecation and such a tear may result in an anal fissure. Above the anal valves are the anal sinuses, recesses in the mucosa of the anal wall, which may retain faecal matter. Opening into the anal sinuses are anal glands which, extending superiorly and inferiorly, penetrate deeply into the anal wall. This anatomical arrangement may result in anal gland infection and abscess formation. Below the anal valves, or pectinate line, is a transitional zone limited inferiorly by Hilton's white line which identifies the lower border of the internal anal sphincter. The short segment of anal canal below the transitional zone is lined with skin which possesses sweat and sebaceous glands.

There are two separate anal sphincters: one internal, the other external. The internal sphincter of

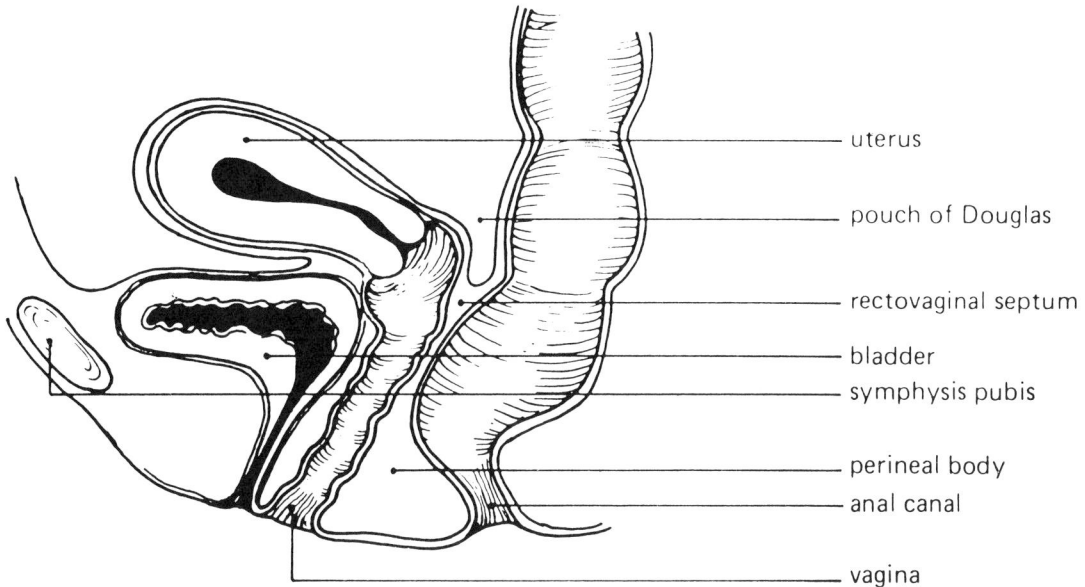

Fig. 2.2 A midline section through the pelvis and perineum.

smooth muscle surrounds the upper two-thirds of the anal canal. It is the thickened lower end of the inner, circular muscle layer of the gut tube and is innervated by the autonomic nervous system via the rectal component of the pelvic plexus. The longitudinal layer of gut muscle become fibrous as it descends the anal canal and eventually fuses with the anal wall below the internal sphincter. The external anal sphincter surrounds the entire length of the anal canal, being separated from the internal sphincter by the fibrous continuation of the longitudinal muscle layer of the gut. The external sphincter is usually described as having subcutaneous, superficial and deep parts (Fig. 2.3). The subcutaneous part surrounds the lowest portion of the anal canal and lies in the same vertical plane as the internal sphincter. The subcutaneous part is separated from the rest of the external sphincter by the peri-anal fascial layer which is reflected from Hilton's white line to the lateral wall of the ischiorectal fossa. The superficial or middle part of the external sphincter forms an elliptical loop around the anal canal, being attached to the tip of the coccyx posteriorly and the perineal body anteriorly. The deep part of the muscle surrounds the commencement of the anal canal and blends with the puborectalis muscle laterally and posteriorly. Anteriorly it fills the gap between the two halves of the puborectalis muscle in front of the anorectal junction and blends with the deep perineal muscles. The integrity of this part of the external sphincter is essential to continence. Deep anterior lacerations of the anal canal during parturition may endanger it. The corrugator cutis ani muscle is formed by thin slips of smooth muscle which radiate from the anal canal into the peri-anal skin. It is part of panniculus carnosus, as is the dartos muscle in the labia majora and platysma in the neck, and is not part of the external sphincter.

The arterial supply to the hindgut portion of the anal canal is by the terminal branches of the superior rectal artery while its terminal part is supplied by the inferior rectal branch of the internal pudendal artery. The muscular wall of the canal is supplied by the middle rectal branch of the internal iliac artery. The venous drainage follows the arterial supply and the anal canal is therefore a site of portal systemic venous anastomosis. The lymphatic vessels also follow the arterial supply to the para-aortic and internal iliac lymph nodes, but the terminal anal canal drains to the superficial inguinal nodes.

The autonomic nervous system supplies the upper part of the anal canal which, although relatively insensitive to pain, is responsive to distention. The lower part of the anal canal is supplied by the

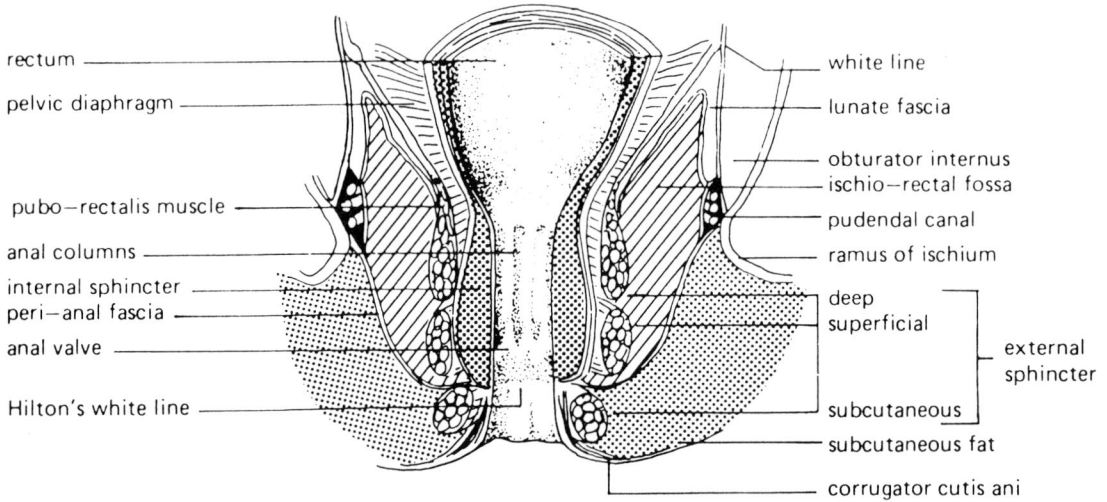

Fig. 2.3 A coronal section through the anal canal and ischiorectal fossae.

inferior haemorrhoidal branch of the pudendal nerve and it is highly sensitive. The external sphincter muscle is supplied by somatic efferent fibres from the second, third and fourth sacral nerves. The inferior haemorrhoidal nerve supplies the sub-cutaneous and deep parts of the muscle while the perineal branch of the fourth sacral nerve supplies the superficial part.

The ischiorectal fossa

This wedge shaped space fills the lateral part of the anal triangle and extends forwards into the urogenital triangle. Its lateral wall is formed by the obturator fascia overlying the lower part of obturator internus muscle. Medially the two fossae are separated by the anococcygeal body, a fibromuscular mass extending to the skin from the anococcygeal raphe, and by the anal canal and perineal body. The pelvic diaphragm forms the roof and the peri-anal fascia the floor. Each fossa is occupied by loose fatty areolar tissue and together they provide dead space for expansion of the anal canal during defaecation (Fig. 2.3).

The peri-anal fascia extends from the anal canal to the lower margin of the lateral wall of the ischiorectal fossa, where it splits to form the pudendal canal. Below the peri-anal fascia lies the subcutaneous peri-anal space. The lunate fascia is a continuation of the peri-anal fascia, extending up the lateral wall of the ischiorectal fossa, medially across its roof and fading out as it descends the medial wall.

The pudendal nerve and internal pudendal vessels leave the pelvis through the greater sciatic foramen below piriformis. Turning forwards immediately, the vessels around the tip of the ischial spine and the nerve around the sacrospinous ligament, they enter the lesser sciatic foramen. In doing so they reach the ischiorectal fossa, in which they run forward, on its lateral wall, within the pudendal canal to gain the urogenital triangle. As the neurovascular bundle proceeds through the ischiorectal fossa, the inferior rectal vessels and inferior haemorrhoidal nerve arise and arch over the lunate fascia to reach the midline structures which they supply. The inferior haemorrhoidal nerve supplies afferent fibres to the terminal part of the anal canal and the peri-anal skin and efferent fibres to two-thirds of the external anal sphincter and to part of the pelvic floor musculature. Since both vessels and nerve arch upwards from their origin on the lateral wall, incisions into the ischiorectal fossa do not endanger them. As it enters the urogenital triangle the pudendal nerve divides into the perineal nerve and dorsal nerve of the clitoris, while the internal pudendal vessels also break up into a number of branches to supply the clitoris and perineum.

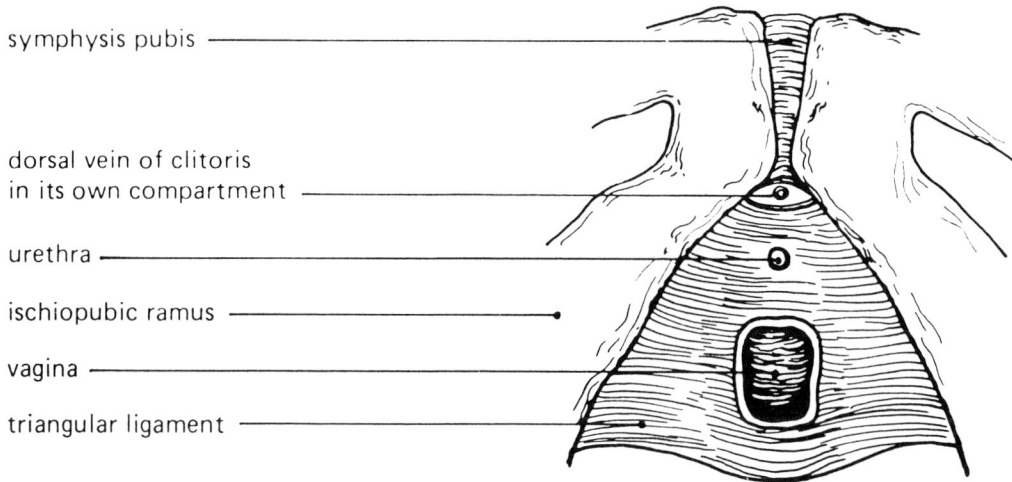

Fig. 2.4 The urogenital diaphragm.

labels on figure:
symphysis pubis

dorsal vein of clitoris
in its own compartment

urethra

ischiopubic ramus

vagina

triangular ligament

THE UROGENITAL TRIANGLE

The urogenital triangle is contained within the sub-pubic arch.

The urogenital diaphragm

The urogenital diaphragm (Fig. 2.4) is a strong fibrous membrane attached to the pubic rami which divides the urogenital triangle into deep and superficial perineal pouches. The urogenital diaphragm is often referred to as the perineal membrane or triangular ligament and it is deficient at three sites in the midline. An apical opening, situated just below the pubic symphysis transmits clitoral vessels and nerves from the deep to the superficial perineal pouch, while the urethra and vagina enter the superficial pouch more posteriorly.

The deep perineal pouch

The deep perineal pouch is bounded by the pelvic floor musculature and pubovesical ligaments above, and the urogenital diaphragm below. On either side lie the ischiopubic rami while posteriorly it is continuous with the ischiorectal fossae. Emerging from each ischio-rectal fossa the pudendal nerve gives the perineal nerve, which divides into deep and superficial branches, and the dorsal nerve of the clitoris. In the same way the internal

pudendal artery gives off a perineal branch, which supplies the perineal body and superficial structures, before entering the deep perineal pouch with the deep branch of the perineal nerve and the dorsal nerve of the clitoris. As the artery traverses the deep pouch it gives off branches to the erectile tissue of the vestibule in the superficial perineal pouch and divides into deep and superficial arteries to the clitoris. Passing through the deep perineal pouch, in the midline, are the urethra and vagina. The vessels and nerves pass forwards on either side of the urethra and vagina. The clitoral branches leave the deep perineal pouch through the apical opening in the urogenital diaphragm. The deep pouch also contains voluntary muscle fibres some of which surround the urethra and vagina while others run transversely into the perineal body behind the vagina.

THE URETHRA

The female urethra is 4 cm long. From the internal urethral orifice it runs downwards and forwards behind the symphysis pubis embedded in the anterior wall of the vagina. After passing through the pelvic floor and perineal membrane it ends at the external urethral orifice, anterior to the vaginal opening, a variable distance behind the glans clitoridis. The

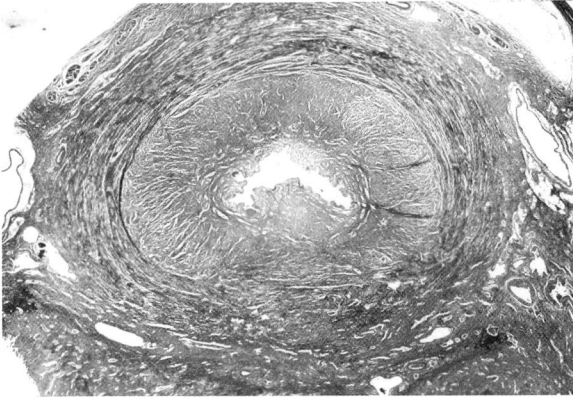

Fig. 2.5 A transverse section through the mid portion of the urethra showing the posterior urethral crest.

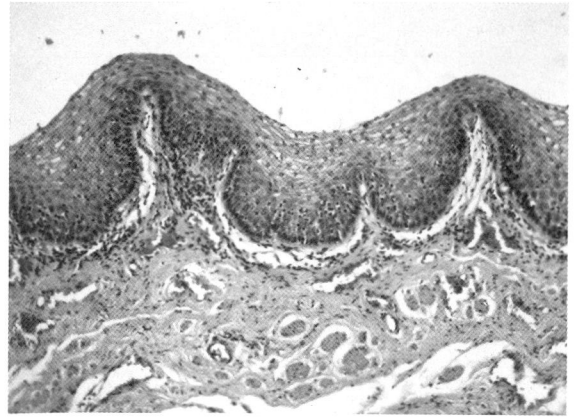

Fig. 2.6 Non-keratinizing stratified squamous epithelium lining most of the urethra.

urethra is fixed at its origin by the pubovesical ligaments, throughout its length by the anterior wall of the vagina, and as it enters the perineum by the perineal membrane.

The walls of the urethra, which are normally in apposition, present longitudinal epithelial folds on their inner aspect. One of these folds, on the posterior wall, is termed the urethral crest since it projects into the lumen rendering it crescentic in cross-section (Fig. 2.5). The urethra possesses an inner epithelial lining supported by a loose vascular lamina propria, and a peripherally situated muscle coat consisting of an outer layer of striated muscle, the external urethral sphincter and an inner layer of smooth muscle.

The striated muscle of the urethra is quite distinct and separate from the pelvic floor musculature. The fibres of this external urethral sphincter are arranged in a circular and an oblique fashion. In the middle third the striated muscle completely surrounds the urethra although the posterior element, between the urethra and vagina, is relatively thin. In the proximal and distal thirds of the urethra the obliquely arranged fibres leave the posterior urethral wall deficient of striated muscle. The thickness of the external urethral sphincter in the female is less than that of the male but its constituent fibres are able to exert tone upon the urethral lumen over prolonged periods, especially in its middle third (Gosling et al 1983). The smooth muscle of the urethra extends throughout its length and consists of slender muscle bundles, the majority of

which are arranged obliquely or longitudinally, although a few on the outer aspect are circularly disposed and blend with the striated muscle of the external urethral sphincter. The urethral smooth muscle is continuous proximally with the detrussor muscle of the bladder and distally with the subcutaneous tissue at the external urethral meatus (Gosling et al 1983).

The lamina propria of the female urethra contains glands and many thin walled veins which give it the appearance of erectile tissue. The glandular tissue is predominantly found in the lower third of the urethra. Groups of these glands, on either side of the urethra, possess common ducts which open on the lateral aspect of the external urethral orifice. These ducts are known as paraurethral or Skene's ducts and they may be the site of infection. The proximal urethral epithelium is transitional and continuous with that of the bladder, while distally and throughout the majority of its length it is non-keratinizing stratified squamous in type (Fig. 2.6). This epithelium becomes keratinizing at the external urethral meatus where it is continuous with the skin of the vestibule.

The blood supply, nerve supply and lymphatic drainage of the pelvic urethra is the same as that for the bladder neck. The perineal urethra is supplied by the pudendal vessels and nerves and the voluntary muscle of the external urethral sphincter is supplied by the perineal branch of the pudendal nerve. The lymphatic drainage of the perineal urethra is to the inguinal nodes.

THE CERVIX UTERI

The cervix uteri does not lie in the perineum but it is an important structure in the female reproductive tract and its secretions have a profound effect upon the vulva.

The cervix uteri comprises one-third of the uterine length, being about 2.5 cm long. It is narrower than the corpus and almost cylindrical in form being broadest in its middle portion. Inferiorly the cervix uteri projects into the vault of the vagina and is enclosed by the vaginal fornices. This anatomical arrangement divides the cervix into supravaginal and vaginal segments. The supravaginal cervix lies below the uterovesical pouch of peritoneum anteriorly and is firmly adherent to the trigone of the bladder. As the ureter approaches the upper angle of the trigone it lies some 2 cm lateral to the supravaginal cervix (Fig. 2.7). At a slightly higher level, the uterine artery, in the base of the broad ligament, begins its ascent of the lateral margin of the uterus. Posteriorly the supravaginal cervix is covered with peritoneum which extends on to the posterior vaginal wall, before sweeping backwards to the rectum to form the rectouterine pouch. The vaginal cervix usually projects downwards and backwards into the vaginal vault. It is bounded by a deep posterior vaginal fornix, a shallow anterior fornix and by lateral fornices of intermediate depth. On its lower surface is a circular aperture, the external os, which gives entry to the cervical canal and the uterine cavity (Fig. 2.2).

The small uterine cavity is divisible into the cavity of the body and the cervical canal. Accurate assessment of the size and shape of the cavity of the corpus uteri has become an important adjunct to the provision of intra-uterine contraceptive devices. Special techniques have been devised to make this assessment (Hasson & Dershin 1981). The cervical canal is narrowed anteroposteriorly. It is continuous above with the cavity of the body through the internal os, and below with the vagina through the external os. The upper third of the cervix is the isthmus uteri; it dilates and is taken up into the corpus uteri as it enlarges during pregnancy.

The uterine artery may arise independently from the anterior division of the internal iliac artery, or from a stem common to it and other branches. The artery and the accompanying veins and nerves constitute the neurovascular pedicle which is enclosed in the condensation of fascia described as the lateral cervical ligament. As the uterine artery approaches the cervix it divides into ascending and descending branches. The large ascending branch is the continuation of the main arterial stem and its numerous medial branches supply the body and fundus of

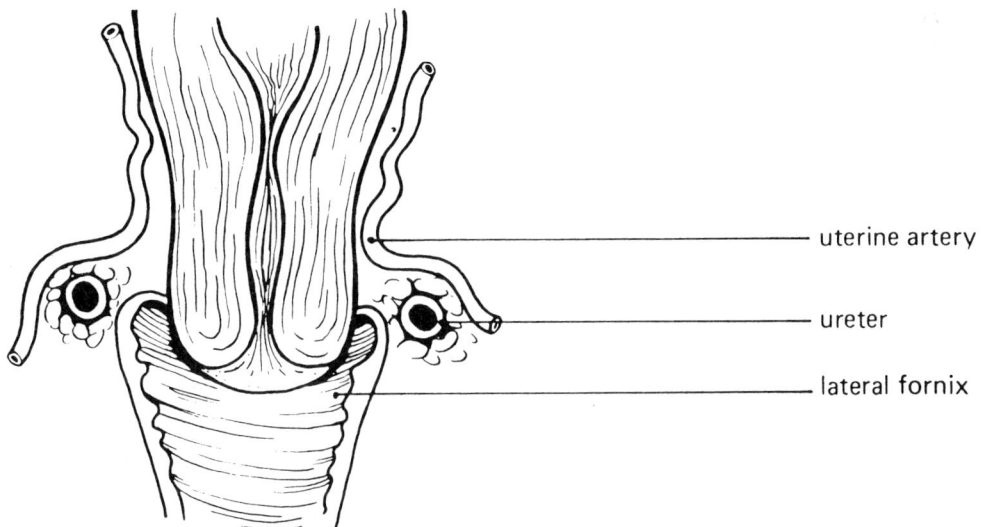

Fig. 2.7 A diagrammatic view of the relationships between the uterine artery, ureter and lateral vaginal fornix.

the uterus as well as the uterine tube. The descending branch of the uterine artery supplies the cervix and upper vagina.

The veins of the corpus, cervix and vagina drain to the uterovaginal venous plexus formed, lateral to the cervix, in the base of the broad ligament. This venous plexus communicates anteriorly with the vesical plexus and posteriorly with the rectal plexus. It drains laterally across the pelvic floor in a number of venous channels which surround the artery and are enclosed with it in the lateral cervical ligament. On the lateral pelvic wall the uterine veins open into the internal iliac veins.

There is evidence from the clinical course of endometrial carcinoma that the human endometrium lacks a lymphatic drainage since lymph node metastases occur only after myometrial involvement and the prognosis, in the absence of myometrial invasion, is very good (Bush 1979). The majority of lymphatics leaving the fundus and upper part of the corpus pass into the upper part of the broad ligament. Here they join lymphatics from the tube and ovary and, travelling with the gonadal vessels, they reach the para-aortic nodes at the level of the second lumbar vertebra. A minority of lymphatics from the fundus, together with some from the uterine tube and ovary, accompany the round ligament of the uterus and drain to the superficial inguinal nodes. The round ligament lies within the broad ligament and runs from the uterotubal junction to enter the deep (internal) inguinal ring. As the round ligament traverses the inguinal canal fibres leave it to fuse with the fibrous and muscular walls of the canal and the remnant emerges from the superficial (external) inguinal ring to fuse with the labium majorus. The round ligament may be accompanied by a peritoneal diverticulum, the canal of Nuck, into the inguinal canal. The lymphatics from the lower part of the body and cervix pass laterally in the base of the broad ligament, in the company of the uterine artery, to reach the nodes alongside the internal iliac vessels. Some of these lymph vessels, however, also drain to the external iliac nodes (Way 1977). Although unusual, umbilical metastasis by lymphatic spread has been reported in a patient with squamous carcinoma of the cervix (Daw & Riley 1982).

Nerve fibres accompany the vessels as they penetrate the walls of the corpus, cervix and vagina.

There is general agreement that almost all of the motor fibres to uterine muscle are sympathetic while afferent innervation of the corpus is sympathetic and of the cervix is parasympathetic.

The cervix exhibits two forms of epithelium: the vaginal surface is covered with stratified squamous epithelium, while the cervical canal is lined by columnar epithelium in which there are numerous mucous secreting cells. The junction between squamous and columnar epithelia may occur at the external os but more often there is a transformation zone of variable extent situated around the external os (Dewhurst 1981).

THE VAGINA

The vagina is a fibromuscular tube which gives access to the cervical canal and uterine cavity from the perineum. It ensheaths the penis during sexual intercourse and the male gametes, after intravaginal ejaculation, begin their ascent of the female reproductive tract through the cervical canal. At delivery the vagina is the birth canal for the emergent infant. These two functions of the vagina demand that it can constrict or be constricted and also dilate.

From its opening between the labia minora the adult vagina extends some 7–10 cm upwards and backwards, to be attached around the periphery of the cylindrical cervix uteri, at some distance above its lower margin. As the vagina ascends from the perineum into the pelvis its long axis forms a right angle with the long axis of the normal anteverted uterus. The cervix therefore projects downwards and backwards into the upper vagina. The circumferential vaginal attachment is achieved by the posterior wall of the vagina being some 2 cm longer than the anterior wall. For ease of description the part of the vaginal cavity surrounding the cervix is divided into anterior, posterior and lateral fornices. The deep posterior fornix is continuous, via the lateral fornices on either side of the cervix, with the shallow anterior fornix. The anterior and posterior walls of the undistended vagina are in contact with each other throughout most of their length, giving the vagina a crescentic or H-shaped appearance in cross section.

The vagina is related anteriorly to the base of the

bladder and to the urethra which is embedded in its anterior wall. Posteriorly the upper part of the vaginal wall is covered with peritoneum. Below the recto-uterine pouch the posterior vaginal wall is directly related to the ampulla of the rectum, while in the perineum the fibromuscular perineal body separates it from the anal canal (Fig. 2.2). The upper vagina gives attachment to the uterosacral ligaments posteriorly, the cardinal ligaments laterally, and the base of the bladder anteriorly, itself supported by the pubovesical ligaments. As the vagina passes through the pelvic floor the most medial fibres of pubococcygeus blend with its walls to form a supporting muscular sling. Below the pelvic diaphragm the vagina is supported by the urogenital diaphragm, the perineal body and the perineal musculature.

The vagina is lined with non-keratinizing stratified squamous epithelium and its walls are made up of smooth muscle and fibroelastic tissue. The outer wall of the vagina accommodates the vascular, lymphatic and nerve plexuses which supply it. The vaginal artery may arise from the internal iliac artery or one of its branches, most commonly the internal pudendal artery (Hollinshead 1971). The uterine artery gives a descending branch to the upper vagina and there is frequently a vaginal branch from the middle rectal artery. The lower vagina is supplied by branches of the internal pudendal artery. These vessels anastomose with each other in or on the vaginal walls. Vessels from the right and left sides anastomose to form unpaired, midline, anterior and posterior azygos arteries. The base of the bladder also receives an arterial supply from this vaginal plexus. The veins of the vagina drain to the uterovaginal plexus which itself communicates with the vesical and rectal venous plexuses. These venous plexuses drain principally to the internal iliac veins. The lymphatic drainage of the upper two-thirds of the vagina is with the cervix uteri to the internal iliac or external iliac lymph nodes. The lower third of the vagina drains with the rest of the perineum to the superficial inguinal nodes.

THE SUPERFICIAL PERINEAL POUCH

The superficial perineal pouch lies below the urogenital diaphragm. Attached to the undersur-

face of lateral margins of the diaphragm and the ischiopubic rami are the crura of the clitoris, each of which is covered by the ischiocavernosus muscle. These crura extend forward as the corpora cavernosa which fuse at the sub-pubic angle to form the body of the clitoris. The clitoral body is attached to the pubic symphysis by a suspensory ligament. Between each clitoral crus and the vaginal opening the erectile tissue of the vestibular bulb is attached to the urogenital diaphragm. These bulbs extend forwards beyond the urethra where they fuse to form a slender band of erectile tissue which is situated on the ventral surface of the clitoris. The vestibular bulbs are covered by the bulbo-spongiosus muscles which extend from the perineal body, around the vagina and urethra, to the clitoris. Just behind the vestibular bulbs, also lying on the urogenital diaphragm, are the greater vestibular glands of Bartholin which open into the vestibule lateral to the vaginal opening. Lying transversely across the base of the urogenital triangle at the posterior margin of the superficial perineal pouch are the superficial transverse perineal muscles (Fig. 2.8). The superficial perineal pouch therefore contains the structural elements of the female external genitalia which, with their skin covering, exhibit the external appearance characteristic of the vulva.

THE VULVA

In common with all other parts of the female reproductive tract the vulva is a target organ for the female sex hormones (Omsjo et al 1984). Although it is insufficient to consider the vulva solely from a dermatological perspective, it is nevertheless a specialised area of skin which undergoes significant change at puberty, during sexual intercourse, pregnancy and labour, at the menopause and during the postmenopausal period. The vulva consists of the mons pubis, the labia majora and minora, the vestibule of the vagina, the hymen, the greater vestibular glands of Bartholin, the clitoris with its prepuce and frenulum, the bulbs of the vestibule and the external urethral orifice. Simple inspection of the perineum will allow only the mons pubis, the labia majora, the margins of the labia minora, the perineal body and the anus to be seen

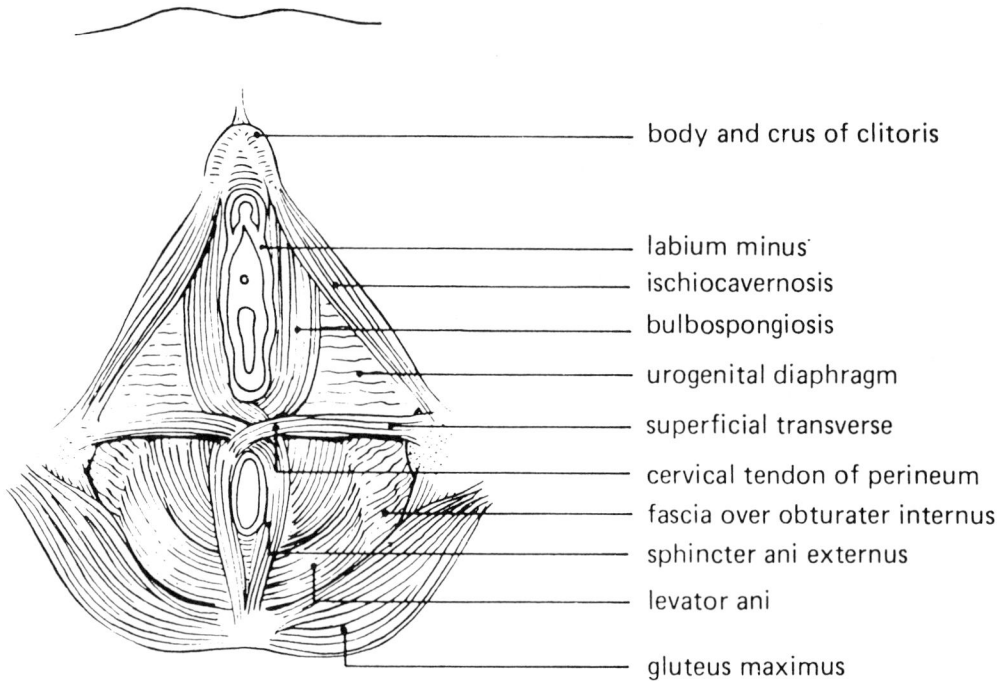

body and crus of clitoris

labium minus

ischiocavernosis

bulbospongiosis

urogenital diaphragm

superficial transverse

cervical tendon of perineum

fascia over obturater internus

sphincter ani externus

levator ani

gluteus maximus

Fig. 2.8 The superficial structures of the perineum.

(Fig. 2.9). Adequate exposure of the vulva requires the separation of the labia majora and minora (Figs. 2.10 and 2.11).

Mons pubis

The mons pubis or mons veneris becomes an identifiable structure at puberty with the deposition of subcutaneous fat and the appearance of pubic hair. In the adult female it forms a prominent cushion of hair-bearing skin and subcutaneous fat overlying the pubic symphysis. Although the character of pubic hair varies with race its distribution rarely extends more than 2 cm beyond the upper limit of the genitofemoral folds (Lunde 1984). This pattern of distribution produces the horizontal upper margin of female pubic hair.

Labia majora

The labia majora are two cutaneous folds which form the lateral boundaries of the pudendal cleft. They originate from the mons pubis anteriorly and merge with the perineal body posteriorly. After puberty the deposition of subcutaneous fat within the labia majora produces a greater degree of prom-

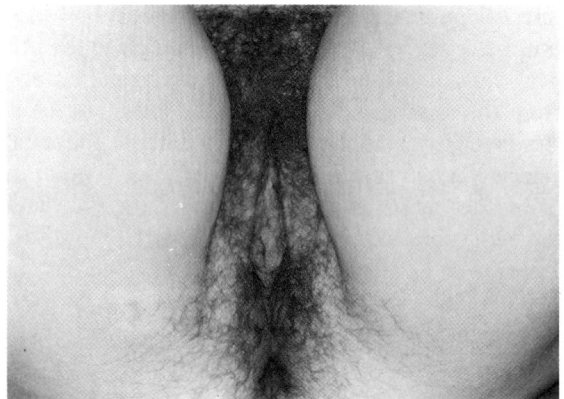

Fig. 2.9 The female perineum.

inence and the presence of pigmentation and hair on their lateral surfaces establishes them as well defined structures. Their lack of definition posteriorly is partially due to the absence of subcutaneous fat in the perineal body and partially to the extension of pigmented and hair-bearing skin to surround the anal opening. The lateral surfaces of the labia majora are adjacent to the medial surfaces of the thighs and are separated from them by a deep groove. The medial surfaces of the labia majora,

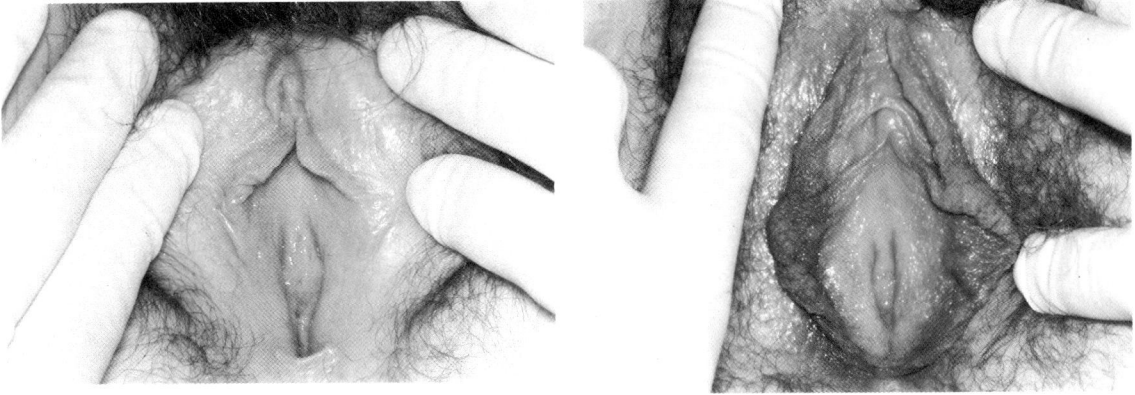

Fig. 2.10 & 2.11 Exposure of the vulva by separation of the labia majora. Note the variable form of the labia minora.

which are hairless and possess numerous sebaceous glands, may be in contact with each other or separated by the protrusion of the labia minora.

The size of the labia majora varies with age, race and parity (Krantz 1977). While asymmetry is not uncommon and is usually of no significance it has been reported as a presenting sign in neurofibromatosis (Friedrich & Wilkinson 1985). After the menopause the labia majora become less prominent. This is associated with a thinning of labial hair due to loss of hair follicles with increasing age (Barmann et al 1969) and a reduction of pigmentation. Conversely, pregnancy, or the use of anovulatory drugs, may cause hyperpigmentation of the labia majora in the sexually mature woman (Parker 1981).

Labia minora

The labia minora are two thin folds of hairless skin, devoid of subcutaneous fat, which are situated between the labia majora on either side of the vaginal and urethral openings. The labia minora are separated from the labia majora by interlabial furrows in which the normal secretions from the adjacent skin surfaces may accumulate in the absence of adequate hygiene. Anteriorly the labia minora divide into lateral and medial parts. The lateral parts unite anterior to the clitoris, in a fold of skin overhanging the glans clitoridis to form the prepuce of the clitoris. The medial parts unite on the under surface of the clitoris to form its frenulum. This anterior division of the labia minora in relation to the clitoris is variable (Figs. 10 & 11). Posteriorly the labia minora fuse to form a transverse fold be-

hind the vaginal opening. This fold, the frenulum of the labia or fourchette, is broken at parturition.

Hypertrophy of the labia minora may be present at birth, be produced intentionally in certain tribal groups or occur as the result of certain sexual practices. Such hypertrophy may be associated with local irritation, discomfort in walking and sitting, problems of personal hygiene or coital difficulty. Surgical removal of excess labial tissue leaving the clitoris and fourchette intact is recommended in such patients (Baruchin & Cipollini 1986). The sequelae of female circumcision as practised in some cultures may cause serious functional disturbance which should not occur after simple labial reduction.

The skin of the labia minora is smooth and pigmented, the pigmentation becoming obvious during adolescence. Being devoid of adipose tissue the labia minora are composed mainly of elastic fibres and blood vessels and possess a rich innervation. The arrangement of blood vessels within the labia minora forms erectile tissue comparable to that in the penile corpus spongiosus, their embryological counterpart in the male. During sexual excitation the blood supply to the labia minora is increased and causes not only a change in colour but also significant enlargement sufficient to induce a minimal degree of traction on the clitoris.

THE VESTIBULE

The cleft between the labia minora is termed the vestibule of the vagina and it extends from the clitoris to the fourchette. Localised within the vestibule are the openings of the vagina, the urethra, the ducts of Bartholin's glands and the minor vestibular glands. That part of the vestibule between the vaginal orifice and the frenulum of the labia minora forms a shallow depression termed the vestibular fossa or fossa navicularis.

Hymen

The junction of the vestibule with the vagina is identified by the presence of the hymen or its remnants. The hymen is normally a thin, incomplete membrane of connective tissue which is easily ruptured. Routine use of tampons and/or regular coitus will reduce the hymen to a series of small irregular deviations around the vaginal opening termed carunculae myrtiformes. Occasionally the hymen may be a rigid structure and will prevent sexual intercourse. Alternatively during coitus a rigid hymen may tear into the vaginal wall and cause severe bleeding.

Bartholin's glands

Bartholin's glands, the eponymous description of the greater vestibular glands, are situated deeply within the posterior parts of the labia majora. Each gland lies just inferior and lateral to the bulbocavernosus muscle and it is normally not palpable. The glandular secretion is clear, mucoid and alkaline and is increased during sexual arousal. Krantz (1977) maintains that these glands "undergo involution, shrink in size and become atrophic after the thirtieth year of life". Nevertheless the glands and their duct may be the site of infection or cyst formation at any age. Bartholin's glands are lobulated and contain multiple acini grouped around the termination of each of the many branching ducts. The acini are lined with cuboidal epithelium and the ducts with stratified transitional epithelium (Kaufman 1981). The main duct of each Bartholin's gland opens at the lateral margin of the vagina just behind the mid-point and superficial to the hymenal ring. Argentaffin cells have recently been described in the epithelial lining of the Bartholin duct system, predominantly in the transitional epithelium of the main excretory duct (Fetissof et al 1985). The same investigators also observed these endocrine cells in the paraurethral glands and, as in

Bartholin's glands, they were distributed randomly among the layers of the transitional epithelium.

Minor vestibular glands

These glands are tubular structures, their acini lined with columnar epithelium and their ducts with transitional squamous epithelium. Robboy et al 1975 found them in 9 out of 19 post-mortem examinations on young women and in numbers varying from 1 to more than 100, the average number being 2–10 and the commonest site being around the fourchette. The opening of the ducts can be seen with the naked eye. They may play a part in the burning vulva syndrome (p. 219).

THE CLITORIS

The clitoris is a specialised structure covered with a stratified squamous epithelium that is thinly keratinized. No sebaceous, apocrine or sweat glands are present (Friendrich & Wilkinson 1982). The body of the clitoris is situated in the midline, at the apex of the vulval cleft. The manner of its formation, from the crura and the vestibular bulbs, has already been described. The whole of the clitoris is composed of erectile tissue and as such is the homologue of the penis. Although uncommon, persistent priapism of the clitoris may occur. A recent report (Melville & Harrison 1985) described its delayed spontaneous resolution in a fit, parous 36 year old woman some nine days after normal marital intercourse. The authors acknowledge that the use of an α-adrenergic agonist, as described by Brindley (1984) for the treatment of priapism in the male, might have achieved an earlier resolution of the problem. Lozano & Castenada (1981) described a case secondary to neoplastic embolism in the corpora cavernosa. The distal portion, or glans clitoridis, can be exposed by upward displacement of the prepuce. Those elements of the labia minora which form the prepuce and frenulum of the clitoris are generously endowed with sebaceous glands and some mucus-secreting glands are also present.

Bulb of the vestibule

As already indicated these erectile tissue masses participate in the formation of the clitoris. Each bulb lies in the superficial perineal pouch adjacent to the lateral wall of the vagina. It is attached to the inferior surface of the urogenital diaphragm by the overlying bulbo-spongiosus muscle. Thus the bulbar erectile tissue embraces the vaginal opening and during sexual arousal its engorgement narrows the vaginal introitus.

THE EXTERNAL URETHRAL MEATUS

The external urethral orifice lies between the vagina and the clitoris. Although always in the mid-line its exact location is variable. Its orifice is usually recognisable but on occasions may be hidden by prolapsing flaps of urethral mucosa.

VULVAL SKIN

The epidermis of the vulval skin and its appendages, hair, sebaceous and sudoriferous glands, are developed from ectoderm. The dermis is developed from mesoderm.

The primitive epidermis is established about the eighth day when ectoderm differentiates within the developing embryo. At this stage the epidermis is a single layer of cells but during the course of the subsequent three weeks specific features of the epidermis develop which set it apart from other epithelia in the body (Holbrooke 1983). A second outer layer develops, the periderm beneath which the primitive epidermis begins the process of stratification. When keratinization occurs at the end of the sixth month, with the formation of the horny layer, the periderm is sloughed into the amniotic fluid (Lind et al 1969).

Three cell types invade the developing epidermis during the first six months of intra-uterine life. Melanocytes, derived from the neural crest (Niebauer 1968) and Langerhan cells, derived from mesoderm (Breathnach & Wyllie 1965), are present at the end of the third month while Merkel cells, the origin of which is uncertain, are present by the sixth month (Breathnach 1971).

With the exception of the palms and soles the dermal-epidermal junction is flat in all parts of the body until hair and glandular primordia descend from the epidermis into the dermis. Primary hair follicles begin to form during the third month of gestation and the process proceeds in a craniocaudal manner (Pinkus 1958). Secondary follicles form in close association with the primary follicles and it is thought that the full complement of hair follicles is present at birth (Ebling 1968). Sebaceous glands begin to appear during the fourth month and differentiation of the primordial cells into sebum producing cells proceeds rapidly (Holbrooke 1983). The development and function of sebaceous glands before birth and in the neonatal period is thought to be regulated by maternal androgens and endogenous fetal steroids (Solomon & Esterly 1970). Sebaceous gland activity before birth is partly responsible for the formation of vernix caseosa. At birth the glands are large and well developed over the entire body and display the same regional variation in size as is seen in the adult. Postnatally they involute and remain quiescent until puberty. Eccrine sweat glands appear during the third month of prenatal life and their ducts are open to the skin surface by the sixth month. Although eccrine sweat glands are innervated as soon as they develop (Montagna 1960) the premature infant usually shows an absent or limited sweating response (Sinclair 1972). The number of sweat glands, like hair follicles, seems to be complete at birth (Pinkus 1910). The apocrine glands do not develop until the sixth month of intra-uterine life. It has been suggested that apocrine gland primordia develop in association with each hair follicle but regress in all areas except the areola, axilla, scalp, eyelids, external auditory meatus, umbilicus and anogenital region (Serri et al 1982, Hashimoto 1970). Apocrine gland activity begins during the last trimester but ceases soon after birth (Montagna & Parakkal 1974).

The intrinsic components of the dermis originate from mesoderm during the second month of embryonic life. The major cellular component is the fibroblast which synthesizes and secretes the amorphous and structural connective tissue matrix which supports the epidermal appendages and other component tissues. The organization of the dermis is progressive throughout gestation and is not complete until some months after birth. Essential for epidermal function is the process of vascularization and innervation which proceeds pari passu.

The epidermis

The epidermis is a stratified squamous epithelium which varies in thickness in different regions of the body. In stained vertical sections its lower border, at the dermal-epidermal junction, presents an undulating appearance due to the epidermal or rete ridges. Histologically the epidermis is described in four layers (MacKie 1984):

1. a basal layer, or stratum germinativum, the lower border of which rests on the basal lamina,
2. a spinous or prickle cell layer which forms the bulk of the epidermis,
3. a granular layer,
4. a horny layer or stratum corneum.

This descriptive approach is advantageous because of the variations which occur in the prominence of the different layers in different regions. It must not however obscure an appreciation of the progressive differentiation which occurs as a single cell line, the keratinocyte, moves upwards through the various layers to form the tough, protective, flexible outer surface of the skin. A section of epidermis from the labia majora, stained with haematoxylin and eosin (Fig. 2.12), shows a classical basal layer of columnar shaped, darkly staining cells. Immediately above the basal layer are the larger polygonal cells of the spinous layer. The cells of this layer are much less basophilic than those of the basal layer and consequently appear more lightly stained. In this particular section a distinct variation in the thickness of the spinous layer is evident. As the keratinocytes ascend the epidermis they become flatter and broader, deeply staining keratohyalin granules appear in their cytoplasm and they establish the granular layer. Above the granular layer an abrupt change occurs, the cells become anucleate and the horny layer is formed.

The epidermis of the labia majora, labia minora and the frenulum of the clitoris is of the type illustrated in Fig. 2.12 in which both the granular and horny layers are relatively inconspicuous. Towards the hymen, the skin on the medial aspects of the labia minora is devoid of granular and horny layers and is often described as a mucous epithelium.

Epidermal derivatives

The mons pubis, the lateral and exposed aspects of the labia majora and the perianal area are covered with hair bearing skin. The hair follicle, the hair, the sebaceous gland, the arrectores pilorum muscle and the apocrine glands form a distinct functional unit throughout these areas of the perineal skin. In addition eccrine sweat glands are present and all of these features are usually seen in sections of the labia majora (Fig. 2.13).

The inner aspects of the labia majora, the whole of the labia minora and the frenulum and prepuce of the clitoris are covered with non-hair bearing skin. These areas of skin are richly provided with sebaceous glands which open directly onto the skin

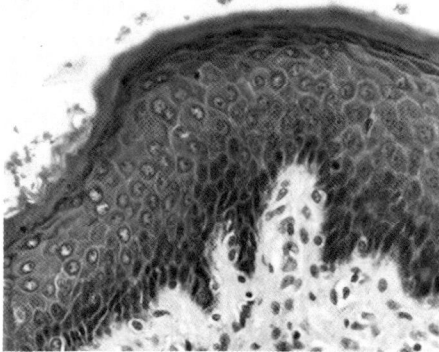

Fig. 2.12 Epidermis from the labium majus showing darkly stained cells in the basal layer above which are lighter stained polygonal cells in the thicker spinous layer. At the surface the granular layer is composed of flatter cells above which is an inconspicuous horny layer (H & E).

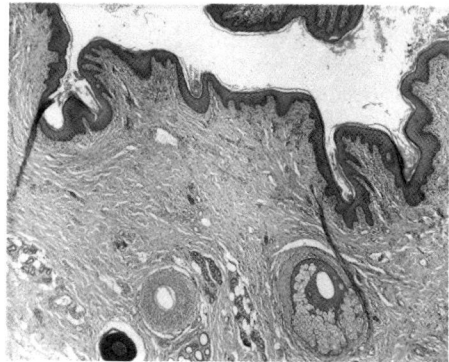

Fig. 2.13 A section of skin from the labium majus showing hair, hair follicles, sebaceous glands, apocrine glands and eccrine sweat glands (H & E).

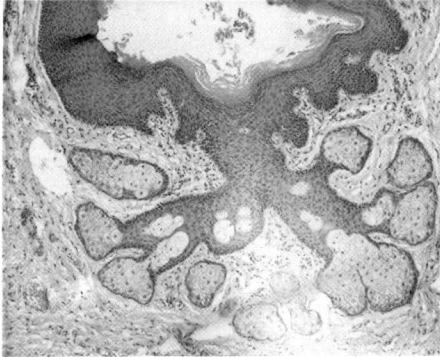

Fig. 2.14 A section of skin from the labium minus showing sebaceous glands opening directly on to the skin (H & E).

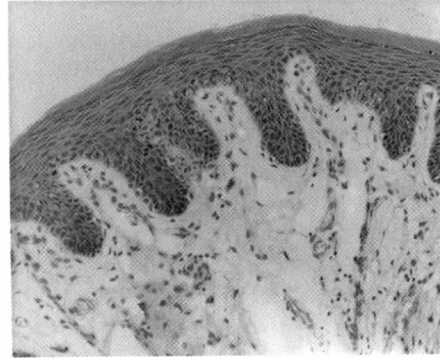

Fig. 2.15 A section of skin from the labium minus showing melanocytes, rounded cells with clear cytoplasm, in the basal layer of the epidermis and a vascular dermis (H & E).

(Fig. 2.14). Because these sebaceous glands are not associated with hair follicles they frequently form tiny elevations visible on the skin surface which are referred to as Fordyce spots. These areas are devoid of apocrine glands and indeed eccrine glands are rarely seen (Fig. 2.15).

Epidermal symbionts

This term is used to describe three cell types, within the epidermis, for which there is evidence of reciprocal supportive function (MacKie 1984).

Melanocytes. The melanocytes or pigment-producing cells are situated mainly in the basal layer of the epidermis. In haematoxylin and eosin stained paraffin sections they appear as rounded cells with clear cytoplasm (Fig. 2.15). Their numbers show regional variations but they are normally present in a ratio between 1:10 and 1:5 of the epidermal basal keratinocytes (Hu 1981). Melanocytes convert the amino acid tyrosine to melanin which protects the dermis from the harmful effects of ultraviolet light. From matched sites negroes and caucasians have comparable numbers of melanocytes per unit area of skin. The dark colour of negro skin is produced by the increased quantity of melanin pigment synthesised and its dispersal as melanin granules amongst the adjacent basal cells. Hormones profoundly influence melanin pigmentation in man although their precise action at the cellular level is obscure. There is also a marked regional variation in the sensitivity of melanocytes to specific hormones. Thus during pregnancy oestrogens and progestogens stimulate increased melanogenesis in the areolae, nipples and perineum and to a lesser extent in the face and midline of the anterior abdominal wall. Facial hyperpigmentation of pregnancy usually diminishes after delivery but it is likely to recur with subsequent pregnancies. The facial hyperpigmentation associated with anovulant contraceptives is accentuated by exposure to ultraviolet light and may not resolve completely after they are discontinued (Parker 1981). It must be admitted that the role of melanin as a protector of the perineal dermis is unlikely to be of great importance in normal circumstances.

Langerhans cells in the epidermis were once thought to be 'effete' melanocytes en route to desquamation (Medawar 1953). They are now recognised as bone-marrow-derived dendritic cells, present in all layers of the epidermis, and intimately involved in the body's immune defence mechanisms. They can be visualised by light microscopy using the gold chloride method or with histochemical or immunological techniques. These later techniques exploit the fact that Langerhans cells are the only cells in the epidermis capable of expressing Fc and C3 receptors as well as HLA-DR antigens (Steinman 1981). The immunological function of Langerhans cells involves the activation of T-lymphocytes which circulate freely through the skin. Such activation is essential in any immune response initiated at the surface of the body. Immunological responses of this type are particularly important at the squamous epithelial surfaces of the female genital tract, surfaces which may be exposed

to allogeneic spermatozoa (see p. 63) as well as to
the potentially oncogenic human papilloma virus.
Indeed, reports suggest that the papilloma virus may
induce changes in Langerhans cells in the cervix
(Morris et al 1983, Tay et al 1987, a & b) and skin
(Gatter et al 1984). A recent quantitative study of
healthy tissue (Edwards & Morris 1985) has shown
the distribution of Langerhans cells in the lower
female genital tract to be 19 per 100 basal squamous
cells in the vulva, 13 per 100 basal squamous cells in
the cervix and 6 per 100 basal squamous cells in the
vagina.

Langerhans cells are often described as antigen-
presenting cells because they associate physically
with epidermal lymphocytes during the course
of an allergic skin reaction (Edelson & Fink 1985).
In addition the dendritic processes of basal
Langerhans cells penetrate the basement membrane and make contact with subepithelial stromal
capillaries (Morris et al 1983). This arrangement
indicates transfer of antigenic information from
Langerhans cells to endothelial cells and this
accords with the suggestion that vascular endothelium is also involved in the process of cell mediated
immune responsiveness. Although much of the recent research on Langerhans cells has concentrated
on their role in the immune system there is some
evidence from experimental animals that they may
also be involved in the control of keratinisation
(Mackie 1984). The interdependence of the skin
and the immune system is further supported by the
increasing evidence that keratinocytes perform
a significant role in the post-thymic maturation of
T-lymphocytes (Patterson & Edelson 1982).

Merkel cells. These epidermal neuroendocrine
cells were described by Merkel in 1875. They are
found throughout the skin, situated singly or in
clusters in the basal layer of the epidermis. Not
only do their dendritic cytoplasmic processes surround adjacent keratinocytes (Winkelmann 1977)
but their cell bodies are intimately associated with
contiguous nerve fibres (Winkelmann & Breathnach 1973). Immunohistochemical studies have
shown that Merkel cells in man, as well as in many
other species, contain vasoactive intestinal polypeptide (VIP) (Gould et al 1985). The precise role
of Merkel cells in the skin is obscure but it has been
suggested that they function as paracrine regulators
of surrounding epidermal and adnexal structures

in a manner comparable with their gastrointestinal
and bronchopulmonary counterparts (Gould et al
1985). Malignant neoplasms of epidermal Merkel
cells may occur (p. 289).

The dermis

The dermis is divisible into papillary and reticular
parts. The papillary dermis projects upwards into
the rete ridges and is composed of fine collagen
fibres, running at right angles to the surface
together with reticular and elastic fibres. This fibre
arrangement supports vascular and lymphatic
channels as well as nerve terminals. The reticular
dermis lies below the papillary dermis and is composed of coarse collagen fibres lying parallel with
the surface. Accompanying the collagen fibres are
thicker elastic fibres which prevent the dermal
collagen from being overstretched. The vascular
and lymphatic plexuses which drain the papillary
dermis lie within the reticular dermis which also
contains the nerve fibres associated with the papillary nerve terminals.

Blood supply

The arterial supply of the perineum is provided
bilaterally by branches of the internal iliac and
femoral arteries. The internal pudendal artery, a
branch of the internal iliac artery, leaves the pelvis
through the greater sciatic notch below the piriformis muscle (Fig. 2.1). Lying on the tip of the ischial
spine it turns forwards through the lesser sciatic
foramen to enter the anal triangle of the perineum
posteriorly. Within the anal triangle it runs forwards on the side wall of the ischiorectal fossa enclosed by the fascia of the pudendal canal. During
its course through the ischiorectal fossa it gives off
the inferior rectal artery which arches over the
fascial roof of the fossa to reach and supply the
anococcygeal raphe, anal canal and perineal body. Entering the urogenital triangle the internal pudendal
artery gives off the perineal branch to the perineal
body and the structures situated more posteriorly
in the superficial perineal pouch. The parent artery
enters the deep perineal pouch and supplies the
erectile tissue of the vestibule, by perforating
branches into the superficial perineal pouch, and
the clitoris by way of its deep and superficial

terminal branches. The latter vessel reaches the body of the clitoris by entering the superficial perineal pouch through the apical deficit in the urogenital diaphragm.

Within the femoral triangle the femoral artery gives off the superficial and deep external pudendal arteries. The superficial external pudendal artery pierces the deep fascia of the thigh anteriorly, to overlie the round ligament of the uterus. It runs medially to supply the mons pubis and labia of the vulva. The deep external pudendal artery pierces the deep fascia of the thigh medially to enter the labia of the vulva. Within the superficial perineal pouch the terminal branches of the internal and external pudendal arteries anastamose with one another.

The venous drainage of the perineum is similarly arranged and eventually reaches the femoral and internal iliac veins. The internal iliac veins drain a rich venous plexus in the pelvic floor which, at least in part, drains all the pelvic viscera. Thus the venous drainage of the terminal gastrointestinal tract is partially to the pelvic plexus but principally to the portal system via the superior rectal and thence the inferior mesenteric vein. The pelvic venous plexus therefore provides a portal systemic anastomoses and portal hypertension predisposes to distention and even thrombosis of the pelvic, rectal, vaginal and vulval veins. Vulvo-vaginal varices however are most common during pregnancy although they may occur in patients with endometriosis, pelvic inflammatory disease, or pelvic tumours. Since many women develop vulval varices during the first trimester of pregnancy the underlying cause is probably not obstructive but hormonal and indeed progesterone is known to cause increased venous distensibility (Gallagher 1986). In the non-pregnant patient, particularly those using anovulent contraceptives, vulval varices may undergo cyclic change during the menstrual cycle (Gallagher 1986).

Lymphatic drainage

Lymphatic capillaries arise in the extracellular tissue spaces and form larger channels which drain to the regional lymph nodes. Efferent vessels leave these regional lymph nodes and the lymph passes through a series of intermediate lymph nodes before returning to the blood via the thoracic duct. Although the lymphatic system forms an essential part of the vascular and immune systems the clinical relevance of regional lymph drainage is in the management of patients with malignant neoplasia.

The regional lymph nodes of the perineum are situated in the groin at the base of the femoral triangle. These superficial lymph nodes subsequently drain to deep nodes in the pelvis and ultimately to para-aortic nodes on the posterior abdominal wall. Any mid-line structure, and especially an anatomical region as well defined as the perineum, has bilateral lymphatic drainage. Thus the lymphatic drainage of either labium minus is to both the ipsilateral and contralateral superficial lymph nodes (Iversen & Aas 1983). Although the lymphatic drainage of the vulva is regularly reviewed (Figge et al 1985) this account is derived principally from Way (1977).

The femoral triangle is a gutter-shaped depression below the groin, with its apex situated medially and inferiorly. Its base is formed by the inguinal ligament, the lower free aponeurotic margin of the external oblique muscle of the anterior abdominal wall. The inguinal ligament extends from the anterior superior spine of the iliac bone laterally to the tubercle on the body of the pubic bone medially. Inferiorly the inguinal ligament gives attachment to the fascia lata, the deep fascia of the thigh. Midway between the pubic symphysis and the anterior superior iliac spine the external iliac artery becomes the femoral artery as it enters the femoral triangle deep to the inguinal ligament and the fascia lata. Medial to the artery is the femoral vein and medial to the vein is the femoral canal, created by the downward extension of the abdominal fascia around the femoral vessels. The long saphenous vein ascends the leg in the superficial fascia and at the medial end of the inguinal ligament passes through the saphenous opening in the fascia lata to enter the femoral vein. The regional lymph nodes of the perineum are arranged in two groups at the base of the femoral triangle. A variable number of lymph nodes lie transversely in the superficial fascia of the thigh, immediately below the medial two-thirds of the inguinal ligament. Another more vertically disposed group lie adjacent to the termination of the long saphenous vein and are referred to as the superficial femoral or subinguinal lymph nodes. This latter group, varying from three to twenty in number, are arranged on both the medial and lateral aspects of the long saphenous vein. Those on the lateral side send efferent lymphatics, through the saphenous opening, to the external iliac group of deep lymph nodes. The superficial lymph nodes of the femoral triangle communicate freely with one another and drain the whole of the perineum, including the lower third of the urethra, of the vagina and of the anal canal.

The external iliac lymph nodes are described with reference to their relationship with the external iliac vessels. The medial group of three to six nodes lie on the medial side of the commencement of the external iliac vein. The lowest node of this group frequently projects into the femoral canal and is the mis-named node of Cloquet (Way 1977). The anterior group is inconstant and when present comprises no more than three nodes lying in the sulcus between the external iliac artery and vein. The lateral group of two to five nodes lies on the lateral side of the external iliac artery. The nodes of the external iliac group communicate freely with one another and with the obturator node. This large constant node, so named because of its proximity to the obturator nerve, lies below the external iliac vessels on the side wall of the pelvis and probably belongs to the external iliac group.

The efferent lymphatics from the external iliac group drain to the common iliac nodes situated on the lateral side of the common iliac artery. The external and common iliac nodes drain, either directly or indirectly, the lower limb, the lower anterior abdominal wall, the perineum and some of the pelvic viscera. Many small nodes lie close to each pelvic viscus and these drain into the numerous nodes embedded in the extraperitoneal tissue on the walls of the pelvis. These pelvic nodes are situated alongside the branches of the internal iliac artery and many groups are named according to the vessels with which they are associated. Such classifications, however, are not helpful since the nodes are so widely scattered that extensive stripping of the pelvic walls is necessary to identify them. All lymphatics from the pelvis eventually drain to the para-aortic nodes.

Innervation

The perineum has both somatic and autonomic innervation and in each there are sensory and motor components. Since the future perineum is the most caudal part of the developing embryo its somatic innervation is from the most caudal segmental spinal levels S1, 2, 3, 4. The lower abdominal wall however is formed by the migration of body wall tissue into the area between the umbilicus and genital tubercles. Thus the nerve supply of the perineal area anteriorly is supplemented by input from the upper lumbar segments i.e. L1, 2. The autonomic or visceral innervation of the perineum is entirely from the most caudal elements of both the sympathetic and parasympathetic systems. The sympathetic outflow from, and input to, the central nervous system is restricted to the region between the first thoracic and second lumbar levels of the spinal cord. The sympathetic innervation of the perineum is located therefore at L1, 2. It reaches the perineum via post-ganglionic grey rami communicantes, arising from the first two lumbar and all four sacral ganglia of the sympathetic trunks. These fibres are distributed with the first and second lumbar segmental nerves and the first, second, third and fourth sacral segmental nerves. In addition other sympathetic fibres from L1, 2 leave the sympathetic trunk as the hypogastric nerves (lumbar splanchnics, presacral nerves) and descend into the pelvis to be associated with the autonomic pelvic plexuses which are distributed with the blood vessels. The parasympathetic outflow from, and input to, the central nervous system consists of cranial and caudal portions. The cranial portion is associated with four of the cranial nerves while the caudal portion is associated with the second and third, or third and fourth sacral segments of the spinal cord as the nervi erigentes. These nerves together with the hypogastric sympathetic nerves form the autonomic pelvic plexuses.

The cutaneous innervation of the perineum conveys all modalities of common sensation—touch, pain, itch, warmth and cold, as well as complex sensations such as wetness. In addition these cutaneous nerves carry post-ganglionic sympathetic nerves which are motor to sweat glands, pilomotor units and the adventitia of the microvasculature. No parasympathetic fibres participate in this cutaneous innervation (Odland 1983) which is provided by the terminal or perineal branches of several nerves. The anterior part of the perineum is supplied by two nerves which emerge from the superficial inguinal ring just above the body of the pubic bone. These are the ilioinguinal nerve (L1) and the genital branch (L2) of the genitofemoral nerve (L1, 2). The lateral aspect of the perineum, more posteriorly, is supplied by the perineal branch (S1) of the posterior cutaneous nerve of the thigh (S1, 2, 3). The remainder of the cutaneous innervation of the perineum is supplied by the pudendal nerve (S2, 3, 4) and the perineal branch of the fourth sacral nerve. This latter nerve supplies the skin of the anal margin. The pudendal nerve enters the ischiorectal fossa, close to the tip of the ischial spine on the medial side of the pudendal artery. Running anteriorly on the lateral wall of the ischiorectal fossa it gives off the inferior haemorrhoidal nerve which arches over the roof of the fossa to reach the mid line where it supplies the terminal part of the anal canal and the perianal skin. The pudendal nerve then divides into the perineal branch, which supplies the rest of the perineal skin, and the dorsal nerve of the clitoris which supplies the anterior labia minora and the glans clitoridis.

These sacral spinal nerves also supply motor innervation to the muscles of the perineum. The pudendal nerve, through its inferior haemorrhoidal branch supplies the deep and subcutaneous parts of the external anal sphincter and through its perineal branch the muscles of both deep and superficial perineal pouches, as well as the anterior part of the levator ani muscle and the sphincter of the urethra. The remainder of the levator ani muscle and the superficial part of the external anal sphincter are supplied by the perineal branch of the fourth sacral nerve. Damage to the pudendal nerves may cause loss of muscle tone in the pelvic floor and be associated with problems of incontinence.

The sensory components of the parasympathetic innervation of the perineum mediates the sensation of distention from the anal canal and vagina while its motor component is responsible for the vascular engorgement of its erectile tissue.

CHANGES IN THE VULVA AND VAGINA THROUGHOUT LIFE

The sequential changes that are clinically recognisable in the vulva and vagina throughout life are undoubtedly hormonally dependent since they correlate well with the onset of both puberty and the menopause. During reproductive life additional cyclic changes occur in the female reproductive tract as a result of sequential alterations of ovarian hormone secretion. These changes may be transiently interrupted by pregnancy, which creates its own unique hormonal environment, or by short term use of anovulant drugs. The use of anovulants long term is associated with well recognised clinical problems, the importance of which should not be underestimated since they may affect over 3 000 000 women in England and Wales (Wellings & Mills 1984). The principal hormones involved in these changes are oestrogens and progestogens although the ovary also secretes small amounts of the male sex hormones. Specialised receptors for these steroid hormones have been identified in the female reproductive tract and perineum but the mechanisms of the actions of oestrogen and progesterone at cellular and tissue level are not entirely clear.

Birth to Puberty

During the first few weeks of life the reproductive tract of the female infant is responsive to the sex steroids which she has received transplacentally from her mother. The effects of these hormones are entirely physiological and may be evident for about four weeks or so (Dewhurst 1980). During this period the infant's vagina will be lined with a stratified squamous epithelium rich in glycogen as a direct effect of the maternal oestrogen (Fig. 2.16). There will often be an obvious vaginal discharge which in some cases will be blood stained as the result of the infant's endometrium breaking down as oestrogen levels begin to fall. The external appearance of the vulva during this neonatal period also reflects the effect of the passively transferred oestrogens (Fig. 2.17). Breast development occurs to some extent in infants of both sexes but will disappear, as do the vulval signs, around the fourth post-natal week.

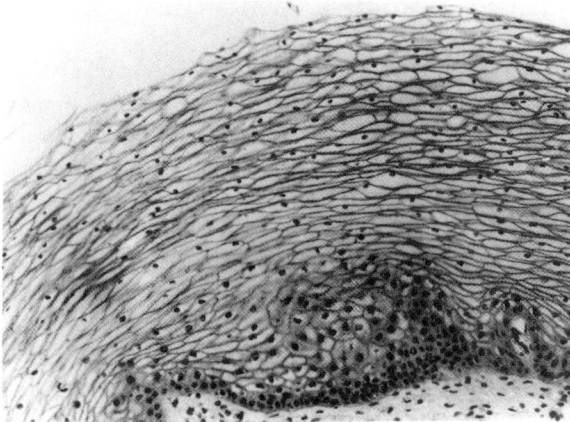

Fig. 2.16 A section from the vagina of a newborn infant showing many layers of cells in the squamous epithelium (From Dewhurst 1980 with permission).

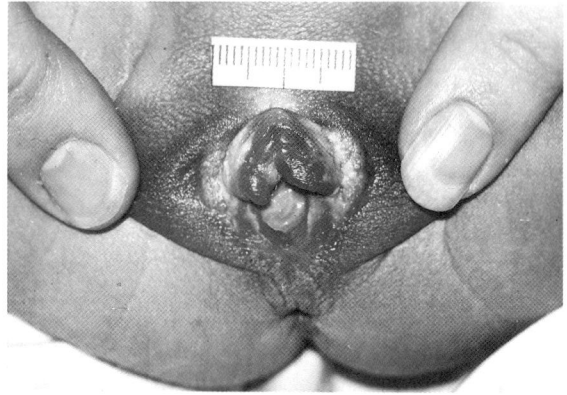

Fig. 2.17 The external genitalia in a newborn female infant (From Dewhurst 1980 with permission).

Thereafter the vaginal epithelium loses its stratification and glycogen and becomes much thinner (Fig. 2.18). These conditions persist until the young girl begins to produce her own oestrogen at puberty. During the prepubertal period the absence of glycogen from the vaginal epithelium restricts the action of lactobacilli, present within 24 hours of birth (Marshall & Tanner 1981), in the acidification of the vaginal environment. The resultant neutrality or alkalinity of the vaginal secretions renders all young girls vulnerable to vulvovaginitis and the possibility of lower urinary tract infections.

Puberty is an ill defined period of time in the life of each individual during which secondary sexual characteristics are being developed. It is also a time when many other physical and psychological changes are taking place. The most important observation concerning the events of puberty is their variability. This applies not only to the age at which they begin but also to the time taken for them to be completed and occasionally the sequence in which they appear. The physical changes associated with puberty in the female are breast development, the appearance of pubic and axillary hair, increase in height and the onset of menstruation.

Breast development has been described in five stages (Tanner 1962):

Stage 1 is the infantile state which persists from the time that the effects of maternal oestrogen have regressed until the changes of puberty begin.

Stage 2 is the 'bud' stage during which the breast tissue appears as a small mound beneath an enlarged areola. This is the first sign of pubertal change in the breast.

Stage 3 establishes a small adult breast with a continuous rounded contour.

Stage 4 is associated with further enlargement of the nipple and areola to produce a secondary projection above the contour of the remainder of the breast.

Stage 5 is the typical adult breast with smooth rounded contour, the secondary projection present in the preceding stage having disappeared.

The first signs of breast development may occur at any age from 8 years onwards and it is unusual for it not to have begun by 13 years of age. Some girls never show a typical Stage 4 passing directly from Stage 3 to 5 while others persist in Stage 4 until the first pregnancy or beyond (Marshall & Tanner 1981). Premature breast development tends to occur more often in Afro-Caribbean girls than in any other ethnic group. The enlargement may occur as early as 4 to 5 years of age but is not accompanied by other evidence of puberty or signs of endocrine disease (Black 1985).

The development and growth of pubic hair is also described in five stages (Tanner 1962) although during Stage 1 there is no pubic hair. In Stage 2 sparse hair appears on the labia majora and on the mons pubis in the midline. There is an increase in quantity and coarseness of the hair, particularly on

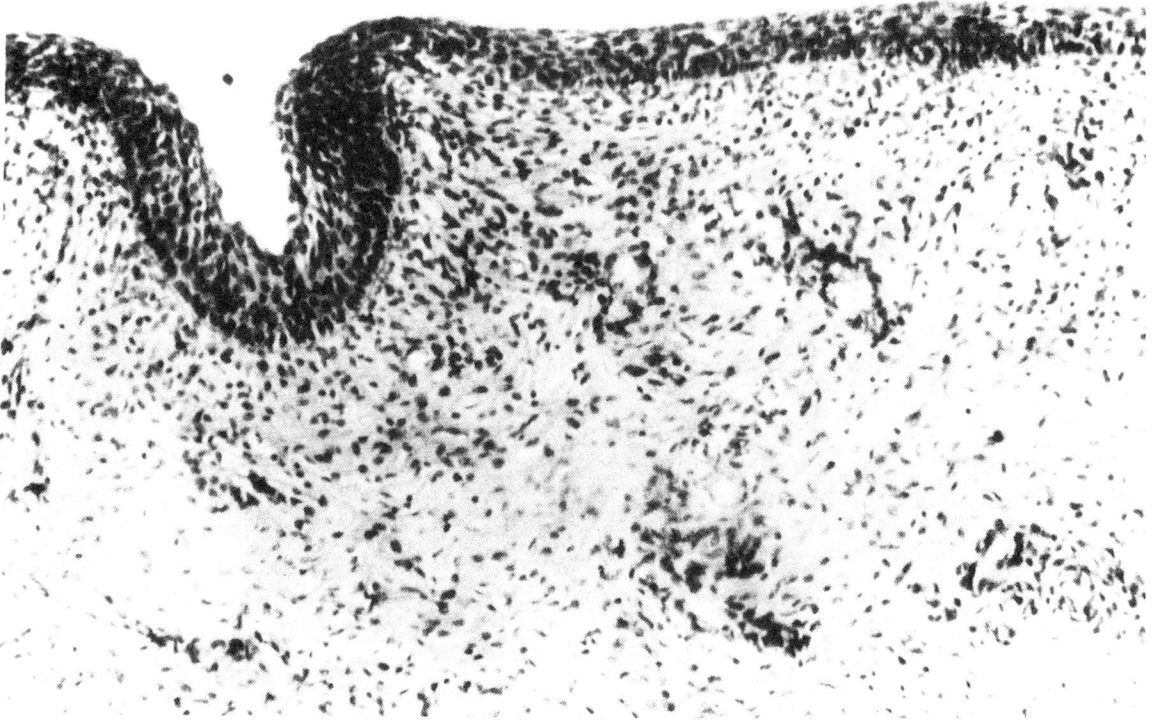

Fig. 2.18 A section from the vagina of a prepubertal female showing a thin epithelial layer (From Dewhurst 1980 with permission).

the mons pubis during Stage 3. Further increase occurs during Stage 4 such that only the upper lateral corners of the usual triangular distribution are deficient. Stage 5 describes the normal adult pubic hair pattern with its extension from the labia on to the medial aspects of the thighs. The adult distribution of pubic hair is usually attained between 12 and 17 years of age.

Axillary hair growth is described in three stages; from a stage at which it is absent, through an intermittent stage to full development. The apocrine glands of the axilla and vulva begin to function at about the time that axillary and pubic hair appear. At the same time the sebaceous glands of the general body skin become more active. The growth of any individual is dictated by a number of factors and Marshall & Tanner (1969) have found that most adolescent girls achieve maximum growth rate between their tenth and fourteenth birthdays.

Menarche occurs near the end of the sequence of changes characteristic of puberty. In the United Kingdom the average age of the menarche is 13.0 years with a standard deviation of approximately 1 year. Thus at the present time 95% of the adolescent female population have the menarche between their eleventh and fifteenth birthdays (Marshall & Tanner 1981). It is very unusual for a girl to menstruate before her breasts have reached Stage 3 and 25% of girls do so while actually in this stage. The majority of girls however begin to menstruate while they are in Stage 4 of breast development but, in about 10% of girls, menarche is delayed until their breasts have reached Stage 5 (Marshall & Tanner 1981). It is not possible to define the maximum interval which may be allowed after the attainment of Stage 5 before it can be assumed that the menarche will not occur. The assessment of skeletal age in these circumstances can be helpful since a bone age in excess of 14.5 'years' is frequently indicative of primary amenorrhoea (Marshall & Tanner 1981). Menarche is not related to the attainment of a particular body weight and it is unlikely that it has any direct relationship to the relative amounts of water, fat, bone or muscle present in the individual (Billewicz et al 1976, Faust 1977, Marshall 1978).

During the two years preceding the menarche

the ovaries increase in size. There is an increase in the number of enlarging follicles although they subsequently regress. This follicular development is associated with increasing levels of oestrogen production which is responsible for the cytological changes evident in the vaginal epithelium. As oestrogen stimulation increases the vaginal epithelium thickens and intracellular glycogen appears. The vagina begins to lengthen and this process continues until after the menarche. During the immediate premenarcheal period the uterine cervix increases in size and develops its adult shape. The cervical canal lengthens and the cervical glands become active. It is during this phase of development that the vaginal fluid increases in quantity and regains its acidity, with a pH of between 4 and 5. At about the same time fat deposition increases the size of the labia majora and the prominence of the mons pubis. The labial skin becomes rugose, the clitoris increases in size, and the urethral orifice more obvious. Coincidentally the vestibular glands of Bartholin begin to secrete and, although the hymen thickens, its orifice increases in diameter.

The Reproductive Years

Ovulation is the significant event of the ovarian cycle and it occurs approximately midway between two successive episodes of menstruation. During the preovulatory or follicular phase of the cycle oestrogen secretion increases to reach a peak a day or two before ovulation. Ovum release probably occurs as a result of coincident surges in the secretion of luteinising hormone and follicle stimulating hormone. During the post ovulatory or luteal phase of the ovarian cycle progesterone, from the corpus luteum, is the predominant hormone, while oestrogen secretion is sustained at a level below that of the preovulatory peak. These cylic changes in ovarian hormone secretion influence the female reproductive tract so as to create the appropriate environment for internal fertilisation and implantation of the embryo.

Uterus

During the preovulatory phase of the cycle the effect of oestrogen on the endometrium is to stimulate mitotic activity and thereby regenerate the endometrial lining, to replace that shed during the previous menstrual flow. After ovulation the endometrium becomes progressively more vascular under the influence of progesterone. However, the cyclic changes in both the quantity and quality of the mucus secreted by the endocervical glands, as a result of these hormonal changes, are of more significance in interpreting the vulval signs of ovarian function. Mucus production is oestrogen dependent and is therefore usually minimal immediately after menstruation. As the preovulatory surge of oestrogen production approaches the secretion of mucus increases and qualitatively it becomes transparent, more viscous and more elastic. These characteristics are maximal just before ovulation when oestrogen secretion is maximal (Ross & Vande Weile 1981). Women interpret these changes as a sensation of vulval 'wetness' (Etchepareborda et al 1983). Studies on the enzymatic content of cervical mucus indicate significant changes in the composition of a number of enzymes during this period of vulval wetness (Blackwell 1984). Two days after ovulation the sensation of vulval wetness disappears as the result of increasing progesterone secretion, which reduces the quantity of mucus produced and alters its characteristics so that it resembles the mucus which preceded the preovulatory surge.

Vagina

The stratified squamous epithelium of the vagina is exquisitely responsive to the influence of ovarian steroids. Both in childhood and after the menopause, in the absence of oestrogen, the vaginal epithelium is thin and undifferentiated. Oestrogen causes a thickening of the epithelium and its differentiation into the well recognised basal, intermediate and superficial layers characteristic of the reproductive years. The percentage of superficial cells present in a vaginal smear is an indicator of the amount of oestrogenic activity. Progesterone produces a relative decrease in the number of superficial cells while increasing the number of intermediate cells (Friedrich 1976).

The vaginal epithelium, under the influence of oestrogen, contains a great deal of glycogen. The normal vaginal flora is mixed but lactobacilli and corynebacteria, which predominate, utilise the glycogen to produce lactic acid and a low vaginal pH.

This protective environment usually precludes the overgrowth of *Candida* species which are also present in the vagina. This delicate balance may be disturbed by the use of antibiotics, such as oxytetracycline in the treatment of acne, although other antibiotics are also capable of inhibiting the lactobacilli and corynebacteria and allowing candidal overgrowth. The acidity of the vaginal environment may be reduced by the alkaline secretions of the cervical glands, particularly in the presence of a large eversion of the endocervix, by the alkaline menstrual flow and by frequent acts of coitus, since both the vaginal transudate and the ejaculate are alkaline. A more subtle change takes place in the vagina when the effects of oestrogen are moderated by a relative dominance of progesterone such as occurs during pregnancy and with the use of anovulant contraceptives. In these situations glycogen is not so readily available because of a reduction in the numbers of cells in the superficial layer of the vaginal epithelium. The same relative lack of epithelial glycogen occurs in women with diabetes mellitus due to increased glycogenolysis associated with disordered carbohydrate metabolism (Friedrich 1983).

Urethra and Vulva

The epithelial lining of the urethra is also influenced by the ovarian hormones and the character of exfoliated urethral epithelial cells changes with the phase of the ovarian cycle. Properly stained smears of epithelial cells in fresh urinary sediment reflects cyclic alterations in oestrogen and progesterone levels in sexually mature women. These cells are more accessible than vaginal epithelial cells in young girls and may be examined for diagnostic purposes when excessive oestrogen production is suspected (Ross & Vande Wiele 1981). Vulval epithelium is also responsive to the cyclical changes in ovarian hormone levels. Changes corresponding to those in the vaginal epithelium may be observed in the epithelium lining the inner aspects of the labia minora (Tozzini et al 1971).

As already noted the most obvious physiological vulval change that occurs during a woman's reproductive years is the subjective sensation of wetness which is present about the time of ovulation. This vulval symptom is a consequence of the changes in the quantity and quality of the cervical mucus secretion during the ovarian cycle. Many of the other vulval signs and symptoms, both physiological and pathological, are the result of changes in the upper reproductive tract, particularly the cervix uteri and vagina. Sexually transmitted diseases are very common and many women are particularly anxious if they have been exposed to the risk of infection. In these circumstances it is important to recognise that a vaginal discharge does not necessarily mean infection and that attempts at self treatment may worsen the situation and make accurate diagnosis more difficult (Friedrich 1983).

Changes related to coitus and pregnancy

During sexual arousal in the female the breasts enlarge and the nipples become erect. This erectile response also occurs in the clitoris, labia minora and the vestibular bulbs on either side of the vaginal opening. The vascular engorgement of the labia minora and vestibular bulbs reduces the size of the introitus by approximately 50% (Burchell & Wabrek 1981). The upper vagina dilates and the uterus is elevated in the pelvis as a result of pelvic vascular congestion. This vascular congestion, mediated by the parasympathetic nervous system, induces a transudate from the vaginal epithelium which produces the lubrication necessary for coitus. Penetration of the vagina by the penis produces traction on the labia minora and thus additional stimulus to the clitoris. During orgasm rhythmic contraction of the pelvic floor and perineal musculature occurs. This is followed by decongestion of the pelvic viscera and vasculature during the phase of resolution. The physiological events occurring in the female reproductive tract during coitus facilitate spematozoal transport, from the site of ejaculation in the upper vagina to the uterine tubes where fertilisation normally takes place. Such spermatozoal transport occurs only at or about the time of ovulation, when changes in the cervical mucus allow entry of spermatozoa into the cavity of the uterus.

In the event of fertilisation and successful implantation of the embryo the pregnant woman will adapt to a unique hormonal environment created by the steroid and protein hormones produced by the placenta. Blood flow through the pelvic circulation is increased five-fold during the first two months of pregnancy and doubles again during the third month (Barrow 1957). Progesterone causes an increase of venous distensibility (Gallagher 1986) and the progesterone-dominant state of pregnancy predisposes to vulval varicosities. In addition the diminished availability of glycogen from the vaginal epithelium renders the vagina more likely to candidal overgrowth which is reported to be 10–20 times more common in pregnant than non-pregnant women (Wallenberg & Wladimiroff 1976). The situation is undoubtedly exacerbated by the host's altered immune responsiveness during pregnancy, perhaps to ensure the survival of the fetal allograft, and these alterations appear to make the pregnant woman more susceptible to primary infection, reinfection and reactivated infection (Brabin 1985).

Injury to the genital tract and vulva may occur during delivery of the infant. Rupture of vessels outside the wall of the genital tract may lead to para-genital haematoma formation, in which case a significant distinction must be made between those which lie above and below the levator ani muscle (Beazley 1981). Infra-levator haematomas may occur as the result of an inadequate episiotomy repair which allows a continual ooze into the surrounding tissues. In this way a great quantity of blood can escape into the ischiorectal fossa or paravaginal tissues. Of more direct relevance, in the present context, are injuries to the vaginal wall and vulva which affect the perineum and may occur spontaneously or as a result of episiotomy. These will usually be identified at the time of delivery and appropriately treated; if not they may be associated with serious functional disturbances at a later date.

The menopause and old age

The menopause, or cessation of menstruation, occurs at a median age of 50.1 years but may take place physiologically between 40 and 53 years of age (Frommer 1964). The age of the menopause does not appear to depend on socio-economic conditions, geographical location, race, marital status or any physical attribute (MacMahon & Worcester 1966). Ageing of the ovaries is eventually associated with the inability to secrete sufficient of the hormones necessary to produce endometrial shedding.

When menstruation has ceased for at least one year the woman is said to be postmenopausal (Davey 1981). Thereafter oestrogen and progesterone levels remain low while gonadotrophin levels increase and may remain elevated for perhaps 20–30 years (Davey 1981).

The postmenopausal changes in the genital and urinary tracts are related to cessation of ovarian hormone secretion but also to the normal ageing process. The body of the uterus is reduced in size, the myometrium is partially replaced by fibrous tissue, the endometrium becomes thin and atrophic and cervical glandular secretion is reduced. The vagina becomes less rugose, narrower and drier and the vaginal epithelium more easily damaged. Microscopically the epithelial layers are reduced in number and the cells lack glycogen, while the stroma is infiltrated with lymphocytes and plasma cells. As a consequence of these changes the vaginal environment becomes alkaline (Davey 1981). Some time later the vulval skin becomes atrophic and, as a result of the loss of subcutaneous fat, the labia majora and mons pubis are reduced in size and the introitus may gape. Loss of muscle tone encourages the possibility of vaginal and uterine prolapse. Changes comparable to those in the vaginal epithelium also occur in the transitional epithelium of the urethra and bladder with the consequent increased risk of recurrent urethritis and cystitis.

Ovarian failure may occur in relatively young women as the result of treatment for other pathological conditions, some of which are life threatening. It has recently been suggested, on the basis of urinary hormone assays, that oestrogen deficiency may even follow tubal ligation in some women (Cattanach 1985).

INCONTINENCE

Incontinence, defined as the inadvertent or uncontrolled passage of faeces or urine or both, is a disability associated with profound social consequences (Swash 1985). In the female it will also have significant clinical effects upon the perineum which may be difficult to interpret if incontinence is not suspected. Urinary incontinence is present in about 12% of women over 65 years of age and in as many as 9% of younger women (Thomas et al 1980).

Faecal incontinence is perhaps less common although half of the patients investigated for diarrhoea in one study were in fact suffering from faecal incontinence (Leigh & Turnberg 1982).

Neurological causes of incontinence include multiple sclerosis, Parkinson's disease and disorders of the spinal cord or cauda equina. It may also occur in patients with peripheral neuropathy, especially when autonomic nerves are affected, as in diabetes mellitus (Swash 1985). Although local causes of incontinence include urinary or anal fistulae the commonest local cause is stress incontinence. It now seems evident that although both urinary and faecal stress incontinence can occur following muscle injury associated with childbirth, the most likely cause of both types of incontinence is nerve injury (Snooks et al 1984). Such nerve injury is associated with repeated straining during defaecation (Parks et al 1977) or childbirth (Snooks et al 1984). The nerves involved are those which innervate the levator ani muscle and the external anal sphincter.

IMMUNE RESPONSIVENESS

Immunological factors are of significance in many aspects of the physiology and pathophysiology of the lower genital tract, and are reviewed by Fox (1987).

In particular, a local secretory immune system is situated in the cervix, and responds to antigenic stimulus by the production of antibodies which are predominantly of the IgA class.

This secretory IgA becomes linked with secretory component, a glycoprotein synthesised in the epithelial cells; this substance appears to facilitate transepithelial transport of the IgA. Secretory IgA has many useful properties (Doe 1982); it can activate components by the alternative pathway, is bactericidal in the presence of lysozyme and complement, and can agglutinate bacteria and opsonize them for phagocytosis, as well as blocking entry of antigens by forming non-absorbable complexes. In addition it can inhibit the adhesiveness of organisms to the mucosa and has a capacity to neutralise virus.

Large numbers of allogeneic spermatozoa enter the female reproductive tract during coitus and some penetrate the tissues of the female host (Hafez 1976, Zamboni 1971). The invading spermatozoa are destroyed by an immune response which generates cytolytic T-lymphocytes specifically effective against the alloantigens expressed by the spermatozoa (McLean et al 1980). This coital immune response is limited by the immunosuppressive function of seminal fluid to the immediate post-coital period (Thomas & McLean 1984). Thus the conceptus, which expresses paternal alloantigens (Heyner 1983), is not subject to immune attack during implantation. Protection against viral infection also requires an effective cytolytic T-lymphocyte response and any limitation of this response will increase the possibility of an oncogenic virus in the ejaculate escaping destruction. Seminal fluid, by virtue of its physiological role in reproduction, may limit the anti-viral response and thereby predispose the female genital tract to viral infection. An additional factor which may render sexually active young women more vulnerable to such infection is the reduced immune responsiveness associated with anovulant contraceptives (Gerretsen et al 1980). It is also generally agreed that a woman is at greater risk of infection when pregnant. This is in part due to a reduced immune responsiveness during pregnancy (Brabin 1985). Therapeutic immunosuppression of renal allograft recipients renders them more susceptible to malignant neoplasia. This was demonstrated in a recent report of squamous cell carcinoma of the vulva in two of two hundred such female patients; the two women concerned were both in their early twenties (Caterson et al 1984).

REFERENCES

Barmann J M, Astore J, Pecoraro V 1969 The normal trichogram of people over 50 years. In: Montagna W, Dobson R L (eds) Advances in Biology of Skin Vol IX Hair Growth. Pergamon Press, Oxford

Barrow D W 1957 The clinical management of varicose veins. 2nd edn Hoebner, New York

Baruchin A M, & Cipollini T 1986 Vaginal Labioplasty. British Journal of Sexual Medicine 13: 32

Beazley J M 1981 Maternal Injuries and Complications. In: Dewhurst J (ed) Integrated Obstetrics and Gynaecology for Postgraduates 3rd edn Blackwell Scientific Publications, Oxford

Billewicz W Z, Fellowes H M, Hytten C A 1976 Comments on the critical metabolic mass and the age of menarche. Annals of Human Biology 3: 51–59

Black J 1985 Afro-Caribbean and African families. British Medical Journal 290: 984–988

Blackwell R E 1984 Detection of ovulation. Fertility and Sterility 41: 680–681

Brabin B J 1985 Epidemiology of infection in pregnancy. Reviews of Infectious Diseases 7: 579–603

Breathnach A S, Wyllie L M 1965 Electron microscopy of melanocytes and Langerhans cells in human fetal epidermis at 14 weeks. Journal of Investigative Dermatology 44: 51–60

Breathnach A S 1971 Embryology of human skin. Journal of Investigative Dermatology 57: 133–143

Brindley G S 1984 New treatment for priapism. Lancet ii: 220–221

Burchell R C, Wabrek A J 1981 Sexual physiology. In: Philipp E E, Barnes J, Newton M (eds) Scientific Foundations of Obstetrics and Gynaecology 2nd ed. Heinemann, London

Bush R S 1979 Malignancies of the ovary uterus and cervix. Edward Arnold, London

Caterson R J, Furber J, Murray J, McCarthy W, Mahony J F, Sheil A G R 1984 Carcinoma of the vulva in two young renal allograft recipients. Transplantation Proceedings 16: 559–561

Cattanach J 1985 Oestrogen deficiency after tubal ligation. Lancet i: 847–849

Davey D A 1981 The menopause and climacteric. In: Dewhurst J (ed) Integrated Obstetrics and Gynaecology for Postgraduates, 3rd edn. Blackwell Scientific Publications, Oxford

Daw E, Riley S 1982 Umbilical metastasis from squamous carcinoma of the cervix. Case Report. British Journal of Obstetrics and Gynaecology 89: 1066

Dewhurst J 1980 Practical Pediatric and Adolescent Gynecology. Marcel Dekker, New York

Dewhurst J 1981 In: Dewhurst J (ed) Integrated Obstetrics and Gynaecology for Postgraduates 3rd edn. Blackwell Scientific Publications, Oxford

Doe W F 1982 Immunological aspects of the gut. In: Lachmann P J, Peters D K (eds) Clinical Aspects of Immunology. Blackwell Scientific Publications, Oxford, p 985

Ebling F J G 1968 Embryology. In: Rook A, Wilkinson D S, Ebling F J G (eds) Textbook of Dermatology Blackwell Scientific, Oxford

Edelson R L, Fink J M 1985 The immunologic function of skin. Scientific American 252: 34–41

Edwards J N T, Morris H B 1985 Langerhans cells and lymphocyte subsets in the female genital tract. British Journal of Obstetrics and Gynaecology 92: 974–982

Etchepareborda J J, Rivero L V, Kesseru E 1983 Billings natural family planning method. Contraception 28: 475–480

Faust M S 1977 Somatic development of adolescent girls. Monographs of the Society for Research into Child Development 42: 1–90

Fetissof F, Berger G, Dubois M P, Arbeille-Brassart B, Lansac J, Jm-Giao M, & Jopard P 1985 Endocrine cells in the female genital tract. Histopathology 9: 133–145

Figge D C, Tamimi H K, Greer B E 1985 Lymphatic spread in carcinoma of the vulva. American Journal of Obstetrics and Gynaecology 152: 387–394

Fox H 1987 Immunopathology of the female genital tract. In: Fox H (ed) Haines and Taylor's Obstetrical and Gynaecological Pathology. Churchill Livingstone, London, p 944

Friedrich E G 1985 Vaginitis. American Journal of Obstetrics and Gynecology 152: 247–251

Friedrich E G, Wilkinson E J 1982 The vulva. In: Blaustein A (ed) Pathology of the Female Genital Tract 2nd edn. Springer Verlag, New York

Friedrich E G 1983 Vulvar Disease 2nd Edn. Saunders, Philadelphia

Friedrich E G, Wilkinson E J 1985 Vulvar surgery for neurofibromatosis. Obstetrics and Gynecology 65: 135–138

Frommer D J 1964 Changing age of the menopause. British Medical Journal 2: 349–351

Gallagher P G 1986 Varicose veins of the vulva. British Journal of Sexual Medicine 13: 12–14

Gatter K C, Morris H B, Roach B, Mortimer P, Fleming K, Masson D Y 1984 Langerhans cells and T-cells in human skin tumours: an immunohistological study. Histopathology 8: 229–244

Gerretsen G, Kremer J, Bleumink E, Nater J P, de Gast G C, The T H 1980 Immune reactivity of women on hormonal contraceptives. Contraception 22: 25–29

Gosling J A, Dixon J S, Humpherson J R 1983 Functional Anatomy of the Urinary Tract. Churchill Livingstone, Edinburgh

Gould V E, Moll R, Moll I, Lee I, Franke W W 1985 Biology of disease. Laboratory Investigation 52: 334–352

Hafez L S E 1976 Transport and Survival of Spermatozoa in the Female Reproductive Tract. C V Mosby, St Louis

Hashimoto K 1970 The ultrastructure of the skin in human embryos. Acta Dermatovenereologia 50: 241–251

Hasson H M, Dershin H 1981 Assessment of uterine shape by geometric means. Contraceptive Delivery Systems 2: 59–76

Heyner S 1983 Alloantigen expression on mouse oocytes and early mouse embryos. In: Wegmann T G, Gill T (eds) Immunology of Reproduction Oxford University Press, New York

Holbrooke K A 1983 Structure and function of the developing human skin. In: Goldsmith L A (ed) Biochemistry and Physiology of the Skin. Oxford University Press, Oxford

Hollinshead W H 1971 Anatomy for Surgeons 2nd edn. Harper & Row, New York

Hu F 1981 Melanocyte cytology in normal skin. In: Ackerman A B (ed) Masson Monographs in Dermatology-1. Masson, New York

Iversen T, Aas M 1983 Lymph drainage from the vulva. Gynecologic Oncology 16: 169–179

Jensen S T 1985 Comparison of podophyllin application with simple surgical excision in clearance or recurrence of perianal condylomata acuminata. Lancet ii: 1146–1148

Kaufman R H 1981 Anatomy of the Vulva and Vagina. In: Gardner H L, Kaufman R H (eds) Benign Diseases of the Vulva and Vagina. Hall, Boston

Krantz K E 1977 The anatomy and physiology of the vulva and vagina. In: Philipp E E, Barnes J, Newton M (eds) Scientific Foundation of Obstetrics and Gynaecology, 2nd edn. Heinemann, London, pp 65–78

Last R J 1959 Anatomy Regional and Applied 2nd edn. Churchill, London

Leigh R J, Turnberg L A 1982 Faecal incontinence: the unvoiced symptom. Lancet i: 1349–1351

Lind T, Parkin F M, Cheyne G A 1969 Biochemical and cytological changes in liquor amnii with advancing gestation. Journal of Obstetrics and Gynaecology of the British Commonwealth. 76: 673–683

Lozano G B L, Castenada P F 1981 Priapism of the clitoris. British Journal of Urology 53: 390.

Lunde O 1984 A study of body hair density and distribution in normal women. American Journal of Physical Anthropology 64: 179–184

MacKie R M 1984 Milne's Dermatopathology 2nd edn. Arnold, London

Macmahon T, Worcester J 1966 National Centre for Health Studies Series II. Washington, DC

Marshall W A 1978 The relationship of puberty to other maturity indicators and body composition in man. Journal of Reproduction and Fertility 52: 437–443

Marshall W A, Tanner J M 1969 Variation in the pattern of pubertal changes in girls, Archives of the Diseases of Children 44: 291–303

Marshall W A, Tanner J M 1981 Puberty. In: Davis J A, Dobbing J (eds) Scientific Foundations of Paediatrics 2nd edn. Heinemann, London

McLean J M, Shaya E I, Gibbs A C C 1980 Immune response to first mating in female rat. Journal of Reproductive Immunology 1: 285–295

Medawar P B 1953 The microanatomy of the mammalian epidermis. Quarterly Journal of Microscopical Science 94: 481–506

Melville H, Harrison N 1985 Persistent priapism in a normal woman. British Medical Journal 291: 516

Montagna W 1960 Cholinesterases in the cutaneous nerves in man. In: Montagna W (ed) Advances in Biology of Skin Vol 1 Pergamon Press, New York

Montagna W, Parakkal P F 1974 Apocrine glands. In: Montagna W, Parakkal P F (eds) The Structure and Function of skin 3rd edn. Academic Press, New York

Morris H H B, Gatter K C, Sykes G, Casemore V, Masson D Y 1983 Langerhans cells in the human cervical epithelium: effect of wart virus infection and intraepithelial neoplasia. British Journal of Obstetrics and Gynaecology 90: 412–420

Niebauer G 1968 Dendritic cells of the skin. Karger, New York

Odland G F 1983 Structure of the skin. In: Goldsmith L A (ed) Biochemistry & Physiology of the Skin. Oxford University Press, Oxford

Omsjo I H, Wright P B, Bormer O P 1984 Estrogen and progesterone receptors in normal and malignant vulvar tissue. Gynecologic and Obstetric Investigation 17: 281–283

Parker F 1981 Skin and hormones In: Williams R H (ed) Textbook of Endocrinology. W B Saunders Company, Philadelphia

Parks A G, Swash M, Urich H 1977 Sphincter denervation in anorectal incontinence and rectal prolapse. Gut 18: 656–665

Patterson J A K, Edelson R L 1982 Interaction of T-cells with epidermis. British Journal of Dermatology 107: 117–122

Pinkus F 1910 Development of the integument. In: Keibel F, Mall F P Manual of Embryology. Lippincott, Philadelphia

Pinkus H 1958 Embryology of hair. In: Montagna W, Ellis R A (eds) The Hair Growth. Academic Press, New York

Robboy S J, Ross J S, Prat J, Keh P C, Welch W R 1978 Urogenital Sinus origin of mucinous and ciliated cysts of the vulva. Obstetrics and Gynecology 51: 347–351

Roberts W H, Krishingner G L 1967 Comparative study of human internal iliac artery based on Adachi classification. 'Anatomical Record 158: 191–196

Ross G T, Van De Wiele R L 1981 The Ovaries. In: Williams R H (ed) Textbook of Endocrinology. Saunders, Philadelphia

Serri F, Montagna W, Mescon H 1962 Studies of the skin of the fetus and child. Journal of Investigative Dermatology 39: 199–217

Shuttleworth K 1977 Urinary continence in the female. In: Philipp E E, Barnes J, Newton M (eds) Scientific Foundations of Obstetrics and Gynaecology. Heinemann, London, pp. 84–86

Sinclair J D 1972 Thermal control in premature infants. Annual Review of Medicine 23: 129–148

Snooks S J, Setchell M, Swash M, Henry M M 1984 Injury to innervation of pelvic floor sphincter musculature in childbirth. Lancet ii: 546–550

Solomon L M, Esterly N B 1970 Neonatal Dermatology 1: The newborn skin. Journal of Pediatrics 77: 888–894

Steinman R M 1981 Dendritic cells. Transplantation 31: 151–155

Stingl L G, Tamaki K, Katz S I 1981 Origin and function of epidermal Langerhans cells. Immunology Review 53: 149–174

Swash M 1985 New concepts in incontinence. British Medical Journal 290: 4–5

Tanner J M (1962) Growth at Adolescence 2nd edn. Blackwell, Oxford

Tay S K, Jenkins D, Maddox P, Campion M 1987a Subpopulations of Langerhan's cells in cervical neoplasia. British Journal of Obstetrics and Gynaecology 94: 10–15

Tay S K, Jenkins D, Maddox P, Singer A 1987b Lymphocyte phenotypes in cervical human papillomavirus infection. British Journal of Obstetrics and Gynaecology 94: 16–21

Thomas I K, McLean J M 1984 Seminal plasma abrogates the post-coital T-cell response to spermatozoal histocompatibility antigen. American Journal of Reproductive Immunology 6: 185–189

Thomas T M, Plymar K R, Blannin J, Meade T W 1980 Prevalence of urinary incontinence. British Medical Journal 281: 1243–1245

Tozzini R, Sobrero A J, Hoovise E 1971 Vulvar cytology. Acta Cytologica 15: 57–60

Wallenburg H C S, Wladimiroff J W 1976 Recurrence of vulvovaginal candidosis during pregnancy. Obstetrics & Gynecology 48: 491–494

Way J 1977 The lymphatics of the pelvis. In: Philipp E E, Barnes J, Newton M (eds) Scientific Foundations of Obstetrics & Gynaecology. Heinemann, London, pp. 118–126

Wellings K, Mills A 1984 Contraceptive trends. British Medical Journal 289: 939–940

Wendell-Smith C P, Wilson P M 1977 Musculature of the pelvic floor. In: Philipp E E Barnes J Newton M (eds) Scientific Foundations of Obstetrics & Gynaecology. Heinemann, London

Winkelmann R K 1977 The Merkel cell system and a comparison between it and the neurosecretory or APUD cell system. Journal of Investigative Dermatology 69: 41–46

Winkelmann R K, Breathnach A S 1973 The Merkel cell. Journal of Investigative Dermatology 60: 2–15

Zamboni L 1971 Fine Morphology of Mammalian Fertilisation. Harper & Row, New York

3

Principles of examination, investigation and diagnosis
C M Ridley

INTRODUCTION

Women with vulval lesions may present themselves to general practitioners, dermatologists, gynaecologists and specialists in genitourinary medicine, and thereby offer opportunities not only of interdisciplinary co-operation but of confusion and mismanagement. It should be possible often to avoid the adverse outcome by discussion and by correlation of different viewpoints on terminology. There are other less easily negotiable difficulties, those inherent in the conditions themselves, and co-operation is important in this respect too. The United Kingdom is fortunate in its efficient network of clinics for sexually transmitted diseases, staffed by specialists in genitourinary medicine and able to deal with the necessary screening and contact tracing. The reports of figures submitted to the Central Medical Office of the Department of Health and Social Security are valuable sources of information on trends of incidence of sexually transmitted diseases. The role of the pathologist must be stressed. He it is who often has the final word in diagnosis and with whom co-operation and understanding are essential. The gynaecologist tends to lean more heavily on the pathologist, and gives him a greater responsibility in comparison with the dermatologist. The latter is more likely to have his own ideas on histology, to want to discuss the sections and to refer problems to a dermatological histopathologist. The general pathologist will be confused if the clinicians cannot agree on the terms they use. The pathologist who specialises in gynaecological pathology will be of invaluable help if he is interested in vulval, cutaneous, pathology, but not if his sphere has been restricted to more proximal parts of the genital tract.

Vulval clinics, usually staffed by a dermatologist and a gynaecologist, have been advocated for many years, especially in the United States. They have been run successfully and yielded useful information.

The International Society for the Study of Vulvar Disease, founded in 1970, and designed to include all specialist interests in vulval problems, has proved valuable in coordination. It has 'task forces' on controversial subjects and is currently dealing with the classification and clarification of terminological problems. There is a need to remember the epidemiological, geographical and cultural differences which will affect the clinical material any one doctor sees, and an international society is of particular value in this respect.

THE CONSULTATION

As in many dermatological consultations the history may be virtually unnecessary to diagnosis, or all important; most clinicians would see the patient before the examination as a matter of courtesy and be prepared to amplify the account then given by judicious later questioning in the light of the findings. Certain well-trodden pathways will be traversed—previous medications, general health and so forth; the auditor must be prepared to explore byways if the patient indicates their relevance, and these often lead to evidence of psychological resentments and anxieties. The history will be difficult to obtain in the non-English speaking community, and interpreters, whether hospital staff or relatives (often children and frequently male), can be of limited value in such delicate transactions.

Examination (which normally includes the whole

of the skin and other systems as indicated) can present its own problems, for example, reluctance to be examined by a male doctor; the importance of the examination in psychological terms is discussed on page 214. Physical problems may also arise such as immobility, obesity and poor light. Natural daylight is best for appreciation of colour change but artificial light will often be needed to illuminate the interstices of the anogenital area. The inexperienced will soon learn the inadvisability of examining several patients in succession without recording the findings of each at the time; in most conditions the exact morphology and location of lesions is of vital importance. A routine order in examination of each part of the area is advisable, and a magnifying glass is helpful. Where the problem is clearly dermatological there is little point in routine vaginal

and cervical examination, but this may be indicated if there is a suggestion of an infective lesion since any sexually transmitted disease may be accompanied by others, and it may be indicated to explore the possibility of accompanying vaginal and cervical disease, when most dermatologists would prefer to enlist the help of gynaecological colleagues. Equally, where any obviously dermatological lesion is present, it is wise for the patient to be seen by a dermatologist. Notes can be supplemented by a drawing or a diagram, preferably by a set of diagrams, as shown in Figure 3.1, so that both aspects of the labia minora can be documented. In genitourinary medicine clinics, where gynaecological findings are of obvious relevance, there is a case for a cervical diagram also. This is usually part of the standard pro forma where a clinic is being held

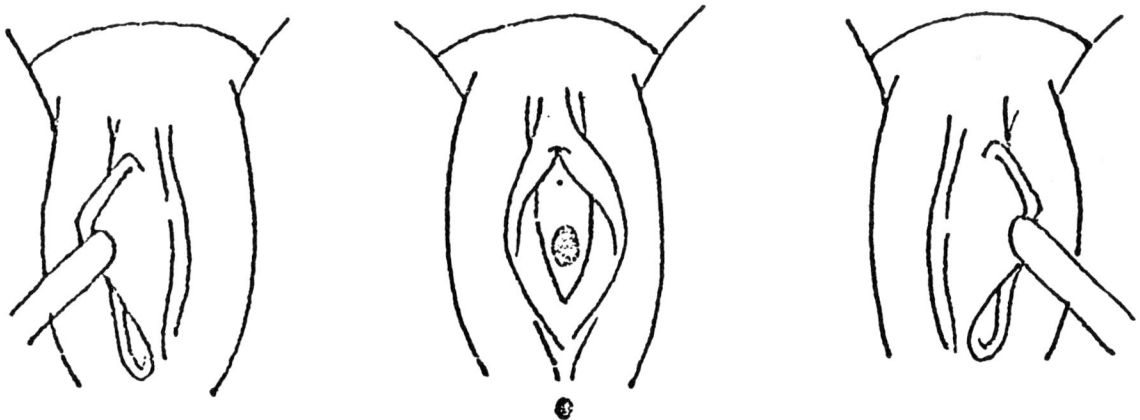

Fig. 3.1 Stylised representation of the vulva. (By courtesy of Dr M. McKay)

Table 3.1 Proforma for vulval clinic.

Dermatological history	Gynaecological history	On examination
Duration:	K—Cycle-	Breasts:
Symptoms i.e. itching	LMP-	Abdomen:
pain	Premenstrual symptoms:	Pelvis:
burning		
	Vaginal discharge:	PV:
Site:	Parity:	PR:
Other sites:	Contraception:	Vulva:
Past history:	Other:	Cervix:
Family history:		
Treatment: Local		
Systemic		
Aggravating factors:		Other sites
General health:		
Drugs:		DIAGNOSIS
Other:		TREATMENT
		APPOINTMENT

with a gynaecologist, and some will like to have the rest of the information standard in such circumstances (Table 3.1) or devise a more elaborate pattern.

Such joint vulval clinics, where a gynaecologist and dermatologist work together, are increasing in number. On balance there is no doubt that they are of great value, but the concept is not without potential drawbacks which must be thought out. The clinics occupy more of the doctors' time for example (although the patient may be saved visits), and it is important to ensure that the patient is not in any uncertainty as to what decisions have been taken and by whom. Not every patient needs to be seen by both specialists, and to some extent the session can be run as two parallel clinics, with discussion on joint patients as necessary. The wide range of conditions and problems attracted to the service, and the demonstration of co-operation between specialities, constitute a rich vein of teaching material. A steady flow of biopsy material from the one source helps to draw the pathologist into the atmosphere of cooperation. Moreover, once a good relationship has been established between the doctors concerned, cases encountered by each separately can be more appropriately dealt with or referred.

INVESTIGATIVE AND DIAGNOSTIC TECHNIQUES

Apart from swabs for specimens taken to culture bacteria, *Candida* and *Trichomonas*, viral transport medium should be at hand for culture of suspected herpetic lesions. Skin scrapings will be required in cases of cutaneous *Candida*, erythrasma or tinea infections. Vulval cytology has a limited role. Smears from material obtained by scraping the inner aspect of the labia majora, using a swab or the blunt end of a blade, to some extent reflect cyclical changes as in the vaginal mucosa (Tozzini et al 1971, Nauth & Haas 1985). Smears may be taken from particular lesions for diagnostic purposes, for example in herpesvirus lesions to demonstrate typical giant cells, or from various neoplasms (but Nauth & Schilke (1982) found positive results in only half of a series of malignant lesions). Nauth & Boon (1983) have devised a morphometric technique which makes

malignant cells easy to recognise even if, as often is the case, the cells are anucleate. Biopsy is, however, at present much more reliable and useful.

Colposcopy

Colposcopy, giving a magnification of six to ten times, is widely used at the cervix to study all aspects of its morphology and has been a notable advance in relating wart virus infection to intraepithelial neoplasia. The vagina, likewise, can be examined. Vulval colposcopy has been less used. It is of little value on keratinised surfaces but can give useful information on the labia minora and vestibule. The patient is examined in the lithotomy position. The technique may be of assistance in localising areas for biopsy. When warts are in question, inspection is aided by the liberal application of acetic acid (usually 5%) using swabs. This stings and the patient should be forewarned. After examination it is washed off. The whiteness which appears with warty or neoplastic tissue correlates with epidermal thickening and abnormality and it throws the vascular morphology into relief. Use of the colposcope also promotes understanding of the morphology of the vestibule; minor vestibular gland orifices and vestibular papillae are clearly visible. Whereas cervical biopsies can be taken through the colposcope without local anaesthesia, vulval tissue unfortunately cannot be so obtained.

The use of 1% toluidine blue (applied then washed off with 5% acetic acid) to delineate 'suspicious', that is, premalignant, areas as a guide to biopsy is not generally recommended, though some workers find it of help still in conjunction with colposcopy. The dye has been thought to be taken up preferentially by the nuclei of highly cellular and aneuploid malignant tissue, but it may in fact rather be taken up by the widened intercellular spaces in malignant tissue. It may give false positive and false negative results (Lancet 1982).

Biopsy

Biopsy is often necessary. For a vulval biopsy, local anaesthesia with 2% lignocaine is rapid and effective, though perhaps because of the softness of the area and rapid diffusion rather more may be needed than in other areas (1–2 ml, however, is usually

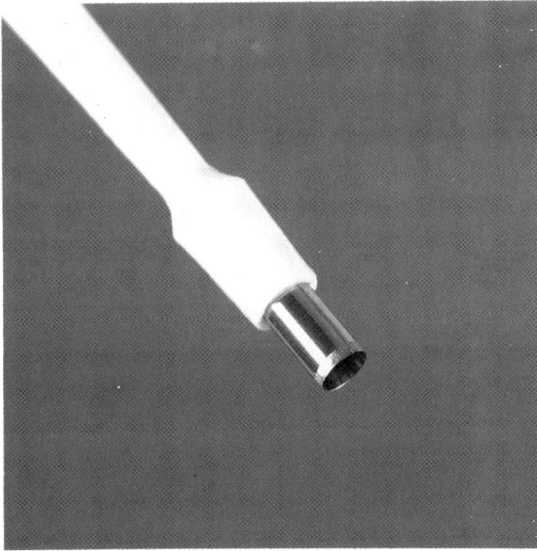

Fig. 3.2 Disposable biopsy punch.

specimens may be called for. For larger or multiple biopsies or specimens from friable non-keratinised areas general anaesthesia may be required, and the gynaecologist may be better able to obtain them than the dermatologist. For punch biopsy 4 mm and 6 mm disposable punches (fig. 3.2) are readily available. They are used to drill out a core of tissue which can then be removed with a pair of sharp scissors and, if necessary, a fine-toothed forceps—using minimal trauma. Haemostasis is with cautery or a silver nitrate stick. It is wise to put the specimen on an absorbent card (or paper) before putting it into the bottle of fixative, to facilitate orientation by the pathologist. Small punch biopsy sites can be allowed to heal without suturing. Infection is rare but, if wished, an antiseptic such as povidone iodine ointment may be prescribed.

For routine histology the tissue is fixed in formalin. However, other techniques are now often called for. When immunoperoxidase staining is required, the type of fixative needed to give the best results should be discussed with the pathologist. The usual alternatives are formalin or snap freezing in liquid nitrogen. Specimens for direct immunofluorescence, for example in bullous diseases, (biopsies should be perilesional) are put into a special transport medium or in a flask containing liquid nitrogen, and material for DNA hybridisation is also snap frozen in liquid nitrogen. Material for electron microscopy should be put into 2% glutaraldehyde at 4°C and sent at once to the laboratory.

adequate). The puncture mark should be squeezed slightly if it is not already evident as a drop of blood since it provides a useful marker for the area anaesthetised, which otherwise is easily 'lost'. On some occasions one will need a formal biopsy, an ellipse with sutures. On others, a punch biopsy will suffice. A compromise is to cut out with a scalpel blade an ovoid strip over a needle introduced under the skin. In both instances, multiple

REFERENCES

Lancet (editorial) 1982 Clinical stains for cancer. Lancet i: 320–321
Nauth H F, Boon M E 1983 Significance of the morphology of anucleated squames in the cytologic diagnosis of vulvar lesions. A new approach in diagnostic cytology. Acta Cytologica 27: 230–236
Nauth H F, Haas M 1985 Cytologic and histologic observations

on the sex hormone dependence of the vulva. Journal of Reproductive Medicine 30: 667–674
Nauth H F, Schilke E 1982 Cytology of the exfoliative layer in normal and diseased vulvar skin. Correlation with histology. Acta Cytologica 26: 269–283
Tozzini R, Sofrero A J, Hoovis E 1971 Vulvar cytology. Acta Cytologica 15: 57–63

4

Diagnosis of human papillomavirus and herpesvirus infections: specialised techniques
D J McCance

The human papillomaviruses (HPV) produce the clinically recognisable lesion condyloma acuminatum, and have recently been associated with other subclinical lesions of the lower genital tract (McCance & Singer 1985). The other common viral infection is caused by *Herpes simplex* virus (HSV) types I and II. This section will deal with laboratory diagnosis with special reference to the recent molecular techniques available to differentiate virus types within the two groups.

CHEMICAL AND PHYSICAL PROPERTIES

Human papillomaviruses (HPV)

There are at present at least 40 types of HPV which are differentiated not by serological means but by the homology of their respective DNA molecules, that is, how similar the DNA sequence or nucleotide pairings of the DNA of one HPV is to. that of another. This technique will be described later. The DNA of these viruses is circular and has a molecular weight of 5×10^6 u with approximately 8000 base pairs, coding for eight to ten proteins. The virion (a complete virus particle) is composed of this DNA (the genome) surrounded by a protein coat (capsid) in an icosahedral symmetry. The virus particle is 45 nm in diameter (Fig. 4.1a).

Herpes simplex virus (HSV)

There are two HSV virus types, I and II. The linear DNA of HSV is large with a molecular weight of 100×10^6 u containing approximately 150 000 base pairs and capable of coding for perhaps up to 100 proteins. The virion is composed of a capsid, sur-rounding the DNA, which has an icosahedral sym metry and outside this a lipid envelope (Fig. 4.1b). This lipid layer is acquired as the virus matures by budding through the nuclear membrane. Viral-coded glycoproteins (gB, gC, gD, gE, gG) are inserted into this lipid envelope and so are exposed on the surface of the virions. The glycoproteins of HSV type 1 are differentiated from type 2 by adding the relevant numeral, for example gC-1 or gC-2.

VIRAL REPLICATION

HPV

Papillomaviruses are host specific and epitheliotropic, usually infecting stratified squamous epithelium. During the replicative cycle of papillomaviruses fully infectious virus particles are found only in the most differentiated cells, that is, the outer cells of the epithelium. Viral DNA may also be detected in lower layers of the epithelium where no viral structural proteins are detected. The close alignment of papillomavirus replication with epithelial differentiation has constantly hampered attempts to produce infectious virus in cell cultures, as such differentiating systems have not been successfully reproduced in vitro.

Replication may be episomal, when HPV DNA replicates in the nucleus free and unassociated with chromosomal DNA and the genome replicates and segregates independently of chromosomal DNA during cell division; or with integration of DNA, when HPV DNA is inserted into chromosomal DNA by covalent bonding, and replicates with the chromosomal DNA.

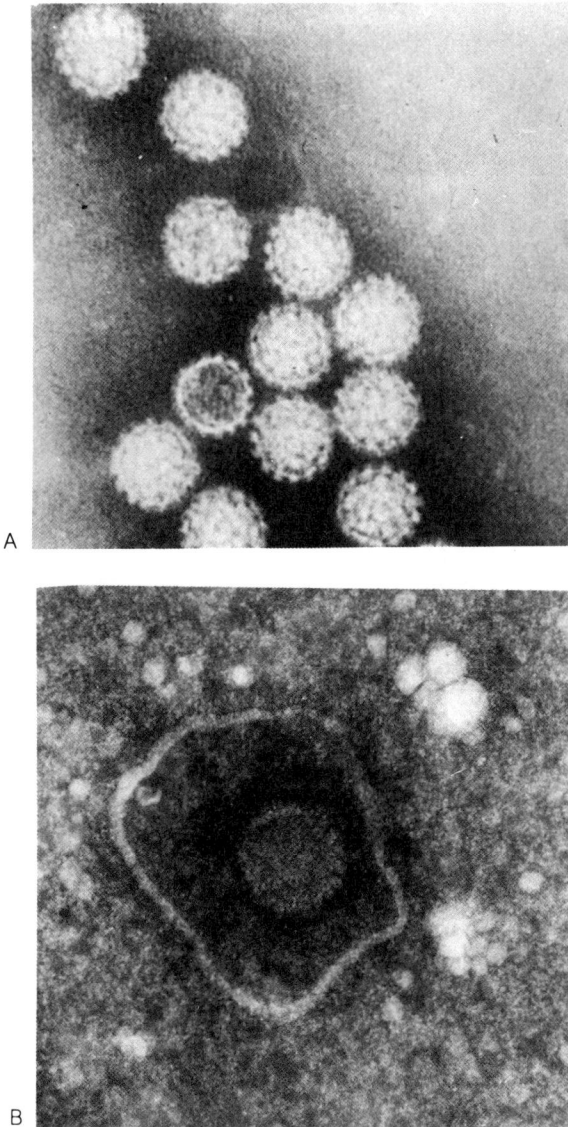

Fig. 4.1 Electromicrographs of (a) human papillomavirus type 6 (× 228 000) (courtesy of Dr J D Oriel); and (b) Herpes simplex virus (× 150 000). (Courtesy of Dr I L Chrystie)

HSV

HSV types I and II infect only humans but can be grown in many cell types in vitro and so much more is known of the replicative cycle and proteins produced. The viral DNA replicates and the capsid is assembled in the nucleus of the cell.

The envelope of the virus and the glycoproteins found inserted into the envelope are acquired as the virus buds through the nuclear membrane. The virus is transported from the nucleus to the outside of the cell via the Golgi apparatus and glycoproteins can also be inserted into the lipid envelope during this process.

HSV is usually isolated in the laboratory from vesicular fluid taken from lesions. The fluid has to be handled carefully and either put into viral transport media, refrigerated and taken to the laboratory as soon as possible, or, ideally, cells may be brought to the clinic and inoculated with the fluid immediately it has been taken.

DIAGNOSTIC TECHNIQUES

Serology: serum antibody measurements

HPV infections

At the moment there is no routine serological test for identification of serum antibodies to HPV types. This situation is due to the inability to produce infectious virus in cell cultures and so produce a ready supply of antigen for such tests. However, one report (Baird 1983) has used detergent-disrupted bovine papillomavirus particles to detect antibodies to papillomaviruses in serum from various individuals. Bovine papillomavirus particles were used as bovine warts are large and give a plentiful supply of virions. The virions were purified on a caesium chloride density gradient, disrupted with detergent and used as the antigen source to detect serum antibodies. Antibodies raised to these disrupted particles in experimental animals detect an antigen common to both human and animal papillomaviruses. This common antigen is a component of the virus capsid (protein coat), which is normally hidden in the assembled particle. Using this antigen source antibodies were found in 95%, 60% and 93% of patients with anogenital warts, cervical intra-epithelial neoplasia (CIN) and cervical cancer respectively, and in 6.6% of patients attending a genitourinary medicine clinic for other sexually transmitted diseases, but none was found in the control group which included children and adults without genital warts. These results are interesting, but need to be confirmed by other groups.

Herpesviruses

It is difficult to differentiate between antibodies in serum to HSV type I from those to HSV type II and this has been one of the criticisms of results showing an association between infection with HSV type II and carcinoma of the cervix. Firstly, over 80% of any population will have antibodies to HSV I and, secondly, there is extensive cross-reactivity between antigens of HSV I and II using polyclonal antibodies. The following two methods have been used to differentiate between HSV I and II serum antibodies (Vonka et al 1984):

1. Microneutralisation test, which detects differences in the ability of serum to neutralise each of the types. Since most people will have antibodies to type I their serum will neutralise HSV type I at higher dilutions than type II. Individuals with antibodies to HSV type II only will neutralise HSV II at greater dilutions than type I, while those with antibodies to both types will neutralise both viruses at similar dilutions. A ratio of the neutralisation titres (II/I) is calculated and from previous research (Rawls et al 1970) it has been shown that an index of II/I greater than 80 indicates infection with HSV type II. It must be emphasised that this is necessary because in any population over 80% of the population will have been infected with HSV type I and that there is considerable cross-reactivity between antigens of HSV I and II. This is not an absolute test and is open to subjective interpretations.

2. A radio-immunoassay or enzyme-linked immunosorbent assay (ELISA) test using as antigen-purified surface glycoprotein C (gC) has been developed by Vonka et al (1984). This antigen detects type specific antibodies but has not been widely used and so its usefulness remains to be assessed. There are other glycoproteins of HSV I and II which may also be type specific and one area of herpes research is to identify these compounds. Recent research suggests that the glycoprotein gG-2 (from HSV II) can differentiate between antibodies to type I and II (Lee et al 1985).

Immunochemical methods

This section deals with the detection of viral antigens, either in histological sections from biopsy material in the case of HPV infections or, in the case of HSV, in tissue culture cells infected with HSV isolated from a lesion.

HPV

As mentioned there have been difficulties in raising antibodies against HPV types, owing to the lack of antigen as a result of the small numbers of virions in infected tissue and because the virus cannot be replicated in cell culture.* However, at the moment an antibody against a common papillomavirus antigen is used to detect HPV antigen in lesions. This antibody is raised against disrupted bovine papillomavirus extracted from bovine warts. The antibody detects a common antigen of the papillomavirus group which is normally masked in the completely assembled virus particle.

The antibody can be used in two types of immunochemical staining techniques; the principle of the test is the same. The tissue to be investigated can either be formalin fixed or snap frozen in liquid nitrogen. Sections cut from snap frozen blocks can then be fixed in methanol at $-20°C$ or acetone at room temperature after cryostat sectioning.

The specific antipapillomavirus antibodies are allowed to interact with the sections, the sections washed and then stained with antispecies antibodies, which are tagged with a reagent which will visualise the specific antibody interactions. Antispecies antibodies are usually tagged with (a) a fluorescent dye, for example fluorescein isothiocyanate or rhodamine, (b) alkaline phosphatase or peroxidase. The latter two give the greater sensitivity and also make tissue definition much easier since fluorescent dyes are seen only against a dark background. Figure 4.2 shows a section from a cervical biopsy showing positively stained nuclei in the outer one-third of the epithelium stained by the alkaline phosphatase method. Note that the positive cells are in the peripheral layers of the epithelium and these cells are producing structural antigens

---

*Open reading frames (ORFs) of HPV are being cloned into bacterial expression vectors with the aim of producing HPV specific proteins and so raise type specific antibodies for detection of HPVs in diseased tissues. Open reading frames are areas of viral DNA that have a start signal for commencement of mRNA production and then somewhere along the DNA (downstream) a stop signal for termination of transcription. These areas can be predicted from the DNA sequence of the HPV genome.

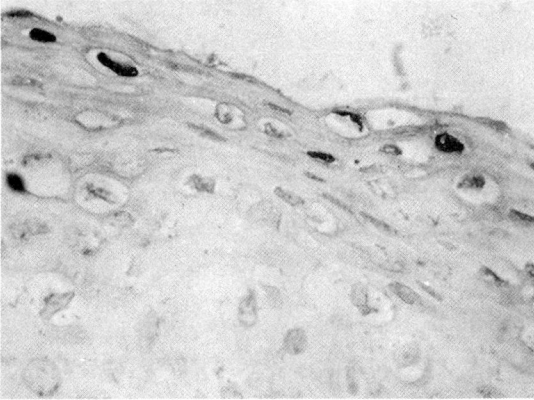

Fig. 4.2 A section from a biopsy reacted with the rabbit anti-papillomavirus antiserum, which detects the papillomavirus common antigen, and subsequently stained with antirabbit antibodies tagged with alkaline phosphatase. A pink/red colour develops using the appropriate enzyme substrate but the positively staining nuclei appear dark in this black and white plate. Note the positive cells are found in the outer part of the epithelium. (courtesy of Mr P G Walker)

and mature virus particles. The staining is confined to the nucleus.

The rate of detection of HPV antigens by this method in vulval and cervical condylomata acuminata and CIN lesions is variable between studies, but 30–50% of biopsies exhibit positive staining with the antibody against the common structural antigen. Few studies have looked at the antigen staining in intra-epithelial neoplasias of the vulva but our preliminary work (Drs D. Jenkins and S. K. Tay) and that of others (Braun et al 1983) suggest a similar pattern as at the cervix. In cervical intra-epithelial lesions there is a reduction in the percentage positive between CIN I, CIN II, CIN III and carcinoma in situ (CIS), with the complete absence of detectable antigen in the latter grade of lesion. This is due to the fact that mature particles are seen in the most differentiated cells of the epithelium; in CIS lesions there is complete disruption in polarity of the epithelium, and no differentiated cells are seen in the outer cell layers of the epithelium. Newer techniques will permit of DNA/DNA hybridisation studies (see below) on fixed tissue (Burns et al 1987, Collins et al 1987).

HSV

Herpes antigens can be detected directly in cells from lesions but it is more usual to grow the virus

and detect antigen in the cells by either of the methods mentioned above. Using monoclonal antibodies to glycoproteins such as gD, the isolated virus types can be differentiated. From such studies it is now clear that an increasing number of genital isolates are type I; in the UK nearly a third are so accounted for.

DNA–DNA Hybridisation

HPV

(a) Principle. Viral DNA can be detected in a piece of tissue using an identical or partially identical viral DNA which has been previously isolated and purified. This latter DNA, called the probe, is usually labelled with a radio-isotope before mixing with the tissue DNA. Since both DNAs are double stranded a denaturation step to produce single strands is carried out before mixing the two sets of DNA. A simple method of denaturation involves heating the DNA above its melting temperature (T_m), that is, that temperature at which the two strands separate, and depends, if environmental conditions are constant, on the deoxyguanosine + deoxycytidine triphosphate ratio (% G + C) of the DNA. The single strands are separated, and when the single-stranded probe is mixed with the single-stranded total DNA from the tissue and the temperature dropped to below the T_m of the DNA homologous single strands will re-anneal. If any DNA in the tissue is homologous to the probe it can be detected since the probe strand is radiolabelled. This is the principle of all DNA–DNA hybridisation experiments, but in practice certain steps are taken to simplify the method and allow visualisation of re-annealed DNA by autoradiography. As well as detecting HPV DNA in tissues this DNA hybridisation method is used to type new HPVs when isolated. HPV types, to be categorised as new, must have a genome with < 50% homology to other types isolated.

(b) Practice.

(i) Preparation of DNA from biopsy and electrophoresis. Total DNA is extracted from the biopsy by one of the standard techniques. The tissue is usually solubilised in a buffered solution containing a detergent (sodium dodecyl sulphate, SDS) and proteinase K. This latter component is present to inactivate DNAses which will degrade

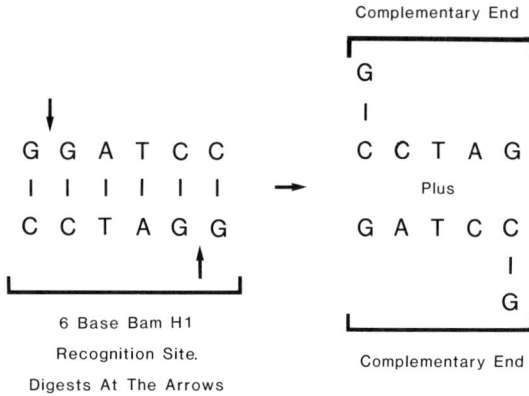

Fig. 4.3 The six base pair recognition site in DNA for the restriction endonuclease *Bam* H1. The enzyme cleaves the DNA at the positions of the arrows leaving two complementary ends.

DNA in the tissues when the various compartments in the cells are solubilised. The DNA when extracted carefully is very viscous due to the high molecular weight of cellular DNA. To make it easier to electrophorese the DNA is digested with restriction endonuclease enzymes, which recognise small specific sequences of nucleotides, usually four or six base pairs in length, and digest or break each DNA strand at this site (Fig. 4.3). Most of the restriction endonucleases produce protruding complementary or 'sticky-ends' at the site of breakage, which has the advantage that the piece of DNA can be joined to another fragment of DNA which is complementary due to digestion with the same enzyme. In this way DNA can be cloned into or joined to plasmid or phage DNA and replicated in bacterial cells to produce multiple copies of inserted DNA. This is a great advantage since papillomaviruses cannot be replicated in the conventional way and it is used to produce sufficient viral probe DNA to carry out many hybridisation experiments.

Some restriction endonuclease enzymes will digest different HPV types into different size bands. The DNA of HPVs is circular; digestion with an enzyme which has only one recognition site results in a linear-molecule-producing band, whereas on digestion with an enzyme with six sites then six bands are produced.

The digested DNA from the biopsy is then subjected to electrophoresis through an agarose horizontal gel, which will separate out the total DNA into various sized fragments with the small ones moving fast and the larger ones running more slowly (Fig. 4.4a). After the gel has been run, usually for 10–15 hours at low voltage, the DNA fragments are denatured by alkali treatment and then transferred to nitrocellulose paper by a process called Southern blotting (Southern 1975; Fig. 4.4b). The capillary flow of the buffer from the reservoir through the gel and up through the paper towels transfers the DNA through the thickness of the gel on to the nitrocellulose filter, where it is trapped. The result is that the nitrocellulose filter becomes a copy of what was on the gel and each band is transferred to the nitrocellulose in the same relationship to other bands as in the gel (Fig. 4.4c). To make sure the DNA is irreversibly stuck to the nitrocellulose the filter is baked at 80°C in a vacuum oven.

(ii) *Radiolabelling the DNA probe.* Searching for small amounts of viral DNA in the total DNA extracted needs probes which are labelled with a relatively high energy emitter at a high specific activity. This can be achieved using ^{32}P(phosphorus)-labelled triphosphates (nucleotide triphosphates ATP, GTP, CTP, TTP); by a process called nick translation (Rigby et al 1977) the labelled triphosphates can replace the unlabelled nucleotides in the DNA probe. This is carried out by using a DNAase enzyme to nick or cut one strand of the DNA and then using a DNA polymerase to add on radiolabelled triphosphates at the site of the nick (Fig. 4.5). This produces a uniformly labelled piece of DNA as the DNAse activity is random along the DNA molecule.

(iii) *Hybridisation.* Before hybridisation can be carried out the probe is denatured by immersion in boiling water for 5 minutes to separate strands. It is then added to the hybridisation solution, which is placed with the nitrocellulose filters in a plastic bag, and hybridisation is carried out over a period of 15 to 48 hours, depending on the concentration of the probe.

After this period the filters are washed to remove the radiolabelled probe not hybridised to DNA on the filter. Hybridisation can be carried out in stringent or non-stringent conditions. This is controlled by the salt concentration and temperature of hybridisation and stringent conditions are those which

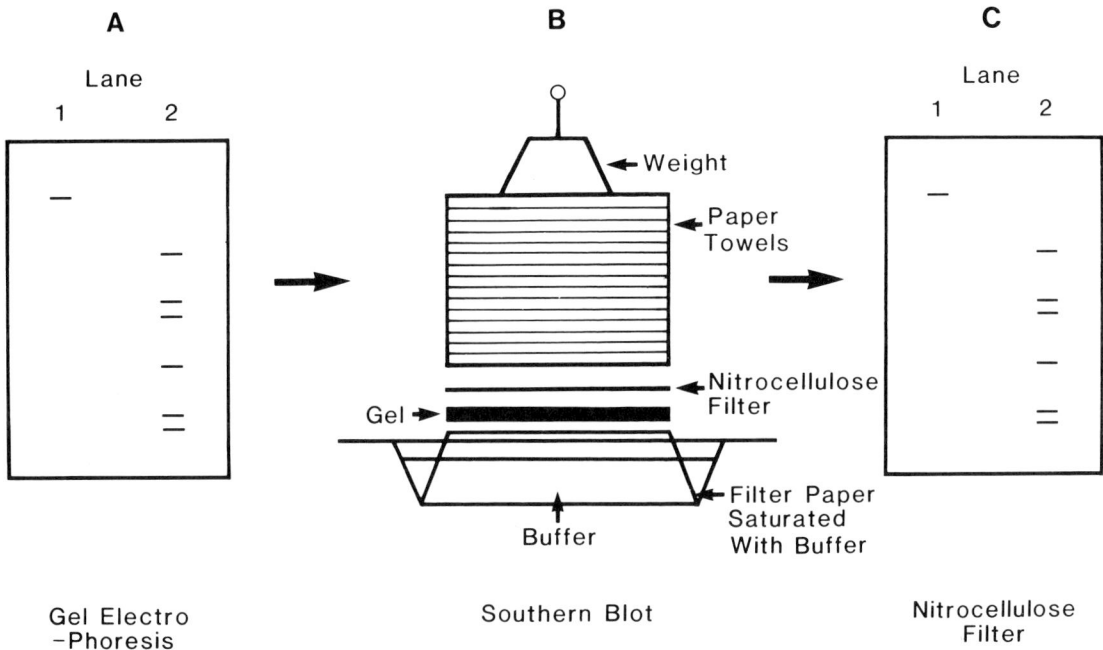

Fig. 4.4 Shows (a) The electrophoresis of biopsy DNA through an agarose gel. (b) The transfer of the DNA from the gel to nitrocellulose filters by the method of Southern (1975). (c) The resulting nitrocellulose filter. The filter can then be used for DNA–DNA hybridisation.

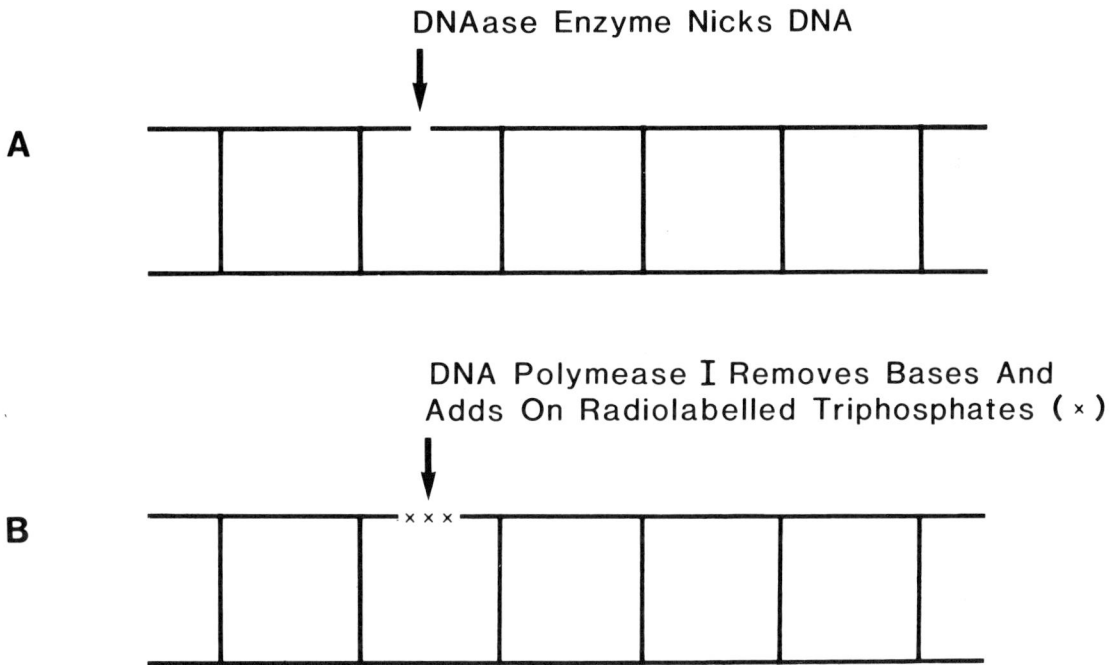

Fig. 4.5 The nick translation process: (a) the enzyme DNAase is used to 'nick' the DNA at random sites; (b) the DNA polymerase I enzyme will digest away triphosphates at the nick site and replace them with triphosphates added into the reaction mixture. If radiolabelled triphosphates are included then the DNA will be labelled accordingly.

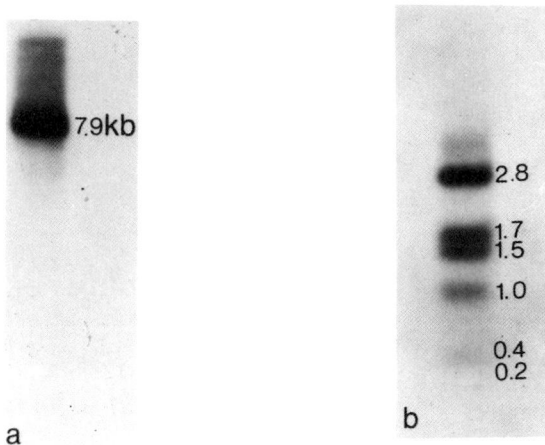

Fig. 4.6 Autoradiograph of HPV16 DNA sequences detected in a vulvar intra epithelial neoplasia, grade III lesion. The total extracted biopsy DNA was digested with the restriction endonuclease *Bam* H1 in (**a**) and *Pst* 1 in (**b**), run on an 0.8% agarose gel and then transferred to nitrocellulose paper by Southern blotting. The filter was hybridised with cloned HPV16 DNA, labelled with [^{32}P]CTP and TTP, at stringent conditions (T_m − 10°C). *Bam* H1 digests HPV16 DNA at one point giving a linear band of 7.9 kilobases (kb), while *Pst* 1 digests the DNA six times giving six bands from 2.8 kb down to 0.2 kb. The smallest band has not shown as bands of this size are inefficiently transferred by Southern blotting and because this was only an overnight exposure, so faint signals will not be easily seen.

allow only identical or almost identical (80% or greater homology) DNA sequences to be detected, while non-stringent conditions allow less closely related DNAs to be identified. If the salt concentration remains constant then the temperature controls stringency; under stringent conditions the hybridisation and wash are usually carried out at temperatures of 10–25°C below the melting temperature of DNA (T_m), whereas under non-stringent conditions the temperature would be 40°C below T_m. As a rough guide to how closely related the DNA detected is to the probe, for every degree below the T_m 1% mismatch is detected, so at

10°C below melting temperature one can detect DNA with 90% homology or greater. Once hybridisation and washing are complete the filter is exposed to X-ray film for a varying period of time to visualise the viral bands that were in the original biopsy material. Figure 4.6 shows the actual HPV16, which was diagrammatically presented in Figure 4.5c, detected in biopsy material. The figure is the developed X-ray and shows viral DNA after digestion by the restriction endonuclease enzymes *Bam* H1 and *Pst*1.

HSV

HSV types can be differentiated at the DNA level using the fact that restriction enzymes will digest type I and II DNA into different bands. The HSV isolated from a vesicular lesion is grown in tissue culture for 2–3 days with the addition of [^{3}H] thymidine, which is incorporated into DNA. The virus is purified from the culture and viral DNA extracted, digested with restriction enzymes and run on a polyacrylamide gel. The number of bands produced varies between HSV type I and II and the different patterns are obvious (Fig. 4.7). Some bands of type I isolates and type II isolates produced by restriction enzymes differ between isolates from different patients, but the overall pattern between type I and II is quite clear.

SUMMARY

Serological tests are the most convenient to carry out as a screening test, but unfortunately so far a type-specific test has not been developed for HPV infections. The testing of antibodies against HSV type I or II has been difficult, in part because of the cross-reactivity between many of the glycoproteins,

Fig. 4.7 An autoradiograph of HSV type 1 and type 2 DNA digested with the restriction enzyme *Kpn* I and run on a 0.6% polyacrylamide gel. The difference in the pattern of bands is obvious between the two viruses and can be used to differentiate between types. Other restriction endonucleases also show band pattern differences between the two HSV types (courtesy of Dr J C M MacNab)

but recently tests have been developed which claim to differentiate between the types. Further studies by several groups will elucidate if this early promise is well founded. At the moment HPV types are classified by DNA–DNA hybridisation, and HSV by growth in vitro followed by restriction endonuclease analysis, or by testing for type specific glycoproteins with monoclonal antibodies.

REFERENCES

Baird, P J 1983 Serological evidence for the association of papillomavirus and cervical neoplasias. Lancet ii: 17–18

Braun L, Farmer E R, Shah K V (1983) Immunoperoxidase localisation of papillomavirus antigen in cutaneous warts and Bowenoid Papulosis. Journal of Medical Virology 12: 187–193

Burns J, Graham A K, Frank C, Fleming K A, Evans M F, McGee JO'D 1987 Detection of low copy HPV DNA and mRNA in routine paraffin sections of cervix by non-isotopic in situ hybridisation. Journal of Clinical Pathology 40: 858–864

Collins J E, Jenkins D, McCance D 1987 The detection of HPV DNA sequences by in situ DNA/DNA hybridisation in CIN and invasive carcinoma: a retrospective study. Journal of Clinical Pathology (in press)

Lee F K, Coleman R M, Pereira L, Bailey P D, Tatsuno M, Nahmias A J 1985 Detection of herpes simplex virus type 2 specific antibody with glycoprotein G. Journal of Clinical Microbiology 22: 641–644

McCance D J, Singer, A 1985 The importance of HPV infections in the male and female genital tract and their relationship to cervical neoplasia. In: Peto R, zur Hausen H (eds) Origins of female genital cancer: virological and epidemiology aspects. Cold Spring Harbor, New York, Banbury Report 21: 311–319

Rawls W E, Iwamoto K, Adam E, Melnick J L 1970 Measurement of antibodies to herpes virus types 1 and 2 in human sera. Journal of Immunology 104: 599

Rigby P W S, Dieckman M, Rhodes C, Berg P 1977 Labelling deoxyribonucleic acids to high specific activity in vitro by nick translation with DNA polymerase I. Journal of Molecular Biology 113: 237–251

Southern EM 1975 Detection of specific sequences among DNA fragments separated by gel electrophoresis. Journal of Molecular Biology 98: 503–517

Vonka J, Kanka J, Hirsch I, Zavadova H, Kocmar M, Suchankova A, Rezacova D, Broucek J, Press M, Domorazkova E, Svoboda B, Havrankova A, Jelinek J 1984 Prospective study on the relationship between cervical neoplasia and herpes simplex type-2 virus. II Herpes simplex type-2 antibody presence in sera taken at enrolment. International Journal of Cancer 33: 61–66

5

Infective conditions of the vulva
J D Oriel

INTRODUCTION

Normal flora of the female genital tract

The normal skin harbours a large population of microorganisms. The common commensals are staphylococci (mainly *Staphylococcus epidermidis*) and diphtheroid bacilli; many other bacteria, and some fungi, may make a transient appearance. The microbial flora of the vulva and fore-arm were compared by Aly et al (1979). Microbial counts were higher on the vulva ($2.8 \times 10^6/cm^2$) than on the fore-arm ($6.4 \times 10^2/cm^2$). Coagulase negative staphylococci, diphtheroids and lactobacilli dominated the vulval flora, but streptococci, coliforms and yeasts were also noted. The skin of the perineum has a higher pH, temperature and humidity than the skin elsewhere on the body, and *Candida albicans* and *Staphylococcus aureus* are commonly present (Aly et al 1979, Noble 1981).

The vaginal fluid contains numerous bacteria. Lactobacilli, *S. epidermidis*, anaerobic streptococci and *Bacteroides* species usually predominate (Corbishley 1977). *Ureaplasma urealyticum* is often present as a commensal; *Mycoplasma hominis* is found in healthy women, but this organism may also be associated with bacterial vaginosis (see p. 105). Neither *Chlamydia trachomatis* nor viruses form part of the normal vaginal flora.

Glycogen is formed in the vaginal epithelium in response to oestrogens. Lactobacilli metabolise glycogen to form lactic acid; this is responsible for the low pH (about 4.5) of the healthy vagina which restricts the growth of many microorganisms (Cruikshank & Sharman 1939). Normally there is a complex flora of interacting microorganisms in the vagina (Corbishley 1977); the stability of this system may be disturbed by events such as pregnancy, diabetes mellitus or the introduction of a pathogen into the lower genital tract.

Sources of infection

In women, infection of the lower genital tract is usually exogenous. Some vulval infections, particularly those caused by fungi or pyogenic cocci, may be transferred to the area by the hands, by fomites, or through immersion in contaminated water. The proximity of the vulva to the anus may allow colonisation of the introitus by coliforms (Fair et al 1970), which may then be inoculated into the urethra and bladder by sexual intercourse and cause urinary tract infection. Organisms such as *Candida* species and threadworms may also reach the vulva and vagina from the anus.

The majority of pathogens reach the lower genital tract of women through sexual contact, either genital to genital (with or without intercourse) or mouth to genital. Bacterial infections such as gonorrhoea, syphilis, chancroid and chlamydial infection, viral infections such as genital warts and genital herpes, and protozoal infections such as trichomoniasis are all introduced in this way. Other infections, for example a recurrent attack of genital herpes, or a further episode of candidosis, may be provoked or aggravated by intercourse.

Host defences

Role of normal flora

In vitro some vaginal commensals, for example lactobacilli and *C. albicans*, inhibit the growth of genital pathogens such as *N. gonorrhoeae* (Hipp et al 1974, Kaye & Levinson 1977), but whether this is of any clinical importance is not known.

Phagocytosis

Polymorphonuclear leucocytes, monocytes and macrophages play an important part in the defence of epithelia. Phagocytosis involving the attachment of microorganisms to the phagocyte and their subsequent ingestion and death has been studied for *N. gonorrhoeae*, *C. trachomatis* and *Trichomonas vaginalis* (Dilworth et al 1975, Wyrick & Brownridge 1978, Rein et al 1980). Little is known about the action of phagocytes on other pathogens.

Humoral immunity

Mucosal antibodies can prevent bacterial attachment, enhance phagocytosis and inactivate viruses. Their action has been reviewed by McNabb & Tomasi (1981). Circulating antibodies to specific microorganisms can be demonstrated in the majority of genital infections but, with the exception of antitreponemal antibodies, there is little evidence that they have any protective effect. Repeated attacks of gonorrhoea, chlamydial infection, genital herpes and trichomoniasis occur despite high titres of circulating antibodies.

Cell-mediated immunity

Patients who have had genital infection by *N. gonorrhoeae*, *T. pallidum*, *C. trachomatis*, Herpes simplex virus and other pathogens show cellular immune responses to specific antigens, but these are not protective against recurrent infection (Kearns et al 1973). In the acquired immune deficiency syndrome (AIDS), the deficient cellular immunity caused by the human immunodeficiency virus (HIV), previously known as the human T cell lymphoma virus III (HTLV III), may result in genital infections, for example by herpes simplex virus and papillomaviruses, of great severity (Siegel et al 1981). Pregnancy is associated with reduced cellular immunity.

Reaction to seminal fluid may be important (p. 63).

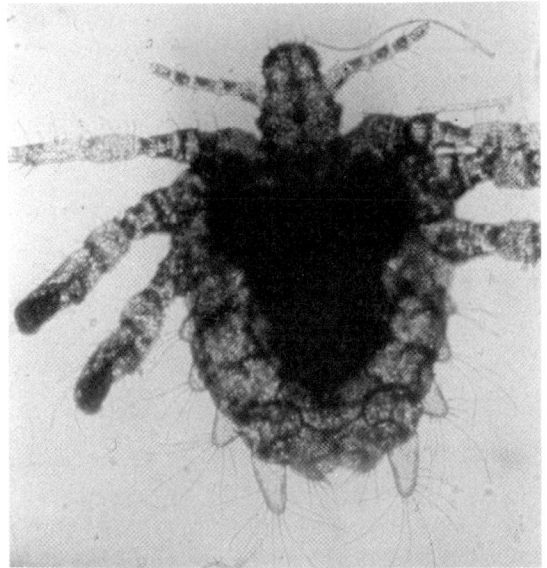

Fig. 5.1 *Phthirus pubis.*

INFECTION WITH ECTOPARASITES

Pediculosis

Phthirus pubis, the crab louse, is an insect of the order Anoplura, and occupies a different genus from *Pediculus humanus* with its two forms, the head and body louse. *P. pubis* is a wingless insect 1–2 mm long, grey in colour and dorsoventrally flattened. The last two pairs of its six legs are modified for grasping hairs (Fig. 5.1). After mating, the female lays eggs which are cemented to hairs near their roots, forming nits. Hatching occurs after 7 days, and the louse reaches maturity 2 weeks later. Adult life expectancy is 3–4 weeks. Crab lice feed almost continuously on human blood, and cannot survive for more than 24 hours away from their host (Nuttall 1918).

Epidemiology

Infection occurs almost invariably through sexual contact. The prevalence of pediculosis parallels that of other sexually transmitted diseases (STDs). In the UK it is reportable from STD clinics, and the number of new cases in women rose from 984 in 1971 to 2748 in 1981 (Chief Medical Officer 1973, 1984). Below the age of 19 years, women are more

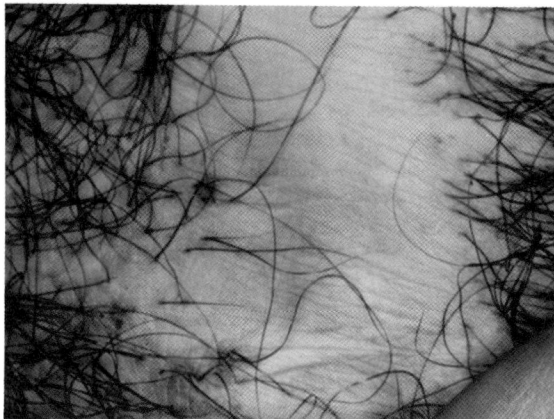

Fig. 5.2 Pediculosis pubis: both pediculi and nits are visible.

often affected than men, but after this age the ratio is reversed (Fisher & Morton 1970). Other STDs are often present in these patients. There has sometimes been speculation that *P. pubis* may act as a vector for other infections, but there is no evidence that this happens.

Clinical features

The incubation period of pediculosis pubis is about 30 days (Fisher & Morton 1970). The commonest symptom is irritation, which is possibly due to sensitisation (Epstein & Orkin 1977); some patients present because they have seen the insects moving, and in others the infection is symptomless (Ackerman 1968). The areas most affected are pubic, perianal and perineal, but occasionally the insects are seen on body or axillary hair or on the eyebrows or eyelashes. Nits are commonly present; their distance from the skin surface indicates the duration of the infection (Fig. 5.2). The scalp is only rarely affected (Elgart & Higdon 1973).

Maculae ceruleae are blue-grey macules on the trunk and thighs which quickly fade; they may be caused by altered blood pigments, or be a product from the louse's salivary glands. Pediculosis pubis may be complicated by pyodermic infection caused by scratching, particularly in people with poor personal hygiene.

Treatment

Since *P. pubis* is sexually transmitted, a search for associated infections should be made before treat-

ment is started: as a minimum, culture for *N. gonorrhoeae* and serological tests for syphilis should be performed. Therapy is quite straightforward, and there is no evidence that *P. pubis* has developed resistance to any of the commonly used pesticides (Gratz 1977). Shaving of the pubic or body hair is unnecessary. After a bath or shower, the patient applies 0.5% malathion lotion to all hairy areas except the scalp. The application is washed off after 24 hours, and personal and bed linen are then changed; discarded items are washed at a temperature of at least 50°C. A second application is necessary only for the heaviest infestations. Patients should be warned that egg cases may remain attached to the hairs for a week or two after therapy, but that their presence does not mean treatment failure. Gammabenzene hexachloride is no longer recommended for the treatment of pediculosis. All sexual contacts of infected women should receive identical treatment as soon as possible.

Scabies

Sarcoptes scabiei is an arachnid of the order Acarina (Johnson & Mellanby 1972). Infection with this parasite causes a widespread and intensely itchy skin eruption. The transmission of scabies requires close and fairly prolonged contact between individuals, and in adults it is regarded as a disease which is predominantly sexually transmitted (Schroeter 1977). Scabies is commonest in the second and third decades of life and, like other STDs, is more often seen in men than in women.

In men with scabies, genital lesions are very common. Surprisingly, vulval scabetic lesions have not been described. According to Mellanby (1972), the distribution of *S. scabiei* in women has not been thoroughly studied.

INFECTION WITH NEMATODES, TAPEWORMS AND FLUKES

Oxyuriasis

Infection with *Enterobius vermicularis* (the threadworm) is common, particularly in children, throughout the world. The worms live in the large

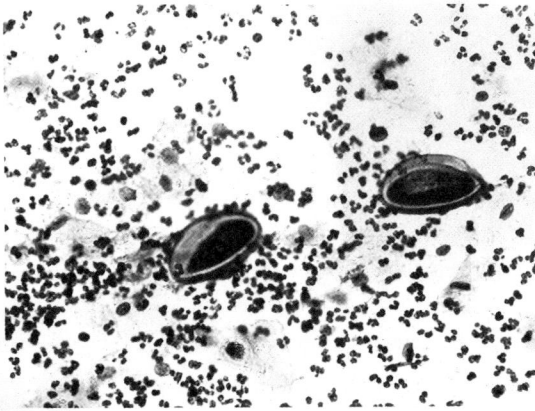

Fig. 5.3 Ova of *Enterobius vermicularis* in cervical smear. (By courtesy of C M Ridley 1975 The Vulva. Major Problems in Dermatology 5. Lloyd Luke)

bowel, and lay eggs on the peri-anal and perineal skin during the night. These ova may then be shed and ingested by another person, or the larvae may hatch and re-enter the anal canal. Pruritus ani, sometimes severe, is a common symptom of infection. Vulval irritation and vulvovaginitis may also occur, and the worms are sometimes found in the vagina (Kacker 1973) (Fig. 5.3).

Threadworms are 3–12 mm long, and may be seen around the anus or between the labia. Identification of the ova is made by applying adhesive tape, conveniently mounted on a slide, to the perineum, preferably in the morning before washing; the eggs adhere to the tape and can be identified by microscopy.

Anthelmintics are relatively ineffective in oxyuriasis, and general measures to prevent self reinfection are important. The hands should be thoroughly washed and the nails scrubbed before meals and after urination and defaecation. If possible, a bath or shower should be taken in the morning to wash off ova deposited during the night. Piperazine salts are the best-known anthelmintics, and should be given to all family members. The dosage for piperazine hydrate is: up to 2 years of age, 50–75 mg/kg; 2–4 years, 750 mg; 5–12 years, 1.5 g; children over 12 years and adults, 2 g. These doses are given daily for 7 days.

Other parasitic worms, *Ascaris lumbricoides* (roundworm) and *Trichuris trichuria* have occasionally been found in the vagina in children (Gardner and Kaufman, 1981).

Filariasis

Wucheria bancrofti and *Brugia malayi* are filarial worms. *B. malayi* is confined to Asia, India and the Pacific islands. The infection is transmitted by mosquitoes: microfilarial in human blood are ingested, and the larvae inoculated into another person. Over a period of years, these develop and reproduce in lymphatic vessels. The subsequent inflammation, if it occurs in inguinal glands, gives rise to genital lymphoedema and elephantiasis.

Filariasis affecting the vulva is usually due to *W. bancrofti*. By the time lymphoedema appears, there is no evidence of active infection. Both sides of the vulva are affected, although the swelling is often greater on one side. The pathological appearances of affected lymph nodes are usually non-specific, but sometimes histology shows parts of dead worms.

The differential diagnosis is from other causes of lymphatic obstruction with vulval swelling: lymphogranuloma venereum, carcinoma, tuberculosis, and following surgery. Diethylcarbamazine is an effective filaricide. Destruction of the microfilaria often induces an allergic response owing to the release of antigen; it is usual to begin treatment with a dose of 1 mg/kg per day, increasing over 3 days to 6 mg/kg per day in divided doses, and this is continued for 3 weeks. Surgical treatment of the elephantiasis may be needed (Lawson 1967).

Onchocerca volvulus is a filarial worm which is endemic in many tropical and subtropical areas. It is transmitted by flies. On the non-genital skin, onchocerciasis causes intensely itchy lichenified eruptions, but the vulva is not affected. The parasite may sometimes be seen in vaginal cytology smears (de Borges 1971) (Fig. 5.4). Treatment is with diethylcarbamazine.

Echinococcosis (hydatid disease)

Echinococcus granularis and *E. multilocularis* are tapeworms which live in the intestines of dogs and other animals. Ova swallowed by humans develop into larvae which enter the blood stream and are carried to distant sites, where hydatid cysts develop. Hydatid cysts of the vulva are rare, but have been described (Anagnostidis 1935, Ricci 1945). They form painless firm or soft subcutaneous swellings; treatment is surgical.

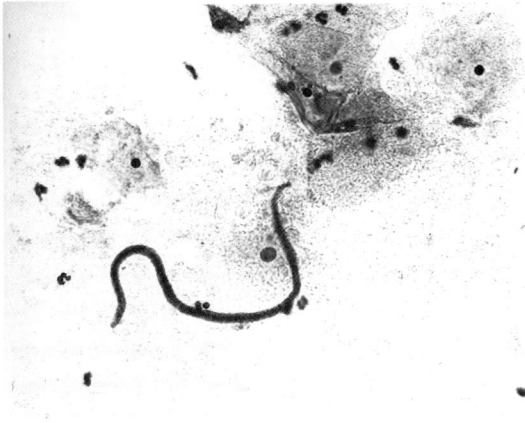

Fig. 5.4 Filarial worm in cervical smear. (By courtesy of C M Ridley 1975 The Vulva. Major problems in dermatology 5. Lloyd Luke)

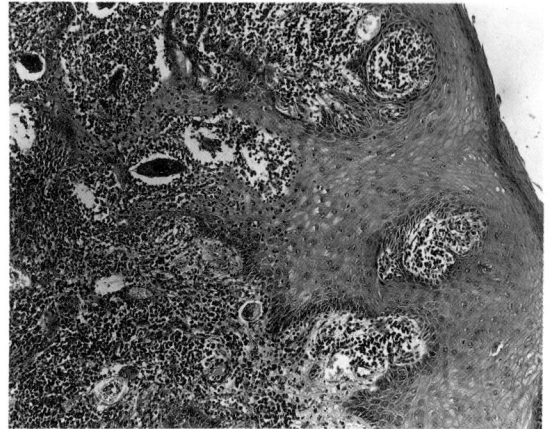

Fig. 5.5 Ova of schistosomiasis ($\times$ 25). (By courtesy of P McKee and the Editor of Clinical and Experimental Dermatology)

Schistosomiasis (bilharzia)

Aetiology

Three main species of the genus *Schistosoma* affect humans: *S. mansoni* in Africa, the Caribbean and South America, *S. japonicum* in the Far East, and *S. haematobium* in Africa and the Middle East. The life cycle is similar for all species, but the intermediate snail host is specific for each. The organisms in the cercarial stage enter the bloodstream via the skin during swimming or wading. The mature stage of male and female parasites is reached in the portal venous system. After copulation, the females migrate to the pelvic venous plexus, *S. mansoni* and *S. japonicum* to the mesenteric, and *S. haematobium* to the vesical plexus. Eggs are laid and penetrate the vessels, reaching surrounding tissues and eventually the skin; the clinical and pathological effects are due to immune reactions to these ova. Some ova are excreted via the urine or faeces and hatch miracidia, which are ingested by the snail host, thus completing the cycle.

Clinical features

Involvement of the female genital tract is usually due to *S. haematobium*, and sometimes to *S. mansoni*. Vulval lesions occur mainly before puberty. They have been described by Charlewood et al (1949) and Boulle & Notelovitz (1964). Recently, McKee et al (1983) have described a series of 16 cases. The disease presents as a chronic granulomatous reaction affecting the labia majora first, and other parts of the vulva later (Fig. 5.5). Lesions resembling condylomata acuminata are seen most often (McKee et al 1983); the masses may coalesce, and sometimes ulcerate. The disease is chronic, and scarring and calcification may occur in fully developed lesions.

Diagnosis

This depends on identification of the ova. The histology of active lesions shows intense inflammation centred on viable miracidia and degenerating forms, and granulomas and numerous eosinophils are present (McKee et al 1983). Ova may also be found in the urine, faeces and vaginal discharge. Biopsy is probably the best procedure for the diagnosis of vulval schistosomiasis; Berry (1971) has described the use of gynaecological cytology for the diagnosis of ulcerative lesions.

The differential diagnosis is from other chronic infective conditions, including condylomata acuminata, lymphogranuloma venereum and amoebiasis, and from carcinoma.

Treatment

Praziquantel is effective against all human schistosomes. A single oral dose of 40 mg/kg is given.

INFECTION WITH PROTOZOA

Trichomoniasis

T. vaginalis is a common human parasite which colonises the lower urogenital tract in men and women. In women it is recovered from the vagina, urethra and bladder, and from accessory ducts such as those of Skene's and Bartholin's glands. Trichomoniasis usually causes symptoms, but can be symptomless.

The organism

T. vaginalis is a motile flagellated protozoan. It is 10 μm × 7 μm in size; organisms from patients with acute symptomatic infections may be smaller than those from patients with silent infections. They have four anterior flagellae, and a lateral undulating membrane. There is a single oval nucleus near the anterior end of the cell, and an axostyle runs through the centre of the organism and protrudes at its posterior end. *T. vaginalis* multiplies by binary fission, and does not form cysts (Honigberg 1978) (Fig. 5.6).

Trichomonads can ingest small particles by phagocytosis, and their nutrition depends on this property. They can also ingest bacteria, which are usually killed within a few hours. It has been claimed that *N. gonorrhoeae* can persist within *T. vaginalis* for long period of time, and thus be protected from the action of gonococcocidal antibiotics (Ovcinnikov et al 1975), but this phenomenon, if it exists, does not seem to cause therapeutic problems in clinical practice.

T. vaginalis grows best under moderately anaerobic conditions. It can easily be cultured in nutrient media with added antimicrobials to suppress the growth of bacteria and yeasts, such as Feinberg–Whittington's or Dimond's media.

Epidemiology

The prevalence of trichomoniasis is variable. In the USA the reported values range from 5% or less in healthy women to 33% in women attending STD clinics (Naguib et al 1966, Sparks et al 1975, Fouts & Kraus 1980). There is no doubt that it is sexually transmissible. Up to 60% of male sex partners of

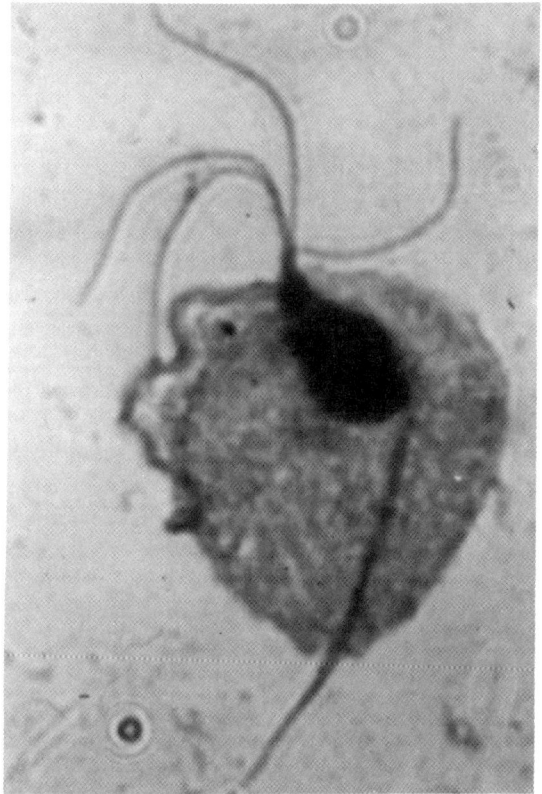

Fig. 5.6 *Trichomonas vaginalis.*

women with trichomoniasis harbour the parasites themselves (Catterall 1977), and many cases of recurrent trichomoniasis can be cured by simultaneous treatment of both partners with antitrichomonal drugs (Lvng & Christensen 1981). The inoculation of *T. vaginalis* into the normal vagina is followed by acute trichomonal vaginitis (Asami & Nakamura 1955). It has been suggested that accidental infection is possible from fomites or in swimming baths, but if this does happen it is infrequent.

Concurrent infection with *T. vaginalis* and other microbes, notably *N. gonorrhoeae*, is common. Gonorrhoea has been reported in 30–46% of women with trichomoniasis (Wisdom & Dunlop 1965, Eriksson & Wanger 1975, Fouts & Kraus 1980), but there is no evidence of any specific association between the two diseases. Several investigators have reported that trichomoniasis is commoner in black than in white women, but this difference may be due to socioeconomic rather than racial factors (Gardner & Kaufman 1981).

Clinical features

The incubation period of trichomoniasis appears to be between 4 and 28 days (Catterall 1972). The clinical picture in women is variable. The classic description is of an acute vulvovaginitis with a frothy malodorous purulent discharge; in severe infections there may be punctate haemorrhages on the ectocervix ('strawberry cervix'). The patient complains of vulval irritation and soreness, and vaginal discharge; these symptoms are often worse during or immediately after menstruation. Recent work indicates that these symptoms and signs are not specifically associated with trichomoniasis (Fouts & Kraus 1980); an aetiological diagnosis of the cause of vulvovaginitis based only on clinical appearances is often wrong (Oriel et al 1972), and laboratory investigation is essential. Between 10 and 50% of women with trichomoniasis are symptomless, and in 15% there is no evidence of vulvovaginitis (Wisdom & Dunlop 1965, Honigsberg 1978, Fouts & Kraus 1980). Although the vagina is almost invariably infected, the urethra and Skene's glands are also colonised in 90% of cases (Whittington 1957). In a small number of women trichomonads can be recovered from the endocervix. Re-infection of the vagina from these other sites accounted for many treatment failures before the advent of the nitroimidazoles. There are no local complications of trichomoniasis, and there is no convincing evidence of any systemic effects. Untreated, the infection runs a prolonged course of months or even years.

Female infants born to women with trichomoniasis can acquire the infection during delivery, although the risk is low (Robinson & Halifax 1961, Bramley 1976). The organisms disappear from the vagina in about 6 weeks, when the influence of maternal oestrogens has waned. McLaren et al (1983) have suggested that the organisms may, rarely, cause neonatal pneumonia.

Diagnosis

The simplest method is microscopy of a drop of vaginal fluid mixed with saline on a slide. Darkfield, phase contrast and bright-field illumination can all be used. At magnification × 400 the irregular jerky movements of the organisms can be seen; higher powers can be used for identifying the flagellae and undulating membrane. It is important that all glassware used is warm and clean and that the preparation is examined as soon as possible, as the organisms rapidly become immobile under adverse conditions.

Most workers believe that culture is more sensitive than direct microscopy for the diagnosis of trichomoniasis. Fouts & Kraus (1980) found that wet mount examination had only half the sensitivity of culture. Others have found much smaller differences in the results obtained with the two methods (Whittington 1957), and no doubt these depend on the culture media used and the skill and experience of the microscopist.

Trichomonads can be identified in smears stained by Giemsa, Papanicolaou, acridine orange and other techniques. During the Papanicolaou staining process the organisms usually lose their flagellae and appear as grey-blue pear-shaped cells with intracytoplasmic granules and small dark grey nuclei (Grubb 1977). The sensitivity of these staining techniques is disputed; results between 44 and 100% of those obtained with other methods have been reported (Hess 1969, Thin et al 1969, Fouts & Kraus 1980). The specificity of staining methods is less than those of microscopy or culture (Perl 1972).

Treatment

The treatment of trichomoniasis was revolutionised by the introduction of the nitroimidazoles, which have now been in general use for a quarter of a century. The best known member of the group is metronidazole, but nimorazole and timidazole are also widely used. There is no evidence that any one member of the group is superior to the others (British Journal of Venereal Diseases 1978). Several treatment schedules have been described. Metronidazole 200 mg three times a day for 7 days was used for many years, but a single oral dose of 2.0 g gives equally good results (Hager et al 1980).

It is usual to treat the male partners of women with trichomoniasis; recurrences are commoner if this is not done (Gardner & Dukes 1955). Single-dose metronidazole regimens have not been thoroughly evaluated in men.

Metronidazole is not recommended during the

first 3 months of pregnancy, but it may safely be given after this (Rodin & Hass 1966). In early pregnancy, there is no alternative to local therapy, although this is not very successful. The best choice is probably a 6-day course of clotrimazole pessaries 100 mg daily, which cures between 61 and 81% of women with trichomoniasis (Legal 1974, Lohmeyer 1974). Metronidazole is not contraindicated in a breastfeeding patient but may affect the taste of the milk.

Metronidazole has an antabuse-like action: alcohol during therapy may induce vomiting and should therefore be avoided. Overgrowth of vaginal yeasts may occur in some patients after a 7-day course of treatment (Beveridge 1962, Hager et al 1980); this is less likely to occur after single-dose therapy. There has been concern about the possible oncogenicity of metronidazole. This arose because the lifetime administration of metronidazole increased the frequency of some naturally occurring tumours in rodents (Rustia & Shubik 1972). However, there is no evidence of any increase in malignant tumours in populations treated with metronidazole (Beard et al 1979), and the risk to an individual woman treated with short term metronidazole must be extremely small.

Treatment failure. Metronidazole therapy is successful in about 90% of women with trichomoniasis. Re-isolation of *T. vaginalis* may be due to re-infection when the male partner has not been treated, but may also be due to poor compliance with multiple-dose therapy, inadequate tissue levels, or to trichomonal resistance. In vitro, it has been shown that some anaerobic organisms, themselves resistant to nitroimidazoles, can inactivate the drugs (Honigberg 1978). Whether this phenomenon also occurs under clinical conditions is uncertain. Resistance of *T. vaginalis* to imidazoles is believed to be uncommon (Meingassner et al, 1978), but it can certainly occur (Thurner & Meingassner et al 1978). It can sometimes be easier to detect resistance if the organisms are cultivated aerobically rather than anaerobically.

When standard courses of treatment have failed and re-infection has as far as possible been excluded it is usual to treat women with relapsing trichomoniasis with higher dosage of metronidazole, for example, 400 mg three times daily for 7–10 days, although this higher dosage may induce vomiting.

Leishmaniasis

Aetiology

Cutaneous leishmaniasis, American mucocutaneous leishmaniasis and visceral leishmaniasis (kala-azar) are all caused by morphologically identical flagellate protozoa; the classification of *Leishmania* associated with different diseases depends on serological, biochemical and cultural features of the organisms, and is not entirely satisfactory (Bray 1974). Genital involvement is commoner in cutaneous leishmaniasis than in the American mucocutaneous variety (Harman 1986). Patients successfully treated for kala-azar with antimony compounds may develop cutaneous lesions called leishmanoids, and vulval leishmaniasis apparently due to sexual transmission of *Leishmania* from these lesions has been described (Symmers 1960).

Epidemiology

Cutaneous leishmaniasis is endemic in countries bordering the eastern Mediterranean, Asia Minor and India, and American mucocutaneous leishmaniasis in virtually every country in Central and South America. Kala-azar occurs in parts of all continents except Australia. Transmission of all these diseases is by sandflies, and there is a reservoir of infection in alternative mammalian hosts.

Clinical features

The incubation period of cutaneous leishmaniasis is between 2 weeks and several months (Marsden 1979). Dissemination of *L. tropica* after inoculation is followed by the appearance of skin lesions which can affect the genitals, although the face and extremities are more commonly involved. Nodular, ulcerative and lupoid forms are described (Feinstein 1978).

Diagnosis

The vulval lesions of leishmaniasis must be distinguished from those of syphilis, pyogenic granuloma and donovanosis as well as from malignant tumours. The diagnosis can be confirmed by identifying the parasites as Leishman–Donovan bodies in smears or tissue sections. *L. tropica* can be cultured in special media, and a leishmanin intradermal test, using an *L. tropica* antigen, becomes positive in the majority of patients.

Treatment

Cutaneous leishmaniasis may heal spontaneously, but if the skin lesions are extensive systemic antimony preparations are usually given. The drug of choice is sodium stilbogluconate; a dose equivalent to 600 mg of pentavalent antimony is given daily by intravenous or intramuscular injection for 10 days. There is no general agreement as to the efficacy of various other local and systemic treatments.

Amoebiasis

Aetiology

Entamoeba histolytica exists in two forms, the motile trophozoite and the cyst. The trophozoite is the pathogenic form, living in the lumen and/or walls of the colon. When diarrhoea occurs, motile trophozoites can be identified in the faeces. In the absence of diarrhoea *E. histolytica* usually forms cysts, which are highly resistant to environmental changes and can be transmitted either directly through oral–anal contact or via flies, food and water.

Epidemiology

Infection with *E. histolytica* is worldwide, being particularly common in tropical and subtropical countries where standards of hygiene are low (Krogstad et al 1978). Cases of amoebic dysentery are usually sporadic, but epidemics, usually waterborne, have occurred.

The frequency with which genital lesions occur in patients with amoebiasis is uncertain, but they are regarded as an unusual complication. Cohen (1973) found that only about 100 cases had been described up to 1971, and in most of these the cervix was affected. Majmudar et al (1976) reported a case of clitoral amoebiasis.

Clinical features

Most lesions begin as cutaneous abscesses which rupture and form painful serpiginous ulcers with a sloughing base, or they present as wart-like lesions. The perineum, vulva and cervix may be affected, and local glands are usually also involved (Gogoi 1969). Intestinal amoebiasis is usually present, causing diarrhoea and sometimes liver abscesses (El Zawahry & El Komy 1973). The vulval and perineal lesions are usually due to a direct extension of intestinal disease, but some are believed to arise through sexual inoculation of the organisms.

Diagnosis

Vulval and perineal amoebiasis must be distinguished from donovanosis, lymphogranuloma venereum, deep mycosis and early syphilis. The diagnosis may be established by identifying motile amoebae in scrapings from the ulcers or from the cervix. Histologically there is an inflammatory reaction, and *E. histolytica* may be seen as a small round eosinophilic body. Trophozoites or cysts may be found in fresh stool specimens.

Treatment

Metronidazole is very effective in cutaneous amoebiasis, and is given in a dosage of 800 mg three times a day for 5 days. Emetine preparations are now rarely used. For chronic infections in which cysts rather than trophozoites are present in the faeces, diloxanide furonate, 500 mg three times a day for 10 days, is the drug of choice.

MYCOTIC INFECTIONS

Vulvovaginal yeast infection

Aetiology

Yeasts may be defined as fungi whose predominant morphological form is unicellular (Lodder 1970). The genera which usually infect the vulva and vagina are *Candida* and *Torulopsis*: although both are yeasts, only *Candida* is able to produce hyphae in culture. The commonest genital yeast is *C. albicans*; other *Candida* species are uncommon. *Torulopsis glabrata* is responsible for a few infections.

All the pathogenic *Candida* and *Torulopsis* species multiply by budding from yeast cells (blastospores). *C. albicans* can form hyphae, which arise by

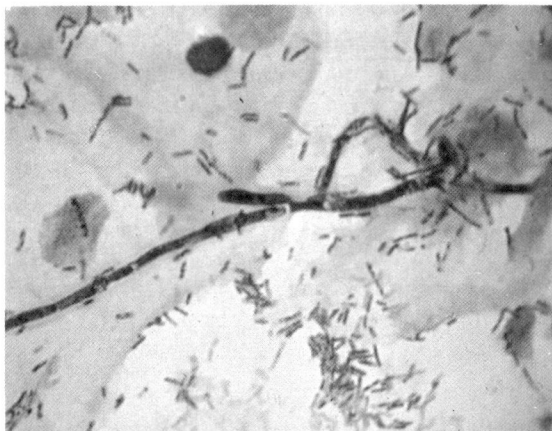

Fig. 5.7 Candidal hyphae.

germination of spores ('germ tubes') or as branches from existing hyphae. A mycelium is an entire fungal aggregate, including a hypha with all its branches. Thus under the microscope *C. albicans* can appear as ovoid budding yeasts, hyphae (Fig. 5.7), and sometimes as refractile chlamydospores; the predominant form in any culture depends on the nature of the growth medium. *T. glabrata* occurs only as blastospores (Odds 1979). Odds et al (1983) have described different strains of *C. albicans* on the basis of nine biochemical tests; the various strains did not appear to differ significantly in terms of clinical behaviour.

Ecology and epidemiology

The skin, mouth, digestive tract and vagina all have an endogenous yeast flora, and candidoses arise when an overgrowth of this flora occurs. *C. albicans* is recovered from the mouth or faeces of up to 20% of unselected women, but in some groups the isolation rate is much higher—for example, *C. albicans* has been recovered from nearly 50% of women attending STD clinics (Rohatiner 1966, Hilton & Warnock 1975, Odds 1979). The isolation rate from the vagina of 'normal' women—that is, those not pregnant or taking oral contraceptives, and free from vaginitis—is under 15% (Lapan 1970). Odds (1979) has calculated the mean isolation rates for *C. albicans* in women with and without vaginitis as 29% and 21% respectively. Vaginal

yeasts are most prevalent in women of childbearing age (Anyon et al 1971).

Genital yeasts are sexually transmissible. Men whose sex partners are colonised are four times more likely to yield yeasts from the penis than those with uninfected partners (Davidson 1977). Oriel et al (1972) found mycotic balanoposthitis in 10% of male partners of women with vaginal candidosis. Davidson (1977) recovered yeasts from 80% of female partners of infected men but from only 32% of partners of uninfected men. Vaginal yeast infection can occur either through spread of the organisms from the anus or through sexual transmission, but it is unlikely that the latter is of major epidemiological importance (Thin et al 1977).

Neonatal candidosis is much commoner in babies born to women with vaginal candidosis than in babies born to uninfected mothers (Hurley & de Louvois 1979).

Pathogenesis of candidosis

Predisposing factors. In 'normal' women, colonisation of the vagina by yeasts is a stable equilibrium between host and parasite. If this equilibrium is disturbed, clinical disease (candidosis) may develop. It has been said: '*Candida albicans* is a better clinician, and can discover abnormalities in persons much earlier in the course of the development of these abnormalities, than we can with our chemical tests' (Odds 1979). Pregnancy, antimicrobial therapy, oral contraception, diabetes mellitus and any cause of depressed cell-mediated immunity are all common predisposing factors for vaginal candidosis.

Colonisation of the vagina by yeasts is greater in pregnant than in non-pregnant women, and symptomatic candidosis may develop in up to 55% of women during the third trimester (Hopsu-Harvu et al, 1980). In pregnancy, the margin between simple colonisation by yeasts and clinical disease appears to be narrow. Carroll et al (1973) found that 86% of pregnant women who yielded *C. albicans* from the vagina showed clinical evidence of vulvovaginitis. Why pregnancy should predispose to vaginal candidosis is uncertain. It has been suggested that yeasts may overgrow because of increased glycogen in the vaginal epithelium during pregnancy (Cruickshank 1934), but lowered cell-mediated immunity to

C. albicans may be responsible (Brunham et al 1983).

The prevalence of yeasts in the vagina is increased by the administration of broad spectrum antibiotics (Winner & Hurley 1964), and symptomatic vulvovaginitis may follow. Although an effect of these agents on the vaginal flora is postulated as the cause, its exact nature has not been determined. Metronidazole also predisposes to genital yeast infection (Beveridge 1962).

Vaginal colonisation by yeasts is greater in users than in non-users of oral contraceptives; this effect is more marked with oestrogenic than with progestagenic preparations (Lapan 1970, Anyon 1971, Spellacy et al 1971). It is not agreed whether, as well as increasing the prevalence of yeasts, oral contraceptives predispose to vulvovaginitis (Odds 1979).

Both the carriage of yeasts and candidal vulvovaginitis are common in diabetics, and indeed vaginitis can be the presenting symptom of diabetes mellitus. The cause may be high vaginal glycogen levels, as in pregnancy. *Candida* infections are common in the immunosuppressed. Vulval lesions may occur in chronic mucocutaneous candidosis (Higgs & Wells 1972).

Host defences. Neutrophils can attach themselves to yeast hyphae and subsequently destroy them (Diamond & Krezesicki 1978), and both neutrophils and monocytes can phagocytose candidal blastospores. Circulating antibodies against and cell-mediated immunity to *C. albicans* have both been demonstrated, but their role in limiting infection is uncertain (Odds 1979). The bacterial flora of the vagina may act as a defence against candidosis by inhibiting candidal multiplication and germ tube formation (Auger & Joly 1980).

The relationship between colonisation of the vagina by yeasts and the development of vulvovaginitis is poorly understood. *C. albicans* is dimorphic, and some studies have indicated an association between mycelium formation and the symptoms and signs of infection. There is no real evidence that this is a factor in the appearance of vaginal candidosis; furthermore, *T. glabrata*, which is also a vaginal pathogen, does not have a filamentous form. It is no longer believed that the appearance of hyphae is an indication of infection rather than colonisation.

The concentration of *C. albicans* in the vagina appears to be unrelated to the development of clinical signs of infection (Mursic 1975). It is probable that the transition of *Candida* and *Torulopsis* from commensalism to parasitism is conditioned for the most part by changes in the host which make it easier for the organisms to adhere to and subsequently damage epithelial cells. It is unlikely that hypersensitivity is a major factor in the development of mycotic vaginitis, because the inflammatory exudate in the vagina is composed of neutrophils rather than eosinophils. The ways in which the predisposing factors described above facilitate candidosis have not yet been satisfactorily explained, and in some cases of recurrent candidal vulvovaginitis none of these factors appears to be operative.

Clinical manifestations

The vulva and vagina are involved together. The cardinal symptom is pruritus, but women also complain of burning, dysuria, vaginal discharge and superficial dyspareunia. On examination, the vulva may show swelling, erythema and scaling, and sometimes excoriation and fissures (Fig. 5.8). The

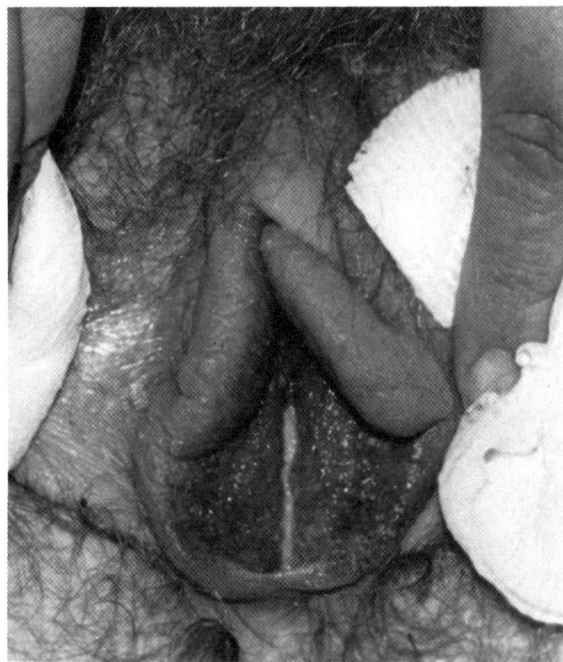

Fig. 5.8 Candidal vulvo vaginitis.

vagina too is erythematous, and a curdy discharge is often present, with plaques of exudate adherent to its walls. The vaginal secretions are not malodorous, and their pH is <4.5.

This classical picture is seen in some patients, but others show a milder disease and many women who are colonised by yeasts show no related symptoms or signs. Carroll et al (1973) have pointed out, however, that at least during pregnancy careful examination will show that the great majority of infected women have some vaginal morbidity. The clinical differentiation between candidosis and other forms of vaginitis such as trichomoniasis is not reliable, and laboratory investigation is always needed (Oriel et al 1972).

Laboratory diagnosis

Vaginal yeast infection may be diagnosed by microscopy and culture. Three methods may be used for microscopy. A specimen of vaginal fluid may be mixed with a drop of normal saline on a slide, or it may be mixed with a drop of 10% KOH and warmed, or it may be spread on a slide and stained by Gram's method. Which of these procedures is used is a matter of personal choice, but none has more than 50% of the sensitivity of culture.

Culture for yeasts is performed on a peptone–glucose–agar medium such as Sabouraud's medium; isolates are confirmed as *C. albicans* by demonstrating germ tube formation by incubation in serum. Other infections may co-exist with *Candida* and should be excluded by appropriate tests.

Treatment

Women with symptomatic candidosis certainly require treatment, but opinion is divided on the management of symptomless yeast carriers. Some physicians leave them untreated unless symptoms develop, but others fear that they may infect their sex partners, or accept the arguments of Carroll et al (1973) concerning vaginal morbidity in symptomless yeast infections, and treat all women with antimycotics if they have positive cultures.

In managing women with vulvovaginal candidosis it is important to diagnose, and treat if possible, any correctable predisposing factors such as

diabetes mellitus. It is generally recommended that constrictive underwear and tights should be avoided, and that cotton is preferable to synthetic material next to the vulval skin. Potential irritants such as bath oils and vaginal deodorants should not be used. Rashid et al (1984) have shown that *Candida* can survive laundering processes, but the clinical relevance of this fact is uncertain.

Most antimycotics fall into one of two groups: the polyenes, for example, nystatin and amphotericin B, or the imidazoles, e.g. clotrimazole and miconazole. Imidazoles are usually preferred to polyenes for therapy; the formulation, that is, cream or pessary, is less important (Odds 1977). Clotrimazole intravaginally, 100 mg at night for 6 nights, or equivalent dosage of other imidazoles, will give cure rates of about 90% (Odds 1977). Clotrimazole therapy can be shortened to 200 mg daily for 3 days, or even to 500 mg as a single application, without loss of efficacy (Masterson et al 1977, Milsom & Forssman 1982). Polyenes are still sometimes useful when imidazoles have given poor results. Nystatin pessaries 100 000 units daily for 14 days, continuing during menstruation, were formerly much used and cure rates of about 80% were obtained (Odds 1977). In addition to intravaginal therapy it is customary to prescribe an antimycotic cream such as clotrimazole or nystatin for application to the vulva twice daily, particularly if there is vulval irritation.

Ketoconazole is an imidazole which can be given orally for the treatment of vaginal candidosis; a dosage of 200 mg once daily for 14 days may be given. The drug has been associated with fatal hepatotoxicity and patients who are receiving it require clinical and biochemical monitoring.

Penile colonisation with yeasts is not uncommon in sex partners of women with vaginal candidosis (Davidson 1977), and it has been suggested that an untreated male partner may contribute to recurrent infection in some women. Recurrent vaginal candidosis can be a major problem in therapy. A search should be made for possible predisposing factors; among these the possibility of re-infection from the partner may be considered, although it has never been shown that the application of antimycotics to the partner's penis improves the prognosis for the woman. Resistance to polyenes and imidazoles does not seem to be a significant problem, and frequent

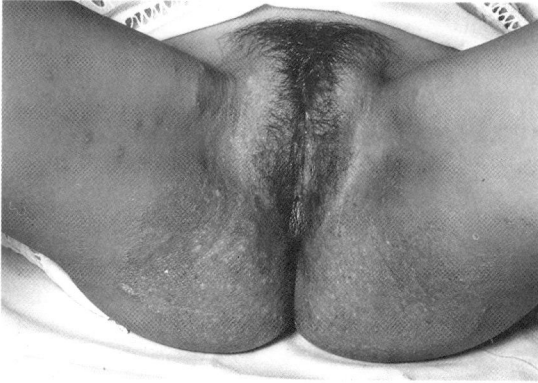

Fig. 5.9 Tinea cruris. (Reproduced from Beilby and Ridley 1975 by courtesy of the authors and publisher)

changes from one antimycotic to another are unhelpful. Intermittent long term prophylactic treatment can be effective (Davidson & Mould 1978). Although yeasts may often be recovered from the anorectum of women with vaginal candidosis, oral nystatin therapy does not appear to improve the efficacy of vaginal antimycotics (Milne & Warnock 1979). *Candida* as an agent in skin lesions of the area and napkin rashes, and its role in vulvodynia, are discussed elsewhere (pp. 163, 194, 219).

Tinea cruris

Aetiology

Tinea cruris is a fungal infection which is common in men but uncommon in women (Ingram 1955, Blank & Mann 1975). The usual cause is *Trichophyton rubrum* or *Epidermophyton floccosum*. Heat and humidity are provoking factors, and tinea cruris is most prevalent in people who wear tight occlusive underwear, particularly during warm weather.

Clinical features

Tinea curis begins as a small erythematous scaly patch which spreads peripherally and tends to clear in the centre (Fig. 5.9). The groins are chiefly affected, but the disease may encroach on the vulva or spread towards the perineum and peri-anal area, either as a continuous rash or as inflamed areas separated by normal skin. Where topical corticosteroids have been applied, the typical features may

be masked. A focus of infection is often present elsewhere, for example on the feet.

Diagnosis

This may be made by microscopy of scrapings from the edge of the eruption suspended in 10% KOH, when the mycelium can be seen, or by culture of the same material (the scrapings can be sent, preferably on black paper for ease of vision, to a suitably experienced laboratory). The main differential diagnoses are flexural psoriasis, which is not usually circinate, erythrasma and cutaneous candidosis. Erythrasma has a brownish colour, is more uniformly scaly, and gives a coral-red fluorescence in Wood's light. Candidal lesions appear more inflamed than those of tinea cruris, and they have a peripheral sodden fringe; these two fungal diseases will readily be differentiated by culture if microscopy is not diagnostic.

Treatment

Imidazole creams have largely replaced benzoic acid preparations, as they are more effective and less messy (Clayton & Connor 1973). Clotrimazole cream 1% may be applied twice daily, and should be continued for a week or two after apparent clinical clearance.

Pityriasis versicolor

Aetiology

Pityriasis versicolor (tinea versicolor) is caused by a *Pityrosporum*, usually *P. orbiculare* (*Malassezia furfur*). It has maximum prevalence in the hot and humid conditions of the tropics, but is common worldwide.

Clinical features

Brownish scaly macules appear, principally on the chest, abdomen and back, and may be accompanied by some itching. The genital area usually escapes, but may be involved if the eruption is widespread (Bumgarner & Burke 1949). Strikingly hypopigmented lesions may occur in the napkin area of black infants (Jelliffe & Jacobson 1954).

Diagnosis

Abundant fungal hyphae and spores can easily be seen by microscopy of skin scrapings suspended in 10% KOH; culture is unnecessary. Pityriasis versicolor must be distinguished from seborrhoeic dermatitis, pityriasis rosea and secondary syphilis.

Treatment

Clotrimazole cream is effective. Selenium sulphide 2.5% suspension is also effective, but should not be applied to the vulva. Ketoconazole orally is effective but not now justifiable because of its potential hepatotoxicity.

Phycomycosis

The various forms of phycomycosis are caused by fungi of the class *Phycomycetes*. Subcutaneous phycomycosis occurs in children and young adults, and is caused by *Basidiobolus ranarum*; it has a worldwide distribution. Deep granulomatous masses appear beneath an intact but inflamed epidermis. Infection of the vulva has been described (Lawson 1967, Scott et al 1985).

Chromomycosis (chromoblastomycosis)

This chronic fungus infection usually affects the leg or foot in bare-footed farm labourers. Kakoti and Dey (1957) described a patient in whom *Hormodendrum compactum* was isolated from a verrucous vulval lesion and from inguinal lymph glands.

Piedra (trichomycosis nodularis)

Black and white varieties of this fungal condition are recognised. The causative organisms are *Piedraia hortai* and *Trichosporon beigelii*. Nodules are seen on the hair. The pubic area, as well as other hairy areas, may be involved; in women, however, this is so much less often than in men (Kalter et al 1986). Microscopy and culture on Sabouraud's medium will prove the diagnosis. The differential diagnosis is from trichomycosis nodosa (of bacterial origin) and pediculosis pubis.

Treatment is by cutting off the hair and applying an antifungal compound; recurrence is common.

BACTERIAL INFECTIONS

Gram positive cocci

Staphylococci

S. aureus is present on the skin and in the nose of up to 30% of healthy people, but can cause many pyogenic infections, which often occur in sites and tissues with lowered host resistance, for example after injury. The organisms produce enzymes such as coagulase, and toxins which help to establish them in the host tissues.

On the vulva, *S. aureus* may cause furuncles and folliculitis. Folliculitis may follow minor trauma such as shaving of perigenital hair, and is usually transient (Fig. 5.10). Secondary infection by *S. aureus*, often in conjunction with other organisms, may complicate pediculosis pubis, molluscum

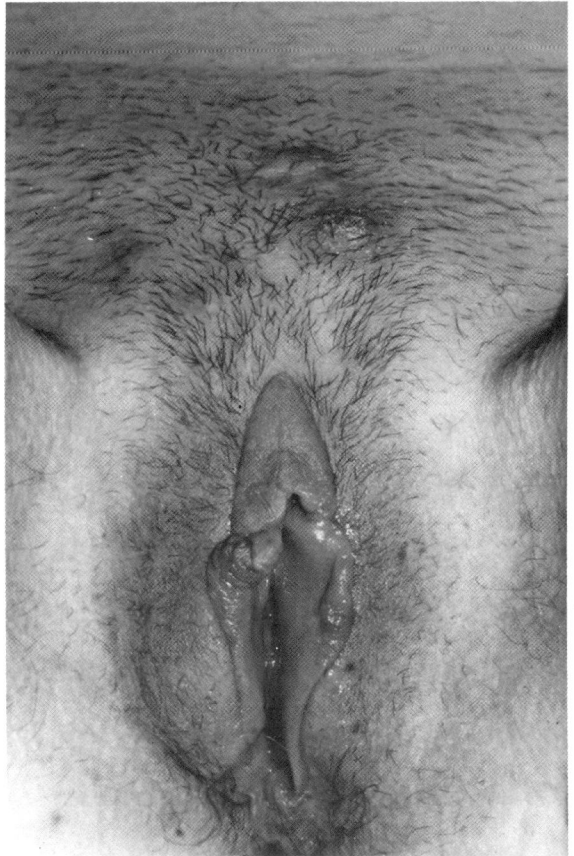

Fig. 5.10 Folliculitis of vulva. Most of these pyogenic lesions are on the mons pubis.

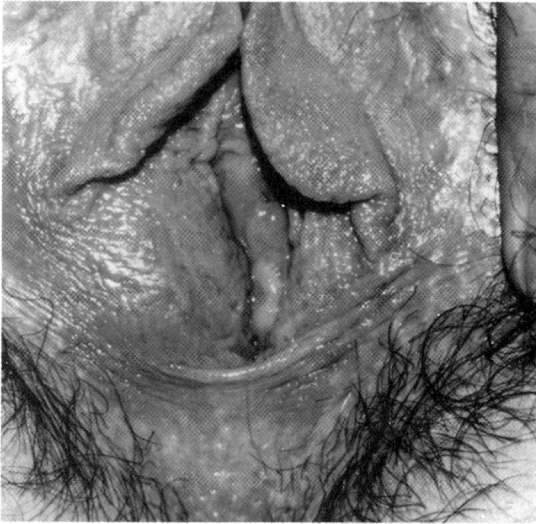

Fig. 5.11 Abscess of Bartholin's gland. These abscesses are commonly due to pyogenic cocci or to *Neisseria gonorrhoeae*.

contagiosum and indeed almost any variety of vulvitis or vulval dermatosis, the organisms often being introduced by scratching. Furuncles are not uncommon on the vulva. Despite treatment and preventive measures they may recur; multiple furuncles may be associated with diabetes mellitus, immune deficiency or other debilitating disorders. It has been suggested that *S. aureus* can sometimes cause vulvovaginitis (Lang et al 1958, Gardner & Kaufman 1981).

S. aureus is a cause of acute infection of the duct of Bartholin's gland, leading to abscess formation; these abscesses may also be associated with *N. gonorrhoeae*, *Pseudomonas aeruginosa*, *E. coli* and *Streptococcus faecalis*, and a few are sterile (Mayer 1972). A tender swelling appears at the affected labium major, and there may be vulval oedema and fever (Fig. 5.11). Some women get recurrent attacks. A cyst of Bartholin's gland duct may precede or follow infection.

Staphylococcus saprophyticus does not form hostile enzymes or toxins, and lacks the pathogenicity of *S. aureus*. It is normally a harmless commensal which colonises the skin, nose and mouth of virtually everyone throughout life. Nevertheless, it can act as an opportunistic pathogen, and has been held responsible for up to 30% of acute urinary tract infections in young women (Gillespie et al 1978). It is not pathogenic to the vulva or vagina.

Streptococci

Most streptococcal infections are caused by the B haemolytic streptococcus of Lancefield's group A – *Streptococcus pyogenes*. The commonest infection caused by this organism is acute tonsillitis/pharyngitis; at one time puerperal sepsis was often due to *S. pyogenes*, although today other organisms are usually responsible. On the vulva, *S. pyogenes* may cause two kinds of infection: erysipelas or cellulitis, and pyoderma.

Erysipelas is a spreading inflammation of the dermis characterised by local redness, heat and swelling, often with a sharp border. It is not essentially distinguishable from cellulitis in which the inflammation extends more deeply, that is in subcutaneous tissue, and which is sometimes more chronic. Fissures and operation wounds may predispose to such infection (Norburn & Coles 1960), which is well recognised to occur as a complication, often recurrent, of lymphatic obstruction of all types, and itself to lead to lymphatic obstruction. Cutaneous infection with *S. pyogenes* is sometimes followed by acute glomerulonephritis; impetigo or pyoderma may be caused by streptococci, although usually in the UK classical impetigo is caused by *S. aureus* (Noble et al 1974, Noble 1981).

Group B streptococci are associated with several human infections which include abscesses, wound infections and septic abortion. They also have a major role in neonatal infection (Baker 1977). Two clinical entities are described: the first and early onset fulminating septicaemia with a high mortality, and the second a meningitis syndrome occurring in infants over the age of 10 days. The source of infection for the first of these is thought to be the maternal genital tract, but for the second may be nosocomial. Asymptomatic colonisation of the vagina by group B streptococci is known to occur during pregnancy, and the use of prophylactic penicillin has been advocated for women found to be colonised. These organisms are not thought to be a cause of vaginitis.

Treatment of vulval infection by pyogenic cocci

Minor degrees of folliculitis and single furuncles do not usually require systemic antibiotics (Rutherford et al 1970), but local antiseptics may limit their spread to surrounding skin. Severe furunculosis or extensive folliculitis merit systemic therapy. Since many staphylococci are penicillinase producing, erythromycin 250 mg or flucloxacillin 250 mg should be given four times a day for 5–7 days. A similar regimen can be used for the immediate treatment of acute infection of Bartholin's glands, but material for culture should be taken first and the antibiotic regimen modified if necessary when the results are available. Abscesses of Bartholin's glands require adequate marsupialisation or other surgical treatment, with histological examination in middle-aged women because malignancy is otherwise often missed.

Oral or parenteral penicillin is rapidly effective for erysipelas; erythromycin is a satisfactory alternative for patients who are allergic to penicillin. Streptococcal pyodermatous lesions respond well to systemic penicillin or erythromycin, combined with the removal of crusts with 0.05% chlorhexidine solution. Again, a specimen for microbiology should be taken before treatment is started.

Gram negative cocci

Neisseria gonorrhoeae

N. gonorrhoeae is a Gram negative coccus whose kidney-shaped cells usually occur as diplococci. Some gonococci bear pili, hair-like appendages which appear to affect pathogenicity (Punsalang & Sawyer 1973). N. gonorrhoeae is a delicate organism, but in appropriate cultural conditions grows well in the laboratory. In women, the organism initially infects the urethra, cervix and anorectum, and from these sites may spread to involve para-urethral glands, Bartholin's glands and the Fallopian tubes, or the infection may disseminate and cause septicaemia.

Epidemiology. Gonorrhoea is one of the commonest infectious diseases in the world. In Europe and the USA its incidence rose markedly in the 1960s, but since the late 1970s has shown a slight decline. In England, the number of new cases of gonorrhoea in women seen in hospital clinics fell from 91.72 to 77.94 per 100 000 population between 1977 and 1981 (Chief Medical Officer 1984a); in 1981, 18 746 cases were seen in hospital clinics in England. Gonorrhoea is commonest among women in their late teens, and in those who are unmarried, of low socio-economic status and who began sexual intercourse at a young age.

The risk of a woman acquiring gonorrhoea from a single sexual contact with an infected man is not known, but about 90% of women who have had intercourse with men with gonorrhoea become infected (Thin 1970). It has also been reported that 16% of women who have fellatio with an infected partner develop gonococcal pharyngitis (Wallin 1975). Whether the use of oral contraceptives increases the risk of a woman contracting gonorrhoea is uncertain (McCormack & Reynolds 1982). Transmission by non-sexual contact can occur in infants but is extremely rare in adults.

Symptoms and signs. The cervix is the commonest site to be infected by N. gonorrhoeae, but the urethra is colonised in about 75% of cases (Barlow & Phillips 1978, Thin & Shaw 1979), and in a few patients may be the only site infected. The rectum is infected in up to 50% of women who have gonococcal infection at any site, and is the sole infected site in 5% (Kinghorn & Rashid 1979, Thin & Shaw 1979). The adult vagina is not usually infected by N. gonorrhoeae, although recovery of gonococci from the vaginal vault in a woman who had had a hysterectomy has been recorded (Judson & Ruder 1979). About 50% of women with uncomplicated gonorrhoea are symptomless (King et al 1980). The remainder have the symptoms of lower genital tract infection: dysuria, vulval irritation or discomfort and vaginal discharge. In some women, these symptoms are due to associated infections, for example trichomoniasis, rather than to gonorrhoea. Women who do become symptomatic usually do so within a few days of infection (Wallin 1975).

Examination may show no abnormality. In some women there is cervical congestion with a mucopurulent exudate, and sometimes purulent material can be expressed from the urethra. Vaginitis is not a feature of gonorrhoea unless there are associated vaginal infections such as trichomoniasis. Proctoscopy may show congestion of the rectal mucosa and a mucopurulent exudate.

Local complications. Acute gonococcal vulvitis is rare in adults, although it can occur in children. Infection of the para-urethral glands of Skene may cause oedema of the urinary meatus, and

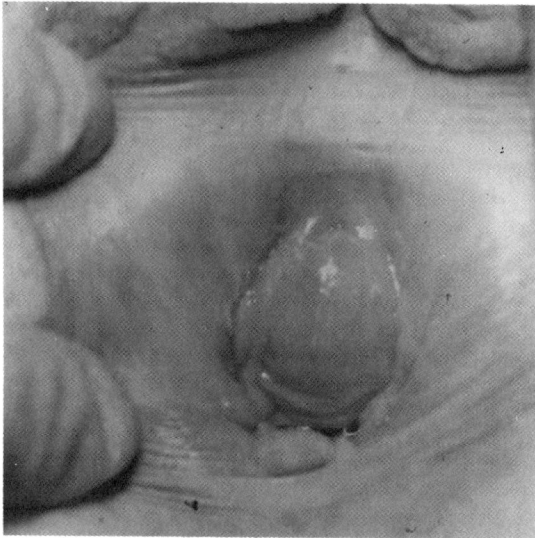

Fig. 5.12 Peri-urethral abscess. This abscess was caused by infection by *N. gonorrhoeae*.

sometimes a small abscess forms which can be palpated through the anterior wall of the vagina (Fig. 5.12). Peri-urethral abscesses can occur, but are rare (King et al 1980).

N. gonorrhoeae has been isolated from the ducts of Bartholin's glands in 28% of a group of women with gonorrhoea, and one-third of these had enlargement and tenderness of the gland (Rees 1967). It may be possible to express a bead of pus from the opening of the duct. If untreated, infection of Bartholin's gland can progress to abscess formation.

The most important complication of gonorrhoea in women is acute salpingitis, which occurs in 10–15% of those with lower genital tract infection; salpingitis often has an adverse effect on both health and fertility. A further serious complication is disseminated gonococcal infection, which occurs in 1% of women with untreated mucosal infections.

Gonorrhoea in children. In adults, the vagina is rarely infected by *N. gonorrhoeae*, but in prepubertal girls vaginal infection can occur, presenting as an acute vulvovaginitis with a variable amount of mucopurulent or purulent exudate. The usual cause of infection is sexual assault; 'accidental' infection, or infection from fomites, is very rare (Farrell et al 1981).

Diagnosis. The diagnosis of gonorrhoea in women depends entirely on the results of laboratory tests. It is important that specimens are collected from all potentially infected sites: the urethra, cervix, anorectum and pharynx. If only one of these is to be sampled it should be the cervix, but it must be recognised that the urethra, anorectum and pharynx may each be the sole site of infection in approximately 5% of women with gonorrhoea. Specimen collection from all these sites is therefore advisable, together with specimens from other areas such as the ducts of accessory glands if indicated. If negative results are obtained the tests are repeated. Examination of a high vaginal swab for *N. gonorrhoeae* has no place in the diagnosis of gonorrhoea, as almost one case in three will be missed if it is so used (Bhattacharyya et al 1973).

Specimens for culture are taken with cotton-wool-tipped swabs. While direct inoculation of culture plates is preferable, transport media such as Stuart's or Ames' can be used, but these should reach the laboratory within 24 hours. Specimens are cultured on selective media which contain antibiotics to reduce the growth of unwanted organisms. It is important to differentiate *N. gonorrhoeae* from other *Neisseriae* which may be present in the genital tract or the pharynx by either sugar fermentation or immunofluorescence (Stokes & Ridgway 1980).

The examination of Gram-stained specimens from the genital tract for the presence of intracellular Gram negative diplococci is a method of diagnosis which is rapid but lacking in sensitivity (Rothenberg et al 1976, Barlow & Phillips 1978); only 50–70% of endocervical infections with *N. gonorrhoeae* give positive results on microscopy. Although antibodies to *N. gonorrhoeae* can be detected by various techniques, there is at present no serological test which is sufficiently sensitive and specific to be of value in diagnosis.

Treatment. *N. gonorrhoeae* has shown decreasing sensitivity to penicillin for many years; in some strains this chromosomally mediated resistance is so high that penicillin cannot be used for therapy. In 1977 a further problem appeared, because penicillinase-producing strains of *N. gonorrhoeae* (PPNG) began to emerge which were totally resistant to penicillin. This type of resistance is plasmid mediated, and PPNG have now become widely prevalent, particularly in developing countries, where they may comprise > 50% of isolates. In many European countries and most areas of the USA penicillin can still be used for the treatment of gonorrhoea; for uncomplicated mucosal infections the following schedules are recommended:

1. Aqueous procaine penicillin G 2.4–4.8 mega units intramuscularly, with probenecid 1.0 g orally.
2. Ampicillin 2.0–3.5 g in a single oral dose, with probenecid 1.0 g orally.

Patients who are not cured by the above regimens, including those infected with PPNG, should receive:

3. Spectinomycin 2.0 g intramuscularly, or:
4. Cefotaxime 1.0 g intramuscularly.

Up to 50% of women with gonorrhoea have a concomitant cervical infection by *C. trachomatis* (Oriel & Ridgway 1982). Because of this, it is recommended that after single-dose treatment for gonorrhoea a course of a tetracycline, for example tetracycline hydrochloride 500 mg four times a day for 7 days, should be given (MMWR 1985).

After the treatment of gonorrhoea at least two follow-up examinations, with cultures for *N. gonorrhoeae*, should be arranged to confirm cure. In addition, all patients should have serological tests for syphilis performed on their first attendance and again 3 months after the date of the original exposure. The tracing and investigation of male sex partners is of course mandatory.

Gram positive bacilli

Corynebacteria

Erythrasma. Erythrasma is caused by *Corynebacterium minutissimum* or related species (Sarkany et al 1961); the ultrastructure of these organisms has been described by Montes & Black (1967). *C. minutissimum* is part of the normal skin flora, but can cause disease in warm humid conditions or if the subject is debilitated, for example by diabetes mellitus (Somerville et al 1970).

Erythrasma affects flexural areas such as the axillae, between the toes, the groins and the natal cleft. It is usually symptomless except in the groins, where there may be some itching. Well-defined brownish-red scaly patches appear in the affected areas. The differential diagnosis is from tinea cruris, intertrigo, seborrhoeic dermatitis and flexural psoriasis. Under Wood's light erythrasma shows a characteristic coral-red fluorescence, caused by the presence of a porphyrin. It is possible to culture *C. minutissimum* in special media, specimens being readily obtained by scraping.

The treatment of choice is oral erythromycin, 250 mg four times a day for 2 weeks. It is effective but recurrence is common. Clotrimazole cream is useful for long term local treatment.

Trichomycosis (nodosa). Trichomycosis (not, in spite of its name, a fungal infection) was formerly attributed to *Corynebacterium tenuis*, but is now known to be caused by at least three species of corynebacteria (Freeman et al 1969). Small nodules of various colours—yellow, red or black (White & Smith 1979)—are attached firmly to the hairs of the axillae or pubic area, and clothing may be stained. Electron microscopy has shown that the bacteria may inflict some damage to the shafts of the hairs (Orfanos et al 1971) and can elaborate a cement-like substance (Shelley & Miller 1984).

Trichomycosis must be differentiated from piedra and from the nits of pediculosis pubis. This can be done by microscopy of the affected hairs, or by examination under Wood's light, when variably coloured fluorescence is seen in trichomycosis, or by culture. The condition is treated by clipping off the affected hair and applying an antiseptic.

Cutaneous diphtheria. Diphtheria, caused by *Corynebacterium diphtheriae*, usually presents as a localised inflammation of the throat with a greyish adherent exudate, accompanied by severe toxaemia. Nowadays it is a rare disease in developed countries. Infection of the skin by *C. diphtheriae* is common in tropical countries, and can occur elsewhere. It presents as multiple punched-out ulcerated lesions, often covered with a greyish membrane. Regional lymph nodes may be enlarged. Vulval infection has been described, occurring either alone or, less often, accompanying respiratory diphtheria (Gardner and Kaufman, 1969). Cases in children have been reported by Hunt (1954), and in adults by Parks (1941) and Machnicki (1953). Toxaemia may be severe. An occasional case of vulvovaginitis in children has been attributed to *C. diphtheriae*, although true infection must be distinguished from the prodromal vulvo-vaginitis of many fevers, including diphtheria.

The diagnosis is made by culture of *C. diphtheriae* on blood tellurite agar. The infection is treated by intramuscular injections of diphtheria antitoxin, and in addition full dosage of penicillin, erythromycin or clindamycin should be given.

Gram negative bacilli

Chancroid (Haemophilus ducreyi)

Aetiology. Chancroid is an acute STD caused by *H. ducreyi*. This is a small Gram negative rod; in the past the organism has been difficult to culture in the laboratory, but much improved growth media have been developed recently (Hammond et al 1978, Ronald 1986).

Epidemiology. Until recently it has been difficult to identify *H. ducreyi*, particularly in those localities where the disease is common; further, many genital ulcers have a polymicrobial flora, and organisms other than *H. ducreyi* can cause ulcers which closely resemble chancroid (Chapel et al 1978). For these reasons, the epidemiology of bacteriologically confirmed chancroid is largely unknown.

It has been estimated that throughout the world chancroid is many times commoner than syphilis and, in some places, commoner than gonorrhoea (Gaisin & Heaton 1975, Nsanze et al 1981). Chancroid is most common in tropical and subtropical developing countries, but bacteriologically confirmed outbreaks have occurred in Western industrialised societies (Ronald et al 1983). The prevalence of chancroid is much greater in men than in women. This implies that many infected women are not being diagnosed, but whether they have symptomless ulceration or can act as carriers of *H. ducreyi* is not known.

Clinical features. The incubation period is usually between 3 and 10 days. Small tender papules appear which soon break down to form ragged, tender non-indurated ulcers (Fig. 5.13). About 50% of cases have only one ulcer. Sometimes the lesions remain pustular—so-called dwarf chancroid (Gaisin & Heaton 1975). In women the majority of chancroidal lesions are on the labia, fourchette, perineum and peri-anal areas, but

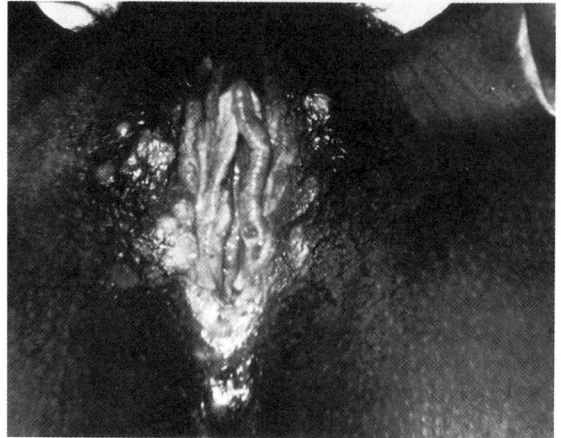

Fig. 5.13 Chancroid: multiple painful ulcers are present.

vaginal and cervical ulcers can also occur (Hammond et al 1978). In up to 50% of women inguinal adenitis develops. This is usually unilateral, and often progresses to form abscesses which may rupture spontaneously. Mild constitutional symptoms may occur in chancroid, but the infection does not disseminate.

Diagnosis. The differential diagnosis is from other causes of the genital ulceration/lymphadenopathy syndrome, in particular syphilis, genital herpes, lymphogranuloma venereum and secondarily infected traumatic lesions. Some patients have genital ulceration of multiple aetiology. The laboratory diagnosis of chancroid depends on the isolation of *H. ducreyi* from the ulcers or from pus from buboes (Ronald 1986). Microscopy of stained smears of clinical material is difficult to interpret (Borchardt & Hoke 1970). No satisfactory serological test is available.

Treatment. Chancroid used to respond to penicillin, but this treatment has now been abandoned because of the emergence of B-lactamase-producing strains of *H. ducreyi*. The tetracyclines have been effective, but resistance has become common in some places (Marmar 1972). Recent work has shown that good results can be obtained with either trimethoprim-sulphamethoxazole (160 mg trimethoprim and 800 mg sulphamethoxazole twice daily), or erythromycin (500 mg four times a day), treatment being continued for 7–10 days (Carpenter et al 1981, Fast et al 1983). Fluctuant lymph nodes should be aspirated.

Donovanosis (Calymmatobacterium granulomatis)

Aetiology. The cause of donovanosis (granuloma inguinale) is *C. granulomatis*, a Gram negative encapsulated rod of uncertain bacteriological status. In tissue smears the organisms can be demonstrated in the cytoplasm of large mononuclear cells, and occasionally in polymorphonuclear leucocytes (Dodson et al 1974). *C. granulomatis* has not been grown on artificial media.

Epidemiology. Donovanosis occurs in tropical and subtropical countries; it is virtually extinct in Europe and North America, but is endemic in parts of South-East Asia, southern India and New Guinea. Although donovanosis is usually classified as an STD (Lal & Nicholas 1970), this has been disputed. Another opinion is that the organisms normally inhabit the intestinal tract; in conditions of poor hygiene, inoculation into genital or anal tissue by coitus may lead to the development of the disease (Goldberg 1964).

Clinical features. The incubation period of donovanosis is uncertain, but may be between 7 and 30 days (Lal & Nicholas 1970). In women, the labia minora, fourchette and mons veneris are the commonest sites initially infected. The lesions are papular or nodular, and the overlying skin breaks down to form soft granulating ulcers. These progressively spread and may eventually involve a large area including the perineum and anus (Fig. 5.14). Concurrent fibrosis may lead to lymphoedema. Regional lymphadenitis does not occur, although granulomatous lesions may appear in the skin overlying the lymph nodes. Vulval granulation may extend into the vagina and affect the cervix; conversely, an initial infection of the cervix may spread to involve the vagina and vulva. Autoinoculation may lead to lesions in the mouth, but systemic spread is rare (Rajam & Rangiah 1954). In long-standing infections urethral, vaginal or anal stenosis may develop.

Diagnosis. This depends on the demonstration of the infecting agent in tissue smears; the best specimens are biopsy or curettings of the ulcer base, stained with Leishman or Giemsa stain (Plummer et al 1984). Histological examination is valuable both for diagnosis and for excluding malignancy (Sowmini 1983). Perigenital and perianal donovanosis lesions may resemble the con-

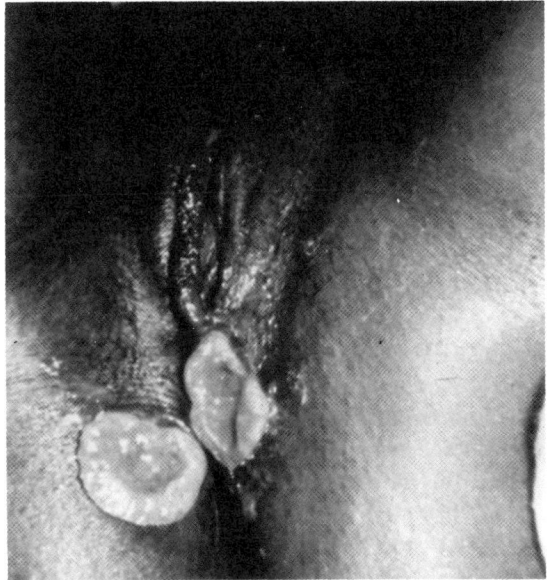

Fig. 5.14 Vulval donovanosis.

dylomata lata of secondary syphilis, so serological tests for this disease should always be performed. Other infections are common in women with donovanosis, who should therefore be carefully screened before treatment.

Treatment. Many antibiotics have been used for therapy, but there has been wide variation in their effectiveness according to locality. The following regimens have been recommended:

1. Tetracycline hydrochloride 500 mg orally four times a day for at least 10 days (Sowmini 1983).
2. Streptomycin 1.0 g intramuscularly twice daily for 10 days (Lal 1971); there is a risk of ototoxicity with prolonged courses of this antibiotic.
3. Ampicillin 500 mg four times a day for 2 weeks (Breschi et al 1974).

Mycobacteria

Tuberculosis (Mycobacterium tuberculosis)

Although the lung is most commonly infected with the chronic granulomatous and caseating lesions of tuberculosis, other sites, including the genitalia, may be infected either directly or by spread from other areas.

Epidemiology. Although in Western industrialised societies the incidence and mortality of tuberculosis has markedly declined in the last two decades, it remains one of the most important infectious diseases in the world. Tuberculosis of the female genital tract is still not uncommon in developing countries. In comparison with infection of the upper genital tract, vulval tuberculosis is rare (Moore 1954). It may occur: (1) as a primary exogenous infection through contact with sputum from a sex partner with pulmonary tuberculosis or with genital secretions when he has renal or epididymal tuberculosis (Bjornstad 1947), (2) by distal spread from the upper genital tract, or (3) by haematogenous infection from tuberculous foci elsewhere.

Clinical features. In a true primary tuberculous complex the initial lesion is an inconspicuous brown-red papule, but this may be missed so that the clinical picture is dominated by inguinal or femoral adenopathy (Stewart 1967). The primary tuberculous lesion usually heals after a few months, but the enlarged glands may persist and break down.

In other forms of vulval tuberculosis cutaneous and/or mucosal lesions appear either as nodules which break down to form ulcers with soft and ragged edges, or as indurated fungating masses. In the chronic stage, fibrosis leads to scarring and there may be persistent sinuses. Involvement of regional lymph nodes may lead to caseation and scarring, or to vulval lymphoedema (Ashworth 1974).

Infection of Bartholin's glands, which is usually unilateral, may be secondary to a tuberculous focus elsewhere (Schaefer 1959); it presents as a painless hard vulval swelling, or as a 'cold' abscess.

Diagnosis. Tuberculous lesions of the vulva must be distinguished from chronic diseases such as lymphogranuloma venereum, donovanosis, hidradenitis and from carcinoma. Histological examination of biopsy material may show tubercles and caseation. Tubercle bacilli may be demonstrated by microscopy of pus or tissue sections stained by a Ziehl–Nielsen technique. Suspected tuberculous material may be cultured for *M. tuberculosis*. It is important to differentiate the organism from opportunist mycobacteria.

Treatment. Treatment of vulval tuberculosis follows the general principles of chemotherapy for this infection (Garrod et al 1981).

Leprosy (mycobacterium leprae)

Various forms are described. Cutaneous lesions range between lepromatous and tuberculoid types, with borderline lesions between them, and indeterminate lesions in early transitory states (Jopling & Harman 1986).

The female genital tract can be infected by *M. leprae*. The ovary is most commonly involved, followed by the cervix, uterus and Fallopian tubes (Bonar & Rabson 1957); infection of these sites is haematogenous. Direct infection of the vulva can also occur, particularly in the nodular and borderline types of leprosy, although this has not been thoroughly studied (Grabstold & Swan 1952).

Actinomycosis (actinomyces israelii)

Actinomycosis is an uncommon chronic granulomatous disease. *A. israelii* is a commensal in the mouth, but in the tissues it causes a subacute or chronic granulomatous infection characterised by the formation of abscesses which drain to the surface through sinuses.

Genital tract infection is rare. It usually arises through extension of bowel disease (Wagman 1975), but several cases have been described which have been associated with intra-uterine contraceptive devices (Lomax et al 1976, Purdie et al 1977). In these, the uterus and adnexa have been infected, but Daniel & Mavrodin (1934) reported three cases of vulval actinomycosis. The chemotherapy of actinomycosis can be difficult; penicillin is probably the antibiotic of choice.

Spirochaetes

Syphilis (Treponema pallidum)

During the last century the morbidity of syphilis has been declining, although there have been periodic increases coinciding with wars, social and political unrest and population movements. After the introduction of antibiotics 40 years ago the incidence of early syphilis declined steeply and late syphilis has become a rare disease in industrialised societies. Nevertheless, syphilis is still an important infection and case finding, diagnosis and treatment remain important.

Aetiology. The species of the genus *Treponema*

which are pathogenic to humans are *T. pallidum*, *T. pertenue*, *T. carateum* and *T. pallidum* var *Bosnia*, which cause venereal syphilis, yaws, pinta and endemic syphilis respectively. These organisms are morphologically and serologically indistinguishable. They have not yet been propagated in vitro, although limited replication of *T. pallidum* has been achieved in a medium containing rabbit epithelial cells (Fieldsteel 1981).

T. pallidum is a slender spiral organism, $6-15\mu$m in length and less than 0.25μm wide. It is too narrow and has too little protoplasm to be visible by light microscopy in an unstained preparation, but dark-ground microscopy reveals it as a slender spiral organism which undergoes characteristic rotatory movements, and changes of shape which include angulation and coil compression and expansion. Electron microscopy shows an electron-dense axial bundle surrounded by several spirally wound filaments, and there appears to be an outer membrane (Ovcinnikov & Delektorskij 1968). Although a life cycle has been demonstrated in non-virulent treponemes, this has not been observed for *T. pallidum*. The organism multiplies by transverse fission every 30 hours (Turner & Hollander 1957).

In clinical practice *T. pallidum* is usually identified by dark-ground microscopy. Staining procedures are much less satisfactory, as it is difficult to differentiate the organisms from their background. Silver impregnation has been successfully used to identify treponemes in tissues, and an immunofluorescent staining method has also been developed for the detection of *T. pallidum* in early syphilitic lesions (Wilkinson & Cowell 1971).

Epidemiology. In industrialised countries the incidence of early syphilis had reached a high level immediately after World War II, but subsequently showed a marked decline, probably because of the introduction of antibiotics. During the 1950s and 1960s the incidence remained low, but recently there has been an increase in cases of early syphilis in men reported in both Europe and the USA, the majority of these infections occurring in male homosexuals. In contrast, the incidence of early syphilis in women has remained steady at a low level for the last decade. The number of new cases in women reported from STD clinics in England was 1.42 per 100 000 population in 1971 and 1.44 per 100 000 population in 1981 (Chief Medical Officer 1973, 1984b). The incidence of syphilis in women in the USA is believed to be at least five times higher than it is in England.

Pathology. *T. pallidum* probably gains entry to the tissues through small abrasions produced during sexual intercourse. The organisms multiply locally, and at the same time some reach the regional lymph nodes. Polymorphonuclear leucocytes are first attracted to the area, and these are followed by thymus-dependent lymphocytes and macrophages (Lukehart et al 1980). Proliferation of blood vessels and endarteritis occur in the area, and the whole complex is now a primary chancre. Ulceration of its surface is due to perivascular infiltration and endarteritis. Similar cellular changes in the regional lymph nodes result in their enlargement.

Circulating antibodies appear early. Reagin is an immunoglobulin which is present in syphilis and some other diseases. It is detected by either complement fixation tests such as the Wassermann or by flocculation tests such as the Venereal Disease Research Laboratory (VDRL) and rapid plasma reagin (RPR) tests. These tests are negative during the incubation period of syphilis, but usually become positive with, or shortly after, the appearance of the chancre. Specific treponemal antibodies can be detected by the fluorescent treponemal antibody (absorbed) (FTA-ABS) test, the *Treponema pallidum* haemagglutination assay (TPHA) test, and the *Treponema pallidum* immobilisation (TPI) test. The first two of these are in current use, but the TPI test is obsolete. The FTA-ABS test is the first of these to become reactive, and is positive in the majority of cases of primary syphilis. The TPHA and TPI tests are slower to respond, but the TPHA test is positive by the end of the primary stage in most patients.

The operation of cell-mediated and humoral immunity in untreated primary syphilis leads to the slow resolution of the primary chancre and the enlarged regional glands. The immune response is, however, incomplete because although the local disease is contained treponemes reach the bloodstream and are disseminated to other organs and tissues; 4–6 weeks after the primary chancre has appeared, this treponemal septicaemia is expressed clinically as secondary syphilis. This persists, with exacerbations and remissions, for up to 9–12 months, after which all the clinical signs of the infection disappear. But again, although it has been contained it has not been eradicated, and true immunity has not developed. During the whole course of secondary syphilis all serological tests are strongly positive.

A period of latency of variable duration now follows. Incomplete suppression of infection may lead to a partial return of the lesions of secondary syphilis, or even of the primary chancre (chancre redux), but eventually all physical signs die away, although the serology remains positive.

Less than a third of patients with untreated early syphilis progress to late syphilis; in the remainder, latency is prolonged for life. Tertiary syphilis presents, 3–20 years after the original infection, as gummas, cardiovascular syphilis and neurosyphilis. A gumma is a granuloma whose histology shows infiltration with lymphocytes and mononuclear cells, with endarteritis, which causes central necrosis or superficial ulceration; partial healing leads to extensive scarring. Gummas may be due to a hypersensitivity reaction to persisting treponemal antigen; it is difficult to demonstrate treponemes in these lesions. Patients with gummas nearly always have reactive reagin tests, and the specific tests are invariably positive (King et al 1980).

During the course of primary, secondary and early latent syphilis occurring during pregnancy, the infection can be transmitted to the fetus transplacentally. The resulting clinical manifestations of the disease in neonates are protean. The lesions of the first 2 years of life resemble those of adult secondary syphilis; from the third year onwards they are of gummatous type. They have been described in detail by King et al 1980.

Vulval lesions in early syphilis. The incubation period of syphilis is 10–90 days, commonly about 2 weeks, and the untreated primary stage lasts for 3–8 weeks. The first lesion is a macule, which soon becomes papular then ulcerates to form a primary chancre. A classical chancre is an indurated painless ulcer with a dull red base. In the majority of cases the regional lymph nodes enlarge within a week of the appearance of the chancre; they are usually painless, firm and smooth.

The symptoms and signs of early syphilis are variable, and some physicians suggest that nowadays the 'classical' chancre may be unusual (Chapel 1978). Multiple chancres are common, and they

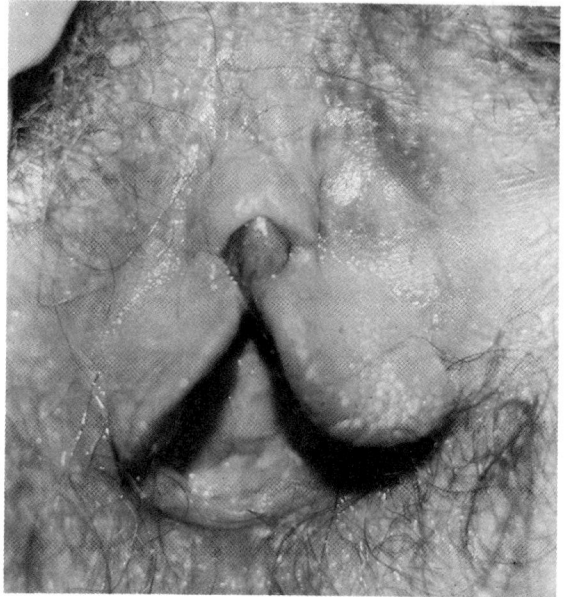

Fig. 5.15 Primary chancre of clitoris: note oedema of clitoral hood.

may be tender because of secondary infection. In some series, only a minority of women with primary syphilis show regional lymph node enlargement (Duncan et al 1984). In developing countries the difficulty of diagnosing primary syphilis is increased because of multiple infections, particularly of syphilis and chancroid (Duncan et al 1984).

Fournier (1906) reported that 46% of chancres were on the labia majora, 22% on the labia minora and 5% on the cervix. Davies (1931) believed that the majority of chancres were on the cervix, but modern experience is that the vulva is much more commonly affected than the cervix (King et al 1980, Duncan et al 1984) (Figs. 5.15, 5.16). Vulval lesions may cause marked labial oedema. Enlargement of the inguinal lymph nodes may be unilateral or bilateral; overlying erythema occurs only if the glands become secondarily infected.

The commonest clinical features of secondary syphilis are constitutional symptoms such as malaise and fever, lesions of skin and mucous membranes, and generalised lymphadenopathy. The vulva is affected by skin eruptions, including condylomata lata, and by mucous patches. The skin rashes of secondary syphilis may be macular, papular, papulosquamous and pustular, and any of

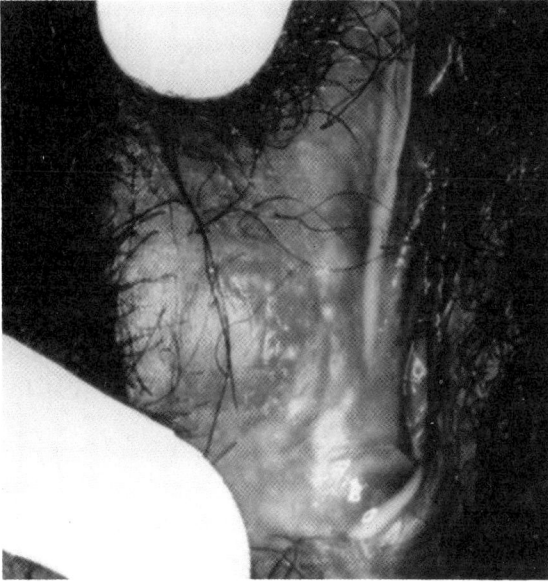

Fig. 5.16 Primary chancre of labium minor.

these may appear on the vulva. Condylomata lata are a variant of the papular syphilide. They develop at the periphery of the vulva and around the anus, and are confluent soft spongy masses with flat tops and broad bases; they may become eroded and exude highly infective serum. Mucous patches usually appear at the same time as maculopapular skin lesions; they are painless, round, greyish-white eroded areas, affecting the labia minora.

Vulval lesions in late syphilis. These are very rare today. Gummas affecting the skin of the vulva occur as squamous psoriasiform lesions, or as sub-cutaneous nodules which may coalesce or enlarge and ulcerate through the skin. Cases have been described by Davies (1931), Matras (1935) and Konrad (1936).

Vulval lesions of congenital syphilis. In early congenital syphilis bullous, papular and papulo-squamous lesions occur on the vulva as part of the syphilitic dermatosis. Mucous patches and moist erosions also occur. Vulval condylomata lata develop later, typically towards the end of the first year of life (Nabarro 1954).

Diagnosis. Primary chancres in women need differentiation from other causes of vulval ulceration including genital herpes, pyogenic lesions, infected

injuries and, in developing countries, chancroid, lymphogranuloma venereum and donovanosis. Rarer causes of genital ulcers include fixed drug eruptions, Behçet's disease and squamous cell carcinoma. Clinical impressions of the cause of vulval ulceration are often inaccurate, and laboratory investigation is always necessary. Herpetic lesions are painful, are not usually indurated, and some may be vesicular. The ulcers of chancroid are painful, vascular and non-indurated; if the regional lymph nodes are infected there is overlying erythema, and suppuration often occurs. Vulval ulcers in lympho-granuloma venereum are small and inconspicuous, while adenopathy is marked. Appropriate laboratory investigations will help to differentiate these conditions from syphilis. It must be remembered that vulval ulcers may have a multiple aetiology, particularly in developing countries.

The vulval lesions of the generalised rash in secondary syphilis may resemble those of many dermatoses. The macular rash may be mistaken for seborrhoeic dermatitis, drug eruptions or exanthemata, and the papular rash may resemble papular urticaria, pityriasis rosea or lichen planus. As regards specifically vulval lesions, condylomata lata may be confused with condylomata acuminata, and mucous patches with primary chancres, genital herpes, fixed drug eruptions and Behçet's syndrome. Women with the vulval manifestations of secondary syphilis are likely to show other clinical features of the disease.

The laboratory diagnosis of early syphilis depends on dark-ground examination for *T. pallidum* and serological tests. Dark-ground microscopy is a valuable and highly specific technique which can be used in early syphilis when there are ulcers or papular lesions of skin or mucous membranes. The area to be examined is first cleaned with 0.9% saline. If the lesion is moist, enough serum for examination may be obtained by squeezing. If the lesion is dry, it must first be scarified at the edge so that it bleeds; after this blood has clotted, a drop of serum is examined. Specimens are examined with dark-ground illumination at magnification × 400 or × 900 to detect motile treponemes. If no organisms are seen on examination of a suspicious lesion, microscopy should be repeated daily for 2–3 days. If the suspect chancre is healing, or has been treated with local antiseptics, it may be possible to aspirate fluid from enlarged regional lymph nodes for dark-ground microscopy.

Serological tests for syphilis should always be performed. The VDRL or RPR test is positive in 50–70% of patients with primary syphilis (Wende et al 1971), and is invariably positive at high titre in secondary syphilis. After this the titre slowly declines, and eventually the test may become negative; in late syphilis, however, it is usually positive. A fall in titre occurs after the successful treatment of early syphilis; most patients have negative reagin tests 1 year after treatment of primary syphilis and 2 years after treatment of secondary syphilis (Fiumara 1980). The FTA-ABS is the most sensitive of the specific treponemal tests, and is reactive in 70–90% of patients with primary syphilis (Duncan et al 1974). The TPHA test is reactive in 64–87% of patients with primary syphilis; both the FTA-ABS and TPHA tests are positive in virtually all cases of secondary syphilis, and thereafter remain positive indefinitely in more than 95% of untreated patients (King et al 1980).

Treatment. *T. pallidum* is still highly sensitive to penicillin, which is the antibiotic of choice for the treatment of syphilis. The WHO (1983) recommends the following regimens for the treatment of early syphilis:

1. Benzathine penicillin G, 2.4 million units in a single session by intramuscular injection, or:
2. Aqueous procaine penicillin G 600 000 units daily by intramuscular injection for 10 consecutive days.

Patients who are allergic to penicillin should receive:

3. Tetracycline hydrochloride 500 mg by mouth four times a day for 15 days, or:
4. Erythromycin 500 mg by mouth four times a day for 15 days.

Experience of the treatment of syphilis with non-penicillin regimens is limited, and the surveillance of patients treated in this way must be very careful.

Late syphilis requires prolonged therapy, and the following is recommended for the treatment of vulval gummas: aqueous procaine penicillin G 600 000 units by intramuscular injection daily for 15 days.

The prognosis of early syphilis if treated with the above regimens is very good; the skin and mucosal lesions heal quickly, and the enlarged lymph nodes slowly regress. Clinical or serological relapse occurs in about 5% of patients (Schroeter et al 1972), often in circumstances where it is difficult to exclude the possibility of re-infection. Patients treated for early syphilis should be assessed clinically and serologically at the end of treatment, then monthly for 3 months, then three-monthly for at least a year. Early syphilis rapidly becomes non-infectious with antibiotic therapy, and intercourse may safely be resumed on the completion of treatment. It is clearly important to locate, examine and if necessary treat sex partners of all women with early syphilis.

Genital mycoplasmas

The first isolations of mycoplasmas from the human genital tract were in 1937, when *M. hominis* was recovered from a Bartholin abscess, and in 1954, when *Ureaplasma urealyticum* was isolated from a man with non-gonococcal urethritis. The role of these organisms in human genitourinary disease has been reviewed recently (Taylor-Robinson & McCormack 1980, International Symposium 1983).

Colonisation of the female genital tract by mycoplasmas is related to sexual experience. The organisms are infrequently recovered from the vagina of women who have not had intercourse, whereas *M. hominis* is present in 20%, and *U. urealyticum* in 75%, of women who have had several sex partners (McCormack et al 1972). For this reason studies of the role of these organisms in genital tract disease need to be carefully controlled.

Bartholin's abscess

Although the first isolation of *M. hominis* was from an abscess of Bartholin's gland (Dienes & Edsall 1937), there is no evidence that genital mycoplasmas cause the disease. Lee et al (1977) examined aspirates from 34 intact Bartholin's abscesses and isolated *M. hominis* from only one, and *U. urealyticum* from none, although the organisms were present in the vagina in most of the patients.

Vaginitis

Non-specific vaginitis, now more often called bacterial, or anaerobic, vaginosis, is discussed on

p. 105. Although *M. hominis* is isolated more often from women with than from women without the condition (Paavonen et al 1983), the role of the organism has not yet been defined.

Other diseases

There is good evidence that *M. hominis* is a cause of salpingitis (Møller 1983). *M. hominis* is also probably a cause of postpartum and postabortion fever (McCormack & Taylor-Robinson 1980). No definite conclusions have been reached on the suggestion that mycoplasmas, particularly *U. urealyticum*, may be a cause of infertility by affecting spermatozoal motility or endometrial function (Gump et al 1984), or on whether the organisms affect the outcome of pregnancy (Taylor-Robinson & McCormack 1980). The role, if any, of genital mycoplasmas in spontaneous abortion is controversial (Stray-Pedersen et al 1978, Harrison et al 1982). Some studies have suggested that *U. urealyticum* may be associated with low birth weight but this issue too is undecided (McCormack & Taylor-Robinson 1984).

Chlamydia trachomatis

Chlamydiae are specialised intracellular Gram negative bacteria. They have a complex life cycle. The infectious particle is the elementary body (EB), which after entry into susceptible cells undergoes a series of replicative changes culminating in the formation of a cytoplasmic inclusion which ruptures and releases further EB, which then infect other cells.

C. trachomatis has the following serovars (Grayston & Wang 1975): A–C, which cause trachoma, D–K, which cause oculogenital infections including non-gonococcal urethritis (NGU) and its related disorders, and L1–3, which cause lymphogranuloma venereum (LGV).

Oculogenital infections

Epidemiology. Serovars D–K of *C. trachomatis* are sexually transmissible. In men they cause NGU, postgonococcal urethritis and epididymitis, and in women urethritis, cervicitis and salpingitis (Weström & Mårdh 1982). In both sexes ocular contact with infected genital secretions may lead to inclusion conjunctivitis. Infection from the maternal genital tract during delivery often causes chlamydial disease of the eye and respiratory tract in neonates (Oriel & Ridgway 1982).

Between 35 and 50% of NGU is caused by *C. trachomatis*, and about two-thirds of female sex partners of men with chlamydial infection become infected themselves. Studies in Europe and the USA show that the incidence of genital chlamydial infection in women has been rising for more than a decade, and it is now the commonest sexually transmitted infection (Oriel & Ridgway 1982).

Clinical features. In women the major target for chlamydial infection is the columnar epithelium of the endocervix, but the urethra and probably the ducts of Bartholin's glands are also liable to infection. The vagina, except in neonates, is much less vulnerable, although chlamydial infection of the postmenopausal vagina has been recorded (Goldmeier et al 1981).

Chlamydial infection of the lower genital tract in women may be manifested by vulval irritation and vaginal discharge (Hare & Thin 1983), but more often it is symptomless. Infection of the female urethra is not uncommon (Paavonen 1979). It can occur alone, but usually there is a concomitant infection of the cervix. The relationship between genital chlamydial infection and urinary symptoms is controversial. Stamm et al (1980) studied a group of women with dysuria but without significant bacteriuria and reported an association between urinary symptoms, pyuria and chlamydial infection of the urethra and/or cervix in these patients. Other workers, however, have failed to confirm this association (Felman et al 1986).

The isolation of *C. trachomatis* from the ducts of Bartholin's glands has been recorded (Davies et al 1978), but there is no evidence that chlamydiae infect the glands themselves.

Diagnosis. Specimens from potentially infected sites are collected with cotton-wool swabs and cultured on a monolayer of specially prepared cells; McCoy cells treated with cycloheximide are often used. After 48 hours' incubation the monolayer is stained with iodine, Giemsa or immunofluorescence and the inclusions identified by microscopy (Schachter & Dawson 1978) (Fig. 5.17).

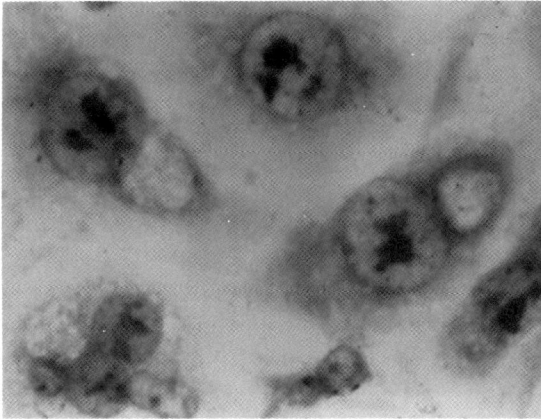

Fig. 5.17 Cell monolayer infected with *Chlamydia trachomatis*: cytoplasmic inclusions.

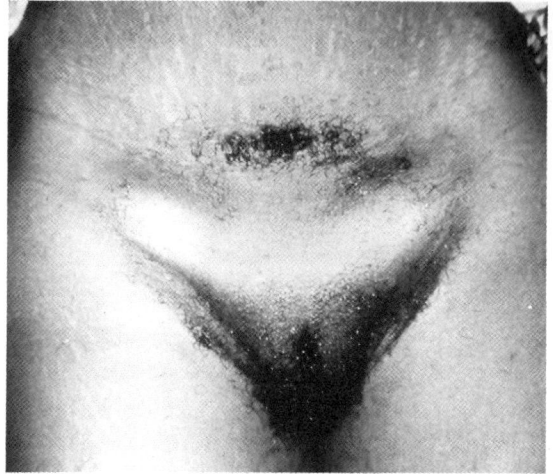

Fig. 5.18 Inguinal lymphadenitis in lymphogranuloma venereum: the primary lesion of LGV is women in usually very inconspicuous.

Recently, antigen detection by direct immuno-fluorescence microscopy and by enzyme-linked immunosorbent assay has become available. While these tests are simpler to perform than culture, both may be less sensitive, particularly in low-risk populations (Smith et al 1987). The Papanicolaou technique is not satisfactory for the diagnosis of chlamydial infection (Schachter & Dawson 1978).

Treatment. *C. trachomatis* is eliminated from the genital tract by tetracyclines. Commonly used therapy is tetracycline hydrochloride 500 mg four times a day for 7 days, or 250 mg four times a day for 14 days. With these regimens cure rates of over 90% can be obtained (Oriel & Ridgway 1982). Women who cannot take tetracyclines because of pregnancy, lactation or intolerance to the drugs may be treated with erythromycin base, stearate or ethyl succinate 250 mg four times a day for 14 days. It is important that male partners of women with genital chlamydial infection are investigated, and treated if necessary.

Lymphogranuloma venereum

The serovars L1–3 of *C. trachomatis* are more invasive than the oculogenital strains and, unlike them, are able to infect lymphatic tissue. The highest prevalence of LGV is in tropical and subtropical regions such as India and West Africa, but it has also occurred in small outbreaks in some temperate regions.

Clinical manifestations. The incubation period of LGV is between 2 and 5 days. The primary lesion is a small painless papule, vesicle or ulcer which rapidly heals. In women this initial lesion is commonest at the fourchette (Greenblatt et al 1959), but it may also occur on the labia, vagina or cervix. Lymphadenopathy, which is a characteristic feature of LGV, develops several weeks later. In women with primary vulval lesions the inguinal glands are affected; they enlarge to form a painful mass which may suppurate and form sinuses (Fig. 5.18). Healing is slow, with extensive scarring, and in some patients the lymphadenopathy persists for months or years.

Late LGV has three components: chronic lymphadenopathy, the anorectal syndrome and genital elephantiasis. The anorectal syndrome is commoner in women than in men. Extension of infection to the wall of the rectum leads to proctocolitis with the passage of mucus, pus and blood (King 1964). Later, rectal strictures, perirectal abscesses and anal fistulae may develop. Vulval elephantiasis is attributed to active chronic infection combined with lymphatic obstruction. Hypertrophic changes appear and there may be polypoid growths and chronic ulceration. Secondary necrosis may lead to much tissue loss ('esthiomene'—from the Greek 'to eat away') (Fig. 5.19).

aspiration, and surgical treatment is usually required for the anorectal syndrome and genital elephantiasis.

MIXED INFECTIONS

Bacterial vaginosis (non-specific vaginitis)

Aetiology

Gardner & Dukes (1955) described a group of women with a grey, homogeneous and malodorous vaginal discharge. There was no laboratory evidence of trichomoniasis or candidosis, but *Gardnerella vaginalis* was recovered on culture. They attributed the syndrome, then called 'non-specific vaginitis', to *Gardnerella* infection.

  G. vaginalis (formerly called *Haemophilus vaginalis*, then *Corynebacterium vaginale*) is a Gram variable coccobacillus with fastidious growth requirements. In up to 50% of healthy women the vagina is colonised with *G. vaginalis*, but in women with 'non-specific vaginitis' the proportion infected, and the colony count, is much higher, the organisms predominating in the vaginal flora (Pheifer et al 1978). This does not prove that *G. vaginalis* causes the disorder, and in recent years attention has been directed towards the role of other organisms.

  Spiegel et al (1980) recovered *Bacteroides* species and *Peptococcus* species from women with 'non-specific vaginitis', and showed by gas-liquid chromotography that in this disease the succinate/lactate ratio is increased; several amines not normally present in the vagina, including putrescine and cadaverine, occur and give the secretions their characteristic smell (Pheifer et al 1978, Hill 1985). After treatment with metronidazole, which is very active against anaerobes but only moderately so against *G. vaginalis*, the vaginal flora and biochemistry return to normal. Anaerobes are not the only organisms associated with the condition, because both *M. hominis* and a motile rod now named *Mobiluncus* have been isolated (Easmon 1986). It may be concluded that 'non-specific vaginitis' is the result of a disturbed relationship between anaerobes, *G. vaginalis* and other organisms. Why this should occur, and the role, if any, of host factors are alike unknown. The disease has now been renamed bacterial vaginosis, or anaerobic vaginosis.

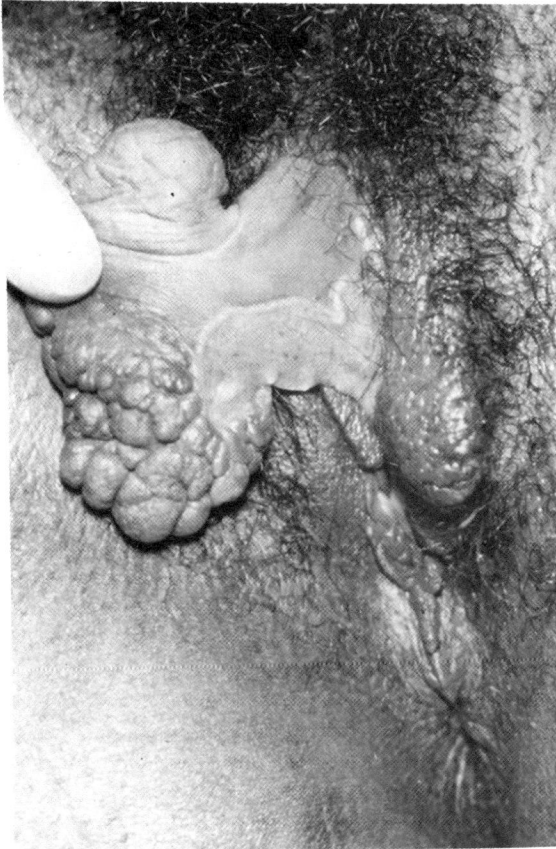

Fig. 5.19 Vulval elephantiasis with esthiomene: notice superficial ulceration. (By courtesy of Baillière Tindall Ltd: Slides of Sexually Transmitted Diseases)

Diagnosis. LGV must be differentiated from other causes of genital ulceration and lymphadenopathy, particularly syphilis. The best diagnostic laboratory test is cell culture for *C. trachomatis*; specimens from any site may be examined, but aspirated pus is the best material. The LGV complement fixation test (LGVCFT) is widely used. It becomes positive within a week or two of infection (Alergant 1957). It is usually impracticable to look for rising titres of antibodies, and if the clinical signs of LGV are present, a titre of >64 is regarded as confirmatory (Schachter & Dawson 1978).

  Treatment. LGV responds well to tetracyclines; for initial treatment tetracycline hydrochloride 1–2 g daily in divided doses for 10 days to 3 weeks has been recommended (Schachter & Dawson 1978); more prolonged therapy may be needed for extensive disease. Sulphonamides and erythromycin have also been used. Inguinal abscesses need

Epidemiology

Bacterial vaginosis is probably commoner than any other vaginal disorder, including trichomoniasis and candidosis (Amsel et al 1983, Blackwell et al 1983). It seems to be confined to sexually active women, but whether sexual transmission of an infecting agent, for example *G. vaginalis*, initiates the disease is uncertain (Pheifer et al 1978); *G. vaginalis* is not known to cause any disease in men (Bowie et al 1977).

Clinical features and diagnosis

Women usually complain of a malodorous vaginal discharge, and sometimes of mild vaginal or vulval irritation, but some are symptomless (Amsel et al 1983). Examination shows a homogeneous grey vaginal discharge, without excessive vaginal erythema. Vulvitis (which is a major feature of vaginal infections such as trichomoniasis and candidosis) is not present. The vaginal pH is >4.5. A fishy amine odour can be smelt when the secretions are mixed with a drop of 10% KOH on a slide. A wet mount shows few leucocytes, but numerous bacteria are present, and some epithelial cells are covered with bacteria so that their outline is obscured ('clue cells'). Culture for *G. vaginalis* and anaerobes is not necessary for the diagnosis of bacterial vaginosis (Easmon 1986).

Treatment

The nitroimidazoles are effective for the treatment of bacterial vaginosis. Metronidazole 200 mg three times a day for 7 days is usually curative. Ampicillin is less effective (Lee & Schmale, 1973) and tetracyclines and erythromycin are both ineffective (Spiegel et al 1980). Sulphonamide creams are obsolete, and have been abandoned (Spiegel et al 1980). At present there is no evidence that investigation or treatment of male sex partners of women with bacterial vaginosis is necessary.

Erosive vulvitis

Bacteroides species are Gram negative anaerobes which are often associated with salpingitis, septic abortion, postpartum infection and other septic conditions of the female genital tract. *B. melaninogenicus* is largely responsible for a form of oropharyngeal ulceration called Vincent's angina; this disease was formerly attributed to a mixed infection with an anaerobic spirochaete *Borrelia vincentii* and a fusiform bacillus *Leptotrichia buccalis*, jointly referred to as 'Vincent's organisms'. Erosive balanitis and erosive vulvitis probably have an aetiology similar to Vincent's angina.

Erosive balanitis is quite common, often occurring as a complication of other infections, as a result of poor subpreputial hygiene, or as an iatrogenic condition. Erosive vulvitis is rarer, but has comparable predisposing causes. Erosive vaginitis is a rare complication of tissue necrosis and retained secretions in seriously ill women (Gardner & Kaufman 1981).

Erosive vulvitis is treated by frequent bathing with 0.9% saline, combined with a course of metronidazole 200 mg three times a day for 7 days for the anaerobic infection. Predisposing causes should be corrected.

Synergistic bacterial gangrene, postoperative progressive gangrene: (necrotising fasciitis)

These conditions are not clearly separable, being progressive and often fatal infections of the superficial fascia and subcutaneous tissues. Necrotising fasciitis is a misnomer according to some and the alternative terms are preferable (Stone & Martin 1972).

The initiating lesion may be an operation or a trivial injury, or even be inapparent. The infection spreads centrifugally through the subcutaneous tissues, and the superficial fascia may be destroyed. Toxaemia is profound. The condition has a varied polymicrobial aetiology, involving many combinations of aerobic micro-aerophilic and anaerobic organisms (Rea & Wyrick 1970). Factors which predispose to the disease and worsen the prognosis are diabetes mellitus, arteriosclerosis, debilitating diseases and irradiation for malignancy.

The earliest sign is an erythematous or violaceous discoloration of the skin, with subcutaneous induration and oedema and marked tenderness.

Later, bullae and subcutaneous necrosis develop. Gas formation can commonly be detected clinically and, more often, radiologically (Fisher et al 1979). The patient becomes very ill, with fever and toxaemia, and the prognosis is poor, particularly if treatment is delayed.

The vulva is a site of election. Cases involving the vulva have been described by Stone & Martin (1972), Borkawf (1973), Hammer & Wanger (1977), Shy & Eschenbach (1981), Meltzer (1983) and Addison et al (1984). The cases of Ewing et al (1979) where three out of four patients who developed oedema post-partum died may fall into this group. Roberts & Hester (1972) described four patients with progressive synergistic bacterial gangrene which originated in abscesses of the vulva or Bartholin's glands; all were diabetic, and three of them died.

Successful treatment requires early diagnosis, wide débridement of infected tissues and appropriate antibiotic therapy.

It is important to distinguish these conditions from pyoderma gangrenosum (p. 142), (Hutchinson et al 1976); in past reports they have probably often been confused.

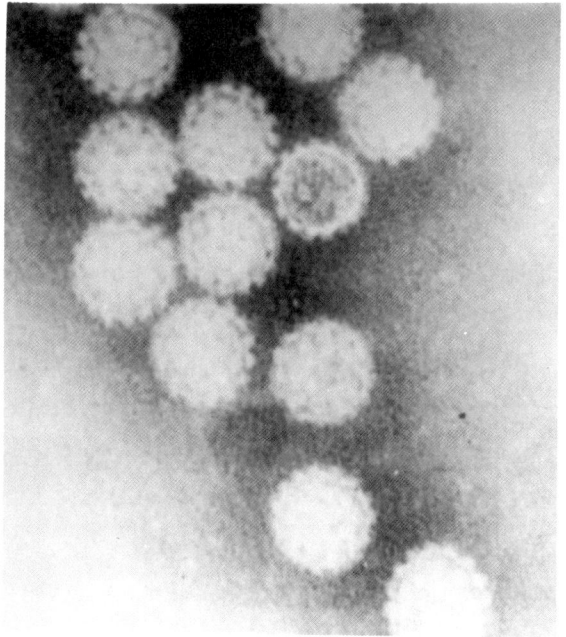

Fig. 5.20 Papillomavirus particles.

Hidradenitis (see p. 153)

INFECTION WITH VIRUSES

Genital papillomavirus infection

Aetiology

The genus Papillomavirus contains many species specific viruses which induce benign skin and mucosal tumours in a wide range of animals. The species which infects humans is designated human papillomavirus (HPV). The virion is 50–55 nm in diameter; the capsid shows icosahedral symmetry and is composed of 72 capsomeres. The genome is a single molecule of double-stranded DNA (Fig. 5.20).

It has been difficult to study papillomaviruses because it has not been possible to induce replication in tissue culture, but recently genetic manipulation techniques have been successfully applied to the study of viral DNA in tissues and viral extracts and knowledge has rapidly increased. By applying these techniques to HPV it has been possible to identify viral types according to the homology of their DNA molecules. If an HPV has less than 50% homology with a virus already isolated it will be put in a new group. According to these criteria there are more than 40 types of HPV. Eight of these have been recovered from the genital tract: HPV6 and HPV11 are particularly associated with condylomata acuminata, flat condylomas of the cervix, cervical intraepithelial neoplasia (CIN), and juvenile laryngeal papillomatosis; HPV16 and HPV18 are present for the most part in the cells of carcinoma in situ and invasive cancer of the penis, vulva and cervix, and HPV31, 33, 34 and 35 have been isolated from small numbers of premalignant and malignant genital lesions (McCance 1986). HPV16 sequences have been demonstrated in the cervix of women without cytological signs of neoplasia (Toon et al 1986).

Oncogenicity of papillomaviruses. The majority of lesions induced by papillomaviruses are benign, but malignant transformation has been observed in some of them. The cottontail rabbit is subject to a papillomavirus infection which causes benign skin warts; 25% of these become malignant, and the development of malignancy is hastened by the application of tar (Syverton 1952). In cattle, bovine papillomavirus type 4 causes benign oesophageal and intestinal papillomas; these become malignant if the animals are fed with bracken (Jarrett et al 1981). In humans, epidermodysplasia verruciformis (EV) is a rare autosomal recessive skin disease characterised by the appearance of widespread plane warts and scaly erythematous patches. One-third of patients with EV develop squamous cell skin cancers, particularly in scaly lesions exposed to sunlight; malignancy is most likely in lesions containing HPV5 DNA sequences (Jablonska & Orth 1983). In the case of verrucous carcinoma the co-factor may be radiation used in therapy. These models suggest that malignant transformation of benign viral proliferative lesions can occur, and that such transformation is conditioned, at least in part, by the viral type present and by the operation of a co-factor.

Pathology of genital lesions caused by HPV. The commonest result of infection by HPV is the formation of warts. The histological features of these lesions are familiar (Lever & Schaumberg-Lever 1975). The dermal papillae are elongated. The basal cell layer is intact, and the spinous or prickle cell layer is hyperplastic (acanthosis). The granular cell layer is often well developed, and contains large vacuolated cells; some of these have cytoplasmic eosinophilic inclusions composed of abnormal keratin, and others have nuclear basophilic inclusions composed of aggregates of papillomavirus particles. Morphologically, four basic types of wart can be distinguished: the common wart (verruca vulgaris), the plantar wart (verruca plantaris), the plane wart (verruca plana) and the anogenital condyloma acuminatum. In the last of these acanthosis is marked, while the stratum corneum usually consists of only a layer or two or parakeratotic cells (Fig. 5.21).

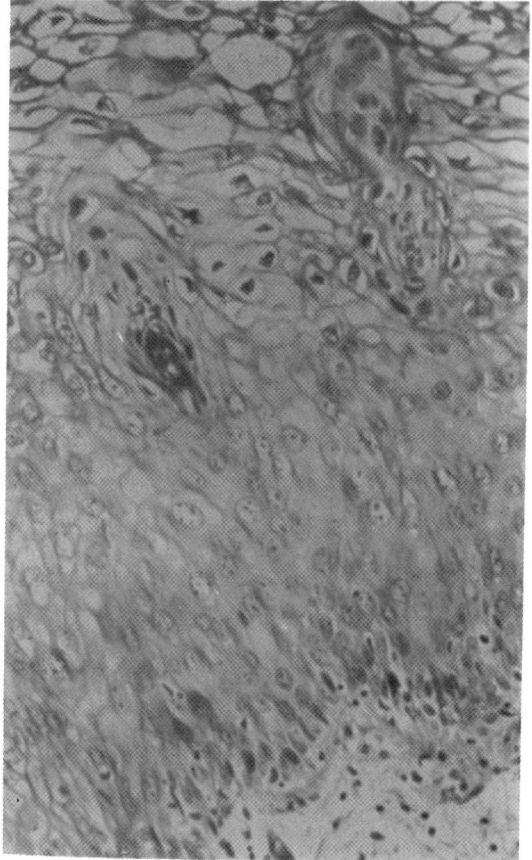

Fig. 5.21 Condyloma acuminatum histology: the section shows acanthosis and superficial vacuolated cells.

Gross et al (1982) sought correlations between the infecting HPV types and the histology of the resulting warts. They found that common warts contained HPV1, HPV2 and HPV4, while plantar warts contained only HPV1. HPV3 was found exclusively in plane warts, and HPV6 only in genital condylomata acuminata. The histological features of the latter were: (1) various degrees of parakeratosis and hyperkeratosis, (2) pronounced acanthosis and papillomatosis, (3) marked perinuclear vacuolation in the outer cell layers, (4) moderate granular layer prominence and (5) increased mitosis in the basal layers.

It is possible to demonstrate the presence of HPV in the cells of genital warts. In about 50% of lesions virus particles can be seen by electron microscopy, and viral antigen can be demonstrated, by immunochemical methods, in the nuclei of infected cells. These techniques will give positive results only in the superficial cell layers of warts. However, the technique of DNA–DNA hybridisation can be used to demonstrate viral DNA in all parts of the lesions (McCance 1986).

Immunology. Studies with immunosuppressed patients show the importance of immune responses in limiting disease caused by HPV. Skin warts are common in immunosuppressed individuals (Spencer & Andersen 1979) (Fig. 5.22). Women who are immunosuppressed after renal transplantation are liable to condylomata acuminata, and women with lymphomas, who often have defective cell-mediated immunity, are liable to vulval warts, which are not only difficult to cure but may progress to intra-epithelial neoplasia (Shokri-Tabibzadeh et al 1981, Schneider et al 1983).

The study of circulating antibodies to HPV has been hampered by the lack of viral antigen imposed by inability to propagate the virus, but these antibodies have been detected in patients with cutaneous warts, particularly when they are regressing (Pyrhonen & Johansson 1975). Antibodies to the 'genital' types, HPV6 and HPV11, have not been studied, but Baird (1983) measured antibodies to a group antigen, obtained from bovine papillomaviral lesions, by an ELISA technique. He found that women with vulval warts, CIN or cervical carcinoma had antibodies present, and to a higher titre, more often than women without these diseases; this suggests that antibody production does occur in women with genital warts despite the small amount of virus often present in these lesions. The question is discussed also on page 71.

Epidemiology

Genital HPV infections are sexually transmissible, with an infectivity of about 60%; the incubation period of genital warts appears to be between 3 weeks and 9 months or more (Oriel 1971). The peak age of onset in women is between 19 and 22 years, and women with genital warts admit to an earlier age of first intercourse and more sex partners than those without the disease (Syrjanen et al 1984). Women with vulval warts, whether seen in STD clinics or in dermatological practice, often have other STDs (Kinghorn 1978; Fairris et al 1984). There is no evidence of an epidemiological link between genital and cutaneous warts. Genital warts are reportable from STD clinics in England, and the incidence appears to be increasing. In 1972 5570 new cases in women were reported, an incidence of 23.42 per 100 000 population; the corresponding figures for 1982 were 12 704 new cases, an incidence of 52.90 per 100 000 population (Chief medical officer, 1974, 1984a).

Vulval warts were formerly uncommon in prepubertal children, but in recent years they seem to be occurring more often (Stumpf 1980). Several modes of infection are possible. Infants can acquire an HPV infection from a mother with genital warts during delivery (Patel and Groff 1972); the resulting disease may not be apparent for several months. One infant reported by Tang et al (1978) actually had genital lesions present at birth, possibly due to an ascending infection or to haematogenous spread of the virus. Conceivably, vulval HPV infection in children could be caused by close non-sexual contact with a family member (Stumpf 1980), or virus

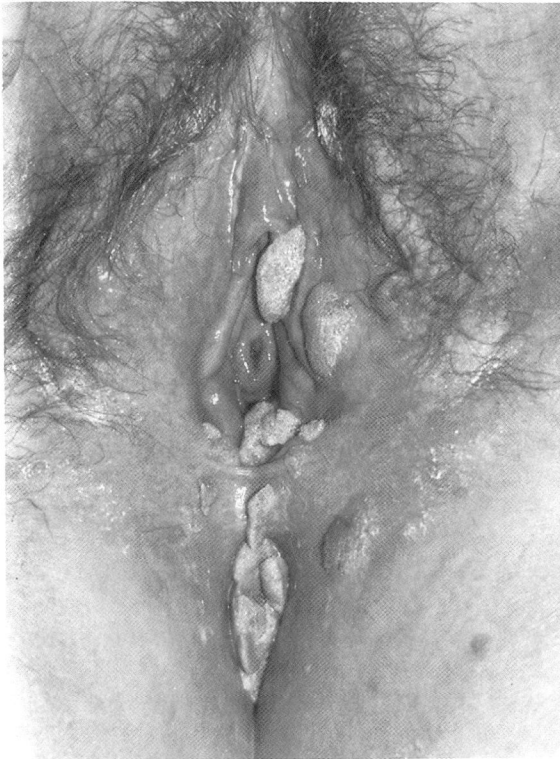

Fig. 5.22 Condylomata acuminata in an immunosuppressed woman.

from warts on the child's or the mother's hands be accidentally transferred to the genital area (Bender 1986). However, it is believed that up to 80% of childhood condylomata acuminata result from sexual molestation (Seidel et al 1979, McCoy et al 1982, de Jong et al 1982, Schachner and Hankin 1985).

Recently, genital tract papillomas in four girls, aged 2–8 years have been examined for HPV by molecular hybridisation, and DNA sequences of HPV6, HPV11 and HPV16 were found to be present (Rock et al 1986). Since these sequences are also present in genital condylomas there is a clear implication that the virus infecting these children was derived from adults with genital warts. This does not prove sexual abuse, as the virus could have been transferred in some other way. The presentation of a child with anogenital wart disease raises difficult medical and social problems (Bender 1986). It is obvious that doctors and other health care workers must identify sexual molestation if it is occurring. It is also important that the desire to protect the child should not result in an innocent adult being wrongly accused of sexual assault. Schachner and Hankin (1985) have listed a series of criteria which may be helpful in making a decision on the matter of sexual abuse in these cases. They include the medical history, the physical findings (including the presence of other sexually transmitted infections) and behavioural and psychological abnormalities. When more is known about the natural history of genital HPV infections in children it may also be possible to use virological procedures.

In female children condylomata acuminata may affect the labial, vaginal and perianal regions (Fig. 5.23). A large lesion of the urethra in a 2½-year-old girl has been described by Zamora et al (1983).

The possibility that laryngeal papillomatosis may develop in infants born to women with genital HPV lesions is important. In one report, two-thirds of the mothers of children with this disease had had genital warts during pregnancy (Quick et al 1980). The infectivity of maternal HPV infection to the baby is not known, but is probably low (Cohn et al 1981). Both HPV6 and HPV11, which are commonly associated with vulval and cervical condylomas, have been recovered from juvenile laryngeal papillomas (Gissmann et al 1983). The epidemiolo-

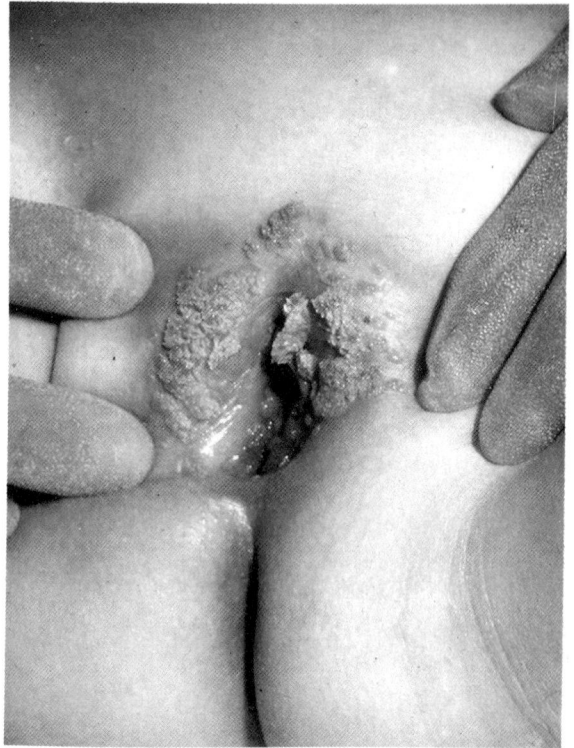

Fig. 5.23 Condylomata acuminata in a child. (Reproduced from Beilby and Ridley (1987) by courtesy of the authors and publisher)

gy of HPV infections in neonates has recently been reviewed by Mounts and Shah (1984).

Clinical features

HPV can infect any part of the vulva, but the earliest lesions most often appear on areas traumatised during coitus such as the fourchette and adjacent labia. Warts are commonly seen on the labia majora and minora, around the urethra and above the clitoris. They often extend into the lower part of the vagina, and sometimes the whole of the vagina is involved. The disease can spread backwards to affect the perineum and peri-anal area and the anal canal (Fig. 5.24). Lesions may also appear in the genitocrural folds and in the pubic area. HPV infection of the vulva is usually expressed as condylomata acuminata, but sometimes as flat lesions resembling plane warts, and a few patients exhibit lesions closely resembling common warts as seen on non-genital areas. If the vulva is treated with 5%

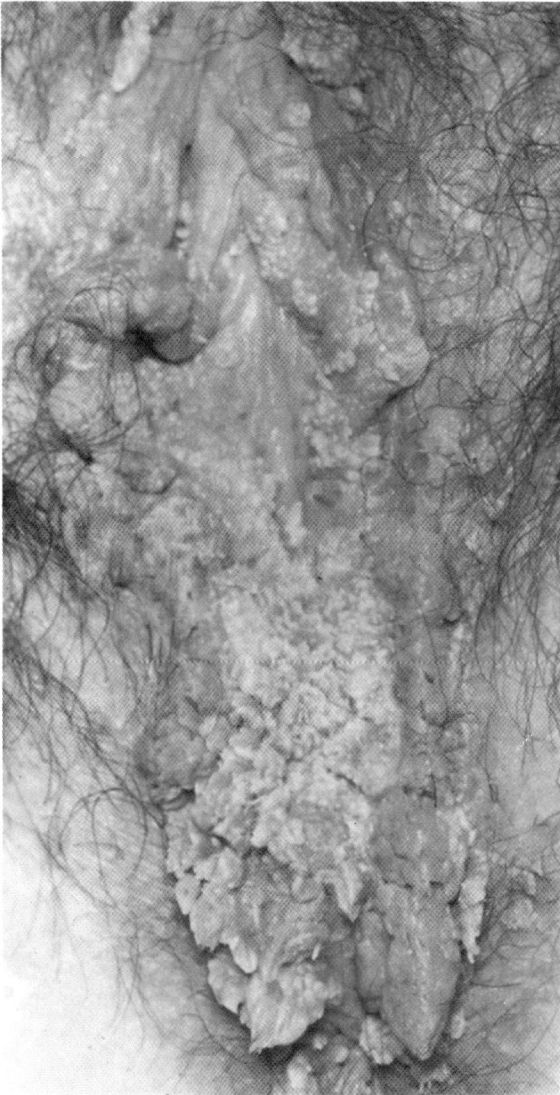

Fig. 5.24 Condylomata acuminata: this patient has extensive vulval disease extending on to the perineum. (By courtesy of Baillière Tindall Ltd: Slides of Sexually Transmitted Diseases)

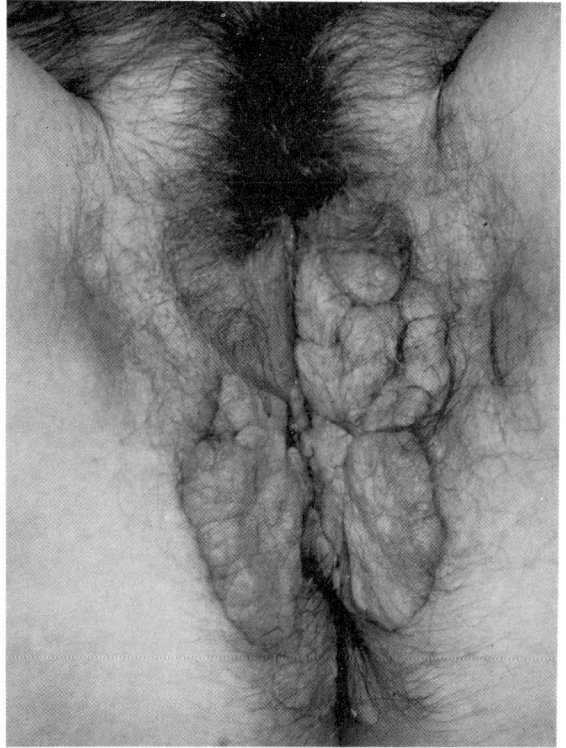

Fig. 5.25 Large condylomata acuminata: in a middle-aged woman. (Reproduced from Beilby & Ridley (1987) by courtesy of the authors and publisher)

acetic acid and then examined with a colposcope, it is apparent that the area involved in HPV infection is considerably greater than naked eye inspection would suggest, and that small lesions are scattered over wide areas of the labia and around the urethra. Subclinical warty lesions may be found in benign dermatoses, for example lichen sclerosus et atrophicus—findings which are as yet of uncertain relevance. With age, warts tend to become hyperkeratotic and in middle-aged women, while

remaining histologically benign, may appear as vast warty masses (Fig. 5.25).

About 15% of women with vulval warts show cervical condylomata acuminata, 'exophytic condylomas', which can be seen by the naked eye. Recent research has shown that HPV infection of the cervix is much commoner than had been thought because in many women it is expressed as 'non-condylomatous wart virus infection' (Reid et al 1980), appearing on colposcopy as a flat shiny-white epithelium, often with a raised and roughened surface (Fig. 5.26). These 'flat condylomas' were previously in many cases misdiagnosed as mild dysplasia, but there is no doubt that they are viral (Meisels et al 1982). Cervical HPV infection is associated with a characteristic cytological appearance, of which the presence of vacuolated koilocytic cells is the most important (Meisels et al 1977). Cytological and colposcopic studies have shown that as many as 50% of women with vulval

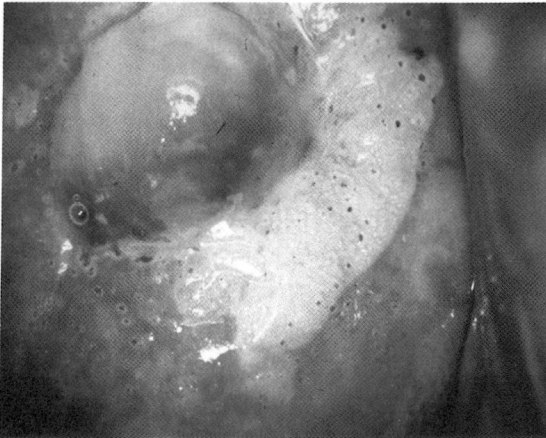

Fig. 5.26 Flat condyloma of cervix: these lesions can be seen by colposcopy after the application of 5% acetic acid. They cannot be identified with the naked eye.

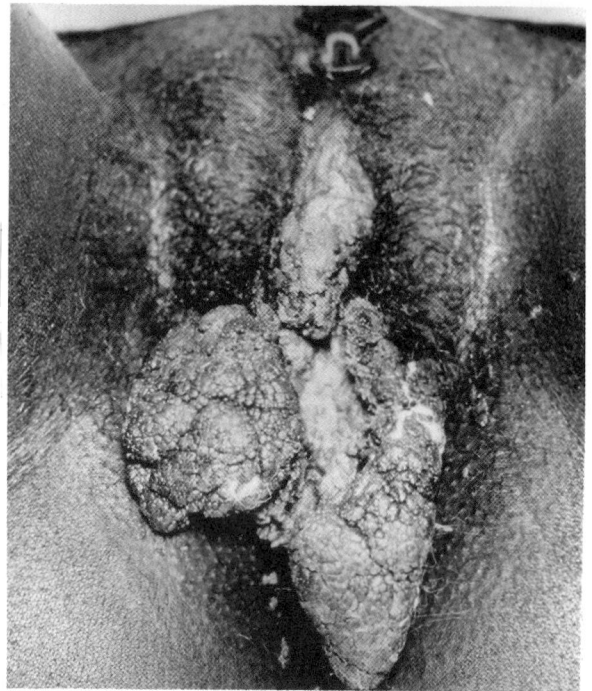

Fig. 5.27 Large condylomata acuminata in pregnancy: these lesions regressed completely after delivery without treatment

warts show evidence of HPV infection of the cervix (Walker et al 1983). Similar 'non-condylomatous' lesions affect the vagina (Roy et al 1981).

Histologically, the majority of vulval HPV lesions are typical condylomata acuminata (Schmauz & Owor 1980). Mature papillomavirus particles can be identified by electron microscopy in about 50% of vulval warts (Oriel & Almeida, 1970), and in a similar proportion papillomavirus antigens have been identified by immunochemical techniques (Woodruff et al 1980, Kurman et al 1981). The viral types most commonly found in vulval warts are HPV6 and HPV11 (Gissmann et al 1983).

HPV infection during pregnancy. Physiological depression of cell-mediated immunity occurs during pregnancy, and this may be the reason for the large vulval condylomata acuminata seen in pregnant women; exceptionally, they may cause problems in delivery because of obstruction of labour and haemorrhage (Wilson 1973) (Fig. 5.27). After delivery these enlarged vulval warts regress, and may disappear completely (Oriel 1971). There is no evidence that the outcome of pregnancy is affected by the presence of condylomata acuminata (Chuang et al 1984).

Infants born to women with vulval warts may develop genital condylomata acuminata, particularly of the vulva, but the possibility of laryngeal papillomatosis is of much greater importance.

Complications

Giant condyloma. This is a rare tumour which was first described by Buschke & Loewenstein. Some say it is identical to verrucous carcinoma. In most reported cases the penis has been affected, but vulval giant condyloma has been described (Baird et al 1979). The disease starts as an apparently straightforward viral wart, but this relentlessly enlarges and causes much tissue destruction (Fig. 5.28). Clinically, it appears to be malignant, but histologically it is benign, resembling condyloma acuminatum; the tumour does not metastasise. Occasionally giant condyloma is further complicated by the development of squamous cell carcinoma (Trope et al 1982). The nature of giant condyloma, and the reasons for its aggressive behaviour, are not understood. Recently Gissmann et al (1982) identified HPV6 DNA in each of three tumours; presumably other factors are involved; what these are is unknown.

Vulval intra-epithelial neoplasia. This term

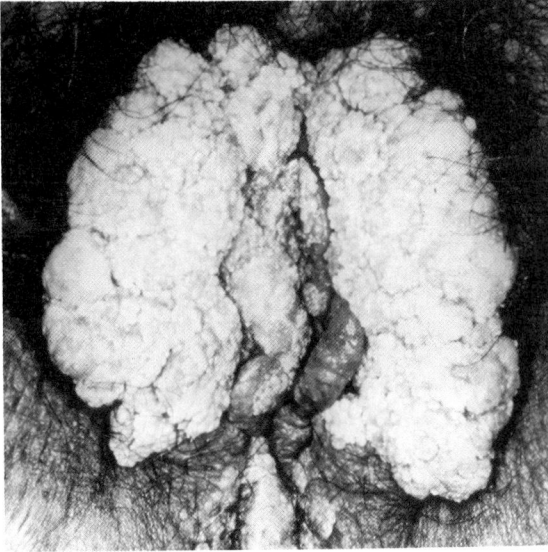

Fig. 5.28 Giant condyloma of vulva.

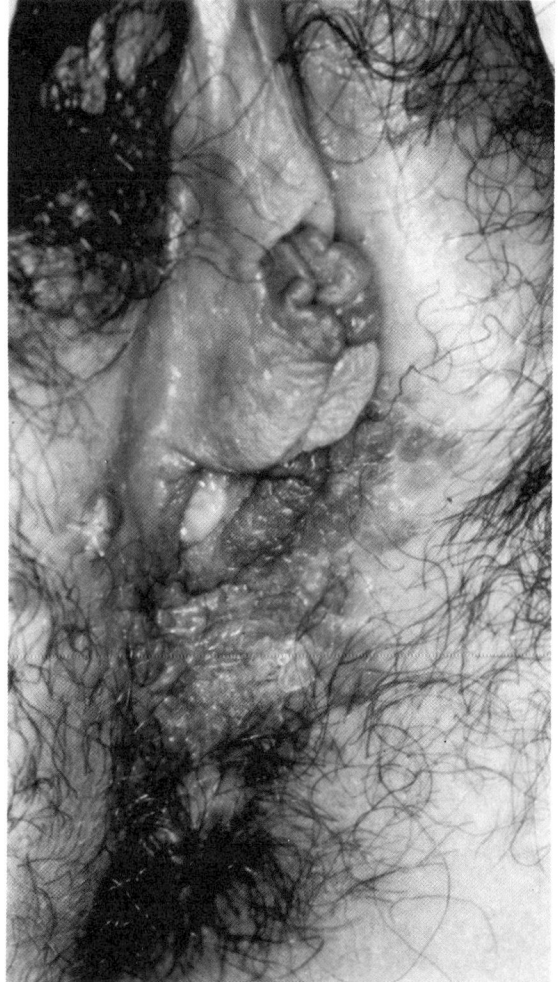

Fig. 5.29 (a) and (b) Bowenoid papulosis (VIN): it is important to distinguish these premalignant lesions from condylomata acuminata.

(VIN) comprises a group of lesions—single or multiple, papular or erosive, pigmented or non-pigmented—previously designated with familiar eponyms including Bowen's disease, Bowenoid papulosis and erythroplasia of Queyrat as well as carcinoma in situ (Fig. 5.29). Histologically, VIN lesions are now graded 1–3 according to the amount of epithelial pleomorphism (Ridley 1984); they are usually aneuploid (Fu et al 1981). VIN, particularly VIN3, is often associated with neoplasms in other parts of the genital tract, particularly the cervix (Campion et al 1985).

VIN is often associated with HPV infection. Clinically, vulval warts may precede or accompany Bowenoid papulosis, carcinoma in situ or even invasive cancer (Laohadtanaphorn et al 1979, Shafeek et al 1979, Wade et al 1979). In premenopausal women the majority of VIN is multifocal, and often accompanied by overtly condylomatous lesions of the vulva (Stanbridge & Butler 1983). In virological studies Kimura et al (1978) identified papillomavirus particles by electron microscopy of some Bowenoid papulosis lesions, and HPV antigen has been detected in Bowenoid vulval lesions by immunochemical techniques (Braun et al 1983, Guillet et al, 1984). Crum et al (1982a, b) looked for HPV antigen in 68 VIN lesions, of which 39

were also tested for viral DNA content. Of the 68 VIN specimens, 4 (6%) gave positive results for HPV. Of the 39 specimens tested for DNA, 35 were aneuploid and one of these 35 contained HPV; 4 were polyploid, and 2 of these 4 contained HPV. It was suggested that HPV is detected infrequently in aneuploid lesions because epithelial maturation is needed for viral assembly; further, abnormal mitoses and atypical nuclear enlargement may be specific predictors of aneuploidy and therefore be reliable for distinguishing condyloma acuminatum from VIN.

Belief in a causal association between HPV and

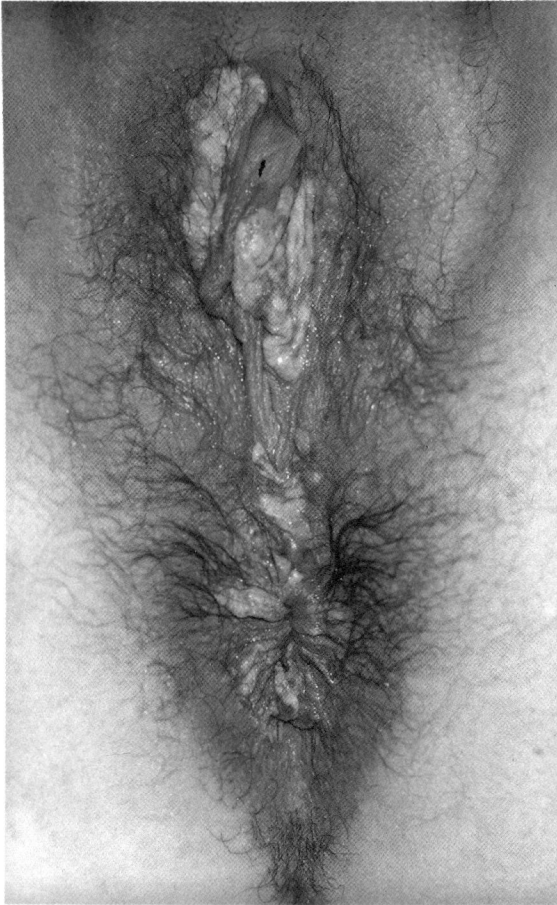

B

VIN has been strengthened by recent developments in molecular virology. HPV6 and HPV11 are present in most condylomata acuminata, and in the majority of non-condylomatous infections of the cervix; they are also associated with CIN grades 1–3 (Gissmann et al 1982, zur Hausen et al 1984, McCance et al 1983). In contrast, HPV16 and HPV18 are consistently associated with carcinoma of the cervix (zur Hausen et al 1984). These findings are paralleled in recent studies of VIN. HPV DNA is present in at least 50% of cases of Bowenoid papulosis (Zachow et al 1982), and Ikenberg et al (1983) have detected HPV16 DNA and related sequences in six out of ten biopsies of Bowen's disease and in eight of ten of Bowenoid papulosis. Campion and Singer (1987) have shown in molecular hybridisation studies that HPV16 DNA sequences were present in over 70% of biopsy specimens from VIN3 and in over 50% of those

from vulval carcinomas. The histopathology of VIN was reviewed in detail by Buckley et al (1984) and is discussed further on p. 267, treatment is considered on p. 334.

Opinions on the natural history of HPV infection of the female genital tract, and its relationship to CIN, vaginal intra-epithelial neoplasia (VAIN), VIN and invasive cancer of the cervix and vulva are developing rapidly (Ridley 1986). A hypothesis can be made that women infected by HPV6 or HPV11 develop vulval, vaginal or cervical lesions which do not progress to malignancy, and indeed may regress spontaneously; on the other hand, women infected by HPV16 or HPV18 may be at greater risk of vulval or cervical intra-epithelial neoplasia and cancer. It seems very probably that co-factors are also involved, since the number of individuals infected with these viral types far exceeds the number who develop premalignant and malignant tumours. Among these co-factors may be Herpes simplex virus infection (zur Hausen 1986). This hypothesis will need validation by further research, but in the mean time the multifocal nature of both benign and malignant HPV infection of the lower female genital tract must influence clinicians in their management of these disorders.

Diagnosis

Vulval warts must be distinguished from other papular conditions of the area. Fibroepithelial polyps should give no difficulty. Altmeyer et al (1982) and Friedrich (1983) described vulval lesions which resembled hirsutes papillaris penis (p. 199) and which might be mistaken for warts, especially of the 'non-condylomatous' type. Among infective diseases to be distinguished from warts are molluscum contagiosum, the papules and condylomata lata of secondary syphilis (see p. 101) and the vulval lesions of donovanosis. Benign vulval tumours such as fibroma, lipoma, hidradenoma, adenoma and endometrioma are usually diagnosed histologically after biopsy.

The distinction of vulval warts from VIN and invasive carcinoma is of great importance but may be difficult, particularly since the diseases may occur together. Biopsy of all vulval lesions whose nature is uncertain, and of condylomata acuminata which are responding poorly to treatment, is mandatory.

Some physicians would go further and recommend that all papular vulval lesions should be biopsied before treatment.

Treatment

Before treatment of vulval HPV-induced lesions is undertaken it is necessary: (1) to confirm that they are benign (see above), (2) to determine the extent of the disease, using vulval/cervical colposcopy, cervical cytology and biopsy as required, and (3) to exclude associated infections. It is important that sex partners of these patients should be examined, as they often have HPV lesions of the genitals (Levine et al 1984). In view of the widespread involvement of the lower genital tract, the frequent concurrence of other infections (Fairris et al 1984) and the need for contact tracing, there is a good case for the initial management of vulval warts being in the hands of genitourinary physicians.

Owing to the spontaneous remission of some genital warts, and the lack of well-controlled clinical trials for most forms of therapy, the treatment of the disease requires sound clinical judgment. The following methods are in use:

Chemotherapy.

Podophyllin. Podophyllin resin is extracted from the rhizomes of *Podophyllum peltatum* and *P. emodi*, and contains several cytotoxic agents of variable potency. A 20–25% solution in ethanol or benzoin tincture is applied to the warts and allowed to dry. Initially, it is washed off after 4 hours, but this interval can be lengthened to 24 hours with successive applications. Treatment is continued once or twice weekly until the lesions have regressed.

Podophyllin has several disadvantages, and in some countries it is not used at all. Its composition is not standardised, and response to therapy is variable and often very poor. It is irritating to normal skin, which means that it must be applied by medical or paramedical personnel and not by the patient. Further, it is potentially toxic. Small quantities are well tolerated, but liberal application to large wart masses has been followed by absorption and systemic effects which include dizziness, vomiting, peripheral neuritis and even coma and death (Montaldi et al 1974). These effects are particularly important during pregnancy, when intrauterine death may occur (Chamberlain et al 1972).

A further possible problem is that in some circumstances podophyllin may be teratogenic (Karol et al 1980). For these reasons, not more than 0.5 ml of 25% solution should be applied during one treatment session, prolonged treatment avoided, and the agent not used at all during pregnancy or for the treatment of cervical lesions. Microscopic differentiation of its cytotoxic effects from neoplasia is possible (King & Sullivan 1947, Wade & Ackerman 1979).

5-fluorouracil. This cytotoxic agent has been used as a 5% cream for the treatment of vulval warts, and successes have been claimed (Handojo & Pardjono 1973). Its action is difficult to control, and it may irritate normal vulval skin; it has not come into general use.

Interferons. Interferons (IFN) inhibit DNA viruses and stimulate local immunity. Their use in the treatment of vulval warts has been reviewed by Kinghorn (1986). Intramuscular injections of fibroblast interferon have been given for up to 6 weeks for vulval and vaginal condylomas, and good results have been reported (Alewattagama & Kinghorn 1984, Schonfield et al 1984). Intralesional IFN alpha-2b has been shown to be an apparently effective treatment for condylomata acuminata in a randomised double-blind study (Eron et al 1986). Side effects of IFN therapy include influenzal symptoms and blood dyscrasias. The place of IFN in the treatment of vulval papillomavirus lesions will require further study.

Surgery. Cryotherapy with liquid nitrogen or a nitrous oxide probe is useful for the treatment of isolated vulval warts, particularly if they are keratinised. Electrocautery, or coagulation with a 'Hyfrecator', under local anaesthesia is an effective outpatient procedure, but it is not suitable for extensive disease. For this, and for warts which are recalcitrant to other forms of therapy, destruction under general anaesthesia is necessary, and a carbon dioxide (CO_2) laser is now often used.

Like cautery, diathermy and the cryosurgery probe, the CO_2 laser causes thermal destruction. Its advantage over the other techniques is its precision: the depth of destruction can be accurately measured, and the loss of normal tissue adjacent to the infected areas is minimal (Ferenczy 1983). Healing is more rapid than after cautery or diathermy (Grundsell et al 1984). If laser therapy of vulval condylomas is performed under colposcopic control, any associated cervical disease can be assessed at the same time and if necessary treated similarly. Bellina (1983) found results with the laser were improved if follow-up was prolonged, with retreatment if necessary, and if male sex partners were examined and treated. Kaufman & Friedrich (1985) preferred the laser to electrosurgery on the grounds of thoroughness and time. Electrosurgery was, however, better for large masses of warts.

Recently, Ferenczy et al (1985) have detected papillomavirus sequences in histologically normal skin adjacent to genital warts, and noted that recurrences after laser therapy of the warts occurred in some of these patients. This raises the possibility that extension of the field of therapy may reduce the risk of recurrence. This approach has been used by Reid (1985) in treating extensive lesions of the vulva, vagina and cervix.

Autogenous vaccine therapy. Autogenous vaccines were first used for the treatment of genital warts many years ago, and encouraging results have been reported in uncontrolled trials. Powell et al (1970) described the successful treatment of lesions which had proved refractory to conventional measures. They suggested that HPV is relatively isolated from the immune system in the superficial layers of the epithelium, and that systemic injections of wart extracts might provoke an enhanced immunological response.

Uncertainty about the content of these vaccines and concern about the oncogenic potential of HPV has limited the use of this form of treatment. Its efficacy is in any case unproved; one controlled trial showed no difference between the response of patients with condylomata acuminata to vaccine or placebo therapy (Malison et al 1982).

Treatment of vulval warts during pregnancy. Recent advances in the epidemiology of HPV infections have posed some problems concerning the treatment of condylomas during pregnancy. On the one hand, vulval warts usually regress after pregnancy, so that although they may become large it may be best to leave them untreated, or with minimal treatment; this is the traditional view. On the other hand, infection may be transmitted to infants, causing genital warts or, much more seriously, laryngeal papillomatosis; although the risk of these diseases is probably low, their existence may

suggest that an interventionist and aggressive treatment policy should be pursued. Until more is known about the natural history and complications of genital warts during pregnancy, decisions about treatment remain a matter of personal opinion.

Podophyllin should not be used during pregnancy because of its potential toxicity, but CO_2 laser therapy is safe, and has largely replaced cautery or diathermy (Ferenczy 1984). Some obstetricians perform caesarian section if there is extensive condylomatous vulvovaginal disease (Goldman 1977), but the indications for this have not yet been defined.

Genital herpesvirus infection

Genital herpes

The first description of genital herpes was given by the French physician Jean Anstruc in 1736. By the end of the 19th century it had become quite common; Unna said in 1883 that he had seen 200 cases in 4 years in prostitutes attending an STD clinic in Hamburg. Herpes simplex virus (HSV) was first grown in the laboratory in the mid 1920s. Lipschutz pointed out in 1921 the clinical and epidemiological differences between oral and genital herpes, and 40 years later it was reported that there were two antigenic types of HSV, and that the viral type recovered was related to the site of the lesions. These discoveries paved the way for subsequent studies of the natural history of genital herpes.

Aetiology

All herpesviruses have a similar structure. The core is composed of double-stranded linear DNA, and this is surrounded by an icosahedral protein capsid composed of 162 subunits. Outside this is an impermeable envelope composed of glycoproteins (Nahmias & Roizman 1973) (Fig. 5.30). The two subtypes HSV1 and HSV2 can be differentiated by serological and cultural methods (Nahmias & Dowdle 1968); the nucleic acids from HSV1 and HSV2 show approximately 50% base sequence homology (Ludwig et al 1972). Roizman & Buchman (1979) have shown that analysis of DNA nucleotide sequences with restriction endonucleases indicates that

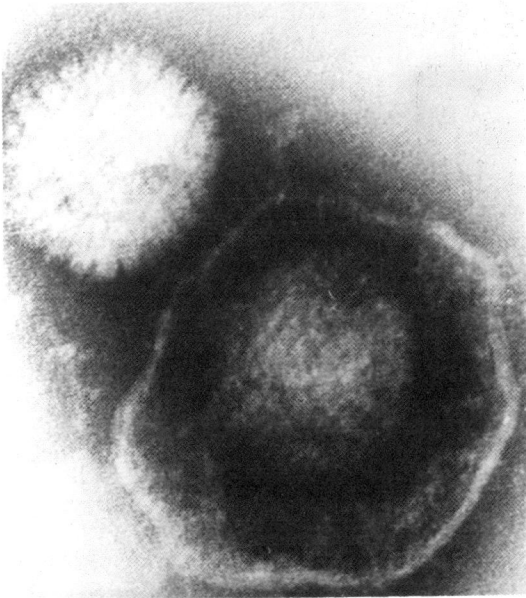

Fig. 5.30 Herpes simplex: virus particles.

there are different strains of both HSV1 and HSV2. It is possible for a person to be infected by different strains at different times, and re-infection by a strain other than the original one is possible.

Life cycle of herpes simplex virus. The virus is introduced directly into epithelial cells; for genital herpes this occurs during intercourse or orogenital contact. A productive phase of infection then develops. After entry into the host cell, the capsid of the virion is uncoated in the cytoplasm and the core DNA enters the nucleus, where viral DNA synthesis and transcription of messenger RNA occur. The messenger RNA then migrates to the cytoplasm and is translated into various virus-specific proteins which then return to the nucleus. Assembly of new virus particles now occurs, and the process culminates in the death and lysis of the host cell and the release of the virus particles. The whole process occurs within 5–6 hours of the entry of the virus (Raab & Lorincz 1981).

Experimental studies in mice have shown that about 24 hours after inoculation HSV begins to spread from the infected epithelium along sensory nerves to regional sensory ganglia (Cook & Stevens 1973). In the case of human genital herpes HSV2, and less often HSV1, has been recovered from the nerve root ganglia of S3 and S4 (Barringer 1974).

Once the virus has reached the ganglia a productive infection ensues, lasting about 2 weeks; after this the stage of latency begins. During latency, infectious HSV cannot be recovered from the ganglia, and no viral antigen can be detected by immunofluorescence; however, if the ganglia are removed and cultured, infectious virus can be isolated in 4–6 days (Stevens & Cook 1971).

The biological mechanisms through which latency is established are not completely understood (Docherty & Chopan 1974). Latency can follow both symptomatic and asymptomatic primary infections, and recurrences of clinical disease can likewise be symptomatic or asymptomatic. There are two theories to explain the reactivation of infection. The first is the 'ganglion trigger' hypothesis. According to this, a stimulus such as stress, fever or menstruation disturbs the balance between virus and host ganglionic cells, so that the virus emerges from the latent state and moves down the sensory nerve to infect epithelial cells where it may, or may not, cause skin lesions. In contrast, the 'skin trigger' hypothesis is that small amounts of virus are often formed in the ganglia and travel to the skin. Normally, these microfoci are eliminated, but sometimes changes in the skin, for example after intercourse, either stimulate virus replication or temporarily suppress local immunity so that lesions develop. There is evidence for and against both these theories, and the issue has not yet been decided (Docherty & Chopan 1974, Hill & Blyth 1976).

Pathology. The lesions of primary and recurrent herpes are histologically identical. Initial dermal congestion, with intracellular and extracellular oedema, culminates in the formation of an epidermal vesicle which ruptures to form a shallow ulcer. The intra-epidermal vesicles do not extend below the basement membrane, so do not lead to permanent scarring.

The nuclei of infected cells contain inclusions which are initially basophilic but later eosinophilic. Both vesicles and ulcerated areas contain multinucleated giant cells, some of whose nuclei also contain inclusions. The inflammatory infiltrate around the herpetic lesion is initially composed of mononuclear cells, but later polymorphonuclear leucocytes preponderate.

Immunology. Antibodies to HSV can be

detected by several techniques, of which complement fixation (CF) and neutralisation have been the most studied (Nahmias et al 1970, Eberle & Courtney 1981). CF and/or neutralising antibodies can be detected in convalescent sera from 95% of patients with primary genital herpes and these antibodies persist after the attack has resolved; their presence does not appear to have any influence on the development of recurrent infections (Douglas & Couch 1970). It is more likely that circulating antibodies play a part in the prevention of infection. The presence of antibodies to HSV1 appears to mitigate the severity of first episodes of genital (HSV2) infection, and indeed may prevent them (Corey et al 1978) (see also p. 72).

An intact cell-mediated immune (CMI) system appears to be essential in preventing severe HSV disease, and in effecting recovery. Cytotoxic T cells, natural killer cells, lymphoproliferative responses and T suppressor cell responses all play a part (Hirsch et al 1970, O'Reilly et al 1977, Ching & Lopez 1979). Immunocompromised individuals such as those receiving immunosuppressive drugs, and those with T cell dysfunction such as patients with the acquired immune deficiency syndrome (AIDS), can experience atypical genital HSV infections (Naraqi et al 1977, Meyers et al 1980). Nevertheless, although CMI has an important influence on the severity of a primary attack its role in recurrent infections is more uncertain. Recent studies of otherwise normal patients who are having frequent attacks of genital herpes have not shown any evidence of defective CMI (Shillitoe et al 1977, Rasmussen & Merigan 1978). The numerous factors which influence the frequency and duration of recurrent attacks of genital herpes will require further study.

Epidemiology

Genital herpes is reportable from STD clinics in the UK, but in most other countries data on national incidence are not available. None the less, there is evidence that the prevalence of these infections has increased in recent years. In England, the number of new cases in women attending STD clinics increased from 3.95 to 18.80 per 100 000 population between 1971 and 1981 (Chief Medical Officer 1973, 1984a). In Auckland, New Zealand, the re-

ported incidence of genital HSV infections nearly doubled each year between 1968 and 1973 (MacDougall 1975). Corey (1984) states that in some parts of the USA the prevalence of evidence of HSV infection in cytological cervical smears showed a marked increase throughout the 1970s, but in other areas the prevalence remained constant. While the available data suggest that genital herpes is being diagnosed more often in some population groups, Corey is uncertain whether there is a true increase in prevalence, or simply an increased awareness of the disease and availability of diagnostic facilities.

Genital herpes affects mostly young adults (Wolontis & Jeansson 1977, Brown et al 1979). Reports from several countries indicate that symptomatic disease most often occurs in single, well-educated white people (Jeansson & Molin 1974, Corey 1984). One study showed that in 60% of patients the HSV infection was the first STD they had had, and in 39% of patients with primary herpes the source contact was a new sex partner (Corey 1984).

The majority of genital herpes is caused by HSV2, but in various studies HSV1 has been recovered from 7–37% of patients with primary infections (Kalinyak et al 1977, Corey 1984). HSV1 infection of the genitals can be attributed to oral sex, and there is evidence that infections of this kind are seen more often in younger age groups, in whom oral sex is said to be more popular (Wolontis & Jeansson 1977).

Circulating antibodies to HSV1 are present in children, and their prevalence appears to be related to socio-economic status. In one study from the USA, Porter et al (1969) detected antibodies in 40% of children aged 8–14 years in a private paediatric group but in 80% of children of the same age attending a public clinic. Exposure to HSV1 in childhood may be declining; Smith & Peutherer (1967) reported a fall in the prevalence of antibodies to HSV1 in children aged 3–15 years from 85% in 1953 to 41% in 1965. Circulating antibodies to HSV2 are not present before puberty, and thereafter their prevalence is related to sexual activity, ranging from 80% in prostitutes to 3% in nuns (Nahmias et al, 1970, Duenas et al 1972, Nahmias & Roizman 1973). In England, Roome et al (1975) reported the detection of antibodies of HSV2 in

7–20% of male and female blood donors, compared with 60% of blood donors who were confined to prison.

The incidence of genital herpes, at least in upper socio-economic groups, appears to be increasing, whereas the prevalence of non-genital HSV1 infection is falling. These phenomena may be linked, since prior HSV1 infection confers partial immunity against HSV2. The increasing incidence of genital herpes due to HSV2 may be due not simply to increased promiscuity, as is commonly assumed, but to a decline in exposure to HSV1 in childhood because of improved living standards.

Transmission of herpes simplex viruses. Asymptomatic carriers play an important part in the epidemiology of genital herpes. Mertz et al (1985) studied a group of source contacts of patients with first-episode genital herpes. They reported that one-third gave no history suggestive of herpes, and although many of the remainder gave a history of herpes, they were unaware that they might be infectious. Shedding of HSV into saliva, cervical secretions and semen can occur in people without symptoms. Genital infection by HSV1 has been recorded as developing after oral sex with partners who, although symptomless, had infected saliva (Embil et al 1981). Adam et al (1980) reported the isolation of HSV2 from the cervix in five of 50 women with a history of genital herpes, but who had had no attacks for at least 6 months and who had no symptoms or signs of infection at the time of virus isolation. The source of the virus which is shed into the genital tract of symptomless men is uncertain (Centifano et al 1972, de Ture et al 1978). It may be concluded that a primary attack of genital herpes may follow sex contact with a partner who has a mild clinical attack of herpes at the time of coitus (a severe attack would usually prohibit intercourse because of pain), but that in many cases the disease follows sexual contact with a partner who is shedding virus without symptoms or signs of infection.

Clinical Manifestations

These are affected by the viral type, previous exposure to HSV1, a past history of genital herpes and by various host factors. The proportion of episodes of genital herpes which are symptomless is not

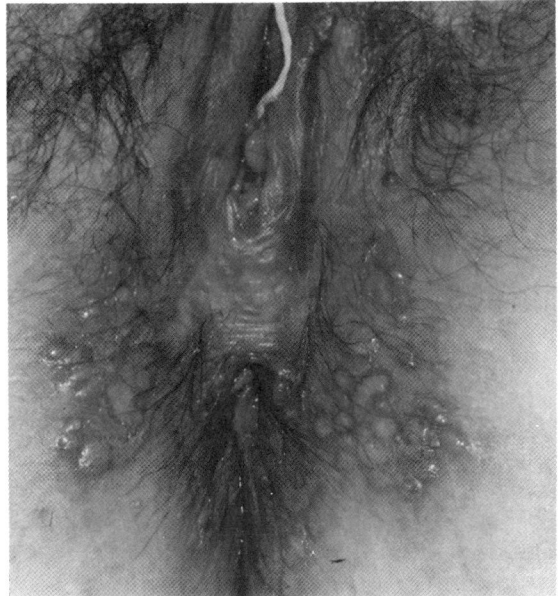

Fig. 5.31 Genital herpes. Vesicular and ulcerative lesions are both visible.

known (Nahamias & Roizman 1973). The incubation period of symptomatic primary infections is usually 3–7 days. Genital or perigenital burning or itching may precede the appearance of genital lesions by 2 or 3 days. The lesions themselves are at first erythematous, but rapidly become vesicular, then rupture to form single, multiple or grouped shallow ulcers, 1–2 mm in diameter. These may coalesce to form larger ulcerated areas. The ulcers themselves are painful, tender and non-indurated (Fig. 5.31). Lesions can appear on any part of the vulva and adjacent structures, but are commonest on the labia majora and minora, the fourchette, perineum and anus. Oedema of the labia is not unusual, and the pain of a severe attack may make it almost impossible to examine the genital area thoroughly. In women, dysuria is a common symptom which is due either to contact of urine with inflamed peri-urethral lesions or to the development of herpetic urethritis or cystitis. Moderate enlargement of inguinal and/or femoral lymph nodes occurs in the 2nd week of the illness. The nodes are tender but almost never suppurate.

The symptoms of primary genital herpes reach a maximum after 7–10 days, and thereafter gradually resolve. The ulcers on the labia majora and perineum begin to crust (mucosal ulcers do not crust) and after 14–21 days healing is virtually complete. However, new lesion formation occurs in 75% of patients with primary genital herpes, and these will slow recovery. The duration of viral shedding from vulval lesions is about 12 days; Corey (1984) estimates the mean time from the onset to complete re-epithelialisation of all lesions as 19 days.

About 90% of women with primary vulval herpes due to HSV2, and 70% of those infected with HSV1, have a concomitant herpetic infection of the cervix (Corey et al 1983); this may be symptomless, or cause a vaginal discharge (Josey et al 1966). The cervix appears congested and multiple shallow ulcers, or even areas of necrosis, can be seen. The duration of viral shedding from the cervix is similar to that from lesions of the vulva.

Pharyngeal infection is commonly associated with primary genital infection by HSV1 and HSV2 (Embil 1981, Lafferty et al 1987). The pharyngitis is usually symptomatic. Examination shows erythema and herpetic ulceration of varying severity (Glezen et al 1975). Most patients with primary genital herpes complain of fever, headache and malaise which are at their worst after 3–4 days, then gradually decline. Severe and prolonged headache may indicate the onset of aseptic meningitis, which occurs in about one-third of women with primary genital herpes (Corey 1984). This meningitis is usually mild, and neurological sequelae are rare. Lumbosacral herpetic radiculitis is a not uncommon complication, indicated by the development of perineal and sacral anaesthesia, constipation and retention of urine (Caplan et al 1977); retention of urine may also be due to severe dysuria from urethral infection. Transverse myelitis is an occasional complication of primary genital herpes (Craig & Nahmias 1973).

Extragenital skin lesions are found in at least one-quarter of women with primary infections (Corey 1984). They occur during the 2nd week of the disease, and mostly affect the thighs and buttocks; they are probably due to auto-inoculation. Disseminated bloodborne infection is rare (Nahmias 1970); multiple vesicles affect the trunk and extremities, and meningitis and rarer complications such as hepatitis, arthritis and thrombocytopenia may appear (Flewett et al 1969, Koberman et al 1980, Shelley 1980).

Bacterial secondary infection of the lesions of genital herpes is uncommon except in immunosuppressed patients, but superinfection by yeasts is common, appearing in the 2nd week of the infection. This may cause vulval irritation or exacerbate any vaginal discharge.

Patients with serological evidence of previous HSV1 infections seem to have a milder disease, with less systemic involvement, a shorter course and fewer complications than those without antibodies to HSV1. There are no clinical differences between primary attacks of genital herpes caused by HSV1 or HSV2.

Recurrent infection. About 50% of women with primary genital herpes caused by HSV1, and 80% with primary infections with HSV2, develop recurrences within the year following infection (Reeves et al 1981). These workers also reported that in women the median time to the first recurrence was 120 days. The subsequent pattern of recurrence is very variable. In one study in the USA two-thirds of patients, regardless of how long they had had genital herpes, were having more than five recurrent attacks a year (Knox et al 1982). The median time between recurrences has been reported as 42 days (Reeves et al 1981). Among the events which are believed to precipitate recurrences are emotional upset, fatigue, fever, menstruation and coitus. Although in some patients these attacks become shorter, and the intervals between them longer, in others there is little change with the passage of time. Women with HSV1 infections have fewer recurrences than those infected with HSV2.

Recurrent genital herpes is usually less severe than first attacks. A smaller area of vulval epithelium is affected, local symptoms are milder, and the duration of the attack is reduced to 7–10 days or less (Chang et al 1974, Corey et al 1983). The duration of viral shedding is reduced to about 4 days. Prodromal symptoms—perigenital aching or local itching, burning or paraesthesia—occur in about 50% of women with recurrent genital herpes (Brown et al 1979). Cervical involvement is much reduced; only 15–30% of women yield HSV from the cervix during recurrent attacks, and there are usually no clinical abnormalities (Guinan et al 1981). Dissemination of virus to other sites does not occur. In the immunosuppressed patient chronic atypical infection of the anogenital area may occur and the virus can be cultured from fissures and erosions.

Genital herpes and pregnancy. Earlier studies suggested that both primary and recurrent herpes could affect the outcome of pregnancy. Nahmias & Roizman (1973) reported that there was a significant increase in spontaneous abortion in women with cervical herpes diagnosed before the 20th week of pregnancy; spontaneous abortion occurred more often in primary than in recurrent infections. Women who had primary cervical herpetic infection after the 20th week of pregnancy showed a 35% rate of premature delivery in comparison with 18% for the general hospital population. More recent studies, however, have emphasised the different effects on pregnancy of primary and recurrent genital herpes. Spontaneous abortion can occur during a primary infection because of an ascending chorio-amnionitis and haematogenous spread of HSV (Hain et al 1980), but it is uncertain whether spontaneous abortion is significantly commoner in women with recurrences (Vontvner et al 1982). Both Grossman et al (1980) and Vontvner et al (1982) found no association between recurrent genital herpes and premature delivery.

Genital herpes and the neonate. Infection of the neonate by HSV during delivery is more likely to occur if the mother has primary herpes than if she has recurrent infection. The risk may be as high as 50% in the first case, but only about 5% in the second (Nahmias et al 1976). It has been reported that 70% of babies with neonatal herpes have been born to mothers with no symptoms or signs at the time of delivery (Whitley et al 1980); Corey (1984) has pointed out that there may nevertheless be a history of genital herpes in the sex partners of these women. In one study from the USA about 25% of neonatal infections were with HSV1 (Whitley et al 1980), and it seems likely that at least some of these were nosocomial.

The many factors involved in the pathogenesis of neonatal herpes include virus type and titre, the level of maternal antibodies, cellular immune responses of the infant and the nature of the environment. Their interaction has been discussed by Tejani et al (1979), Yeager & Zinkham (1980), Parvey & Ch'ien (1980) and Corey (1984). Neonatal herpes is a preventable disease. Antenatal screening is advisable for women who develop clinically suspicious lesions, women with a past history of genital herpes and women whose sex partners have the disease. Cultures for HSV should be taken from the vulva and cervix at the 36th week of pregnancy and should be repeated weekly until delivery.

It has been recommended that if virus is present at or near the time of delivery, or if suspect lesions are present when the mother goes into labour, caesarian section should be performed, preferably before the membranes rupture (Committee 1980, Kilbrick 1980). Recently, Prober et al (1987) have concluded that the risk to a baby born to a woman with recurrent genital herpes is very low, even if she is shedding the virus at the time of delivery, and that this risk should be weighed against the maternal and neonatal morbidity associated with caesarian delivery. If a woman is experiencing her first attack of genital herpes at the time of delivery, caesarian section is probably prudent.

Genital herpes and vulval neoplasia. There is serological and epidemiological evidence that HSV2 may be involved in the pathogenesis of cervical neoplasia. The prevalence of antibodies to HSV2 is highest in women with invasive cervical cancer and progressively lower in those with CIN2 and 1 and in healthy controls (Nahmias & Roizman 1973). In serological and cytological studies, HSV2 infection has been shown to precede CIN (Aurelian et al 1981). HSV2 DNA has been found in a single invasive cervical cancer (Frenkel et al 1972), and HSV2 specific RNA complementary to HSV2 DNA has been reported in biopsies of 60% of women with invasive cancer, but in only 2% of matched controls (Eglin et al 1981). Despite this evidence, the causative role of HSV2 in cervical cancer is not firmly established (Nahmias & Sawanabori 1978, Zur Hausen 1982).

The presence of HSV2-induced protein antigens in squamous cell carcinoma in situ of the vulva has been demonstrated by Kaufman et al (1981), but whether HSV2 is responsible for the malignant transformation of these cells or is only an opportunistic infectious agent is undecided. The natural history of vulval neoplasia has not received the detailed analysis which has been given to CIN, and further epidemiological and virological studies will be needed before the oncogenic potential, if any, of HSV2 infection of the vulva can be decided (Schwartz & Naftolin 1981).

Diagnosis

The differential diagnosis of genital herpes is from other causes of vulval ulceration. Among infective causes, primary and secondary syphilis must always be excluded, even in confirmed cases of herpes, as the two diseases may occur together. In women who live in or have recently travelled to the tropics, chancroid and the initial lesions of lymphogranuloma venereum may resemble genital herpes, and may be differentiated by appropriate laboratory tests. Non-infective causes of genital ulceration includes aphthous ulcers, Behçet's syndrome and Crohn's disease; in these diseases the duration of ulceration is more prolonged, and the ulcers themselves larger and deeper than in genital herpes.

Laboratory diagnosis (see also p. 71 et seq). Several procedures are available. The most sensitive is virus isolation in tissue culture. The best yield of virus comes if specimens of vesicle fluid are collected, but material from ulcerative lesions gives adequate results. It is important to sample the cervix as well as vulval lesions. Specimens are sent to the laboratory in virus transport medium kept at +4°C in crushed ice. They are then inoculated on to tissue culture cells such as human embryonic kidney and baby hamster kidney cells (Cruickshank et al 1975). The preparations are incubated and examined regularly for a cytopathic effect (CPE). If the viral inoculum is large, a typical CPE may be visible in 24 hours, but the median time from inoculation of HSV to the development of CPE is 4 days (Corey 1984). Isolates can be confirmed as HSV by direct immunofluorescence, and differentiation of HSV1 from HSV2 by microneutralisation or immunofluorescence techniques.

Cytology can be used for the diagnosis of HSV infections. Scrapings of vulval lesions, or cervical smears, are stained by Papanicolaou or Wright–Giemsa methods and examined microscopically for intranuclear inclusions and giant cells. These methods are specific but insensitive. In comparison with virus culture, Papanicolaou staining gives 63%, and Wright–Giemsa staining 44%, of diagnoses (Brown et al 1979). Immunological methods of diagnosis include a direct immunofluorescence test; provided enough cells are present in smears from the lesions, its sensitivity is 70–90% that of virus culture (Mosley et al 1981). An immunoperoxidase test has been described whose sensitivity is somewhat greater than the immunofluorescence test (Mosley et al 1981). The development of monoclonal antibodies is likely to improve the sensitivity and specificity of tests of this kind. It is possible to demonstrate HSV virions by electron microscopy; this technique is rapid, but very insensitive (Brown et al 1979). The detection of circulating antibodies against HSV1 and HSV2 is used for research and for sero-epidemiological studies, but is not a procedure of much value for the diagnosis of genital herpes in an individual patient. A single-serum examination is of no value, and attempts to demonstrate seroconversion and rising titres of antibodies have given conflicting results.

Treatment

The treatment of genital herpes is unsatisfactory, and the problems posed by latency and recurrent infection have not yet been overcome.

General measures. It is important to exclude associated infections by appropriate laboratory tests. Women with primary vulval herpes often feel unwell because of viraemia and anxiety about the condition, and rest is important. If the local symptoms are severe, or there is evidence of incipient complications such as meningitis or difficulty in urination, admission to hospital is indicated. A high fluid intake is encouraged, and analgesics given. Frequent bathing with 0.9% saline is soothing. Bacterial secondary infection is unusual, but if it should occur cotrimoxazole (which has no antitreponemal action) is the drug of choice. Candidosis may cause troublesome irritation, and may be treated with antimycotic pessaries.

Retention of urine can usually be avoided if a high fluid intake is maintained and the patient encouraged to urinate, but if it should occur an indwelling catheter will be needed for a few days.

Suprapubic drainage is recommended by some physicians to avoid contamination of the urethra by HSV, but the value of this procedure has not been proved in controlled studies.

Counselling patients with vulval herpes is very important. They are often concerned about recurrent attacks, pregnancy and the possibility of infecting their sex partners. The risk of infecting partners is low once genital lesions have healed, and in general patients with recurrent vulval herpes should be encouraged to lead a normal sex life, avoiding intercourse during attacks until the skin has completely healed. Nevertheless, the risk of infecting others between attacks, although low, exists; the advisability of telling a partner that she has recurrent herpes is a delicate and emotive problem which the patient may like to discuss with her physician.

Antiviral agents. Antiviral therapy for genital herpes has recently been reviewed by Nicholson (1984). Acyclovir has now been thoroughly evaluated, and is regarded as the best of the antiviral drugs for this disease. Treatment with oral acyclovir, 200 mg five times daily for 5 days, has a marked effect on the duration of the symptoms and signs of infection and on the duration of viral shedding (Bryson et al 1983). The application of acyclovir cream 5% 4-hourly also reduces the duration of pain, virus shedding and the time to complete healing (Corey et al 1982a, Fiddian et al 1983); topical therapy has no effect on systemic manifestations such as fever and headache, or on dysuria or vaginal discharge (Corey et al 1982b). Intravenous acyclovir, 5 mg/kg body weight given 8-hourly for 5 days, is highly effective (Mindel et al 1982). Acyclovir therapy for primary genital herpes, however administered, has no influence on the rate of recurrence.

The effects of oral and topical acyclovir therapy on recurrent genital herpes are less marked than on primary infections. If acyclovir cream is applied, the duration of viral shedding is slightly reduced, but there is little effect on the time taken for the lesions to heal (Corey 1982a, Reichman et al 1983). Oral therapy is a little more effective, particularly if it is started during the prodromal period of an attack (Reichman et al 1984). Long term prophylaxis with oral acyclovir has also been studied in controlled trials. There were significantly fewer recur-

rences in those who received acyclovir than in those receiving a placebo (Douglas et al 1984, Mindel et al 1984, Straus et al 1984). A dosage as low as 200 mg twice daily will induce a 50% reduction in the number of recurrent attacks (Douglas et al 1984). When therapy is discontinued, however, the attacks resume their pretreatment frequency. The indications for continuous acyclovir therapy are not clear at present, and there has been concern about the possibility of side effects with prolonged therapy (although none has been described to date) and the emergence of acyclovir-resistant strains of HSV. At present, intravenous acyclovir therapy is reserved for inpatients with very severe or complicated infections, oral therapy is used for the treatment of primary genital herpes, and topical therapy used for mild primary attacks. None of these forms of treatment is very effective if therapy is delayed until the attack is well established.

Many other antiviral agents have been studied for the treatment of genital herpes, but none has been shown in controlled clinical trials to approach the efficacy of acyclovir. They are discussed by Nicholson (1984).

Immune modulators. Levamisole has no value for the treatment of recurrent genital herpes (Chang & Fiumara 1978). Its value in primary infections has not been investigated. Inosine pranobex (isoprinosine) has immune-potentiating properties, and its effect on genital herpes has been studied. Corey et al (1979) reported that primary infections appeared to respond better to the drug than to a placebo. Recently, Mindel et al (1987), is a double-blind trial, found that patients treated with acyclovir healed more quickly and had a shorter duration of viral shedding than those treated with inosine pranobex. There is some evidence that the rate of recurrent herpes simplex infections is reduced by intermittent inosine pranobex therapy (Galli et al 1982). The drug has been discussed in recent reviews (Lancet 1985; Drug Therapeutics Bulletin 1986).

Vaccines. Heterologous vaccines such as vaccinia, BCG and polio vaccines are of no value for the treatment of genital herpes (Tager 1974, Berman 1976). A heat-inactivated HSV vaccine (Lupidon) was available in Europe for many years but was never fully evaluated in controlled clinical trials. Subunit vaccines, prepared from surface proteins of HSV, might be of value for the immunisation of those who may be exposed to infection, and have been advocated for therapy; however, controlled trials have not yet been conducted, and the value of such vaccines is not decided (Mindel 1984).

Prophylaxis. The use of condoms during foreplay and intercourse may reduce the transmission of HSV, although this has not been established by clinical trials. Some spermicides inactivate the virus in vitro, but it is not known whether this has any clinical relevance in prophylaxis. Attempts are currently being made to develop a vaccine against genital herpes. It is clearly important that such a virus vaccine does not itself establish a latent infection, and its safety and efficacy would need to be established by very carefully conducted studies. No vaccine which satisfies these requirements is currently available.

Varicella-zoster

Varicella-zoster virus (Herpesvirus varicellae) causes disease of two clinical types, varicella (chickenpox) mostly in children, and herpes zoster, mostly in adults. Its properties have been reviewed by Andrewes et al (1978). It is believed that the virus lies dormant in the dorsal root ganglia after an attack of varicella and later in life becomes reactivated and causes herpes zoster. Zoster is common in patients with neoplasms, particularly those (such as lymphoma) affecting cell-mediated immunity, and in patients on immunosuppressive therapy, but it can affect healthy people.

Varicella

This is a highly contagious disease, commonest in children aged 5–8 years. The incubation period is 14–21 days. The eruption starts with faint macules which rapidly become vesicular, and successive crops appear over a few days. Eventually all lesions scab and disappear without scarring. Complications are rare.

Vulval lesions can occur as part of the exanthem, but there is no specific association. Congenital varicella has been reported (Freud 1958, Pearson 1964); the route of infection appears to be transplacental rather than via the birth canal.

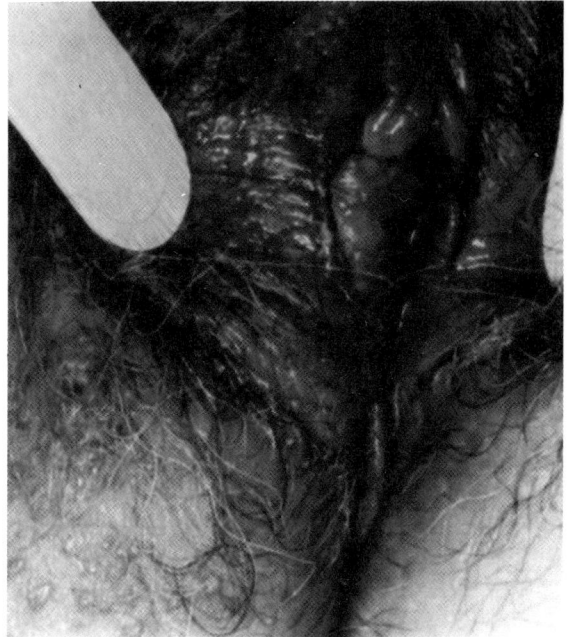

Fig. 5.32 Vulval herpes zoster: the third sacral nerve root is involved.

Herpes zoster

Zoster is a disease of the nerves of the skin and of the tissues which they supply; although cervical and thoracic nerves are usually affected, lumbosacral nerves are involved in 15% of cases. The rash of zoster is often preceded and accompanied by local itching or pain, and is essentially unilateral. Vulval lesions appear if the dermatome of S3 is affected (Fig. 5.32). The eruption is vesicular; after a few days crusts form and eventually separate, leaving no scarring. Vaginal lesions have been recorded (Janson 1959), and transient enlargement of the inguinal glands often occurs.

Neurogenic bladder is often present in patients with anogenital zoster affecting S3, or less often S2 or S4 dermatomes. Hesitancy of urination or even actual retention may occur (Izumi & Edwards 1973, Waugh 1974), but the prognosis is good. Post-herpetic neuralgia in the affected neurotome is not uncommon, particularly in older patients, and may drag on for many months or years.

The histology of the lesions of varicella and zoster is identical. There are intra-epidermal vesicles, with ballooning of adjacent prickle cells. Acidophil intranuclear inclusions and multinucleate giant cells are present, and there is some dermal inflammation.

The diagnosis of vulval zoster is usually easy, but if the lesions are sparse drug eruptions, syphilis and genital herpes may need to be excluded. Genital herpes may readily be distinguished from zoster by culture of vesicle fluid.

Treatment. Vulval zoster is usually a mild disease, and specific antiviral therapy is not often indicated. Several antiviral agents have been evaluated for non-genital zoster, and could be used for vulval disease if necessary. The value of idoxuridine is not agreed. A 40% solution dissolved in dimethylsulphoxide appears to give the best results, but although the time to resolution of inflammation is shortened the duration of pain may not be lessened (Juel-Jensen et al 1970, Wildenhoff et al 1979). No controlled studies of the efficacy of this treatment against vulval zoster have been performed; it would be contra-indicated in pregnancy and the solvent dimethylsulphoride could be irritating to the vulval epithelium. Intravenous acyclovir shortens the course of zoster, but does not prevent postherpetic neuralgia (Peterslund et al 1981, Bean et al 1982). Although it has not been evaluated for genital zoster, oral acyclovir may modify acute herpes zoster and reduce pain (McKendrick et al 1986).

Infectious mononucleosis

Epstein–Barr virus (EBV) is a herpesvirus which is associated with infectious mononucleosis, Burkitt's lymphoma and nasopharyngeal carcinoma. Several mucosal and cutaneous manifestations of infectious mononucleosis are recognised, but genital ulceration is rare (Brown & Stenchever 1977, Lawee & Shafir 1983). Recently, Portnoy et al (1984) have described a young woman who developed painful vulval ulceration during an attack of virologically and serologically confirmed infectious mononucleosis. Genital herpes, chancroid and syphilis were all excluded, and EBV was recovered from the vulval lesions. The ulcers were very painful, and did not heal for over a month. EBV shedding from the cervix has been demonstrated (Sixbey et al 1986, Lancet 1986); sexual transmission is therefore a possibility.

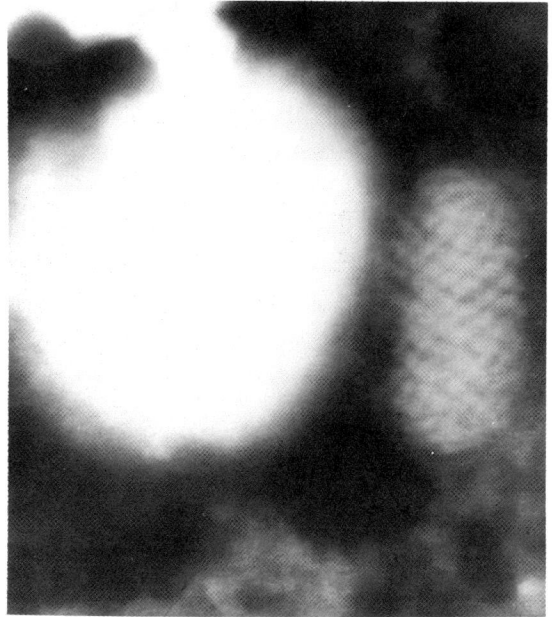

Fig. 5.33 Virus of molluscum contagiosum.

Genital poxvirus infection

Vaccinia

Accidental infection of the vulva with vaccinia virus from a vaccination site used to happen occasionally, and the resulting eruption was sometimes confused with genital herpes. Smallpox is now extinct and all supplies of vaccine have been withdrawn, so vulval vaccinia is of only historical interest. A case, with a review of the literature, was described by McCann et al (1974).

Molluscum contagiosum

Aetiology. The virus of molluscum contagiosum is a brick-shaped particle, 200×100 nm in size; the outer tubular structures are arranged spirally, giving it a 'ball of yarn' appearance (Fig. 5.33). The genome is double-stranded DNA (Parr et al 1977). It has not been possible to propagate the virus in the laboratory.

Epidemiology. The incidence of molluscum is biphasic, with peaks in childhood and in young adult life. In children the lesions appear usually on the face, trunk and limbs; genital lesions may also occur, but the mode of infection in that case is

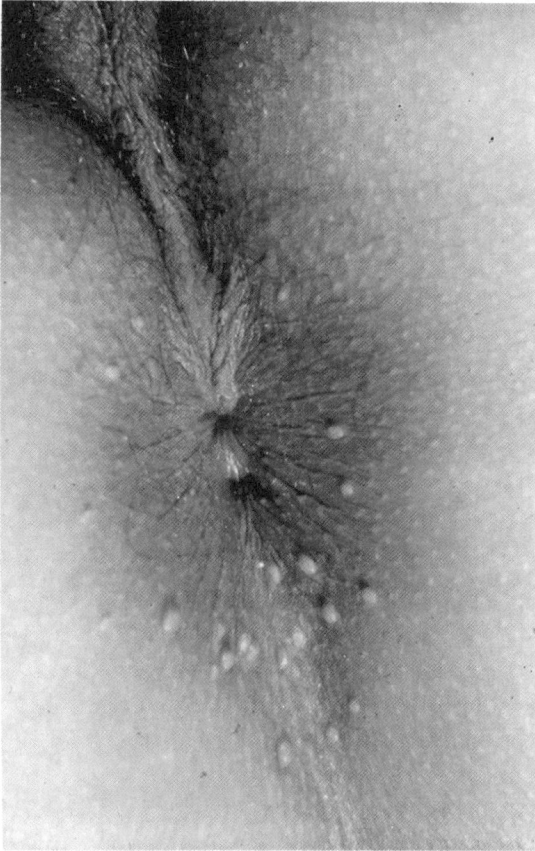

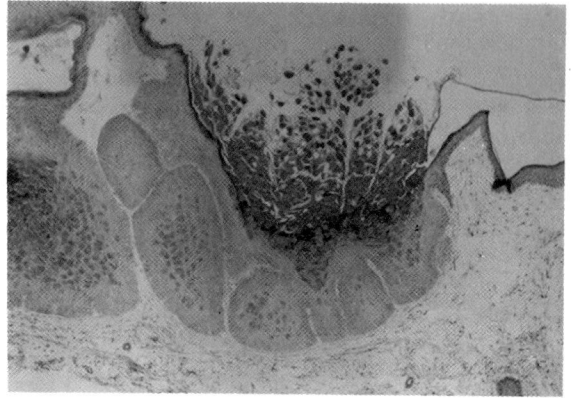

Fig. 5.35 Molluscum contagiosum histology: the section shows acanthosis and numerous amorphous molluscum bodies.

uncertain (Fig. 5.34). In young adults the genitals are predominantly affected and the disease is thought to be sexually transmitted (Cobbold & MacDonald 1970); lesions may be seen in the sex partners of infected individuals, and people with genital molluscum contagiosum often have other STDs (Wilkin 1977, Brown et al 1981). The disease may be becoming commoner; the number of new cases reported in women attending STD clinics in England rose from 0.60 to 2.01 per 100 000 population between 1971 and 1981 (Chief Medical Officer 1973, 1984a).

Pathology. The molluscum lesion is an umbilicated papule. Its base is composed of acanthotic prickle cells; as these move towards the surface cytoplasmic virus particles appear, which replicate to form a large inclusion which displaces the nucleus to the periphery of the cell. Eventually the nucleus disappears completely, and the cell is now entirely occupied by a 'molluscum contagiosum body', which is in effect a 'sack of virus' (Blank & Rake 1955). The central core of the lesion is composed of these bodies, together with cellular debris (Fig. 5.35). Molluscum contagiosum lesions may become inflamed, and occasionally they ulcerate; sometimes this inflammation heralds resolution.

Immunology. Circulating antibodies to the molluscum contagiosum virus can be detected by various techniques; their role is uncertain (Brown et al 1981). The release of virus into the dermis, either spontaneously or through trauma, may produce a cell-mediated immune response (Postlethwaite 1970). This could explain the eczematous reaction seen in many patients with molluscum contagiosum, and explain the resolution of many lesions following trauma (de Oreo et al 1956).

Clinical features. The incubation period of molluscum contagiosum is between 2 and 6 weeks (Felman & Nikitas 1980). The lesions are firm pearly hemispheric papules, usually between 2 and 5 mm in diameter, with a dimpled centre from which cheesy material may be squeezed. The number of lesions present is usually between 1 and 20. In women they appear on the lower abdomen, pubis, labia majora and adjacent skin; they do not occur on the vagina or cervix. They are very numerous in patients with impaired immunity (Pauly et al 1978), and multiple mollusca on the face may be a feature of AIDS. Spontaneous resolution occurs in some women, but in others the lesions persist for years.

Diagnosis. Molluscum contagiosum lesions may be mistaken for genital warts, and at times if solitary may resemble other vulval conditions such as basal cell carcinoma. If they are secondarily infected the lesions may resemble furuncles, and if they ulcerate will have to be distinguished from other forms of genital ulceration.

For laboratory diagnosis biopsy may be performed. A useful alternative diagnostic test is to scrape out the core of the lesion with a small curette and mix the material with a drop of 10% KOH on a slide. At magnification × 400 molluscum bodies appear as irregular masses about 35 μm in diameter.

Treatment. The simplest treatment is to introduce pure liquid phenol into the centre of the lesions with a sharpened applicator. Alternatively they may be curetted under local anaesthesia, or treated with cryotherapy. Since molluscum contagiosum in adults is predominantly an STD, it is important to exclude associated infections.

Orf

Orf is a worldwide disease of sheep and lambs, caused by a poxvirus. It causes haemorrhagic pustules, often with a central depression. Human meat handlers may become infected with orf on their hands, arms and face (Hodgson-Jones 1951). A putative case of vulval orf in a child who lived on a farm and played with an infected animal has been described by James (1968).

REFERENCES

Ackerman A B 1968 The resurgence of *Phthirus pubis*. New England Journal of Medicine 278: 950–951

Adam E, Dreesman G, Kaufman R H et al 1980 Asymptomatic shedding after herpes genitalis. American Journal of Obstetrics and Gynecology 137: 827–830

Addison W A, Livengood C H, Hill G B et al 1984 Necrotising fasciitis in diabetes. Obstetrics and Gynecology 63: 473–478

Alergant C D 1957 Lymphogranuloma inguinale in the male in Liverpool England 1947–54. British Journal of Venereal Diseases 33: 47–51

Alewattegama A, Kinghorn G R 1984 Systemic interferon in the treatment of resistant genital warts. Lancet i 1468

Altmeyer P, Chilf G-N, Holzmann H 1982 Hirsuties papillaris vulvae (Pseudocondylomata of the vulva). Hautarzt 33: 281–283

Aly R, Britz M B, Maibach H I 1979 Quantitative microbiology of the vagina. British Journal of Dermatology 101: 445–448

Amsel R, Totten P A, Speigel C A et al 1983 Nonspecific vaginitis. Diagnostic criteria and microbial and epidemiologic associations. American Journal of Medicine 74: 14–22

Anagnostidis N 1935 Kyste hydatique de la grande lèvre de la vulve et mécanisme de sa production. Gynécologie et Obstetrique 32: 356–358

Andrewes C, Pereira H G, Wildy P 1978 Viruses of vertebrates, 4th edn. London, Baillière Tindall, p 327

Anyon C P, Desmond F B, Eastcott D F 1971 A study of *Candida* in one thousand and seven women. New Zealand Medical Journal 73: 9–13

Asami K, Nakamura M 1955 Experimental inoculation of bacteria-free *Trichomonas vaginalis* into human vaginae and its effect on the glycogen content of vaginal epithelia. American Journal of Tropical Medicine and Hygiene 4: 254–258

Ashworth F L 1974 Tuberculous lymphoedema. British Medical Journal iv: 167–169

Auger P, Joly J 1980 Microbial flora associated with *Candida albicans*. Obstetrics and Gynecology 55: 397–401

Aurelian L, Manak M M, McKinlay M et al 1981 The Herpes virus hypothesis—are Koch's postulates satisfied? Gynecological Oncology 12: S56–S87

Baird P J 1983 Serological evidence for the association of papilloma virus and cervical neoplasia. Lancet ii: 17–18

Baird P J, Elliott P, Stening M et al 1979 Giant condyloma acuminatum of the vulva and anal canal. Australian and New Zealand Journal of Obstetrics and Gynaecology 19: 119–122

Baker C J, Goroff D K, Alpert S et al 1977 Vaginal colonisation with group B streptococcus: a study in college women. Journal of Infectious Diseases 135: 392–397

Barlow D, Phillips I 1978 Gonorrhoea in women: diagnostic, clinical and laboratory aspects. Lancet i: 761–763

Barringer J R 1974 Recovery of Herpes simplex virus from human sacral ganglia. New England Journal of Medicine 291: 828–834

Bean B, Braun C, Balfour H H 1982 Acyclovir therapy for acute herpes zoster. Lancet ii: 118–121

Beard C M, Noller K L, O'Fallon W M et al 1979 Lack of evidence for cancer due to use of metronidazole. New England Journal of Medicine 301: 519–522

Beilby J O W, Ridley C M 1987 Pathology of the vulva. In: Fox H (ed) Haines' and Taylor's obstetrical and gynaecological pathology, 3rd edn. Churchill Livingstone, Edinburgh

Bellina J H 1983 The use of the carbon dioxide laser in the management of condyloma acuminatum with 8 year follow-up. American Journal of Obstetrics and Gynecology 147: 375–378

Bender M E 1986 New concepts of condylomata acuminata in children. Archives of Dermatology 1121–1123

Berman S M 1976 BCG immunoprophylaxis of recurrent herpes progenitalis. Archives of Dermatology 112: 1410–1412

Berry A 1971 Evidence of gynecologic bilharziasis in cytologic material. A morphologic study for cytologists in particular. Acta Cytologica 15: 482–486

Beveridge M M 1962 Vaginal moniliasis after treatment of trichomonal infection with 'Flagyl'. British Journal of Venereal Diseases 38: 220–222

Bhattacharyya M N, Jephcott A E, Morton R S 1973 Diagnosis

of gonorrhoea in women: comparison of sampling sites. British Medical Journal ii: 748–750

Bjornstad R 1947 Tuberculous primary infection of genitalia—two cases of venereal genital tuberculosis. Acta Dermato-Venereologica 27: 106–109

Blackwell A L, Fox A R, Phillips I et al 1983 Anaerobic vaginosis (non-specific vaginitis); clinical, microbiological and therapeutic findings. Lancet ii: 1379–1382

Blank F, Mann S J 1975 Trichophyton rubrum infections according to age, anatomical distribution and sex. British Journal of Dermatology 92: 171–174

Blank H, Rake H 1955 Viral and rickettsial diseases of the skin, eye and mucous membranes. Churchill Livingstone, London, pp. 182–192

Bonar B E, Rabson A S 1957 Gynecologic aspects of leprosy. Obstetrics and Gynecology 9: 33–38

Borchardt K A, Hoke A W 1970 Simplified laboratory technique for diagnosis of chancroid. Archives of Dermatology 102: 190–196

Borkawf H I 1973 Bacterial gangrene associated with pelvic surgery. Clinical Obstetrics and Gynecology 16: 40–45

Boulle A, Notelovitz M 1964 Bilharzia of the female genital tract. South African Journal of Obstetrics and Gynaecology 18: 48–50

Bowie W R, Pollock H M, Forsyth P S et al 1977 Bacteriology of the urethra in normal men and in men with non-gonococcal urethritis. Journal of Clinical Microbiology 6: 482–488

Bramley M 1976 Study of female babies of women entering confinement with vaginal trichomoniasis. British Journal of Venereal Diseases 52: 58–62

Braun L, Farmer E A, Shah K V 1983 Immunoperoxidase localisation of papilloma virus antigen in cutaneous warts and Bowenoid papulosis. Journal of Medical Virology 12: 187–193

Bray R S 1974 Leishmania. Annual Review of Microbiology 28: 189–199

Breschi L C, Goldman G, Shapiro S R 1974 Granuloma inguinale in Viet Nam: successful therapy with ampicillin and lincomycin. Journal of the American Venereal Disease Association 1: 118–120

British Journal of Venereal Diseases (Editorial) 1978 The nitroimidazole family of drugs. British Journal of Venereal Diseases 54: 69–71

Brown S T, Jaffe H W, Zaidi A et al 1979 Sensitivity and specificity of diagnostic tests for genital infection with Herpesvirus hominis. Sexually Transmitted Diseases 6: 10–13

Brown S T, Nalley J F, Kraus S J 1981 Molluscum contagiosum. Sexually Transmitted Diseases 8: 227–234

Brown Z A, Stenchever M A 1977 Genital ulceration and infectious mononucleosis: report of a case. American Journal of Obstetrics and Gynecology 127: 673–674

Brown Z A, Kern E R, Spruance S L et al 1979 Clinical and virologic course of herpes simplex genitalis. Western Journal of Medicine 130: 414–421

Brunham R L, Martin D H, Hubbard T W et al 1983 Depression of the lymphocyte transformation response to microbial antigens and to phytohaemagglutinin during pregnancy. Journal of Clinical Investigation 72: 1629–1638

Bryson Y J, Dillon M, Lovett M et al 1983 Treatment of first episodes of genital herpes simplex virus infection with oral acyclovir. New England Journal of Medicine 308: 916–921

Buckley C H, Butler E B, Fox H 1984 Vulvar intraepithelial neoplasia and microinvasive carcinoma of the vulva. Journal of Clinical Pathology 37: 1201–1211

Bumgarner F E, Burke R C 1949 Pityriasis versicolor. Atypical clinical and mycological variations. Archives of Dermatology 59: 192–194

Campion M J, Singer A, Clarkson P K, McCance D J 1985 Increased risk of cervical neoplasia in consorts of men with penile condylomata acuminata. Lancet i: 943–946

Campion M J, Singer A 1987 Vulval intraepithelial neoplasia: a clinical review. Genitourinary Medicine 63: 147–152

Caplan L R, Kleeman F J, Berg S 1977 Urinary retention probably secondary to herpes genitalis. New England Journal of Medicine 297: 920–921

Carpenter J L, Back A, Gehle D et al 1981 Erythromycin therapy of chancroid. Sexually Transmitted Diseases 8: 192–197

Carroll C J, Hurley R, Stanley V C 1973 Criteria for diagnosis of Candida vulvovaginitis in pregnant women. Journal of Obstetrics and Gynaecology of the British Commonwealth 80: 258–263

Catterall R D 1972 Trichomonal infections of the genital tract. Medical Clinics of North America 56: 1203–1209

Catterall R D 1977 The sexually transmitted diseases. In: Rook A (ed) Recent advances in dermatology 4. Churchill Livingstone, Edinburgh

Centifanto Y M, Drylie D M, Deardourff S L et al 1972 Herpesvirus type 2 in the male genitourinary tract. Science 178: 318–319

Chamberlain M J, Reynolds A L, Yeoman W B 1972 Toxic effect of podophyllum in pregnancy. British Medical Journal iii: 391–392

Chang T, Fiumara N 1978 Treatment with levamisole of recurrent herpes genitalis. Antimicrobial Agents and Chemotherapy 13: 809–812

Chang T W, Fumara W J, Weinstein L 1974 Genital herpes: some clinical and laboratory observations. Journal of the American Medical Association 229: 544–545

Chapel T A 1978 The variability of syphilitic chancres. Sexually Transmitted Diseases 5: 68–70

Chapel T A, Brown W J, Jeffries C et al 1978 The microbiological flora of penile ulceration. Journal of Infectious Diseases 137: 50–56

Charlewood G P, Shippel S, Renton H 1949 Schistosomiasis in gynaecology. Journal of Obstetrics and Gynaecology of the British Commonwealth 56: 367–370

Chief Medical Officer 1973 Sexually transmitted diseases: extract from annual report of the Chief Medical Officer to the Department of Health and Social Security for the year 1971. British Journal of Venereal Diseases 49: 89–95

Chief Medical Officer 1974 Sexually transmitted diseases: extract from the annual report of the Chief Medical Officer of the Department of Health and Social Security for the year 1972. British Journal of Venereal Diseases 50: 73–79

Chief Medical Officer 1984a Sexually transmitted diseases. Extract from the annual report of the Chief Medical Officer of the Department of Health and Social Security for the year 1982. British Journal of Venereal Diseases 60: 199–203

Chief Medical Officer 1984b Sexually transmitted diseases: extract from the annual report of the Chief Medical Officer of the Department of Health and Social Security for the year 1983. Genitourinary Medicine 61: 204–207

Ching C, Lopez C 1979 Natural killing of Herpes simplex virus type 1-infected target cells: normal human responses and influence of antiviral antibody. Infection and Immunity 26: 49–56

Chuang T-Y, Perry H O, Kurland L T, Ilstrup D M 1984 Condylomata acuminata in Rochester Minnesota 1950–1978 2.

Anaplasia and unfavourable outcomes. Archives of Dermatology 120: 476–483

Clayton Y M, Connor B L 1973 Comparison of clotrimazole cream, Whitfield's ointment and nystatin ointment for the topical treatment of ringworm infections, pityriasis versicolor, erythrasma and candidosis. British Journal of Dermatology 89: 197–199

Cobbold R J C, MacDonald A 1970 Molluscum contagiosum as a sexually transmitted disease. Practitioner 204: 416–420

Cohen C 1973 Three cases of amoebiasis of the cervix uteri. Journal of Obstetrics and Gynaecology of the British Commonwealth 80: 476–480

Chon A M, Kos J T, Taber L H et al 1981 Recurring laryngeal papillomas. American Journal of Otolaryngology 2: 129–132

Committee 1980 Committee on fetus and newborn, committee on infectious disease: perinatal herpes simplex infections. Pediatrics 66: 147–148

Cook M L, Stevens J G 1973 Pathogenesis of herpetic neuritis and ganglionitis in mice: evidence of intra-axonal transport of infection. Infection and Immunity 7: 272–288

Corbishly C M 1977 Microbial flora of the vagina and cervix. Journal of Clinical Pathology 30: 745–748

Corey L 1984 Genital herpes In: Holmes K K, Mårdh P-A, Sparling P F, Weisner P J (eds) Sexually transmitted diseases. McGraw Hill, New York, p 449

Corey L, Reeves W C, Holmes K K 1978 Cellular immune response in genital herpes simplex virus infections. New England Journal of Medicine 299: 986–991

Corey L, Chiang W T, Reeves W L et al 1979 Effect of isoprinosine on the cellular immune response in initial genital herpes virus infection. Clinical Research 27: 41A

Corey L, Benedetti J K, Critchlow C W et al 1982a Double-blind controlled trial of topical acyclovir in genital herpes simplex virus infections. American Journal of Medicine 731A: 326–334

Corey L, Nahmias A J, Guinan M E 1982b A trial of topical acyclovir in genital herpes simplex virus infections. New England Journal of Medicine 306: 1313–1319

Corey L, Adams H G, Brown Z A et al 1983 Genital herpes simplex infection: clinical manifestations, course and complications. Annal of Internal Medicine 98: 958–972

Craig C, Nahmias A 1973 Different patterns of neurologic involvement with herpes simplex virus types 1 and 2: isolation of herpes simplex virus from the buffy coat of two adults with meningitis. Journal of Infectious Disease 127: 365–370

Cruickshank R 1934 Conversion of glycogen of vagina into lactic acid. Journal of Pathology and Bacteriology 39: 213–219

Cruickshank R, Sharman A 1939 The biology of the vagina in the human subject II: The bacterial flora and secretion of the vagina in relation to glycogen in the vaginal epithelium. Journal of Obstetrics and Gynaecology of the British Empire 41: 208–212

Cruickshank R, Duguid J P, Marmion B P, Swain R H A 1975 In: Medical microbiology (12th edition), Churchill Livingstone, Edinburgh, p 219

Crum C P, Braun L A, Shah K V et al 1982a Vulvar intraepithelial neoplasia: correlation of nuclear DNA content and the presence of a human papillomavirus (HPV) antigen. Cancer 49: 468–471

Crum C P, Fu Y S, Levine R U et al 1982b Intraepithelial squamous lesions of the vulva: biologic and histologic criteria for the distinction of condylomas from vulvar intraepithelial neoplasia. American Journal of Obstetrics and Gynecology 144: 77–83

Daniel C, Mavrodin D 1934 L'actinomycose genitale de la femme. Revue Francaise de Gynecologie et d'Obstetrique 29: 1–11

Davidson F 1977 Yeasts and circumcision in the male. British Journal of Venereal Diseases 53: 121–122

Davidson F, Mould R F 1978 Recurrent genital candidosis in women and the effect of intermittent prophylactic treatment. British Journal of Venereal Diseases 54: 176–183

Davies T A 1931 Primary syphilis in the female. Oxford Medical Publications (Oxford University Press), Oxford; Humphrey Milford, London

Davies J A, Rees E, Hobson D et al 1978 Isolation of Chlamydia trachomatis from Bartholin's duct. British Journal of Venereal Diseases 54: 409–413

de Borges R 1971 Findings of microfilarial larval stages in gynaecologic smears. Acta Cytologica 15: 476–480

de Jong A R, Weiss J C, Brent R L 1982 Condylomata acuminata in children. American Journal of the Diseases of Children 136: 704–706

de Oreo G A, Johnson H H, Brinkley G W 1956 An eczematous reaction associated with molluscum contagiosum. Archives of Dermatology 74: 344–348

de Ture F A, Drylie D M, Kaufman H E et al 1978 Herpes virus type 2: study of semen in male subjects with recurrent infections. Journal of Urology 120: 449–451

Diamond R D, Krezesicki R 1978 Mechanisms of attachment of neutrophils to Candida albicans pseudohyphae in the absence of serum and of subsequent damage to pseudophypae by microbicidal processes of neutrophils in vitro. Journal of Clinical investigation 61: 360–365

Dienes L, Edsall G 1937 Observations on the L-organism of Kleinberger. Proceedings of the Society for Experimental Biology and Medicine 36: 740–745

Dilworth J A, Hendley J O, Mandell G L 1975 Attachment and ingestion of gonococci by human neutrophils. Infection and Immunity 11: 512–516

Docherty J J, Chopan M 1974 The latent herpes simplex virus. Bacteriological Review 38: 337–349

Dodson R F, Fritz G S, Hubler W R et al 1974 Donovanosis: a morphologic study. Journal of Investigative Dermatology 62: 611–614

Douglas R G, Couch R B 1970 A prospective study of chronic Herpes simplex virus infection and recurrent herpes labialis. Journal of Immunology 104: 289–294

Douglas J M, Critchlow C, Benedetti J et al 1984 A double-blind study of oral acyclovir for suppression of recurrences of genital herpes simplex virus infection. New England Journal of Medicine 310: 1551–1556

Drug Therapy Bulletin 1986 Inosine pranobex—only for use in controlled trials. Drug Therapy Bulletin 24: 95–96

Duenas A, Adam E, Melnick J L et al 1972 Herpesvirus type 2 in a prostitute population. American Journal of Epidemiology 95: 483–489

Duncan M O, Ballard R C, Bilgeri Y R et al 1984 Sexually acquired genital ulceration in urban black women. Southern Africa Journal of Sexually Transmitted Diseases 4: 23–27

Duncan W C, Knox J M, Wende R D 1974 The FTA-ABS test in darkfield positive primary syphilis. Journal of the American Medical Association 228: 859–860

Easmon C S F 1986 Bacterial vaginosis. In: Oriel J D, Harris W R, (eds) Recent advances in sexually transmitted diseases 3. Churchill Livingstone, Edinburgh

Eberle R, Courtney R J 1981 Assay of typ-- -ecific and type-common antibodies to Herpes simplex virus types 1 and 2 in human sera. Infection and Immunity 31: 1062–1072

Eglin R P, Sharp F, MacLean A B et al 1981 Detection of RNA complementary to Herpes simplex virus DNA in human cervical squamous cell neoplasms. Cancer Research 41: 3597–3603

Elgart M L, Higdon R S 1973 Pediculosis pubis of the scalp. Archives of Dermatology 107: 916

El Zawahry M, El Komy M 1973 Amebiasis cutis. International Journal of Dermatology 12: 305–310

Embil J A, Manuel F R, McFarlane E S 1981 Concurrent oral and genital infection with an identical strain of herpes simplex virus type 1. Sexually Transmitted Diseases 8: 70–72

Epstein E, Orkin M 1977 Pediculosis, clinical aspects. In: Orkin M, Maibach H I, Parish L C, Schwartzman R M (eds) Scabies and pediculosis. Lippincott, Philadelphia, p. 153

Eriksson G, Wanger L 1975 Frequency of N. gonorrhoeae, T. vaginalis and C. albicans in female venereological patients. A one year study. British Journal of Venereal Diseases 51: 192–197

Eron L J, Judson F, Tucker S et al 1986 Interferon therapy for condylomata acuminata. New England Journal of Medicine 315: 1059–1064

Ewing T L, Smale L E, Elliott F A 1979 National deaths associated with postpartum vulvar edema. American Journal of Obstetrics and Gynecology 134: 173–179

Fair W R, Timothy M M, Miller M A et al 1970 Bacteriologic and hormonal observations of the urethra and vaginal vestibule in normal premenopausal women. Journal of Urology 104: 426–431

Fairris G M, Stratham B N, Waugh M A 1984 The investigation of patients with genital warts. British Journal of Dermatology 111: 736–738

Farrell M K, Billmire M E, Shamroy J A et al 1981 Prepubertal gonorrhoea: a multidisciplinary approach. Pediatrics 67: 151–153

Fast M V, Nsanze H, D'Costa L J et al 1983 Antimicrobial therapy of chancroid: an evaluation of five treatment regimens correlated with in vitro sensitivity. Sexually Transmitted Diseases 10: 1–6

Feinstein R J 1978 Cutaneous leishmaniasis. Dermatology 1: 45–50

Felman Y M, Nikitas J A 1980 Genital molluscum contagiosum. Cutis 26: 28–35

Felman Y M, Johnson A, Schoeber P C et al 1986 Etiology of urinary symptoms in sexually active women. Genitourinary Medicine 62: 333–341

Ferenczy A 1983 Using the laser to treat vulvar condylomata acuminata and intraepidermal neoplasia. Canadian Medical Association Journal 128: 135–137

Ferenczy A 1984 Treating genital condylomas during pregnancy with the carbon dioxide laser. American Journal of Obstetrics and Gynecology 148: 9–12

Ferenczy A, Mitao M, Nagai N et al 1985 Latent papillomavirus and recurring genital warts. New England Journal of Medicine 313: 784–788

Fiddian A P, Kinghorn G R, Goldmeier D et al 1983 Topical acyclovir in the treatment of genital herpes: a comparison with systemic therapy. Journal of Antimicrobial Chemotherapy 12 (supp B): 67–77

Fieldsteel A H 1981 Cultivation of virulent Treponema pallidum in tissue culture. Infection and Immunity 32: 908–916

Fishe I, Morton R S 1970 Phthirus pubis infestation. British Journal of Venereal Diseases 46: 326–329

Fisher J R, Conway M J, Takeshita R T 1979 Necrotising fas-

ciitis. Importance of roentgenographic studies for soft-tissue gas. Journal of the American Medical Association 241: 803–807

Fiumara N J 1980 Treatment of primary and secondary syphilis: serological response. Journal of the American Medical Association 243: 2500–2503

Flewett T H, Parker R G, Philip W M 1969 Acute hepatitis due to herpes simplex in an adult. Journal of Clinical Pathology 22: 60–66

Fournier 1906 Quoted by Stokes J H in Modern clinical syphilology 1944 W B Saunders, Philadelphia, p 492

Fouts A C, Kraus S J 1980 Trichomonas vaginalis: re-evaluation of its clinical presentation and laboratory diagnosis. Journal of Infectious Diseases 141: 137–143

Freeman R G, McBride M E, Knox J M (1969) Pathogenesis of trichomycosis axillaris. Archives of Dermatology 100: 90–93

Frenkel N, Roizman B, Cassal E et al 1972 A DNA fragment of Herpes simplex 2 and its transcription in human cervical cancer tissue. Proceedings of the National Academy of Science USA 69: 78–79

Freud P 1958 Congenital varicella. American Journal for the Diseases of Children 96: 730–733

Friedrich E G 1983 The vulvar vestibule. Journal of Reproductive Medicine 28: 773–777

Fu Y S, Reagan J W, Richart R M 1981 Definition of precursors. Gynecologic Oncology 12: S220–S231

Gaisin A, Heaton C L 1975 Chancroid: alias the soft chancre. International Journal of Dermatology 14: 188–197

Galli M, Lazzakin A, Moroni M 1982 Inosiplex in recurrent herpes simplex infections. Lancet ii: 331–332

Gardner H L, Dukes C D 1955 Haemophilus vaginalis vaginitis. A newly defined specific infection previously classified as non-specific vaginitis. American Journal of Obstetrics and Gynecology 69: 962–970

Gardner H L, Kaufman R H 1981 Pediatric vulvovaginitis p 415, trichomoniasis p 243, Staphylococcal vaginitis p 301. In: Benign diseases of the vulva and vagina, 2nd edn. G K Hall

Garrod L P, Lambert H P, O'Grady F 1981 Antibiotic and chemotherapy, 5th edn. Churchill Livingstone, Edinburgh, p 393

Gillespie W A, Sellin M A, Gill P et al 1978 Urinary tract infection in young women with special reference to Staphylococcus saprophyticus. Journal of Clinical Pathology 31: 348–350

Gissmann L, de Villiers E-M, zur Hausen H 1982 Analysis of human genital warts (condylomata acuminata) and other genital tumours for human papillomavirus type 6 DNA. International Journal of Cancer 29: 143–146

Gissmann L, Wolnik L, Ikenberg H et al 1983 Human papillomavirus types 6 and 11 sequences in genital and laryngeal papillomas and in some cervical cancers. Proceedings of the National Academy of Science USA 80: 560–563

Glezen W P, Fernald G W, Lohr J A et al 1975 Acute respiratory disease of university students with special reference to the etiologic role of Herpesvirus hominis. American Journal of Epidemiology 101: 111–121

Gogoi M P 1969 Amebiasis of the female genital tract. American Journal of Obstetrics and Gynecology 105: 1281–1286

Goldberg J 1964 Studies of granuloma inguinale VII some epidemiological considerations of the disease. British Journal of Venereal Diseases 40: 140–145

Goldman L 1977 Spread of condylomata acuminata to infants and children (letter). Archives of Dermatology 113: 1294–1295

Goldmeier D, Ridgway G L, Oriel J D 1981 Chlamydial vulvovaginitis in a postmenopausal woman. Lancet ii: 476–477

Grabstold H, Swan L 1952 Genitourinary lesions in leprosy with special reference to the problem of atrophy of the testis. Journal of the American Medical Association 149: 1287–1291

Gratz N G 1977 Treatment resistance in louse control. In: Orkin M, Maibach H I, Parish L C, Schwartzman R M, (eds) Scabies and pediculosis. Lippincott, Philadelphia, p 179

Grayston J T, Wang S-P 1975 New knowledge of chlamydiae and the diseases they cause. Journal of Infectious Diseases 132: 87–105

Greenblatt R B, Dienst R B, Baldwin K R 1959 Lymphogranuloma venereum and granuloma inguinale. Medical Clinics of North America 43: 1493–1506

Gross G, Pfister H, Hagedorn M, Gissmann L 1982 Correlation between human papillomavirus (HPV) type and histology of warts. Journal of Investigative Dermatology 78: 160–164

Grossman J H 1980 Viral infection in obstetrics and gynecology. Obstetrics and Gynecology Annual 9: 55–76

Grossman J H, Wallen W C, Sever J L 1981 Management of genital herpes simplex virus infection during pregnancy. Obstetrics and Gynecology 58: 1–4

Grubb C 1977 Colour atlas of gynaecological cytopathology. HM + M, Aylesbury, p 23–30

Grundsell H, Larsson G, Bekassy Z 1984 Treatment of condylomata acuminata with the carbon dioxide laser. British Journal of Obstetrics and Gynaecology 91: 193–196

Guillet G Y, Braun L, Masse R et al 1984 Bowenoid papulosis. Demonstration of human papilloma virus (HPV) with anti-HPV immune serum. Archives of Dermatology 120: 514–516

Guinan M E, MacCallum J, Kern E R, Overall J C, Spruance S L 1981 Course of an untreated episode of recurrent genital herpes simplex infection in 27 women. New England Journal of Medicine 304: 759–763

Gump D W, Gibson M, Ashikaga T 1984 Lack of association between genital mycoplasmas and infertility. New England Journal of Medicine 310: 937–941

Hager W D, Brown S T, Kraus S J et al 1980 Metronidazole for vaginal trichomoniasis: seven day vs single dose regimens. Journal of the American Medical Association 244: 1219–1220

Hain J, Doshi N, Harger J H 1980 Ascending transcervical herpes simplex infection with intact fetal membranes. Obstetrics and Gynecology 56: 106–109

Hammar H, Wanger L 1977 Erysipelas and necrotising fasciitis. British Journal of Dermatology 96: 409–419

Hammond G W, Lian C J, Wilt J C 1978 Determination of the hemin requirement of Haemophilus ducreyi: evaulation of the porphyrin test and media used in the satellite growth test. Journal of Clinical Microbiology 7: 243–246

Handojo I, Pardjono A 1973 Treatment of condylomata acuminata with 5% 5-fluorouracil ointment. Asian Journal of Medicine 9: 162–166

Hare M J, Thin R N 1983 Chlamydial infection of the lower genital tract of women. British Medical Bulletin 39: 138–144

Harman R R M 1986 Parasitic worms and protozoa. In: Rook A, Wilkinson D S, Ebling F J G, Champion R H, Burton J L (eds) Textbook of dermatology, 4th edn. Blackwell Scientific, Oxford, chapter 26

Harrison H R, Alexander E R, Weinstein L et al 1982 Epidemiologic correlations of genital infections and outcomes in pregnancy. In: Mårdh P-A, Holmes K K, Oriel J D, Piot P, Schachter J (eds) Chlamydial infections. Elsevier Biomedical, Amsterdam, p 159

Hess J 1969 Review of current methods for the detection of Trichomonas in clinical material. Journal of Clinical Pathology

22: 269–278

Higgs J M, Wells R S 1972 Chronic mucocutaneous candidiasis: associated abnormalities of iron metabolism. British Journal of Dermatology 86, Suppl 8: 88–102

Hill LVH 1985 Anaerobes and Gardnerella vaginalis in non-specific vaginitis. Genitourinary Medicine 61: 114–119

Hill T J, Blyth W A 1976 An alternative theory of herpes simplex recurrence and a possible role for prostaglandins. Lancet i: 397–398

Hilton A L, Warnock D W 1975 Vaginal candidosis and the role of the digestive tract as a source of infection. British Journal of Obstetrics and Gynaecology 82: 922–926

Hipp S S, Lawton W D, Chen N C et al 1974 Inhibition of Neisseria gonorrhoeae by a factor produced by Candida albicans. Applied Microbiology 27: 192–196

Hirsch M S, Zisman B, Allison A C et al 1970 Macrophages and age-dependent resistance to herpes simplex virus in mice. Journal of Immunology 104: 1160–1165

Hodgson-Jones I S 1951 Orf in London. British Medical Journal i: 795–796

Honigberg B M 1978 Trichomonads of importance in human medicine. In: Kreiser J P (ed) Parasitic protozoa, vol. 2. Academic Press, New York, p. 275

Hopso-Harvu V K, Gronroos M, Punnonen R 1980 Vaginal yeasts in parturients and infestation of the newborn. Acta Obstetrica Gynecologica Scandinavica 59: 73–77

Hunt E 1954 Ulcers of the vulva. In: Diseases affecting the vulva, 4th edn. Henry Kimpton, London, p. 122

Hurley R, de Louvois J 1979 Candida vaginitis. Postgraduate Medical Journal 55: 645–649

Hutchinson P E, Summerly R, Lawson R S 1976 Progressive postoperative gangrene: a reminder. British Journal of Dermatology 194: 89–95

Ingram J T 1955 Tinea of vulva. British Medical Journal ii: 1500

International Symposium 1983 International symposium on M. hominis—a human pathogen. Sexually Transmitted Diseases 10: 225–385

Izumi A K, Edwards J 1973 Herpes zoster and neurogenic bladder dysfunction. Journal of the American Medical Association 224: 1748–1750

Jablonska S, Orth G 1983 Human papovaviruses. In: Rook A J, Maibach H I (eds) Recent Advances in Dermatology 6. Churchill Livingstone, Edinburgh, p 1

James J R E 1968 Orf in man. British Medical Journal iii: 804–806

Janson P 1959 Seltere zoster verlaufeformen. Zeitschrift für Haut und Geschlechtskrankheiten 26: 292

Jarrett W F H, McNeil P E, Laird H M et al 1981 Papilloma viruses in benign and malignant tumours of cattle. In: Essex M, Todaro G, zur Hausen H (eds) Cold Spring Harbor Laboratory. Cold Spring Harbor, New York, p 215

Jeansson S, Molin L 1974 On the occurrence of genital herpes simplex virus infection. Acta Dermatovenereologica 54: 479–484

Jelliffe D B, Jacobson F W 1954 The clinical picture of tinea versicolor in negro infants. Journal of Tropical Medicine and Hygiene 57: 290–292

Johnson C G, Mellanby K 1972 The parasitology of human scabies. Parasitology 39: 285–290

Jopling W H, Harman R R M 1986 Leprosy. In: Rook A, Wilkinson D S, Ebling F J G (eds) Textbook of dermatology, 4th edn. Blackwell Scientific, Oxford, ch 23, p. 823

Josey W E, Nahmias A S, Naib Z M, Utley D M, McKenzie W J, Coleman M T 1966 Genital herpes simplex infection in the female. American Journal of Obstetrics and Gynecology 96:

493–501

Judson F N, Ruder M A 1979 Effect of hysterectomy on genital infections. British Journal of Venereal Diseases 55: 434–438

Juel-Jensen B E, McCallum F O, Mackenzie AMR et al 1970 Treatment of zoster with idoxuridine in dimethyl sulphoxide: results of two double-blind controlled trials. British Medical Journal iv: 776–780

Kacker T P 1973 Vulvovaginitis in an adult with threadworms in the vagina. British Journal of Venereal Diseases 49: 314–315

Kakoti L M, Dey N C 1957 Chromoblastomycosis in India. Journal of the Indian Medical Association 28: 351

Kalinyak J E, Fleagle G, Docherty J 1977 Incidence and distribution of herpes simplex virus types 1 and 2 from genital lesions in college women. Journal of Medical Virology 1: 175–181

Kalter D C, Tschen J A, Cernoch P L et al 1986 Genital white piedra: Epidemiology, microbiology and therapy. Journal of the American Academy of Dermatology 14: 982–993

Karol M D, Conner C S, Watabe A S et al 1980 Podophyllum: suspected teratogenicity from topical application. Clinical Toxicology 16: 283–286

Kaufman R H, Friedrich E G 1985 The carbon dioxide laser in the treatment of vulvar disease. Clinical Obstetrics and Gynecology 28: 220–229

Kaufman R H, Dreesman G R, Burek J et al 1981 Herpesvirus-induced antigens in squamous-cell carcinoma in situ of the vulva. New England Journal of Medicine 305: 483–488

Kaye D, Levinson M E 1977 In vitro inhibition of growth of Neisseria gonorrhoeae by genital micro-organisms. Sexually Transmitted Diseases 4: 1–3

Kearns D H, Seibert G B, O'Reilly R et al 1973 Paradox of the immune response to uncomplicated gonococcal urethritis. New England Journal of Medicine 289: 1170–1174

Kilbrick S 1980 Herpes simplex infections at term. Journal of the American Medical Association 243: 157–160

Kimura S, Hirai A, Harada R et al 1978 So-called multicentric pigmented Bowen's disease. Dermatologica 157: 229–237

King A 1964 Recent advances in venereology. J and A Churchill, London, p 304

King A, Nicol C S, Rodin P 1980 Venereal diseases, 4th edn. Bailliere Tindall, London, p 53, 215

King L S, Sullivan M 1947 Effects of podophyllin and of colchicine on normal skin, on condyloma acuminatum and on verruca vulgaris. Archives of Pathology 43: 374–386

Kinghorn G 1978 Genital warts: incidence of associated infections. British Journal of Dermatology 99: 405–409

Kinghorn G R 1986 Treatment of papillomavirus infections. In: Oriel J D, Harris J R W, (eds) Recent advances in sexually transmitted diseases 3. Churchill Livingstone, London, pp 147–155

Kinghorn G R, Rashid S 1979 Prevalence of rectal and pharyngeal infection in women with gonorrhoea in Sheffield. British Journal of Venereal Diseases 55: 408–410

Knox S R, Corey L, Blough H A et al 1982 Historical findings in subjects from a high socioeconomic group who have genital infections with herpes simplex virus. Sexually Transmitted Diseases 9: 15–20

Koberman T, Clark L, Griffin W T 1980 Maternal death secondary to disseminated Herpesvirus hominis. American Journal of Obstetrics and Gynecology 137: 742–743

Konrad, K 1936 Ulceroses Syphilid zwei Jahre nach durchgefuhrer Malariakur. Zentralblatt für Haut-und Geschlechtskrankenheiten 53: 150

Krogstad D J, Spencer H C, Healy G R 1978 Current concepts in parasitology—amebiasis. New England Journal of Medicine 298: 262–265

Kurman R J, Shah K H, Lancaster W D et al 1981 Immunoperoxidase localisation of papillomavirus antigen in cervical dysplasia and vulvar condylomata. American Journal of Obstetrics and Gynecology 140: 931–935

Lafferty W E, Coombs R W, Benedetti J et al 1987 Recurrences after oral and genital Herpes simplex virus infection. Influence of site of infection and viral type. New England Journal of Medicine 316: 1444–1449

Lal S 1971 Continued efficacy of streptomycin in the treatment of granuloma inguinale. British Journal of Venereal Diseases 47: 454–455

Lal S, Nicholas C 1970 Epidemiological and clinical features in 165 cases of granuloma inguinale. British Journal of Venereal Diseases 46: 461–463

Lancet (Leading Article) 1985 Inosine pranobex and mucocutaneous herpes. Lancet i: 200–201

Lancet (Leading Article) 1986 EBV and the uterine cervix. Lancet ii: 1134–1135

Lang W R, Israel S L, Fritz M A 1958 Staphylococcal vulvovaginitis: a report of two cases following antibiotic therapy. Obstetrics and Gynecology 11: 352–354

Laohadtanaphorn S, Hunter J C, Ansell I D 1979 Multicentric pigmented carcinoma-in-situ in the vulva in association with vulval condylomata acuminata. Australian and New Zealand Journal of Obstetrics and Gynaecology 19: 249–252

Lapan B 1970 Is the 'pill' a cause of vaginal candidosis? Culture study. New York State Journal of Medicine 70: 949–951

Lawee D, Shafir M S 1983 Solitary penile ulcer associated with infectious mononucleosis. Canadian Medical Association Journal 129: 146–147

Lawson J B 1967 Chronic lymphoedema and elephantiasis of the vulva. In: Lawson J B, Stewart D B (eds) Obstetrics and Gynaecology in the tropics and developing countries. Arnold, London, p 466

Lee L, Schmale J D 1973 Ampicillin therapy for Corynebacterium vaginale vaginitis. American Journal of Obstetrics and Gynecology 115: 786–790

Lee Y -H, Rankin J S, Alpert S et al 1977 Microbiological investigation of Bartholin's gland abscesses and cysts. American Journal of Obstetrics and Gynaecology 129: 150–153

Legal H-P 1974 The treatment of trichomonas and candida vaginitis with clotrimazole vaginal tablets. Postgraduate Medical Journal 50: 581

Lever W F, Schaumberg-Lever G 1975 Histology of the skin, 5th edn. Lippincott, Philadelphia, p 337–360

Levine R U, Crum C P, Herman E et al 1984 Cervical papillomavirus infection and intraepithelial neoplasia: a study of male sexual partners. Obstetrics and Gynecology 64: 16–20

Lipschutz B 1921 Untersuchungen über die Aetiologie der Krankheiten der herpes Gruppe. Archives von Dermatologie und Syphililologie (Berlin) 136: 428–438

Lodder J 1970 The yeasts: a taxonomic study, 2nd edn. Elsevier North Holland, Amsterdam

Lohmeyer H 1974 Treatment of candidosis and trichomoniasis of the female genital tract. Postgraduate Medical Journal 50: S81

Lomax C W, Harbert G M, Thornton W N 1976 Actinomycosis of the female genital tract. Obstetrics and Gynecology 48: 341–346

Ludwig H O, Biswal N, Benyesh-Mernick M 1972 Studies on the relatedness of herpesviruses through DNA–DNA hybridisation. Virology 49: 95–101

Lukehart S A, Baker-Zander S A, Lloyd R M et al 1980 Characterisation of lymphocyte responsiveness in early experimental syphilis—II Nature of cellular infiltration and *Treponema pallidum* distribution in testicular lesions. Journal of Immunology 124: 461–467

Lyng J, Christensen J A 1981 A double-blind study of the value of treatment with a single-dose tinidazole of partners to females with trichomoniasis. Acta Obstetrica Gynecologica Scandinavica 60: 199–204

McCallum M, Tozer R A 1973 A Survey of selected vaginal flora in Malawian women. Central African Journal of Medicine 19: 176–180

McCance D J 1986 Human papillomaviruses infecting the genital tract. In: Oriel J D, Harris J R W (eds) Recent advances in sexually transmitted diseases 3. Churchill Livingstone, Edinburgh, pp 109–125

McCance D J, Walker P G, Dyson J L et al 1983 Presence of human papillomavirus DNA sequences in cervical intra-epithelial neoplasia. British Medical Journal 287: 784–788

McCann J S, Harris J R W, Mahoney J D H 1974 Vaccinia of the vulva: a case report. British Journal of Venereal Diseases 50: 155–156

McCormack W M, Reynolds G H 1982 Effect of menstrual cycle and method of contraception on recovery of *Neisseria gonorrhoeae*. Journal of the American Medical Association 247: 1292–1294

McCormack W M, Almeida P C, Bailey P E et al 1972 Sexual activity and vaginal colonisation with genital mycoplasmas. Journal of the American Medical Association 221: 1375–1377

McCoy C R, Applebaum H, Besser A S 1982 Condylomata acuminata: an unusual presentation of child abuse. Journal of Pediatric Surgery 17: 505–507

McDougall M L 1975 Genital herpes simplex in the female 1968–1973. New Zealand Medical Journal 82: 333–337

McKee P H, Wright E, Hutt M S R 1983 Vulval schistosomiasis. Clinical and Experimental Dermatology 8: 189–194

McKendrick M W, McGill J I, White J E, Wood M J 1986 Oral acyclovir in acute herpes zoster. British Medical Journal 293: 1529–1532

McLaren L C, Davis L E, Healy G R, James C G 1983 Isolation of Trichomonas vaginalis from the respiratory tract of infants with respiratory disease. Pediatrics 71: 888–890

McNabb P C, Tomasi T B 1981 Host defence mechanisms at mucosal surfaces. Annual Review of Microbiology 35: 477–496

Machnicki S 1953 Diphtheria of the vulva and vagina. Zeitschrift für Haut- und Geschlechtskrankheiten 86: 386

Majmudar B, Chaiken M C, Lee K U 1976 Amebiasis of clitoris mimicking carcinoma. Journal of the American Medical Association 236 i: 1145–1146

Malison M D, Morris R, Jones L W 1982 Autogenous vaccine therapy for condyloma acuminatum. A double-blind controlled study. British Journal of Venereal Diseases 58: 62–65

Marmar J L 1972 The management of resistant chancroid in Viet Nam. Journal of Urology 107: 807–815

Marsden P D 1979 Current concepts in parasitology: leishmaniasis. New England Journal of Medicine 300: 350–355

Masterson G, Napier I R, Henderson J N et al 1977 Three-day clotrimazole treatment in candidal vulvovaginitis. British Journal of Venereal Diseases 53: 126–128

Matras G 1935 Lues III. Ulcer gummosa. Zentralblatt für Haut und Geschlechtskrankheiten 51: 89

Mayer H G K 1972 Pathogénie et traitement des prétendues abces et kystes de la glande de Bartholin. À propos de 109 observations. Journal de Gynécologie Obstetrique et Biologie de la Reproduction 1: 71

Meingassner L, Havelec L, Mieth H 1978 Studies on strain sensitivity of *Trichomonas vaginalis* to metronidazole. British Journal of Venereal Diseases 54: 72–76

Meisels A, Fortin R, Roy M 1977 Condylomatous lesions of the cervix and vagina II Cytologic, colposcopic and histopathologic study. Acta Cytologica 21: 379–390

Meisels A, Morin C, Casas-Cordero M 1982 Human papillomavirus infection of the cervix. International Journal of Gynecologic Pathology 1: 75–94

Mellanby K 1972 Scabies, 2nd edn. Classey, Hampton, England

Meltzer R M 1983 Necrotising fasciitis and progressive synergistic bacterial gangrene. Obstetrics and Gynecology 61: 757–760

Mertz G H, Schmidt O, Jourden J L et al 1985 Frequency of acquisition of first-episode genital infections with Herpes simplex virus from symptomatic and asymptomatic source contact. Sexually Transmitted Diseases 12: 25–32

Meyers J D, Flournoy N, Thomas E D 1980 Infection with herpes simplex virus and cell-mediated immunity after marrow transplant. Journal of Infectious Diseases 142: 338–346

Milne J D, Warnock D W 1979 Effect of simultaneous oral and vaginal treatment on the rate of cure and relapse in vaginal candidosis. British Journal of Venereal Diseases 55: 362–365

Milsom I, Forssman L 1982 Treatment of vaginal candidosis with a single 500 mg clotrimazole pessary. British Journal of Venereal Diseases 58: 124–126

Mindel A 1984 Herpes vaccine. British Journal of Venereal Diseases 60: 204

Mindel A, Adler M W, Sutherland S 1982 Intravenous acyclovir treatment for primary genital herpes. Lancet i: 697–700

Mindel A, Weller I V D, Faherty A et al 1984 Prophylactic oral acyclovir in recurrent genital herpes. Lancet ii: 57–59

MMWR (Morbidity and Mortality Weekly Report) 1985 Sexually transmitted disease treatment guidelines 1985. Centers for Disease Control 34: 4S

Møller B R 1983 The role of mycoplasmas in the upper genital tract of women. Sexually Transmitted Diseases 10: 281–284

Montaldi D H, Giambrone J P, Courey N G et al 1974 Podophyllin poisoning associated with the treatment of condylomata acuminata: a case report. American Journal of Obstetrics and Gynecology 119: 1130–1131

Montes L F 1969 Erythrasma and diabetes mellitus. Archives of Dermatology 99: 674–676

Montes L F, Black S H 1967 Fine structure of diphtheroids of erythrasma. Journal of Investigative Dermatology 48: 342–346

Moore D 1954 Genito-peritoneal tuberculosis—a review of 26 cases. South African Medical Journal 28: 666–673

Mosley R, Covey L, Winter C, Benjamin D 1981 Comparison of viral isolation, direct immunofluorescence and indirect immunoperoxidase for detection of genital herpes simplex virus infection. Journal of Clinical Microbiology 13: 913–918

Mounts P, Shah K V 1984 Respiratory papillomatosis. Progress in Medical Virology 29: 90–114

Mursic V P 1975 Diagnosis, pathogenicity and therapy of candidosis. Munchen Medische Wochenschrift 117: 893–896

Nabarro D 1954 Congenital syphilis. Edward Arnold, London

Naguib S M, Comstock G W, Davis H J 1966 Epidemiologic study of trichomoniasis in normal women. Obstetrics and Gynecology 27: 607–616

Nahmias A J 1970 Disseminated herpes simplex virus infections. New England Journal of Medicine 282: 684–686

Nahmias A J, Dowdle W 1968 Antigenic and biologic differences in herpesvirus hominis. Progress in Medical Virology

10: 110–159

Nahmias A J, Roizman B 1973 Infection with herpes simplex viruses 1 and 2. New England Journal of Medicine 289: 667–673, 719–725, 781–789

Nahmias A J, Sawanabori S 1978 The genital herpes–cervical cancer hypothesis: 10 years later. Progress in Experimental Tumor Research 21: 117–139

Nahmias A J, Josey W E, Naib Z M et al 1970 Antibodies to herpesvirus hominis types 1 and 2 in humans: patients with genital infections. American Journal of Epidemiology 91: 539–546

Nahmias A J, Visintone A M, Reimer C B et al 1976 Herpes simplex virus infections of the fetus and newborn. In: Krugman S, Gershon A A (eds) Infections of the fetus and newborn infant. Liss, New York, p 63

Naraqi S, Jackson G G, Jonasson O et al 1977 Prospective study of prevalence, incidence and source of herpesvirus infections in patients with renal allografts. Journal of Infectious Diseases 136: 531–540

Nicholson K G 1984 Antiviral therapy. Respiratory infections—genital herpes and herpetic keratitis. Lancet ii: 617–621

Noble W C 1981 Microbiology of human skin, 2nd edn. Lloyd Luke, London

Noble W C, Presbury D, Connor B L et al 1974 Prevalence of streptococci and staphylococci in lesions of impetigo. British Journal of Dermatology 91: 115–119

Norburn L M, Coles R B 1960 Recurrent erysipelas following vulvectomy. Journal of Obstetrics and Gynaecology of the British Commonwealth 67: 279–281

Nsanze H, Fast M V, D'Costa J et al 1981 Genital ulcers in Kenya: clinical and laboratory study. British Journal of Venereal Diseases 57: 378–381

Nuttall G H 1918 The biology of Phthirus pubis. Parasitology 10: 383–390

Odds F C 1977 Cure and relapse with antifungal therapy. Proceedings of the Royal Society of Medicine 70 Supplement 4: 24–28

Odds F C 1979 Candida and candidosis. Leicester University Press

Odds F C, Abbott A B, Reed T A G, Willmott F E 1983 Candida albicans strain types from the genitalia of patients with and without Candida infection. European Journal of Obstetrics, Gynecology and Reproductive Biology 15: 37–43

O'Reilly R J, Chibbaro A, Anger E et al 1977 Cell-mediated immune response in patients with recurrent herpes simplex virus infection II Infection-associated deficiency of lymphokine production in patients with recurrent herpes labialis or herpes progenitalis. Journal of Immunology 108: 1095–1102

Orfanos C E, Schloesser E, Mahrle G 1971 Hair destroying growth of Corynebacterium tenuis in the so-called trichomycosis axillaris. Archives of Dermatology 103: 632–636

Oriel J D 1971 Natural history of genital warts. British Journal of Venereal Diseases 47: 1–13

Oriel J D, Almeida J D 1970 Demonstration of virus particles in human genital warts. British Journal of Venereal Diseases 46: 37–42

Oriel J D, Ridgway G L 1982 Genital infection by Chlamydia trachomatis. Edward Arnold, London

Oriel J D, Partridge B M, Denny M J et al 1972 Genital yeast infection. British Medical Journal iv: 761–764

Ovcinnikov N M, Delektorskij V V 1968 Further study of ultrathin sections of Treponema pallidum under the electron microscope. British Journal of Venereal Diseases 44: 1–34

Ovcinnikov N M, Delektorskij V V, Turanova E N et al 1975 Further studies of Trichomonas vaginalis with transmission

and scanning electron microscopy. British Journal of Venereal Diseases 51: 357–375

Paavonen J 1979 Chlamydia trachomatis induced urethritis in female partners of men with nongonococcal urethritis. Sexually Transmitted Diseases 6: 69–71

Paavonen J, Miettinen A, Stevens C E et al 1983 Mycoplasma hominis in nonspecific vaginitis. Sexually Transmitted Diseases 10: 271–275

Parks J 1941 Diphtheritic vaginitis in the adult. American Journal of Obstetrics and Gynecology 41: 714–718

Parr R P, Bennett J W, Garon C F 1977 Structural characterisation of the molluscum contagiosum virus genome. Virology 81: 247–255

Parvey L S, Ch'ien L T 1980 Neonatal herpes simplex virus infection introduced by fetal-monitor scalp electrodes. Pediatrics 65: 1150–1153

Patel R, Groff D B 1972 Condyloma acuminata in childhood. Pediatrics 50: 153–154

Pauly C R, Artis W M, Jones H E 1978 Atopic dermatitis, impaired cellular immunity and molluscum contagiosum. Archives of Dermatology 114: 391–396

Pearson H E 1964 Parturition varicella-zoster. Obstetrics and Gynecology 23: 21–24

Perl G 1972 Errors in the diagnosis of Trichomonas vaginalis infection as observed among 1199 patients. Obstetrics and Gynecology 39: 7–12

Peterslund N A, Seyer-Hansen K, Ipsen J et al 1981 Acyclovir in herpes zoster. Lancet ii: 827–830

Pheifer T A, Forsyth P S, Durfee M A et al 1978 Nonspecific vaginitis. Role of Haemophilus vaginalis and treatment with metronidazole. New England Journal of Medicine 298: 1429–1434

Plummer F A, Kraus S J, Sottnek F O et al 1984 Chancroid and granuloma inguinale. In: Wentworth B B, Judson F N (eds) Laboratory methods for the diagnosis of sexually transmitted diseases. American Public Health Association, Washington, D C, p 204

Porter D D, Wimberly I, Benyesh-Melnick M 1969 Prevalence of antibodies to E B virus and other herpesviruses. Journal of the American Medical Association 208: 1675–1679

Portnoy J, Ahronheim G A, Ghibu F et al 1984 Recovery of Epstein–Barr virus from genital ulcers. New England Journal of Medicine 311: 966–968

Postlethwaite R 1970 Molluscum contagiosum. Archives of Environmental Health 21: 432–438

Powell L C, Pollard M, Jinkins J L 1970 Treatment of condyloma acuminata by autogenous vaccine. Southern Medical Journal 63: 202–205

Prober O G, Sullender W M, Yasukawa L L et al 1987 Low risk of herpes simplex virus infections in neonates exposed to the virus at the time of vaginal delivery to mothers with recurrent genital herpes simplex virus infections. New England Journal of Medicine 316: 240–244

Punsalang A P, Sawyer W D 1973 Role of pili in the virulence of Neisseria gonorrhoeae. Infection and Immunity 8: 255–282

Purdie D W, Carty M J, McLeod T I F 1977 Tubo-ovarian actinomycosis and the IUCD. British Medical Journal ii: 1392

Pyrhönen S, Johansson E 1975 Regression of warts: an immunological study. Lancet i: 592–594

Quick C A, Watts S L, Krzyzek R A et al 1980 Relationship between condylomata acuminata and laryngeal papillomas. Clinical and molecular virological evidence. Annals of Otology, Rhinology and Laryngology 89: 467–471

Raab B, Lorincz A L 1981 Genital herpes simplex—concepts and treatment. Journal of the American Academy of Dermatology 5: 249–263

Rajam R V, Rangiah P N 1954 Donovanosis (granuloma inguinale, granuloma venereum). WHO Monograph Series, 24

Rashid S, Collins W, Corner J, Morton R S 1984 Survival of *Candida albicans* on fabric after laundering. British Journal of Venereal Diseases 60: 277

Rasmussen L, Merigan T C 1978 Role of T lymphocytes in cellular immune responses during herpes simplex virus infection in humans. Proceedings of the National Academy of Science USA 75: 3957–3961

Rea W J, Wyrick W J 1970 Necrotising fasciitis. Annals of Surgery 172: 957–963

Rees E 1967 Gonococcal bartholinitis. British Journal of Venereal Diseases 43: 150–156

Reeves W C, Corey L, Adams H G et al 1981 Risk of recurrence after first episode of genital herpes: relation to HSV type and antibody response. New England Journal of Medicine 305: 315–319

Reichman R C, Badger G J, Guinan M E et al 1983 Topically administered acyclovir in the treatment of recurrent herpes simplex genitalis: a controlled trial. Journal of Infectious Diseases 147: 336–340

Reichman R C, Badger G J, Mertz G J et al 1984 Treatment of recurrent genital herpes simplex infections with oral acyclovir. Journal of the American Medical Association 251: 2103–2107

Reid R 1985 Superficial laser vulvectomy. I. The efficacy of extended superficial ablation for refractory and very extensive condylomas. American Journal of Obstetrics and Gynecology 151: 1047–1052

Reid R, Laverty C R, Coppleson M et al 1980 Noncondylomatous cervical wart virus infection. Obstetrics and Gynecology 55: 476–483

Rein M F, Sullivan J A, Mandell G L 1980 Trichomonacidal activity of human polymorphonuclear leucocytes: killing by disruption and fragmentation. Journal of Infectious Diseases 142: 575–585

Ricci J 1945 One hundred years of gynaecology 1800–1900. Blakiston, Philadelphia, p 470

Ridley C M 1984 Vulval dysplasia. British Journal of Hospital Medicine 159: 223

Ridley C M 1986 Recent advances in vulval disease. In: Champion R H (ed) Recent advances in dermatology 7. Churchill Livingstone, London, p 223

Roberts D B, Hester L L 1972 Progressive synergistic bacterial gangrene arising from abscesses of the vulva and Bartholin's gland. American Journal of Obstetrics and Gynecology 114: 285–290

Robinson S C, Halifax N S 1961 Observations on vaginal trichomoniasis in pregnancy. Canadian Medical Association Journal 84: 984–963

Rock B, Naghashfar Z, Barnett N, Buscema J, Woodruff J D, Shah K 1986 Genital tract papillomavirus infection in children. Archives of Dermatology 122: 1129–1132

Rodin P, Hass G 1966 Metronidazole and pregnancy. British Journal of Venereal Disease 42: 210–212

Rohatiner J J, 1966 Relationship of *Candida albicans* in the genital and anorectal tracts. British Journal of Venereal Diseases 42: 197–200

Roizman B, Buchman T 1979 The molecular epidemiology of Herpes simplex virus. Hospital Practice 95: 104–115

Ronald A R 1986 Laboratory diagnosis of *Haemophilis ducreyi* infection. In: Oriel J D, Harris J R W (eds) Recent Advances in sexually transmitted diseases 3. Churchill Livingstone, Edinburgh, pp 59–69

Ronald A R, Wilt J C, Albritton W C 1983 *Haemophilis ducreyi*. In: Holmes K K, Mårdh P A (eds) International perspectives on neglected sexually transmitted diseases. Hemisphere, Washington, p 93

Roome A P, Montefiore D, Waller D 1975 Incidence of Herpesvirus hominis antibodies among blood donor populations. British Journal of Venereal Diseases 51: 324–328

Rothenberg R B, Simon R, Chipperfield E et al 1976 Efficacy of selected diagnostic tests for sexually transmitted diseases. Journal of the American Medical Association 235: 49–51

Roy M, Meisels A, Fortier M, Morin C, Casas-Cordero M, Robitaille C G 1981 Vaginal condylomata: a human papillomavirus infection. Clinical Obstetrics and Gynecology 24: (2) 461–483

Rustia M, Shubik P 1972 Induction of lung tumours and malignant lymphomas in mice by metronidazole. Journal of the National Cancer Institute 48: 421–428

Rutherford W H, Calderwood J W, Hart D et al 1970 Antibiotics in surgical treatment of septic lesions. Lancet i: 1077–1080

Sarkany I, Taplin D, Blank H 1961 Erythrasma. Journal of the American Medical Association 177: 130–133

Schachner L, Hankin D E 1985 Assessing child abuse in childhood condylomata acuminatum. Journal of the American Academy of Dermatology 12: 157–160

Schachter J, Dawson C R 1978 Human chlamydial infections. PSG, Littleton, Massachusetts, p 122

Schaefer G 1959 Diagnosis and treatment of female genital tuberculosis. Clinical Obstetrics and Gynecology 2: 530–535

Schmauz R, Owor R 1980 Condylomatous tumours of the vulva, vagina and penis. Relationship between histological appearance and age. Journal of Clinical Pathology 33: 1039–1046

Schneider V, Kay S, Lee H M 1983 Immunosuppression as a high-risk factor in the development of condyloma acuminatum and squamous neoplasia of the cervix. Acta Cytologica 27: 220–224

Schonfield A, Schattner A, Crespi M et al 1984 Intramuscular human interferon B injections in the treatment of condylomata acuminata. Lancet i: 1038–1041

Schroeter A 1977 Scabies—a venereal disease. In: Orkin M, Maibach H I, Parish L C, Schwartzman R M (eds) Scabies and pediculosis. Lippincott, Philadelphia, p 56

Schroeter A L, Lucas J B, Price E V et al 1972 Treatment for early syphilis and reactivity of serologic tests. Journal of the American Medical Association 221: 471–476

Schwartz P E, Naftolin F 1981 Type 2 Herpes simplex virus and vulvar carcinoma in situ (leading article). New England Journal of Medicine 305: 517–518

Scott R A, Gallis H A, Livengood C H 1985 Phycomycosis of the vulva. American Journal of Obstetrics and Gynecology 153: 675–676

Šeidel J, Zonana J, Totten E 1979 Condylomata acuminata as a sign of sexual abuse in children. Journal of Pediatrics 95: 553–554

Shafeek M A, Osman M I, Hussein M A 1979 Carcinoma of the vulva arising in condylomata acuminata. Obstetrics and Gynecology 54: 120–123

Shelley W B 1980 Herpetic arthritis associated with disseminated herpes simplex in a wrestler. British Journal of Dermatology 103: 209–212

Shelley W B, Miller M A 1984 Electron microscopy, histochemistry and microbiology of bacterial adhesion in trichomycosis axillaris. Journal of the American Academy of Dermatology 10: 1005–1014

Shelton T B, Jerkins G R, Noe H N 1986 Condylomata acuminata in the pediatric patient. Journal of Urology 135: 548–549

Shillitoe H J, Wilton J M A, Lehner T 1977 Sequential changes in cell mediated immune responses to herpes simplex virus after recurrent herpetic infection in humans. Infection and Immunity 18: 130–137

Shokri-Tabibzadeh S, Koss L G et al 1981 Association of human papillomavirus with neoplastic processes in the genital tract of four women with impaired immunity. Gynecologic Oncology 12: 5129–5140

Shy K K, Eschenbach D A 1981 Fatal perineal cellulitis from an episiotomy site. Obstetrics and Gynecology 54: 292–298

Siegal F P, Lopez C, Hammer G S et al 1981 Severe acquired immunodeficiency in male homosexuals manifested by chronic perianal ulcerative herpes simplex lesions. New England Journal of Medicine 305: 1439–1444

Singer A, Campion M J, Clarkson P K, McCance D J 1986 Recognition of subclinical human papilloma virus infection of the vulva. Journal of Reproductive Medicine 31: 985–986

Sixbey J W, Lemon S M, Pagana J S 1986 A second site for EBV shedding: the uterine cervix. Lancet ii: 1122–1124

Slutchuk M, Scatliff J, Hammond G W et al 1980 Clinical, epidemiological, laboratory and therapeutic features of an urban outbreak of chancroid in North America. Reviews of Infectious Diseases 2: 867–879

Smith I W, Peutherer J F 1967 The incidence of Herpesvirus hominis antibody in the population. Journal of Hygiene (London) 65: 395–404

Smith J W, Rogers R E, Katz B P et al 1987 Diagnosis of chlamydial infection in women attending antenatal and gynecologic clinics. Journal of Clinical Microbiology 25: 868–872

Somerville D A, Seville R H, Cunningham R C et al 1970 Erythrasma in a hospital for the mentally subnormal. British Journal of Dermatology 82: 355–358

Sowmini C N 1983 In: Holmes K K, Mårdh P A (eds) International perspectives on neglected sexually transmitted diseases. Hemisphere, Washington, p 205

Sparks R A, Williams G L, Boyce J M H et al 1975 Antenatal screening for candidiasis, trichomoniasis and gonorrhoea. British Journal of Venereal Diseases 51: 110–115

Spellacy W N, Zaias N, Buhi W C et al 1971 Vaginal yeast growth and contraceptive practices. Obstetrics and Gynecology 38: 343–349

Spencer E S, Andersen H K 1979 Viral infections in renal allograft recipients treated with long term immunosuppression. British Medical Journal ii: 829

Spiegel C A, Amsel R, Eschenbach D et al 1980 Anaerobic bacteria in nonspecific vaginitis. New England Journal of Medicine 303: 601–607

Stamm W E, Wagner K F, Amsel R et al 1980 Etiology of the acute urethral syndrome in women. New England Journal of Medicine 303: 409–415

Stanbridge C M, Butler E B 1983 Human papillomavirus infection of the lower female genital tract: association with multicentric neoplasia. International Journal of Gynecological Pathology 2: 264–274

Stevens J G, Cook M L 1971 Latent herpes simplex virus in spinal ganglia of mice. Science 173: 843–845

Stewart D B 1967 Donovanosis and lymphogranuloma venereum. In: Lawson J B, Stewart D B (eds) Obstetrics and gynaecology in the tropics and developing countries. Edward Arnold, London, p 432

Stokes E J, Ridgway G L 1980 Clinical bacteriology. Edward Arnold, London, p 127

Stone H H, Martin J D 1972 Synergistic necrotizing cellulitis. Annals of Surgery 175: 702–711

Straus S E, Takiff H E, Seidlin M et al 1984 Suppression of frequently recurring genital herpes: a placebo-controlled double-blind trial of oral acyclovir. New England Journal of Medicine 310: 1545–1550

Stray-Pedersen B, Eng J, Reikvam T M 1978 Uterine T-mycoplasma colonisation in reproductive failure. American Journal of Obstetrics and Gynecology 130: 307–311

Stumpf P G 1980 Increasing occurrence of condylomata acuminata in premenarchal children. Obstetrics and Gynecology 56: 262–264

Symmers W StC 1960 Leishmaniasis acquired by contagion. A case of marital infection in Britain. Lancet i: 1276

Syrjänen K, Väyrynen M, Castrén O, Yliskoski M, Mäntyjärri R, Pyrhönen S, Saarikoski S 1984 Sexual behaviour of women with human papillomavirus (HPV) lesions of the uterine cervix. British Journal of Venereal Diseases 60: 243–248

Syverton J T 1952 The pathogenesis of the rabbit papillom-to-carcinoma sequence. Annals of the New York Academy of Science 54: 1126–1140

Tager A 1974 Preliminary report on the treatment of recurrent herpes simplex with poliomyelitis vaccine. Dermatologica 149: 253–255

Tang C K, Shermeta D W, Wood C 1978 Congenital condylomata acuminata. American Journal of Obstetrics and Gynecology 131: 912–913

Taylor-Robinson D, McCormack W M 1980 The genital mycoplasmas. New England Journal of Medicine 302: 1003–1010, 1063–1067

Tejani G, Klein S W, Kaplan M 1979 Subclinical herpes simplex genital infection in the perinatal period. American Journal of Obstetrics and Gynecology 135: 547

Thin R N T 1970 Direct and delayed methods of immunofluorescent diagnosis of gonorrhoea in women. British Journal of Venereal Diseases 47: 27–30

Thin R N T, Shaw E J 1979 Diagnosis of gonorrhoea in women. British Journal of Venereal Diseases 55: 10–13

Thin R N T, Melcher D H, Tapp J W et al 1969 Detection of *Trichomonas vaginalis* in women: comparison of 'wet smear' results with those of two cervical cytological methods. British Journal of Venereal Diseases 45: 332–333

Thin R N T, Leighton M, Dixon M J 1977 How often is genital yeast infection sexually transmitted? British Medical Journal ii: 93–94

Thurner J, Meingassner J G 1978 Isolation of *Trichomonas vaginalis* resistant to metronidazole. Lancet ii: 738

Toon P G, Arrand J R, Wilson L P, Sharp D S 1986 Human papillomavirus infection of the uterine cervix of women without cytological signs of neoplasia. British Medical Journal 293: 1261–1264

Trope C, Grundsell H. Henrikson H et al 1982 Giant condyloma acuminatum with focal malignant degeneration. Acta Obstetrica Gynecologica Scandinavica 61: 93–95

Turner T B, Hollander D H 1957 Biology of the treponematoses. WHO Monograph Series 35, Geneva, p 42

Vontvner L A, Hickok A E, Brown Z et al 1982 Recurrent genital herpes simplex virus infection in pregnancy: infant outcome and frequency of asymptomatic recurrences. American Journal of Obstetrics and Gynecology 143: 75–84

Wade T R, Ackerman A B 1979 The effects of podophyllum resin on condylomata acuminata. Archives of Dermatology 115: 1349

Wade T R, Kopf A W, Ackerman A B 1979 Bowenoid papulosis of the genitalia. Archives of Dermatology 115: 306–308

Wagman H 1975 Genital actinomycosis. Proceedings of the Royal Society of Medicine 68: 228–230

Walker P G, Colley N V, Grubb C et al 1983 Abnormalities of the uterine cervix in women with vulval warts. British Journal of Venereal Diseases 59: 120–123

Wallin J 1975 Gonorrhoea in 1972. A 1-year study of patients attending the VD unit in Uppsala. British Journal of Venereal Diseases 51: 41–47

Waugh M A 1974 Herpes zoster of the anogenital area affecting urination and defaecation. British Journal of Dermatology 90: 235–238

Wende R D et al 1971 The VDRL slide test in 322 cases of dark-field positive primary syphilis. Southern Medical Journal 64: 5–10

Weström L, Mårdh P A 1982 Genital chlamydial infections in the female. In: Mårdh P A, Holmes K K, Oriel J D, Piot P, Schachter J (eds) Chlamydial infection. Elsevier Biomedical, Amsterdam, p 121

White S W, Smith J 1979 Trichomycosis pubis. Archives of Dermatology 115: 444–445

Whitley R J, Nahmias A J, Visintine A M et al 1980 The natural history of herpes simplex virus infection of mother and newborn. Pediatrics 66: 489–494

Whittington M J 1957 Epidemiology of infections with Trichomonas vaginalis in the light of improved diagnostic methods. British Journal of Venereal Diseases 33: 80–91

Wildenhoff K E, Ipsen J, Esmann V et al 1979 Treatment of herpes zoster with idoxuridine ointment, including a multivariate analysis of symptoms and signs. Scandinavian Journal of Infectious Diseases 11: 1–9

Wilkin J K 1977 Molluscum contagiosum venereum in a women's out-patient clinic. A venereally transmitted disease. American Journal of Obstetrics and Gynecology 128: 531–535

Wilkinson A E, Cowell L P 1971 Immunofluorescent staining for the detection of Treponema pallidum in early syphilitic lesions. British Journal of Venereal Diseases 47: 252–254

Wilson J 1973 Extensive vulval condylomata acuminata necessitating Caesarian section. Australian and New Zealand Journal of Obstetrics and Gynaecology 13: 121–124

Winner H I, Hurley R 1964 Candida albicans. Churchill Livingstone, London

Wisdom A R, Dunlop E M C 1965 Trichomoniasis: study of the disease and its treatment in women and men. British Journal of Venereal Diseases 41: 90–96

Wolontis S, Jeansson S 1977 Correlation of herpes simplex virus types 1 and 2 with clinical features of infection. Journal of Infectious Diseases 135: 28–33

Woodruff J D, Braun L, Calavieri R et al 1980 Immunologic identification of papillomavirus antigen in condylomatous tissue from the female genital tract. Obstetrics and Gynecology 56: 727–732

World Health Organisation 1983 Current treatments in the control of sexually transmitted diseases. Report of a WHO Consultative Group, Geneva 1982, WHO/VDT/p 433

Wyrick P B, Brownridge E A 1978 Growth of Chlamydia psittaci in macrophages. Infection and Immunity 19: 1054–1060

Yeager A M, Zinkham W T 1980 Varicella-associated thrombocytopenia. Clues to the etiology of childhood idiopathic thrombocytopenic purpura. Johns Hopkins Medical Journal 146: 270–274

Zachow K R, Ostrow R S, Bender M et al 1982 Detection of human papillomavirus DNA in anogenital neoplasia. Nature 300: 771–773

Zamora S, Baumgartner G, Shaw M 1983 Condyloma acuminatum in a $2\frac{1}{2}$ year old girl. Journal of Urology 129: 145–146

zur Hausen H 1982 Human genital cancer: synergism between two virus infections or synergism between a virus infection and initiating events? Lancet ii: 1370–1372

zur Hausen, H 1986 Intracellular surveillance of persisting viral infections. Lancet ii 489–491

zur Hausen H, Gissmann L, Schlehofer J R 1984 Viruses in the etiology of genital cancer. Progress in Medical Virology 30: 170–186

6

General dermatological conditions and dermatoses of the vulva
C M Ridley

This section is mainly concerned with specific dermatological entities. Those discussed comprise those conditions which have a predilection for the vulva, or are common there and elsewhere, or those which while rare have some particular academic or clinical importance.

For further clinical and histopathological details of these conditions as they occur elsewhere the reader is referred to standard texts, for example Lever & Schaumburg Lever (1983), Mehregan (1986), Rook et al (1986). In most cases it will be advisable for the dermatologist's aid to be enlisted in management.

In practice, many vulval problems presented to the clinician are multifactorial, and one important factor is the local environment. Warmth and moisture lead to maceration. Scaling is less apparent or is pale and soggy rather than crisp and white. These factors become the more important the more lesions on the mucosal rather than keratinised surfaces are concerned, and it is well recognised that, as in the mouth, some conditions are less distinctive both clinically and histologically when they occur at the vulva.

Vulval (labia majora) skin can be shown objectively to differ from skin elsewhere. Compared with fore-arm skin it is more readily irritated by local applications, has an increased transepidermal water excretion (Britz & Maibach 1979a, b) and is more easily penetrated by ^{14}C-labelled hydrocortisone (Britz et al 1980). These findings have obvious relevance to allergic and irritant dermatitis and to the use of local preparations.

Finally, it should be remembered that intra-epithelial neoplastic conditions (extramammary Paget's disease, vulval intra-epithelial neoplasia) may mimic benign dermatoses (Fig. 6.1 a and b).

For this reason biopsy of any lesion not clearly categorised or not responding to simple treatment is essential. Many of the common dermatoses, however, will be easily recognisable to the trained dermatological eye, and in rarer conditions biopsy when desirable (for example to establish immuno-fluorescence findings) will often be from other sites.

VULVAL MANIFESTATIONS OF SYSTEMIC DISEASE

Behçet's disease is considered on page 154.

Amyloidosis

Cutaneous lesions are rare and found only in primary and myeloma-associated disease. They are typically glassy or waxy and may show purpura and telangiectasia (Breathnach 1985). Northcutt & Vanover (1985) have reported an example of nodular cutaneous lesions at the vulva in a woman 53 years of age. In this case the lesions were reddish and ulcerated and clinically simulated malignancy.

Histology shows amyloid of immunoglobulin light chain derivation with typical straight filaments of amyloid on electron microscopy. The amyloid material surrounds vessel walls, accounting for the purpura seen clinically.

Acrodermatitis enteropathica

This condition is related to zinc deficiency, whether genetically determined because of the defect in absorption inherited as a recessive characteristic, or acquired though such causes as total

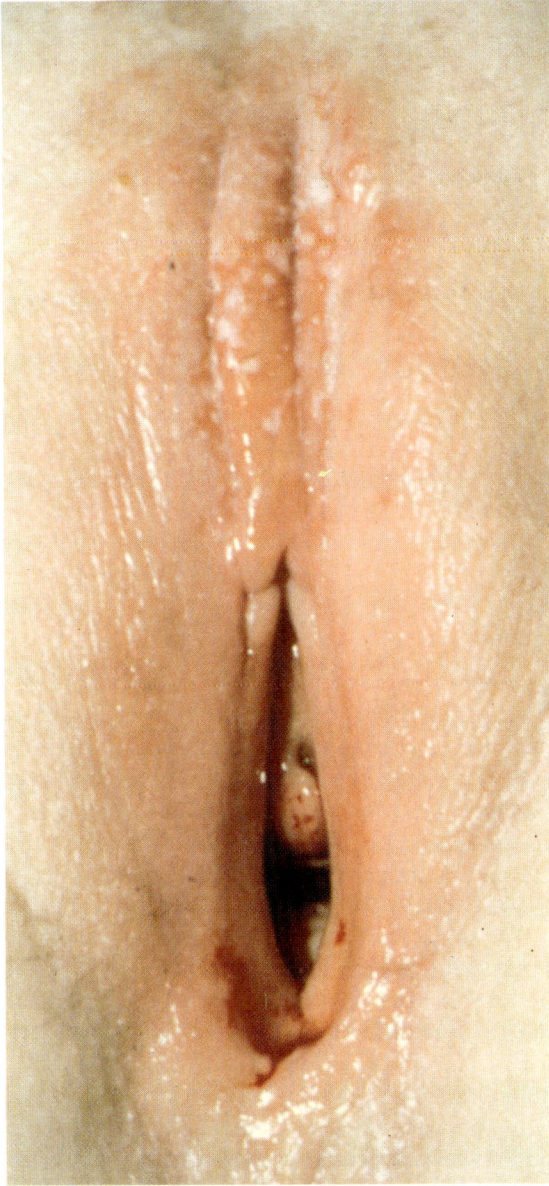

A

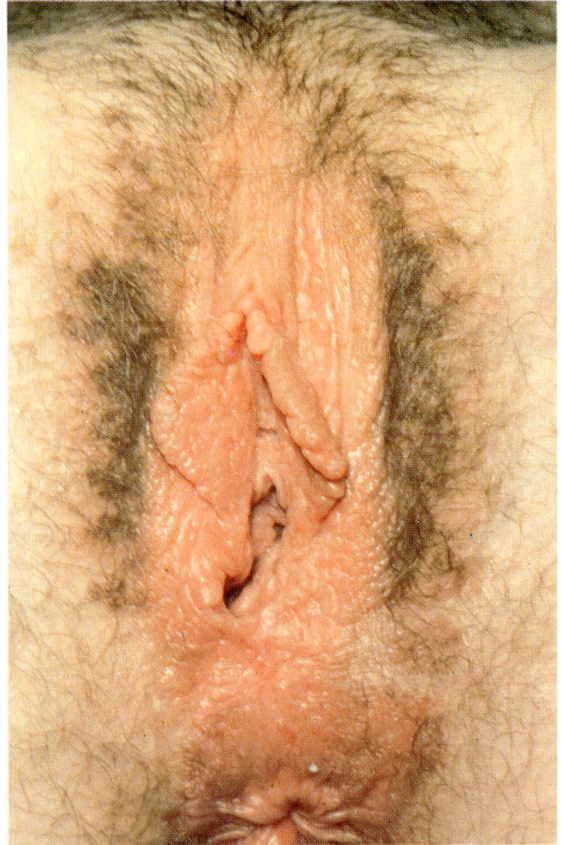

B

Fig. 6.1 (**a**) Extra-mammary Paget's disease (**b**) vulval intraepithelial neoplasia (squamous type)

parenteral nutrition, Crohn's disease (Burgdorf 1981), jejuno-ileal bypass surgery, alcoholism, prematurity, penicillamine given for cystinuria or Wilson's disease, or chelating agents given for iron overload in thalassaemia (Leigh et al 1979, Ridley 1982). The genetically determined examples, and some of the others, are seen in infancy. Adults may suffer from the acquired type, and from relapses of the genetic type, as in the patient of Verburg et al (1974) who developed lesions in pregnancy though previously well controlled on oral zinc therapy. Oral zinc is now the accepted treatment though before its lack was incriminated (Moynahan 1974) di-iodoquine was given with limited success.

The lesions are red, eroded and vesiculopustular; they affect not only the genital area but other parts, particularly the face, and there is loss of hair (Fig. 6.2 a & b). The histology is non-specific so differential diagnosis is on clinical and microbiological grounds from candidosis, seborrhoeic dermatitis, and other banal eruptions, with serum zinc determinations in any case of doubt; a rare differential is Netherton's syndrome, where, in association with ichthyosis, atopy and hair abnormalities, chronic infective anogenital lesions are somewhat similar (Greene & Muller 1985).

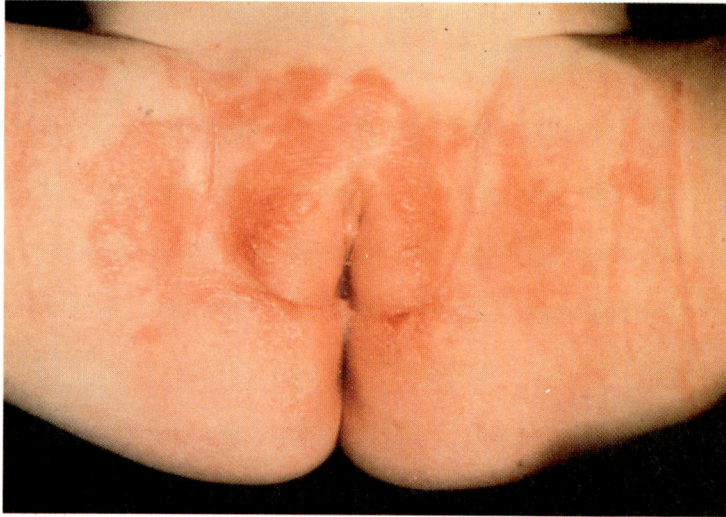

A

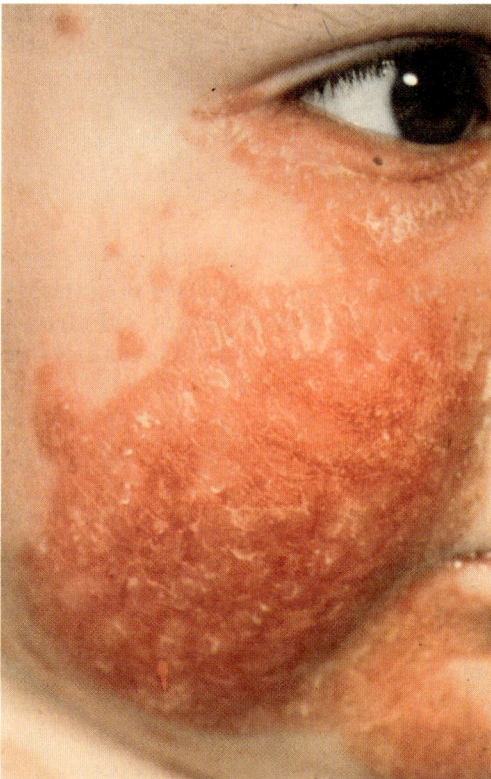

B

Fig. 6.2 Acrodermatitis enteropathica; (a and b) red eroded areas of vulva and face. (By courtesy of Dr D Atherton)

Glucagonoma

This rare pancreatic tumour is strongly associated with a distinctive eruption known as necrolytic migratory erythema and affecting many areas of the body but mainly the genital area. All the first cases (Mallinson et al 1974) showed the rash and so have almost all reported since. The mechanism by which the rash is induced is uncertain (Bloom & Polak 1983).

The subject is usually a middle-aged woman who is ill, with weight loss, stomatitis, glossitis and perhaps diabetes. The lesions are erythematous and bullous, extending and then healing at the edges. The histology shows epidermal necrolysis and a mild lymphocytic dermal infiltrate.

In the differential diagnosis pustular psoriasis, bullous dermatoses and acrodermatitis enteropathica as well as toxic epidermal necrolysis may have to be considered, though the latter is more acute. The clinical picture, however, is usually fairly typical and affords the astute dermatologist an opportunity to diagnose occult abdominal malignancy.

Ulcerative colitis

Anogenital skin lesions are much rarer than in Crohn's disease. Verbov (1973) found only one definite example out of 40 patients. Forman (1966) described a pustular vegetative lesion in the groins

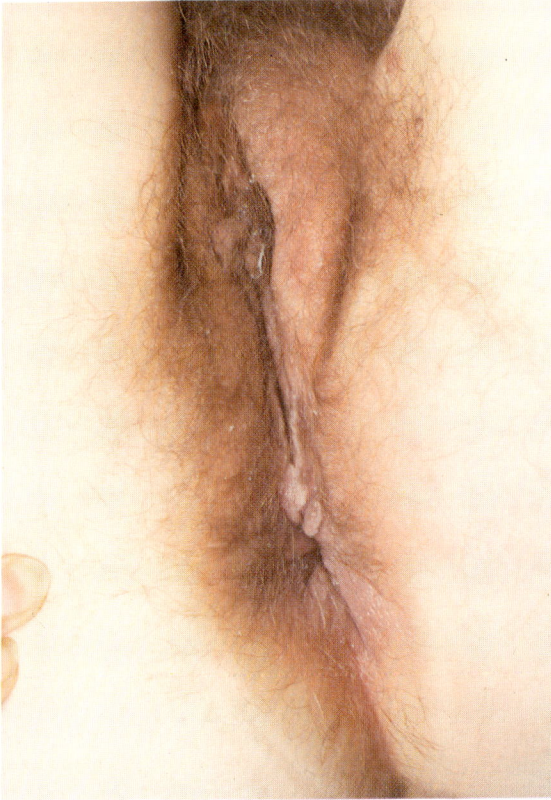

Fig. 6.3 Crohn's disease: unilateral vulval oedema

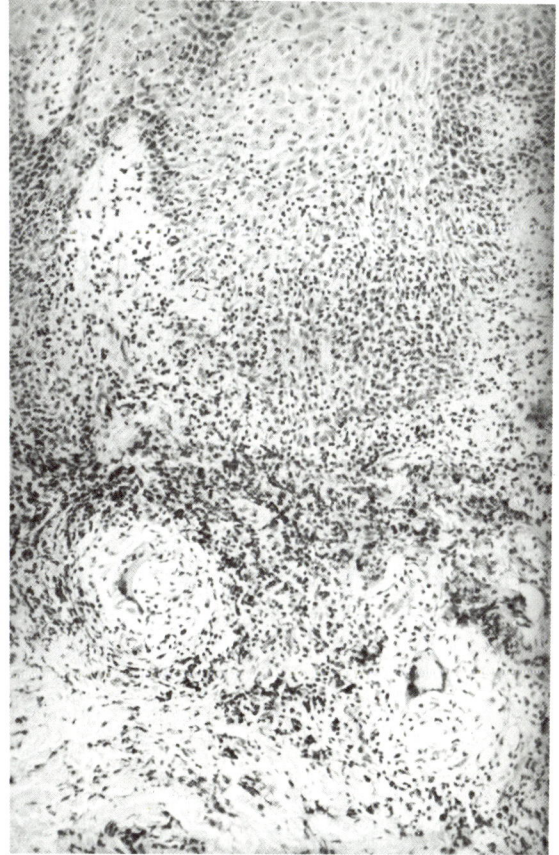

Fig. 6.4 Crohn's disease: granulomatous histology. (By courtesy of Dr C M Ridley The vulva. Major problems in dermatology 5. Lloyd Luke)

in some patients. Although it is suggestive clinically of pemphigus vegetans the histology shows only rare acantholysis and it appears to be distinct. Immunofluorescence is negative. It is best described as pemphigus vegetans, Hallopeau type, or pyodermite végétante.

Crohn's disease

Skin lesions are not unusual and as with oral lesions may be the harbinger of intestinal disease, which they may precede by up to several years. Anogenital manifestations are well recognised. In the series of McCallum & Kinmont (1968), Mountain (1970) and Verbov (1973) up to 30% of patients were so affected. The lesions may be a direct continuation of bowel involvement. If normal skin intervenes, and especially if the lesions are well clear of the anogenital area, they are referred to as metastatic. As regards the anogenital lesions the usual appear-

ance is of ulcers, sinuses which may affect the groin and abdominal wall, fistulae, abscesses and oedematous peri-anal tags, as well as oedema which may be unilateral (Baccaredda-Boy & Crovato 1970, Laugier et al 1971, Ansell & Hogbin 1973, Levantine 1973) and occur alone (Fig. 6.3). Atherton et al (1978) described genital oedema in a boy aged 6 years. Recent reviews are those of Devroede et al (1975), McCallum & Gray (1976) and Burgdorf (1981). Vulval or pelvic lesions may give rise to dyspareunia (Hamilton et al 1977, Brooke 1978). Prezyna & Kalyanaraman (1977) found 'Bowen's disease' in the vulvovaginal lesions of one patient.

Histology shows non-caseating epithelioid granulomata (Fig. 6.4), and the differential diagnosis is from other granulomatous conditions, infective and non-infective, and from hidradenitis in respect of the sinuses and abscesses. Kremer et al (1984) described a florid example of Crohn's disease confined to the anogenital area and listed a scoring system to use in making the diagnosis: epithelioid granulomata with one other feature, or, if no epithelioid granulomata are found, then three features. Features are listed as terminal ileitis, anal ulcers, anal tags, fissures, lymphoid aggregates in the bowel wall and transmural inflammation.

The lesions may respond to medical treatment (steroids, antibiotics, especially metronidazole, immunosuppressive agents, salazopyrine) or surgical treatment of the underlying disease. Bandy et al (1983) discussed the surgical management of associated rectovaginal fistulae. Holland & Greiss (1983) gave detailed and sympathetic consideration to the same problem, and concluded that proctocolectomy is curative, though radical. Local treatment is useful in mild cases; faecal contamination can be a problem but local antiseptics, for example povidone iodine skin wash, may be helpful. A topical corticosteroid has been shown to help in a localised penile lesion (Sumathipala 1984) and corticosteroids in an adhesive base may be of particular value. Limited surgery to tags and sinuses is worth considering. In cases which are resistant to these approaches, vulvectomy may have to be considered (Kao et al 1975) or excision and grafting (Reyman et al 1986). In many cases nutritional deficiencies are present and call for treatment.

Sarcoidosis

Neill et al (1984) recorded a rare example of ulcerated sarcoidosis of the vulva. The patient had proved sarcoidosis, and there was no evidence of Crohn's disease or of any infection which could mimic sarcoidosis. The lesions were extensive, shallow painless ulcers affecting the submammary, peri-anal and labia majora area. Histology was consistent with sarcoidosis. Tatnall et al (1985) reported on a patient with papular lesions of vulva and peri-anal areas. The histology was that of sarcoidosis and the patient had a raised serum angiotensin-converting enzyme, a positive Kveim test and pulmonary lesions. A patient with nodular sarcoidosis affecting the vulva was reported by de Oliveiro Neto (1972) and patients have been reported with sarcoidosis of the Fallopian tubes and uterus.

Other granulomatous lesions

The cases of Larsson & Westermark (1978) and Wagenberg & Downham (1981) describing patients with chronic vulval oedema resembling cheilitis granulomatosa with a granulomatous histology are of uncertain provenance. No mention is made of bowel signs or symptoms but they could have been examples of Crohn's disease, perhaps before the onset of gut signs and symptoms. An example of a patient who had had swollen labia for almost 2 years, and who was found to show a granulomatous histology but without evidence of Crohn's disease after intensive investigation, is illustrated in Figure 6.5 a and b.

Pyoderma gangrenosum

The indolent ulcers of this rare condition may, unusually, affect the vulva. The aetiology is undetermined but there is a strong association with rheumatoid arthritis and ulcerative colitis, and sometimes other conditions, for example Crohn's disease (Burgdorf 1981, Gellert et al 1983). A useful clinical feature is a tendency of pyoderma gangrenosum to show multiple punched out 'pepperpot-like' small ulcers, set in an area of induration. Otherwise the lesion presents as a deep ulcer with a dusky oedematous and overhanging edge. The lesions are often multiple. The histology is usually inflammatory but non-specific. However, there may be evidence of vasculitis.

The differential diagnosis is from infective ulcerations and in particular (Hutchinson et al 1976) from synergistic bacterial gangrene (postoperative progressive gangrene) (p. 106). The correct diagnosis is important to make since treatment of pyoderma gangrenosum is by systemic steroids or azathioprine or dapsone rather than by surgery and antibiotics. The patient of Work (1980) who responded to extensive surgery, and was reported as pyoderma gangrenosum in association with ulcerative colitis, seemed unusual. The lesions had persisted over many years and appeared more like those of Crohn's disease, although histology was nonspecific.

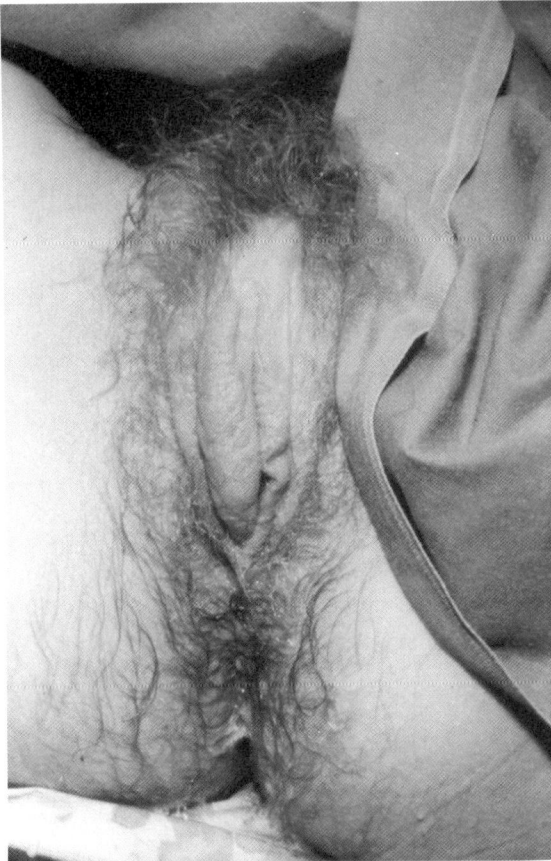

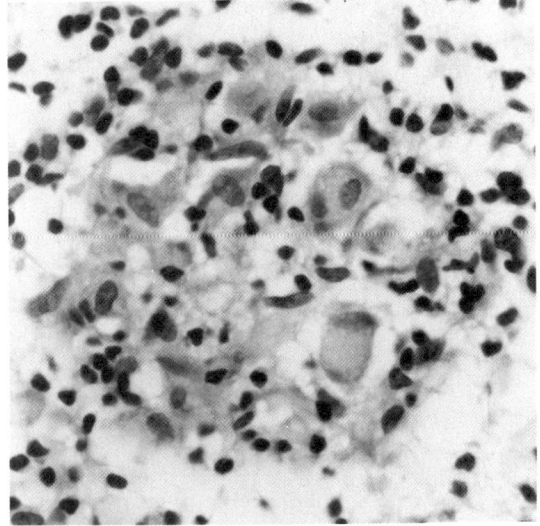

A

B

C

Fig. 6.5 (a) Swollen labia in a patient with no evidence of Crohn's disease; (b) histology showing granulomatous appearance (H & E × 14); (c) (H & E × 30). (By courtesy of Dr M Griffiths)

Acute febrile neutrophilic dermatosis (Sweet's syndrome)

In this rare condition (Sweet 1979) the patient is usually a middle-aged or elderly woman. She suffers an episode which is often recurrent and characterised, as a rule, by fever, malaise, neutrocytosis and the development of erythematous plaques.

Histologically there is intense inflammation with masses of neutrophils, and often eosinophils, and much leucocytoclasis. Prednisolone is usually effective.

Lindskov (1984) reported under this title a woman 50 years of age who had pustules and plaques affecting the limbs and the labia minora. Histology showed leucocytoclasis and dermal pustule formation and the response to prednisolone was good.

Histiocytosis X

This entity was defined in 1953 by Lichtenstein and is a proliferative histiocytic condition which appears in three clinical forms: Letterer–Siwe (acute disseminated), Hand–Schuller–Christian (chronic progressive) and eosinophilic granuloma (benign localised). The cardinal feature is the presence of histiocytosis X cells, which are large and on electron microscopy show racquet-like structures (Langerhans granules) in the cytoplasm together with histiocytes, eosinophils and giant

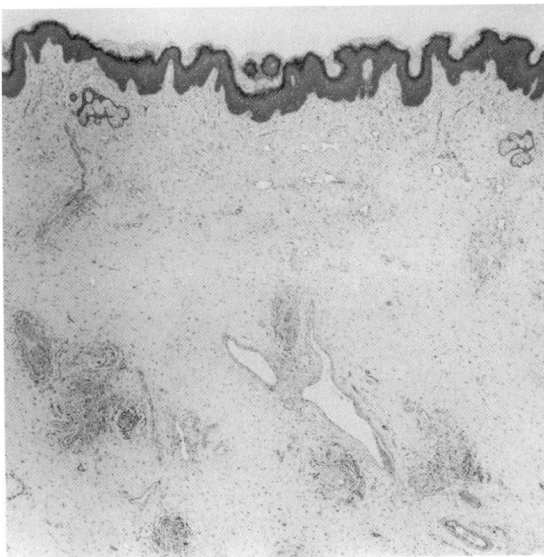

cells. An early proliferative stage merges into stages showing xanthomatous and granulomatous features. All the forms have recently been comprehensively reviewed by Gianotti & Caputo (1985).

Letterer–Siwe disease

Cutaneous lesions are common and usually appear in infancy on the trunk and scalp; in the napkin area the yellowish, often purpuric papules may be mistaken for a banal dermatosis. The bones, lungs, liver and spleen are often involved. Some cases remit but the majority are fatal.

Hand–Schuller–Christian disease

This disease tends to appear between the ages of 1 and 5 years. Bone lesions, exophthalmos and diabetes insipidus are recognised features. A rash appears in about a third of the cases (Fig. 6.6). It is similar to the rash of Letterer–Siwe disease and the course is variable.

Eosinophilic granuloma

This occurs, as a rule, in older patients (often male) and cutaneous lesions are rare, though the genital area may be affected.

Cases under one or other of these headings, where lesions affected the vulva and vagina, have been reported by Kierland et al (1957), Borglin et al (1966), Toth et al (1969), Case Records (1970), Dupree & Lee (1973), Rose et al (1984) and Thomas et al (1986); the latter authors noted a total of 23 cases in the world literature.

Treatment of all forms is with chemotherapy, usually vinblastine sulphate, with or without prednisolone and the results can be good. The diabetes insipidus is treated by vasopressin, and surgery and X-ray therapy may improve bone as well as skin lesions (Greaves 1986).

GENETIC DISORDERS

Some genetic conditions are discussed elsewhere: epidermolysis bullosa and familial benign chronic pemphigus (Hailey–Hailey disease) both on page 159.

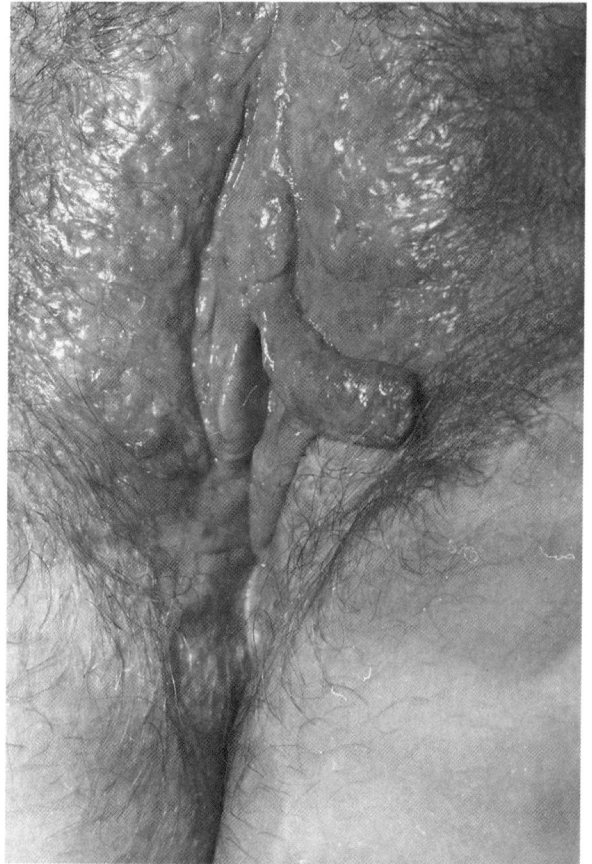

Fig. 6.6 Histiocytosis X: diffuse nodulation and some superficial ulceration. The patient had diabetes insipidus and scalp lesions. (By courtesy of C M Ridley 1975 The Vulva. No. 5 Major Problems in Dermatology. Lloyd Luke)

Von Recklinghausen's disease (neurofibromatosis)

Tumours are discussed elsewhere (p. 251). As well as the commonly noted axillary pigmented macules, similar perineal lesions have been noted (Crowe 1964).

Cowden's disease (multiple hamartoma syndrome)

In this rare condition, probably determined by an autosomal gene and reviewed by Starink & Hausman (1984), hamartomatous lesions involve ectodermal, mesodermal and endodermal tissues. The skin may show acral, facial and oral mucosal lesions. The vulva may be affected by the acral type which are keratotic papillomata, sometimes showing a follicular origin (Burnett et al 1975, Brownstein et al 1979), or by other lesions, for example an apocrine cystadenoma in the case of Salem & Steck (1983). Excision of any troublesome lesion is indicated.

Lawrence Seip syndrome (total lipo-atrophy)

This is a rare condition, probably inherited through an autosomal recessive gene. Clitoral hypertrophy may be found (Janaki et al 1980).

Pseudoxanthoma elasticum

The condition is inherited mainly in an autosomal recessive manner. Its main importance is the serious potential of systemic vascular lesions and lesions of the eye, but the skin is a site of election. Cases where the vagina and vulva were involved have been reported by Kissmeyer & With (1922), Szymanski & Caro (1955), Shaffer et al (1957) and Goodman et al (1963).

The lesions are yellowish papules, confluent in large plaques, often with purpura or telangiectasia. Histologically the main feature is the presence of dystrophic elastic fibres showing deposition of calcium.

Lesions elsewhere on the body are likely and the 'plucked chicken skin' appearance is easy to recognise. No treatment is possible except limited surgical removal if requested.

Facio-digital genital syndrome (Aarskog syndrome)

This is an X-linked recessive determined condition in which affected males show genital abnormalities. Female carriers may show some features of the syndrome but not apparently genital ones (de Saxe et al 1984).

The LAMB syndrome (lentigines, atrial myxoma, mucocutaneous myxomata, blue naevi)

Rhodes et al (1984) described an example of this rare condition in a girl of 13 years, who as well as an atrial myxoma and sundry other lesions had lentigines of the face and vulva, confirmed by histology. Lentigines were not found on the vaginal or anal mucosa. A further case with a review of the literature has been added by Reed et al (1986).

Ehlers Danlos syndrome (EDS) type IV

The EDS is now known to comprise at least nine types, all characterised by different connective tissue abnormalities. In type IV the skin is transparent and fragile but hyperelasticity is slight. Arterial and bowel rupture may be fatal. The fault lies in the production of type III collagen. Rudd et al (1983) studied 20 women in four families with EDS type IV. Ten had been pregnant with a total of 20 pregnancies and five patients had died as a result.

Complications and fatalities had resulted from rupture of bowel, large vessels or uterus, laceration of the vagina and postpartum haemorrhage. Twelve of the 16 live-born babies had EDS IV, and two died during delivery. Two had been aborted deliberately.

This appears to be the only type of EDS in which there are risks in pregnancy. The need for counselling and careful supervision is obvious.

Darier's disease (keratosis follicularis)

The condition is inherited through an autosomal dominant gene. In practice many cases seem to arise as a mutation since a family history is lacking.

The lesions are widespread on the body and the genital area is commonly affected. They appear in late childhood as a rule and steadily worsen (Fig. 6.7). The vagina and the cutaneous and mucosal aspects of the vulva may all show brownish horny papules which are often confluent, macerated and secondarily infected. Herpes infections (and vaccinia) are more severe than expected (Shelley 1974).

The histology is diagnostic (Fig. 6.8). In addition to hyperkeratosis, parakeratosis, acanthosis and sometimes pseudo-epitheliomatous hyperplasia there are lacunae above the basement membrane containing acantholytic cells, some keratinising to form corps ronds which in the upper epidermis are smaller and called grains. Electron microscopic appearances (Caulfield & Wilgram 1963) indicated

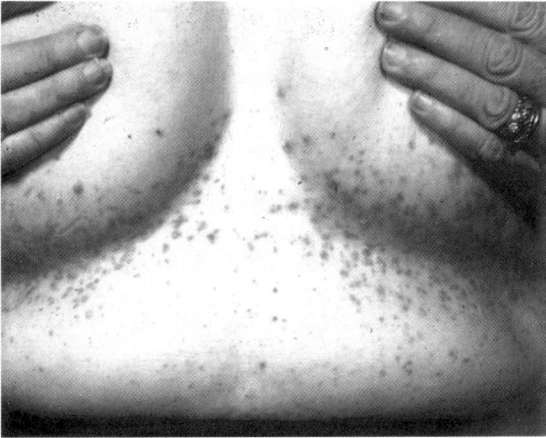

Fig. 6.7 Horny papules of Darier's disease.

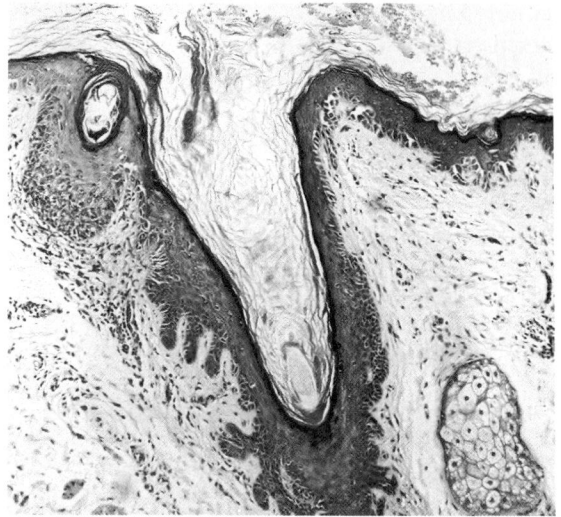

Fig. 6.8 Darier's disease: hyperkeratosis, keratotic plugging, suprabasal cleft and lacuna formation. (H & E × 105) (Reproduced from Beilby & Ridley (1987) by courtesy of the authors and publisher)

a detachment of tonofilaments from desmosomes which then disintegrate. Mann & Haye (1970) believed that the desmosome abnormality could be primary and suggested that the whole of the cell surface may be abnormal, allowing the possibility of various mechanisms in the formation of acantholytic cells.

The histological differential diagnosis is from benign familial chronic pemphigus (Hailey–Hailey disease) and pemphigus but the clinical appearances are distinctive. Clinically the main differential diagnosis is more likely to be from acanthosis nigricans, which has a different histology.

Treatment is unsatisfactory and severely affected patients have a miserable existence with malodorous painful infected masses. Local hygiene is obviously important. Oral etretinate has been beneficial in spite of marked side effects. The main danger is the risk of pregnancy as the drug is highly teratogenic; pregnancy moreover is not safe until a year after treatment has been stopped. Since Darier's disease is inherited by a dominant gene, pregnancy should in any case be discouraged.

Other disorders showing histological features of Darier's disease

Ackerman (1972) classified focal acantholytic dyskeratoses as multiple, whether permanent (Darier's disease) or transient (Grover's disease); and as single, whether clinically inapparent, papular or nodular.

Warty dyskeratoma

This corresponds to the nodular form and lesions are usually isolated and on the head and neck area. Duray et al (1983) reported three examples at the vulva. All were on the labia majora and did not recur following resection.

Papular acantholytic dyskeratosis of the vulva

Under this title, Chorzelski et al (1984) described a woman 23 years of age with papular, dome-shaped, smooth whitish lesions mainly on the labia majora. The histology showed acantholysis and dyskeratosis, together with corps ronds and grains as in Darier's disease.

The author has seen a patient with an identical histological picture (Fig. 6.9) but where there were no visible lesions. Hu et al (1985) have blamed heat and sweat for transient (non-vulval) lesions.

It is possible that cases reported as unusual variants of benign familial chronic pemphigus (p. 159) were in fact in one of these categories. Recent discussion indicates continuing uncertainty (Chorzelski & Jablonska, Coppola & Muscardin, Warkel & Jager, Weedon, and Van der Putte 1986).

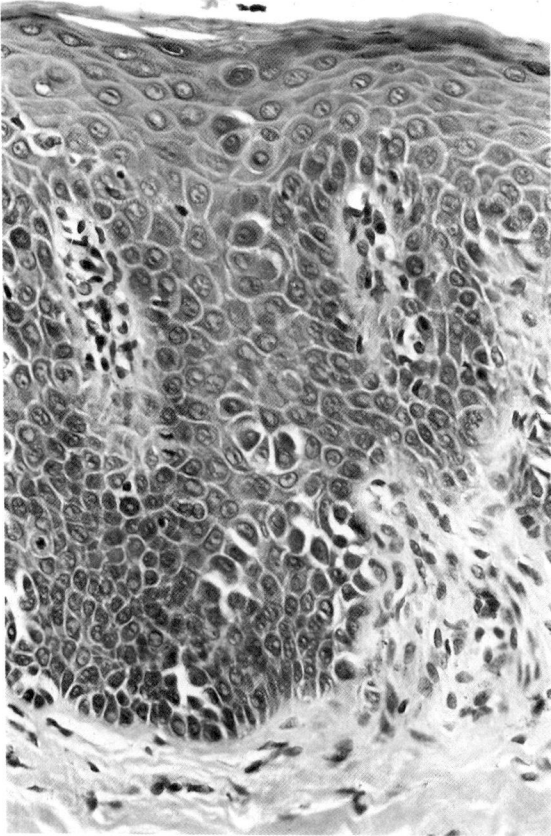

Fig. 6.9 Papular acantholytic dyskeratosis. (H & E × 280) (By courtesty of Dr C H Buckley)

White sponge naevus

White hyperkeratotic lesions of the oral mucosa, often inherited as an autosomal dominant condition, have been described. In some cases, for example those of Dégos & Ebrard (1958), genital lesions have also been present. Jorgenson & Levin (1981) reviewed the literature, and Buchholz et al (1985) reported a new example where the lesion occurred only at the vulva. The histology showed hyperkeratosis and acanthosis, with some vacuolation of the prickle cells.

DISORDERS OF HAIR

Pilonidal sinuses

Vulval lesions are less common than sacrococcygeal ones, but have been noted. Most, if not all, arise in response to penetration of the skin by a hair. Examples have been reported by Betson et al (1962) and by Radman & Bhagavan (1972).

The lesion is painful and may present as an abscess requiring incision. Definitive treatment is by excision. The histology shows a tract lined by granulation tissue and fragments of hair can often be seen.

Folliculitis

This is not uncommon, particularly on the mons pubis. Physical or chemical irritants (such as sugar, sometimes used as a depilatory) or an infection (e.g. after shaving) may be responsible. The lesions are follicular papulopustules. Histology shows inflammatory changes, mainly at the follicular ostium.

It is important not to miss an underlying infection by pediculi at this site.

Treatment is by removing any known irritant, application of local antiseptics such as povidone iodine and possibly short courses of oral antibiotics; a search for carriage of pathogens at the perineum may be indicated if lesions recur.

Pseudofolliculitis pubis

A reaction to ingrowing hair is common in the beard area after shaving. Alexander (1974) reported such a case on the pubic area of a female negro. Similar changes may occur after regrowth of hair following pre-operative shaving or in Muslim women in response to regular shaving, but appear to be rare.

Avoidance of shaving, or instruction in shaving technique, is likely to lead to improvement.

Alopecia areata

Genital hair is lost in alopecia totalis. Occasionally patches of alopecia are seen short of this. The lesion is non-inflamed, round and symptom free (Fig. 6.10). Lesions are usually to be found elsewhere.

Histology (rarely necessary) shows some lymphocytic infiltrate round the hair bulb in early stages, and follicles smaller and higher in the dermis than are normally found.

Treatment is unsatisfactory and rarely called for at this site. A topical corticosteroid is often used but may be of only placebo value.

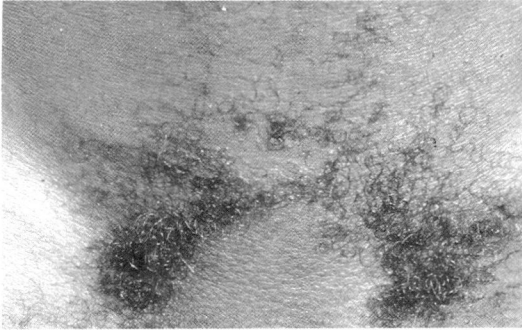

Fig. 6.10 Genital alopecia areata.

Other causes of alopecia

The pubic hair becomes thinner with age, but does not disappear entirely.

Rarely the pubic hair will be lost as part of a general reaction to cytotoxic drugs.

DISORDERS OF PIGMENTATION

Pigmented tumours are discussed elsewhere.

Hyperpigmentation related to haemosiderin

Not all pigmentation is caused by melanin. Haemosiderin is also important. Haemosiderin tends to be reddish brown rather than brownish black, but the two can be difficult to distinguish. Haemosiderin will be found where there has been extravasation of blood from damaged or inflamed or unsupported blood vessels. Thus it is a feature of lichen sclerosus et atrophicus, plasma cell vulvitis of Zoon, caruncles and prolapsed tissue of cervical, vaginal or urethral origin.

Hyperpigmentation related to melanin

Normal variation of diffuse pigmentation is considerable within and between different races and in relation to hormonal status. Minor changes are of no significance. Jones (1979) studied skin in postmortem specimens from the vulva of 35 white women with no clinically apparent pigmentation and was able to detect patches of melanosis histologically.

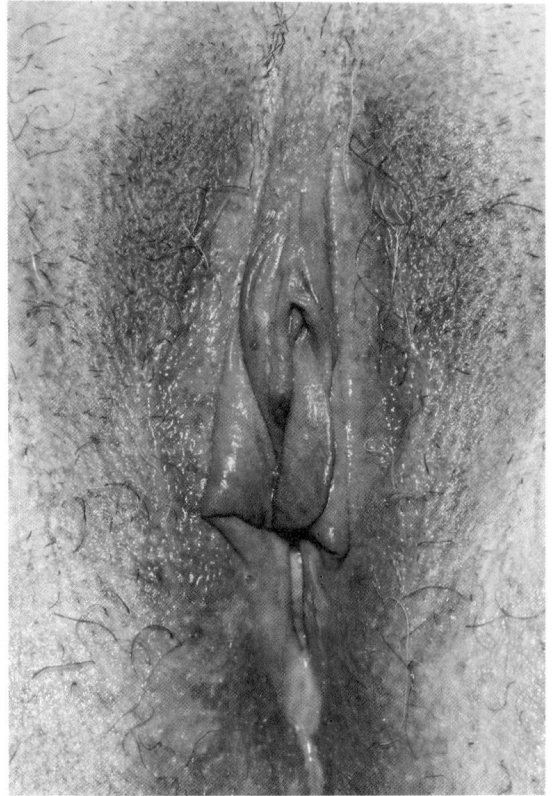

Fig. 6.11 Lentigines: extensive macular pigmentation on lateral aspects of vulva.

Marked diffuse macular hyperpigmentation may occur as a post-inflammatory effect particularly, for example, in lichen planus. Histology in that case will reveal pigmentary incontinence with pigmented macrophages in the upper dermis.

Jackson (1984) has described apparently similar extensive pigmentation which was clinically marked but entirely benign histologically and was not suggestive of post-inflammatory change.

The commonest macular pigmented lesion, single or multiple, is probably a lentigo (p. 295), and multiple lentigines may account for Jackson's findings. Indeed, Sison-Torre & Ackerman (1985) have described under the heading of melanosis of the vulva eight women with extensive pigmentation of this type (Fig. 6.11). They stressed that while it is impossible to distinguish from melanocytic malignancy clinically, yet biopsy will clearly show that such examples of melanosis are benign and analogous to a simple lentigo; the pigmentation is

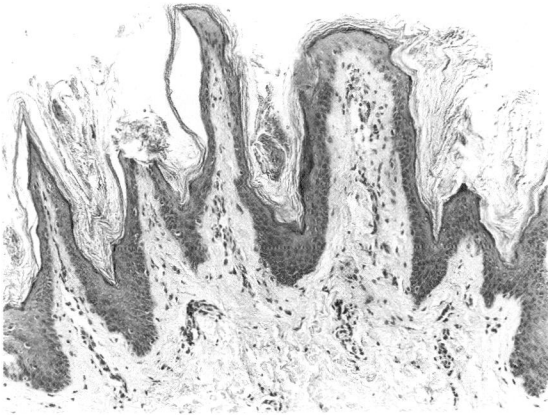

Fig. 6.12 Acanthosis nigricans: hyperkeratosis and papilloma-toses (acanthosis and pigmentation may not be marked). (H & E × 50) (By courtesy of Dr D Jenkins)

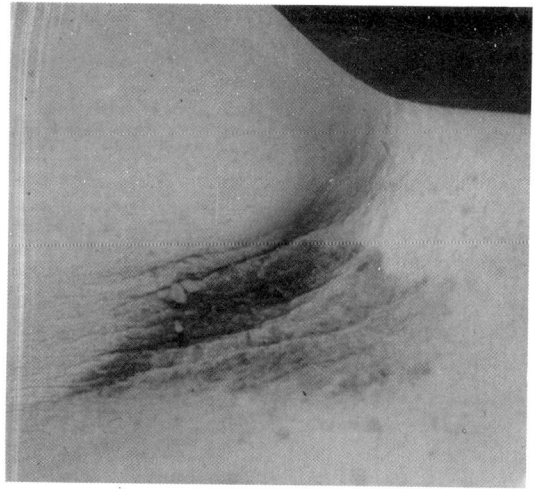

Fig. 6.13 Pseudo-acanthosis nigricans: darkening and tags in a flexure.

caused by proliferation of normal melanocytes arranged in solitary units at the dermo-epidermal junction. There are no atypical melanocytes, and no nests of melanocytes.

All in all, such lesions are an imperfectly understood group which would repay further study.

Any pigmented tumour, fixed solitary pigmented macule or more extensive area of pigmentation should be biopsied or excised to determine its origin.

Acanthosis nigricans

This rare and specific dermatosis may occur in childhood, either alone or as part of rare, often endocrinological syndromes; it will then tend to improve at puberty, although some cases actually begin at that time. More often it occurs in adult life. Unless, as is very infrequently the case, nicotinic acid (Shelley 1972) or triazinate (Greenspan et al 1985) can be incriminated, it is then invariably associated with systemic malignancy. The malignancy is usually an adenocarcinoma but occasionally a lymphoma (Staughton, personal communication), or epithelial carcinoma (Mikhail 1979).

The lesions affect the face, the mucosae and the flexures, and the genital area is a site of predilection. They are dark, at first velvety and then warty. All aspects of the vulva are involved.

The histology (Fig. 6.12) shows hyperkeratosis

and papillomatosis, some acanthosis and pigmentation. Horny inclusions are sometimes present.

Pseudo-acanthosis nigricans (see below) and Darier's disease may be confused with it. In the latter case the histological findings are distinctive.

Treatment is symptomatic and the prognosis poor except in drug-induced cases.

Pseudo-acanthosis nigricans

This name is given to the banal darkening and thickening of flexural skin, often accompanied by skin tags, in obese and darkish skinned patients (Fig. 6.13). The mucosae are not affected. The changes regress if weight is lost. The clinical diagnosis is usually straightforward, but the histology shows acanthosis and pigmentation and is different only in degree from that of true acanthosis nigricans.

Fixed drug eruption

In this condition lesions appear at the same fixed site or sites when a particular drug is ingested. Its mechanism remains unexplained (Ackroyd 1985). It is well recognised on the penis but vulval reports are sparse; Klostermann (1972) had an illustration of such a lesion and Shelley (1972) asserted that vaginal lesions could occur. Sinha (1982) reported a vulval example caused by dapsone, Sehgal &

Gangwani (1986) found two examples (one vaginal and one vulval) in women out of a total of 29 with genital lesions, and Hughes et al (1987) reported two examples at the vulva related to trimethroprim.

The drugs responsible vary with prescribing patterns and are perhaps now mainly sulphonamides, although in the past barbiturates, phenolphthalein and phenazones were often involved (Kauppinen & Stubb 1985).

The lesion is a pigmented plaque which flares up to produce an oedematous or even bullous area when the drug is ingested and then subsides to leave pigmentation which usually persists.

The histology shows epidermal necrosis with dermal inflammation and later deposition of melanin. The clinical differential diagnosis is from herpes or syphilis, or perhaps in the quiescent stage from pigmented vulval intra-epithelial neoplasia or a mole.

Miscellaneous causes of pigmentation

Staining of vulval skin

The proprietary laxative Dorbanex® is excreted in the urine, which may be red, and the skin correspondingly stained. It can also cause irritation and reddish-brown staining of anogenital and thigh skin in those who are incontinent of faeces, having been reduced in the bowel to dithranol, and the vaginal secretions may be orange when this drug is given (Bunney & Noble 1974, Barth et al 1984, Greer 1984).

Trichomycosis (p. 95) and chromhidrosis (p. 151) may lead to some discoloration of the skin.

Hypopigmentation

Patchy hypopigmentation is a common sequela of inflammation in a dark skin and is often to be seen, for example, in a napkin rash (Fig. 6.14).

Vitiligo

In vitiligo (Fig. 6.15) there is complete depigmentation of an area of skin which is in all other respects normal. The patch is well defined and the condition usually symmetrical. If the area is hairy, the hair may or may not retain its colour.

The histology shows melanocytes which are re-

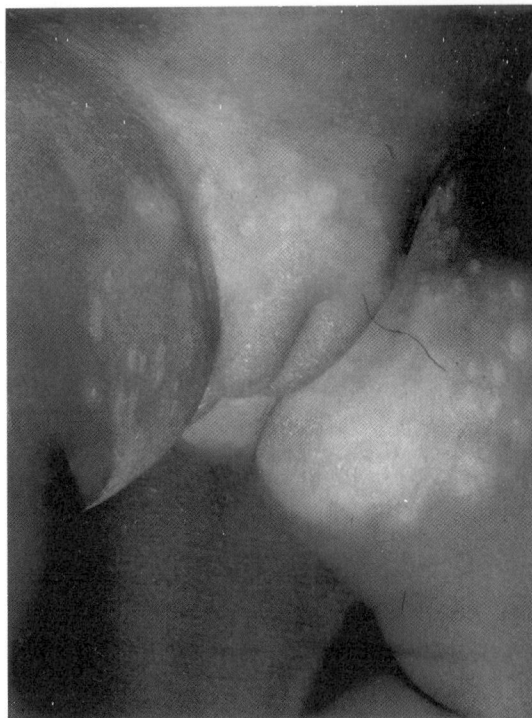

Fig. 6.14 Patchy hypopigmentation following a napkin rash in a dark-skinned child.

duced in number, or apparently normal though non-functional; or they may be absent.

The differential diagnosis from the pale thickening of lichenification (p. 168) is usually easy but to distinguish vitiligo from a mild lichen sclerosus et atrophicus can be difficult and it is then that a biopsy will be helpful. Postinflammatory loss of pigment is usually incomplete and ill-defined. Occupational depigmentation from paratertiary butyl phenol can occur in the genital area in men (Moss & Stevenson 1981), but is unlikely in women.

There is no effective treatment. Measures which might be tried elsewhere are inappropriate at this site.

DISORDERS OF SEBACEOUS GLANDS

Sebaceous glands may be clinically apparent on the labia minora and majora, either as discrete yellowish specks (analogous to the lesions frequently noted on the oral mucosa, the Fordyce condition) or as sheets of aggregated yellowish lesions. Pa-

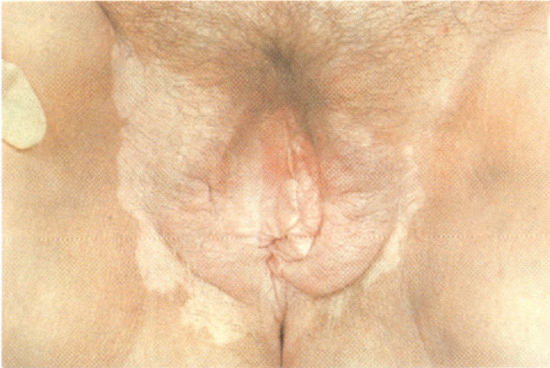

A

Fig. 6.15 Vitiligo: loss of pigmentation in (**a**) an adult; (**b**) a dark-skinned child. (Reproduced from Beilby & Ridley (1987) by courtesy of the authors and publisher)

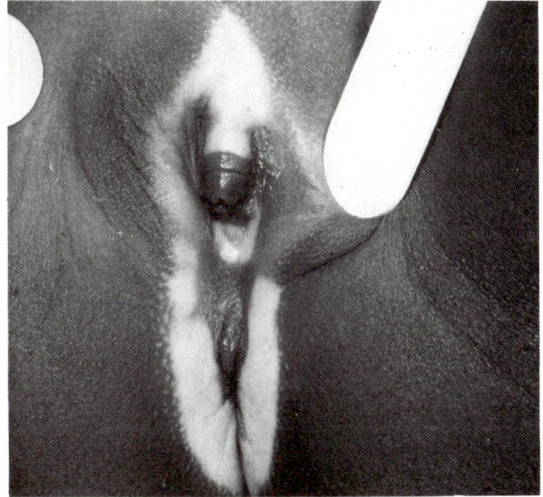

B

tients who notice the appearance require assurance that the condition is a variant of normal.

Blockage of ducts with formation of temporary or permanent yellow papules, nodules and cysts (p. 232) is not rare and, particularly on the labia majora, lesions may be numerous (Fig. 6.16 a and b). If treatment is requested, they may be evacuated.

Acne of the vulva

It is doubtful whether acne of the vulva exists. Deep 'acne conglobata' lesions may affect the buttocks and anogenital area in hidradenitis but may indeed represent part of the apocrine gland disorder rather than true acne although it may be that sebaceous glands are to some extent involved in hidradenitis (Ebling 1986).

Occasionally patients are seen with lumpy painful lesions, varying with the menstrual cycle, in the labia (Fig. 6.17). Such a case was described by Iglesias et al (1984); histology was said to be typical of acne but no details were given.

Some such lesions may well represent blockage and inflammation in sebaceous structures, others a similar process in relation to apocrine glands.

Sebaceous hyperplasia

Rocamora et al (1986) have described a case where sebacous lobules surrounding a central duct formed soft polypoid lesions. They were distinct

from ectopic sebacous glands and neoplasms (pp. 305, 309).

DISORDERS OF SWEAT GLANDS

Eccrine miliaria

Occlusion of the sweat gland orifices, under conditions of heat and humidity, leads to the appearance of papulovesicles. They are encountered mainly in infants. The obstruction may result in a subcorneal vesicle or vesiculation proximal to a deeper obstruction at the dermo-epidermal junction.

Apocrine miliaria

Apocrine miliaria are poorly documented but probably not uncommon, in areas where the glands are present, appearing as transient painful papules often with a cyclical (menstrual) pattern. Grimmer (1968), however, found them in an elderly woman.

Chromohidrosis

This refers to the secretion of coloured sweat, usually arising in apocrine glands. The vulva is not a common site, but Joosse et al (1964) reported lesions there. Areas of pigmentation under the skin were found to be a lipofuscin, probably a normal tissue constituent; however, the granules were larger than normal and more numerous.

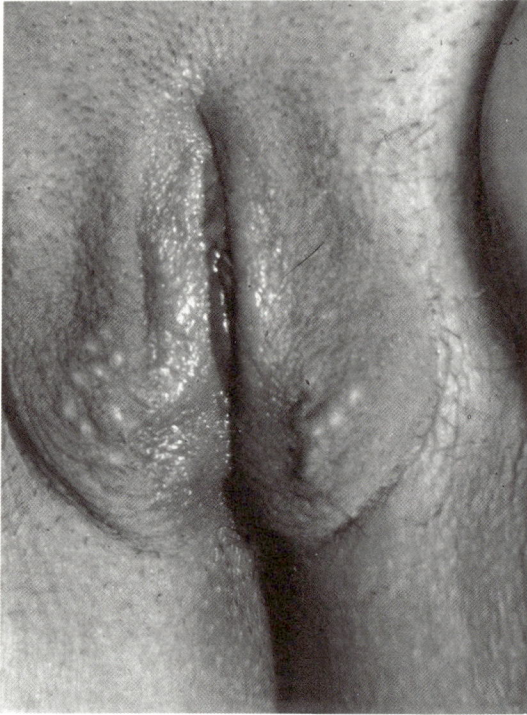

A

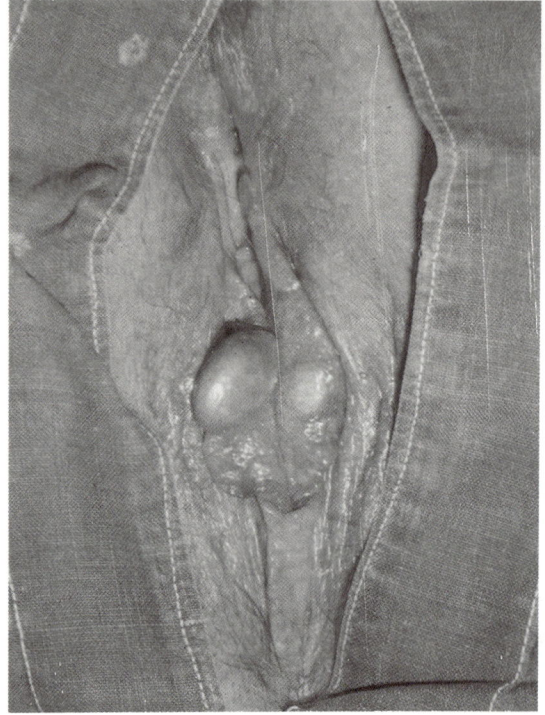

B

Fig. 6.16 (a and b) Yellowish nodules and cysts of sebaceous origin.

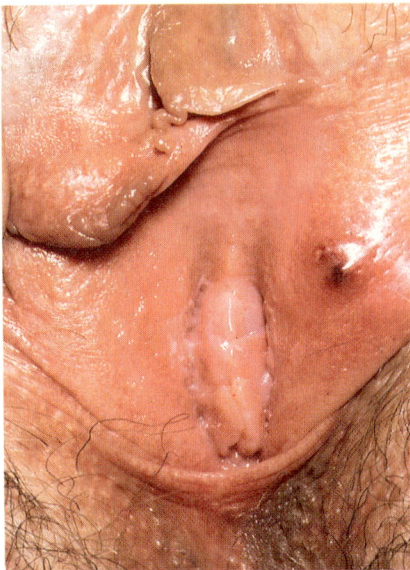

Fig. 6.17 Example of inflammatory lesion with cyclical variation.

Fox Fordyce disease

This rare eruption of unknown aetiology is characterised by close-set itchy skin-coloured or darker follicular papules on the axillae, breasts and anogenital area (Fig. 6.18). They develop after puberty and become more itchy with menstruation, while improving in pregnancy and after the menopause.

Sweat drops are seen in the apocrine ducts and there may be surrounding inflammation and plugging, perhaps with rupture.

The differential diagnosis histologically in Fox Fordyce disease is from apocrine miliaria, and clinically from syringomata (which, however, do not usually itch). Hormonal manipulation, for example the contraceptive pill, may improve the symptoms. Topical corticosteroids may be of some limited value. Surgical measures may be the final resort.

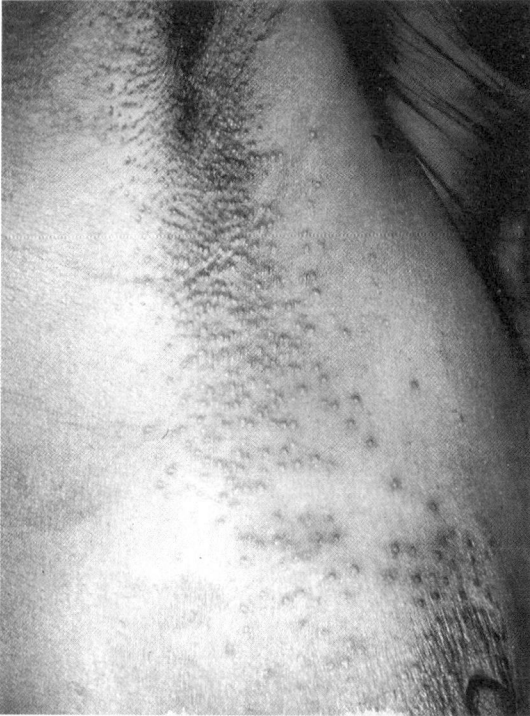

Fig. 6.18 Fox Fordyce disease: typical papules of breast and axilla. (Reproduced from Beilby & Ridley (1987) by courtesy of the authors and publisher)

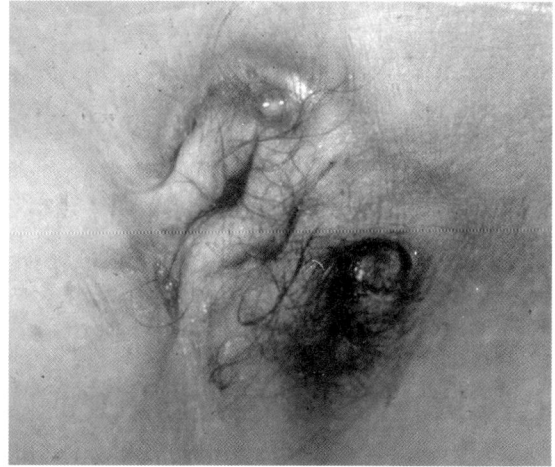

Fig. 6.19 Hidradenitis suppurativa: inflamed and scarred lesions of flexure.

Hidradenitis suppurativa

This inflammatory condition too mainly affects the apocrine glands and so is rare before puberty, and tends to decline after the climacteric. Anogenital lesions are common, being found in the genito-crural folds and on the mons pubis and buttocks. Other lesions may occur in the axillae and on the breasts. Negroes are said to be more commonly affected than those of white races.

The aetiology is unknown. Deodorants and de-pilatories can be exculpated (Morgan & Leicester 1982) though occlusion of the axillary skin has been shown to lead to bacterial proliferation in the affected glands and to a clinical lesion (Shelley 1972). Mortimer et al (1986a) have suggested that androgens are of importance in its mediation; in 42 women patients a significant incidence of endocrine abnormalities was found both clinically (irregular periods, premenstrual exacerbation of disease, acne and hirsutes) and biochemically (the patients had a higher concentration of free testosterone and a higher free androgen index than did normal controls). Such a mechanism would fit in with the limitation of the condition to reproductive years and with the improvement often seen in pregnancy. There has been general agreement that acne is common in hidradenitis; however, Fitzsimmons et al (1985) found otherwise, and these authors also pointed out some evidence of genetic factors.

Tender nodules form, soften and may form an abscess. Surface discharge is rare. Widespread sinuses and induration develop and occasionally fistulae may open into the anus. Sometimes lesions are mild and infrequent, and between attacks are represented by small scars with typical dark plugs or comedones (Fig. 6.19). Mortimer et al (1986b) found these comedones in apocrine sites, not only in diseased areas, and also noted a significant incidence of comedones in the postauricular region, a site where apocrine glands are not expected to be present.

Mixed organisms tend to be found but Highet et al (1980) stressed that *Streptococcus milleri* is of particular relevance in anogenital lesions, and may be missed if it is not sought by appropriate microbiological methods. There may be vaginal carriage of the organism and a reservoir in the gut.

Histology shows distended apocrine ducts which may contain bacteria, with inflammation, fibrosis and perhaps foreign body giant cells. The differential diagnosis is from Crohn's disease, infections caused by fungi, granuloma inguinale and lymphogranuloma venereum. Pseudo-epitheliomatous hyperplasia may be seen and nine cases with true squamous carcinoma have so far been reported (Sparks et al 1985). Two out of the nine were women, with buttock lesions.

Mortimer et al (1986b) in a double blind controlled crossover study found that anti-androgen therapy (ethinyloestradiol 50 μg/cyproterone acetate 50 mg or ethinyloestradiol 50 μg/norgestrel 500 μg) was effective.

Otherwise, or in addition, treatment is with courses of systemic antibiotics, if possible matched to the offending organism, and may include metronidazole (bearing in mind the risks of neuropathy with prolonged courses). With this may be coupled local cleansing agents such as povidone iodine. Etretinate, according to some, is of doubtful value (Dicken et al 1984) but Stewart & Light (1984) found it helpful; both in uncontrolled trials. Norris & Cunliffe 1986 have shown that isotretinoin is of no value. Surgery is often the best treatment, with or without grafting (Bhatia et al 1984). Smaller lesions can be excised with primary closure. It is, however, possible that after removal of such localised small areas others will develop in due course.

BEHÇET'S SYNDROME AND OTHER ULCERATIVE CONDITIONS

Behçet's syndrome

This condition, defined in 1937 as a triad of oral, genital and ocular lesions, is a multisystem disease with several clinical subdivisions: arthritic, neurological, ocular and mucocutaneous. Often it warrants a definite diagnosis only after a long period of unfolding. Cutaneous manifestations include erythema nodosum, pyodermatous lesions, and sterile pustules as well as mucosal ulcers. The aetiology is likely to be viral; probably an immunopathological response to HSV type I infection (Lehner & Barnes 1979, Eglin et al 1982) is involved, and circulating immune complexes (Jorizzo et al 1984) have been demonstrated which may be helpful in diagnosis (Jorizzo et al 1985). The vulval lesions are painful, shallow ulcers of varying sizes which persist over weeks or months (Fig. 6.20).

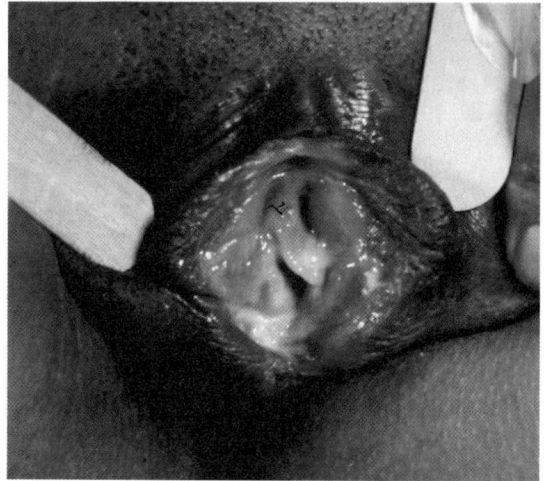

Fig. 6.20 Behçet's syndrome: vulval ulceration. (Reproduced from Beilby & Ridley (1987) by courtesy of the authors and publisher)

Scarring is usual but not inevitable. The commonest site is the labia minora. Oral and ocular lesions may be present.

The histology is often non-specific but sometimes thrombosed arterioles are seen.

Management

Treatment is unsatisfactory. Topically bland preparations and corticosteroids can help. Systemic steroids are also sometimes of benefit. Latterly thalidomide has been put forward (Saylan & Saltik 1982); with due awareness of its dangers and with perhaps restriction to those not of childbearing years this can be of value. In the UK the drug is not now easily available even on a named-patient basis (Lancet 1985).

Other non-infective ulcers

Some patients have painful vulval ulcers often tending to recur. Sometimes they also have oral ulcers. A few may represent early oculo-cutaneous Behçet's syndrome, but some do not.

Oral ulcers are now classified as minor and major aphthous ulcers, and herpetiform ulcers. All may occur singly. In Behçet's syndrome they occur together (Lehner 1968, Cooke 1979). According to Eglin et al (1982) the minor aphthous type is of vir-

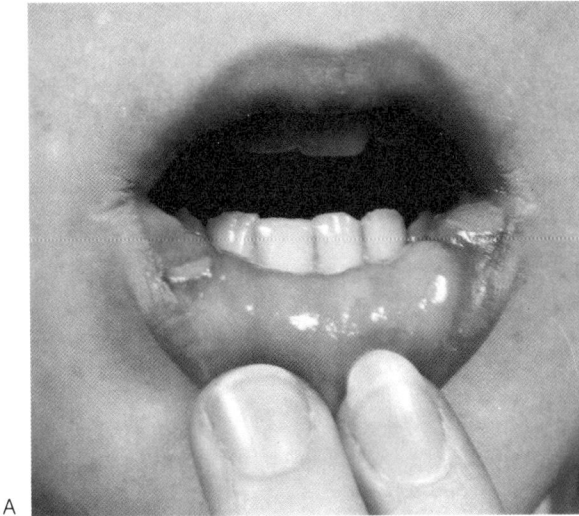

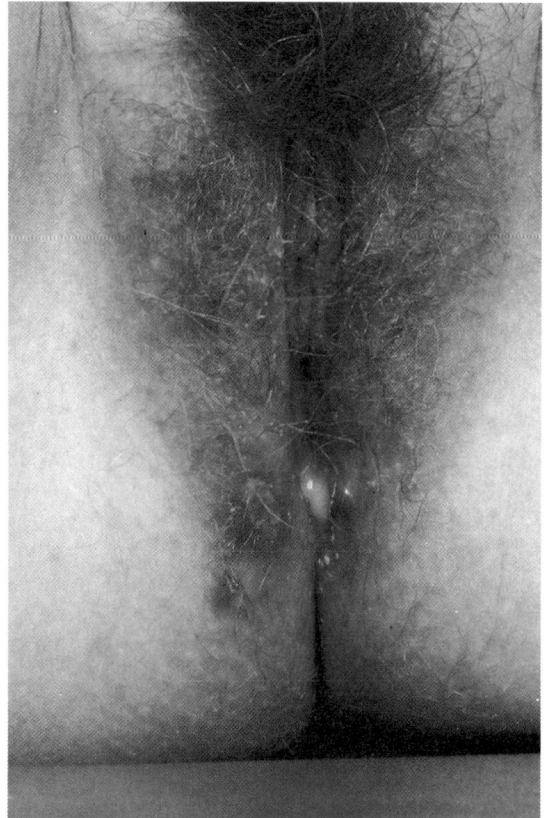

Fig. 6.21 Recurrent major aphthous ulcers: (a) mouth; (b) vulva.

al origin. Vulval ulcers have not been so neatly categorised but may be essentially similar. Older views of aetiology have looked to non-pathogenic Bacillus crassus, a lactobacillus (Lipschutz 1913), a hypersensitivity to bacteria (Barile et al 1963), and an unusual reaction to streptococcus 2A (Donatsky 1976). A more likely cause is the auto-immune phenomena related to viral infection (Lehner 1968, Eglin et al 1982).

Simple aphthous ulcers

These are painful, small, red with a yellow base and usually on the labia majora. They last about a week and rarely scar. There may be oral ulceration at the same time. Perhaps they are the equivalent of minor aphthous ulcers.

Sutton's ulcers (periadenitis mucosa necrotica recurrens)

These ulcers are commoner in the mouth, where they appear to be the type now called major aphthous ulcers, than at the vulva. They are deep, painful, often leave scars and frequently recur. A family history is common with oral lesions, and may be a feature in patients with both oral and genital ulcers (Fig. 6.21).

Lipschutz ulcers (ulcus vulvae acutum)

These were described by Lipschutz in 1913 and comprised ulcers which could be acute with fever and lymphadenopathy, or chronic; they mainly involved the labia minora and the introitus. Both types led to scars. Sometimes a few lesions were seen on the labia majora, when they tended to scar less often. His last two types are probably accounted for under the heading of Behçet's syndrome and aphthosis. The first acute type may be that sometimes seen as a short-lived matter in an adolescent girl with no other lesions, or of the possibly non-specific sort noted in acute fever (van Joost 1971). Ulcers perhaps of the same type have been noted in pityriasis lichenoides (Joulia & le Coulant 1954, Burke et al 1969) and infectious mononucleosis (Brown & Stenchever 1977, and, in penile lesions, Lawee & Shafir 1983). Portnoy et al (1984), however, described such ulcers in infectious mononucleosis from which the Epstein–Barr virus was recovered. Ulceration may be a specific manifestation also in syphilis or diptheritic vulvo-vaginitis (Parks 1941, Machnicki 1953). Boyce & Valpey (1971) reported an outbreak of painful vulval ulcers, which healed rapidly, in women re-united with servicemen returning from Asia who were themselves symptom free. The aetiology remained obscure.

The histology of all these ulcers is non-specific. The differential diagnosis will include infective diseases particularly syphilis, herpes simplex and zoster, and the bullous diseases, since bullae often rupture to leave ulcers.

Management

In chronic cases thalidomide might be considered as in Behçet's syndrome (Bowers & Powell 1983) but the drug is now virtually unavailable. Local or oral corticosteroids are often used together with simple antiseptic applications and oral analgesics; a useful mixture for topical use is 5 ml of triamcinolone acetamide injection (10 mg per ml) mixed with 95 ml of tetracycline syrup (125 mg per ml). Lignocaine gel may be of a little help.

BULLOUS DERMATOSES

The dermatoses characterised by bullae (blisters) are a heterogeneous collection as regards aetiology. Nevertheless, on clinical and histological grounds it is best to consider most of them together. Those which have no predilection for the vulva and rarely affect it will be omitted, so we shall not consider porphyria, pemphigus foliaceus, dermatitis herpetiformis or pemphigoid (herpes) gestationis.

Stevens Johnson syndrome

Mucosal involvement (oral, ocular, genital) is the essential feature of this variant of erythema multiforme, skin lesions not being necessary for the diagnosis. The aetiology may be unknown or attacks may be precipitated by infection, especially herpes simplex, and drugs; except where a drug cause (commonly sulphonamide) can be established and re-ingestion avoided, the outbreaks may recur. The illness is acute and often accompanied by systemic symptoms.

There are painful shallow ulcers of the labia and sometimes of the adjoining skin.

The histology (rarely studied at this site) shows a subepidermal bulla with basal cell necrosis, oedema of the papillae and an inflammatory infiltrate.

The diagnosis is usually obvious except in respect of toxic epidermal necrolysis. It may be difficult, however, to establish if a focus of genital or oral herpes has been, or is, present to account for the eruption.

Good nursing and simple local applications are the mainstay of treatment. Oral steroids are often given in severe cases to suppress symptoms until natural resolution occurs.

Toxic epidermal necrolysis (Lyell's syndrome)

This condition is found in two forms, histologically but not clinically distinct. In children, the usual cause is an exotoxin of certain phage types of *S. aureus*, the so called staphylococcal scalded skin syndrome; whereas in adults a drug is the usual factor, often a butazone or a sulphonamide; although staphylococcal as well as idiopathic (and sometimes recurrent) cases occur (O'Keefe et al 1987). The onset is acute with marked systemic illness and exquisitely painful lesions rapidly showing denudation of the epidermis. The vulval area is often involved in both types with, sometimes, vulvo-vaginal scarring. The soreness and reddening may indeed begin there. The outcome may be fatal. Histologically, the staphylococcal type has an intra-epidermal split below the granular layer. In the drug induced type the whole epidermis is necrotic with a subepidermal bulla and much basal cell destruction. Frozen sections are advised in case of doubt, since the patient may be very ill & treatment differs in the two types. The differential diagnosis from Stevens Johnson syndrome can be difficult or even impossible clinically and histologically in the drug-induced form. The evidence of typical iris lesions of erythema multiforme on the skin is helpful. In the staphylococcal form, treatment is with systemic antibiotics; in the drug induced form by withdrawal of the drug; systemic steroids are contraindicated (Roujeau et al 1986). In both

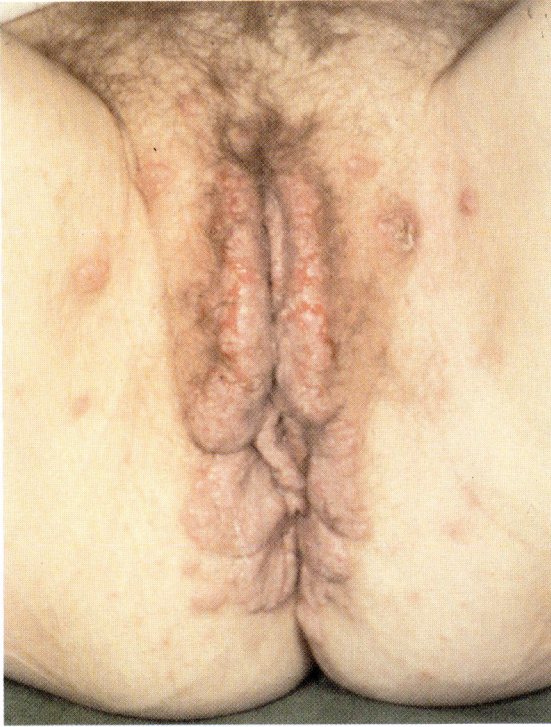

Fig. 6.22 Pemphigus vulgaris, vegetans type: confluent bullous masses. (By courtesy of Dr C M Ridley (1975) The vulva. Major problems in dermatology 5. Lloyd Luke)

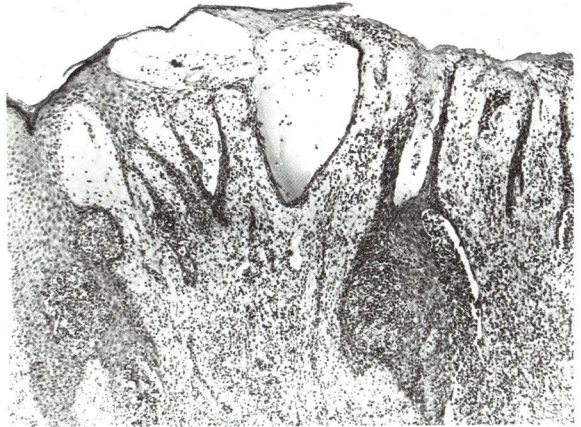

Fig. 6.23 Pemphigus vulgaris, vegetans type, acanthosis, intra-epidermal vesicles, acantholysis and a heavy infiltrate of eosinophils. (H & E × 40) (By courtesy of Dr C M Ridley (1975) The vulva. Major problems in dermatology 5. W B Saunders)

cases symptomatic measures and good nursing are essential. In severe examples the patient should be transferred to a burns unit (Lancet 1984) since the nursing and medical problems are identical to those of severe burns.

Pemphigus vulgaris

A chronic condition of middle life, particularly prevalent in Jewish subjects, pemphigus vulgaris has a predilection for the mucosae and may sometimes affect them exclusively.

Auto-immune phenomena are found and may be causal; HLA associations vary with ethnic groups, even within Jewish populations: A26 and BW38 in Ashkenazi Jews, A26 alone in non-Ashkenazi Jews, and A10 in Japanese for example (Rowell 1984). Lesions suggestive of pemphigus vulgaris and its variants can also be provoked or mimicked by D-penicillamine (Troy et al 1981). The bullae arise from normal skin and are painful, flaccid and eroded at an early stage. In pemphigus vegetans, a chronic and more benign variant of pemphigus vulgaris, heaped-up masses of such lesions are seen (Fig. 6.22). Secondary infection is common. Cutaneous and mucosal aspects of the anogenital area are involved and lesions may affect the vagina (Mikhail et al 1967). Friedman et al (1971) noted lesions on the cervix, showing acantholysis on histological examination.

The histology (Fig. 6.23) is characterised by intra-epidermal bulla formation and acantholysis beginning as mainly suprabasal clefts. In the pemphigus vegetans variant hyperkeratosis, papillomatosis and acanthosis are marked, and eosinophils infiltrate the epidermis. Electron microscopy reveals widening of the intracellular spaces, followed by detachment of cells from each other with retraction of tonofibrils and disappearance of the desmosomes. The basal cells, however, remain attached to the basement membrane.

Direct immunofluorescence reveals IgG deposited on the intercellular substance between the prickle cells; with indirect immunofluorescence, circulating antibodies to intercellular substance are found. The titre corresponds to the severity of the lesions.

Differential diagnosis is rarely a problem given histological and immunofluorescence evidence, together perhaps with the presence of typical lesions elsewhere. Management is difficult in severe cases, even with careful nursing, analgesia and high doses of oral steroids (say 100 mg of prednisolone daily). Maintenance is on a lower dose; azathioprine is often added and gold has been used in a few cases. Plasmaphoresis may be of some value but is not readily available (Swanson & Dahl 1981).

Cicatricial pemphigoid (CP) (benign mucous membrane pemphigoid)

Cicatricial pemphigoid is a rare condition usually affecting the middle aged, but well recorded in childhood (Jolliffe & Sim Davis 1977). Again an auto-immune aetiology seems likely. However, the case with vulval lesions of van Joost et al (1980) appeared to be drug induced, and that reported by Stage et al (1984) as bullous pemphigoid in relation to a drug, also with vulval lesions, was very probably CP (Ridley 1985, Stage 1985). In both cases the drug was a beta blocker. As with pemphigus, D-penicillamine may be involved in the appearance of CP (Shuttleworth et al 1985).

Sometimes the tense scarring bullae are widespread but the more usual picture is of small chronic affected areas of the skin (often scalp) and/or mucosae. Anogenital lesions may be extensive or extremely localised and asymmetrical (Fig. 6.24). The vagina and probably the anal canal may be involved. Scarring and obliteration of sulci leads to dyspareunia and difficulty in micturition; sometimes, however, incipient changes are subtle, with developing sulcal shallowness. Some older patients reported as showing examples of labial adhesions may well have had CP (p. 195).

Histology shows subepidermal bullae without acantholysis, but with some dermal inflammation and, later, fibrosis. Electron microscopy of ocular lesions (Carroll & Kuwabara 1968) showed increased keratofibrils and desmosomes in the conjunctival epithelial cells. Direct immunofluorescence reveals IgG in the basement membrane zone and circulating antibasement-membrane antibodies can be found, though less often. The differential diagnosis is usually from pemphigus or perhaps from erosive and scarring lichen planus, but lesions

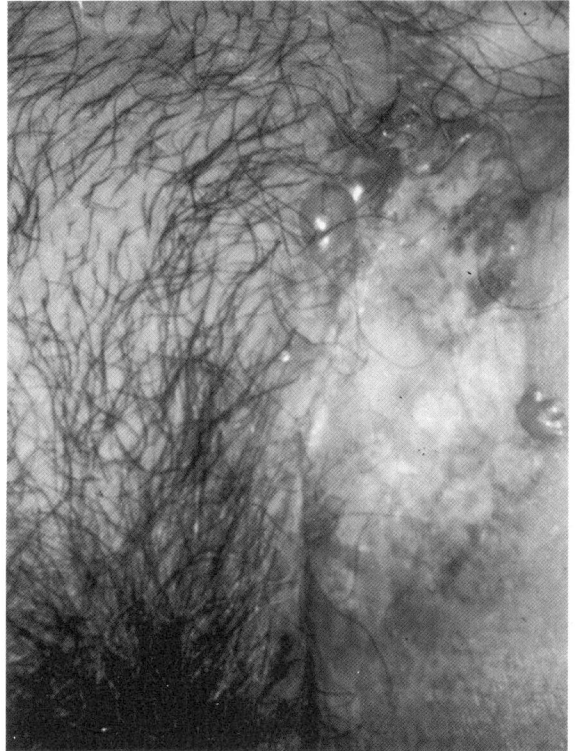

Fig. 6.24 Cicatricial pemphigoid: scarring and tense bullae in genital area. (Reproduced from Beilby & Ridley (1987) by courtesy of the authors and publisher)

elsewhere will give some points of differentiation, while histology and immunofluorescence are usually definitive; sometimes a stenosing lichen sclerosus et atrophicus may have to be considered.

Treatment in mild cases is with topical corticosteroids and more severe cases may call for a trial of systemic prednisolone or dapsone.

Pemphigoid (bullous pemphigoid)

A condition mainly of the elderly, pemphigoid does not as a rule affect the genital area.

De Castro et al (1985) have reported an example in a child where the vulva was the only site involved. Cicatricial pemphigoid could not be excluded, however.

Subcorneal pustular dermatosis

This is a rare chronic condition of unknown aetiology and more often found in women than in men.

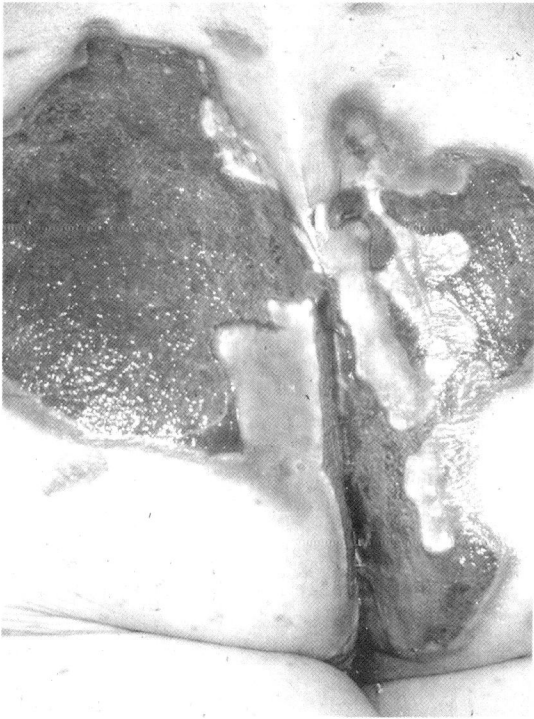

Fig. 6.25 Junctional epidermolysis bullosa: extensive anogenital ulceration.

Waves of superficial pustules with a circinate edge affect any area of the body at intervals of a few days or weeks. The genitocrural area is often involved, though mucosal aspects are spared. Histology shows raised-up subcorneal pustules full of polymorphs. Immunofluorescence is negative.

The only condition likely to be confused with it in the genital area is pustular psoriasis where the pustule is deeper in the epidermis. Treatment with dapsone 50–150 mg daily is effective and the lesions tend to be self limiting. Myeloma, however, has been associated.

Epidermolysis bullosa (EB)

Scarring forms of this genetically determined condition, where the site of cleavage is the basal lamina of the epidermis, may affect the mucosae though the mouth and oesophagus appear to be the sites of election. A case was reported by Shackelford et al

(1982) of a girl with anal scarring leading to constipation and bladder compression, narrowing of the vestibule and partial fusion of the labia; she had vaginal and uterine reflux of urine and repeated urinary tract infections. Examples where cleavage is in the lamina lucida, that is, of the junctional type, can affect the genital area. The case of Steinkampf et al (1987) was probably of this type. Another patient with the junctional type had extensive anogenital bullae and ulcers which caused anal stenosis (Fig. 6.25) as well as extensive lesions elsewhere and typical changes of nail, teeth and hair (Ridley 1982). Only symptomatic treatment is available.

Benign familial chronic pemphigus (BFCP) Hailey–Hailey disease

This is a rare dermatosis inherited as an autosomal dominant condition, although only about 70% of patients give a positive family history. Lesions appear from adolescence onwards and affect keratinised skin of the anogenital area as well as the neck and flexures of the limbs. Cases have been reported confined to the vulva (Thiers et al 1968, Hazelrigg & Stoller 1977), and in a similar case (Lyles et al 1958) the lesions appeared in pregnancy and remitted postpartum. King et al (1978) reported its association (presumably by chance) with syringomata.

The appearance is of moist red plaques with fissuring (Fig. 6.26). The lesions are painful and itchy. Fresh lesions can be triggered off not only by heat and friction, but by bacteria (Chorzelski 1962), contact allergy (Izumi et al 1971), Herpes simplex (Leppard et al 1973) and *Candida* (Burns et al 1967).

Histology (Fig. 6.27) shows suprabasal clefting and striking and extensive intra-epidermal acantholysis, the 'dilapidated brick wall' appearance. Electron microscopy has demonstrated detachment of tonofibrils from desmosomes and suggested an abnormality of intercellular substance in clinically normal skin (Nürnberger & Müller 1967). Immunofluorescence is negative.

The differential diagnosis histologically is from Darier's disease where, however, corps ronds are to be found and the clinical findings are totally different; and from pemphigus vulgaris where acan-

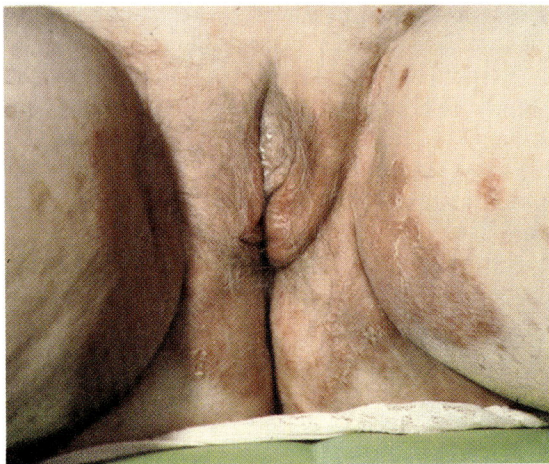

Fig. 6.26 Benign familial chronic pemphigus: moist diffuse scaly and fissured erythema of genitocrural area. (Reproduced from Beilby & Ridley (1987) by courtesy of the authors and publisher)

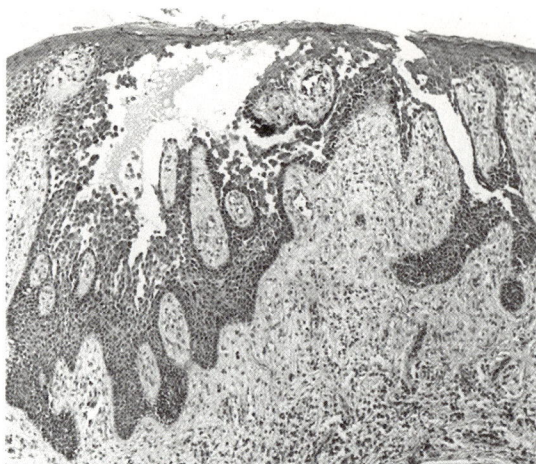

A

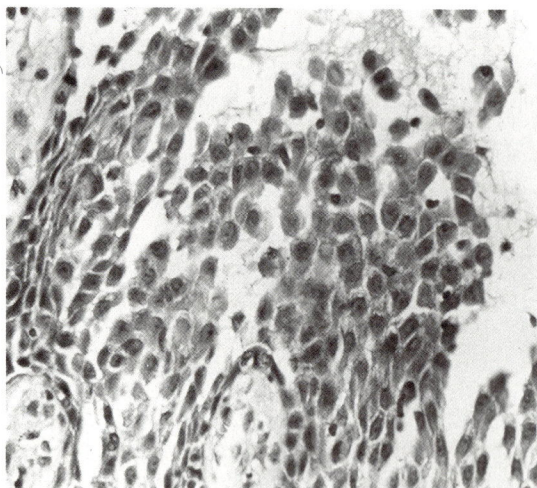

B

Fig. 6.27 (a and b) Benign familial chronic pemphigus: extensive acantholysis leading to the 'dilapidated brick wall' appearance. (H & E × 45) (Reproduced from Beilby & Ridley (1987) by courtesy of the authors and publisher)

tholysis is less extensive but more complete when it occurs; in BFCP the cells appear less severely damaged and some continue to adhere to one another.

The important clinical differential diagnosis is less from other bullous diseases than from banal inflammatory dermatoses. If the fissured appearance, family history, or presence of lesions elsewhere do not raise suspicion, resistance to treatment with simple measures may do so. Histology will then quickly resolve the matter.

Management is largely by local measures. Folds should be kept separated to minimise heat and friction, and local antiseptics or antibiotics employed judiciously together with topical corticosteroids of various strength. Where repeated bacterial infection occurs, long term prophylactic oral antibiotics can be helpful. Any suspicion of a contact sensitivity must be investigated and dealt with promptly. Grenz rays have been shown to help (Sarkany 1959) and sometimes excision and grafting are resorted to. In the case of Bitar & Giroux (1970), grafting was re-employed after the patient had developed a basal cell carcinoma at the site of radiotherapy given for the condition and the grafts then made had remained unaffected by any recurrence.

Relapsing linear acantholytic dermatosis

Vakilzadeh & Kolde (1985) have reported the case of a girl 5 years of age with an extensive unilateral lesion appearing at the age of 3 months, to which they gave this name; anogenital involvement was present. The clinical, histological and electron microscopy findings were similar to those of BFCP, and distinct, the authors felt, from those of Darier's disease. It is possible, however, that it should be considered under that heading (p. 145). The same may apply to the report of Evron et al (1984) of a patient with a solitary vulval plaque of acantholysis.

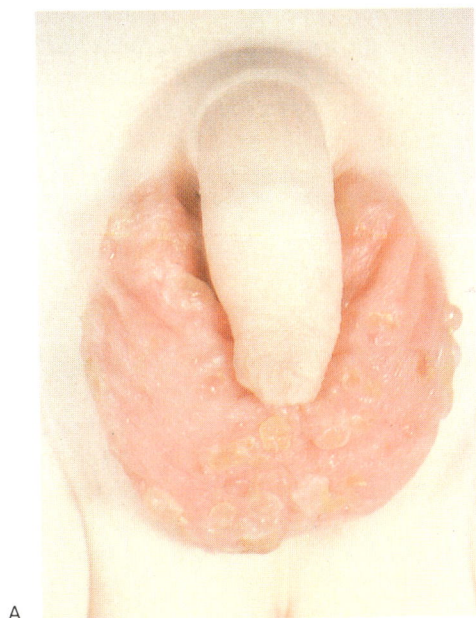

A

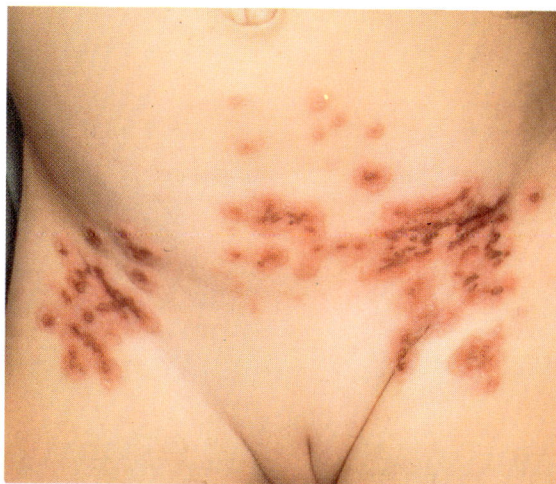

B

Fig. 6.28 Benign chronic bullous disease in childhood: (**a**) bullae of scrotum and peri-anal area in a male; (**b**) bullae of lower abdominal wall in a female

Benign chronic bullous disease of childhood (linear IgA disease of childhood)

A bullous condition affecting the vulva in childhood has long been recognised, but terminology has been confused, and it was originally described as juvenile dermatitis herpetiformis or juvenile pemphigoid. While both dermatitis herpetiformis and pemphigoid may on occasion begin in childhood, they do not in fact affect the vulva and the clinical picture hitherto given these titles is now better called benign chronic bullous disease of childhood (Marsden et al 1980) or linear IgA disease of childhood. The aetiology is unknown though an association with HLA-B8 is found (as in dermatitis herpetiformis).

The lesions are tense bullae, often itching, crusted and secondarily infected (Fig. 6.28 a and b). Clustering of lesions is helpful diagnostically.

The histology is that of subepidermal bullae without acantholysis but with other variable features. Thus some have eosinophils, some show dermal capillary neutrophil microabscesses, while others have neither. Immunofluorescence shows linear IgA. The differential diagnosis is not difficult clinically and the immunofluorescence findings are helpful in that dermatitis herpetiformis has papil-

lary granular IgA and bullous pemphigoid has linear basement membrane IgG.

Treatment with dapsone in doses of the order of 25 mg three times daily is effective but children tend to tolerate it badly as regards haemolysis and anaemia, and sulphapyridine is a safe alternative in a dose of about 500 mg twice daily.

PLASMA CELL VULVITIS OF ZOON

One may begin with descriptions of plasmacytosis orificialis, genital and oral (Schuermann 1960, Korting & Theisen 1963). Zoon (1952) gave the term plasma cell balanitis to lesions localised to the penis. Zoon (1955) described a similar condition in the female, as did Garnier (1954, 1957). Further reports of male examples were given by Brodin (1980) and Stern & Rosen (1982), whereas Crosti & Riboldi (1975), Mensing & Janner (1981) and Davis et al (1983) described lesions of the vulva. It appears to be commoner in men, however, and the report of Souteyrand et al (1981) was of 19 cases in men and only one in a woman.

It is generally agreed that clinically the lesions are fairly striking in the male with glistening red areas, speckled and haemorrhagic on the glans and prepuce, and that in the female lesions are similar but less obvious and are to be found in all areas of

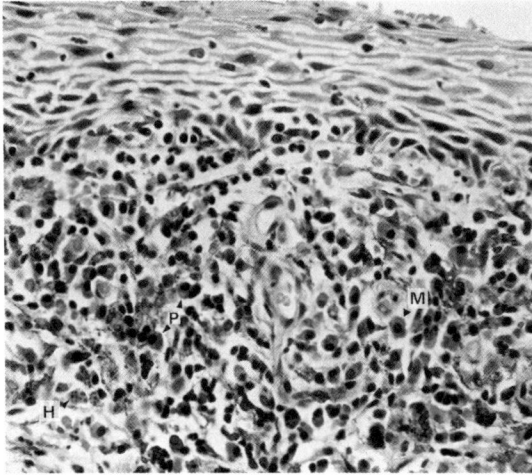

Fig. 6.29 Plasma cell balanitis and vulvitis of Zoon. 'Lozenge keratinocytes' in epidermis, separated by uniform intercellular oedema, loss of granular layer, effacement of rete ridge pattern. Dermal infiltrate with preponderance of plasma cells (P), haemosiderin-laden macrophages (H) and mast cells (M). (H & E × 140). (By courtesy of Dr D R MacDonald et al and the British Journal of Dermatology)

the vulva. Souteyrand et al (1981) gave the most detailed histological account, asserting that the changes are specific and uniform (Fig. 6.29). The features of value were a thinned epidermis with an absence of the horny and granular layer and loss of the rete ridge pattern. The keratinocytes were reduced in numbers and size, and individual cells were lozenge shaped, that is, diamond shaped with the horizontal axis the wider one. Intercellular spaces were widened. There was no evidence of atypia or increased mitoses. In the dermis the blood vessels were proliferative and a notable feature was that single dilated vessels tended to be directed vertically or obliquely. There were extravasated red cells and haemosiderin. The dermis was, as a rule, the site of a dense lichenoid infiltrate usually with a predominance of plasma cells, but in some cases there was a lesser infiltrate with a degree of fibrosis.

The authors considered that the plasma cells were not an essential feature as they were so variable, but that vulvitis of Zoon was indeed an entity. They would also include as vulvitis of Zoon the cases reported by Jonquières & de Lutsky (1980) as lichenoid telangiectatic purpuric balanitis or vulvitis. Aetiologically they considered, as had others, that poor hygiene and friction played a part (in all their male cases the patients were uncircumcised

and circumcision appeared to clear the condition). Nevertheless the position is still somewhat confused. In practice, experienced histopathologists seem reluctant to make the diagnosis and repeat biopsies of doubtful cases often yield even more doubtful verdicts.

Erythematous vulvitis en plaques, inflammation of minor vestibular glands, and focal vulvitis or vestibulitis

Pelisse & Hewitt (1976) reported a group of patients with what they called erythematous vulvitis 'en plaques' where red spots in the posterior vestibule gave rise to dyspareunia and where plasma cells were a prominent feature. Friedrich (1983b) considered that these lesions might be the same as those attributed to inflammation of minor vestibular glands and that all might be considered as plasma cell vulvitis. The minor vestibular glands are situated in the area of the hymeneal ring, lined with transitional epithelium and containing mucus-secreting acini. Robboy et al (1978) noted them in 9 out of 19 autopsy specimens of young women, their numbers ranging from 2 to 10. The orifices are just visible to the naked eye and clearly seen with the colposcope. As described by Friedrich (1983b) and Woodruff & Parmley (1983) they can become inflamed and give rise to dyspareunia. Red dots which correspond to localised symptoms are seen, or diffuse erythema as more glands become involved. Histology shows inflammation in the glands with a plasma cell infiltration. Friedrich (1983b) postulated that in the cases of Pelisse & Hewitt (1976) (noted by the authors to involve, on occasion, the orifices of Bartholin's glands or paraurethral glands) squamous metaplasia had replaced the glandular elements, leaving only an inconspicuous epithelial fold surrounded by an infiltrate rich in plasma cells. Peckham et al (1986) have described as 'focal vulvitis' lesions with rather nonspecific histology but a similar clinical picture; Friedrich (1987) now prefers the term vulval vestibulitis.

It is possible that these conditions account for some cases of the burning vulva syndrome (p. 219). It does not seem likely that they could account for all the cases described as plasma cell vulvitis, particularly if one accepts the criteria of Souteyrand et al (1981). It seems more probable

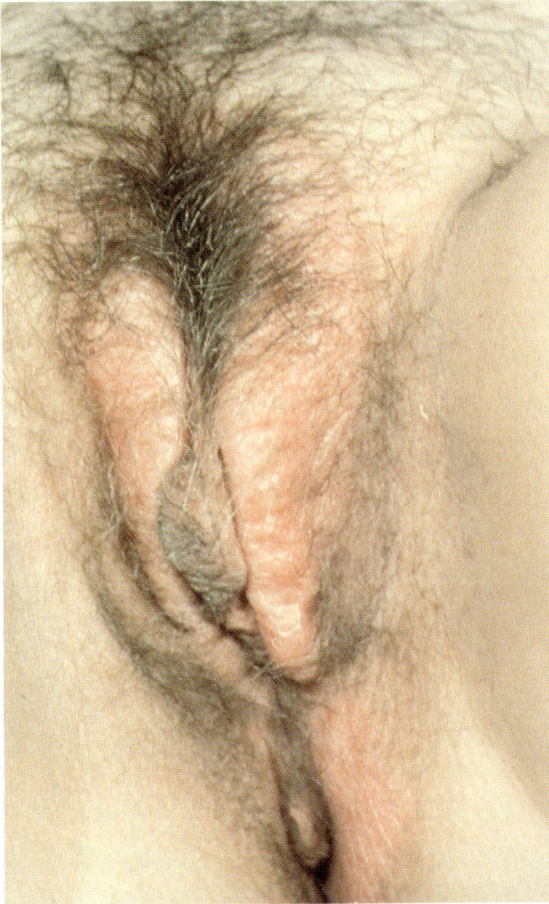

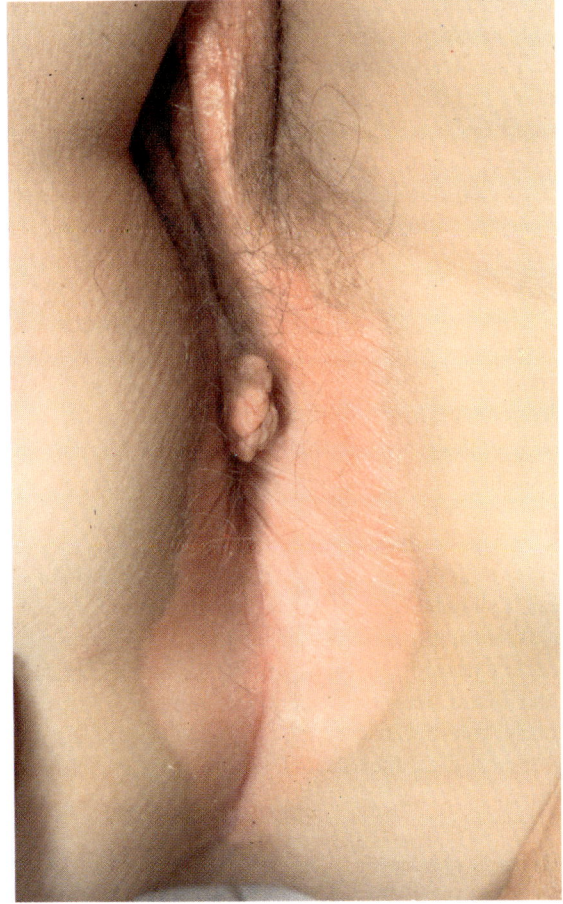

A

B

Fig. 6.30 Psoriasis: well-defined smooth erythema of: (**a**) vulval; and (**b**) peri-anal area. (Reproduced from Beilby & Ridley (1987) by courtesy of the authors and publisher)

that the ubiquitous mucosa-loving plasma cell is confusing the categorisation of not one but several entities.

INTERTRIGO

This inflammation of flexures, brought about by heat, sweating, obesity and friction, is common in the groins, genitocrural area and natal cleft, as it is in the submammary area and under folds of abdominal skin.

The lesions are ill-defined and erythematous. Secondary infection, often with *Candida*, is common and in that event small outlying scaly satellite lesions are often present and the main lesions tend to have a sodden macerated fringe. The histology shows non-specific inflammation.

Intertrigo must be distinguished from flexural psoriasis where the border is much sharper, and from seborrhoeic dermatitis (in both there tend to be lesions elsewhere).

Treatment rests upon dealing with predisposing factors, separation of folds by smooth material such as cotton and the use of mild topical corticosteroids and antiseptics or antibiotics. Miconazole/hydrocortisone is a useful combination.

PSORIASIS

Flexural psoriasis is less common than are lesions on extensor aspects, but nevertheless is frequently encountered. Although psoriasis is genetically determined, various trigger factors will set it off in those with the diathesis, and friction and occlusion may cause or perpetuate such flexural lesions.

The silvery scaling of psoriasis is lost in sheltered areas but the bright erythema and sharp outline remain (Fig. 6.30). A fissure in the natal cleft often bisects lesions there. The mons pubis is often involved and lesions at that site are more scaly. Mucosal aspects of the vulva are not involved except sometimes in the rare pustular form of psoriasis. Itching and anxiety are common.

Histology (Fig. 6.31) shows parakeratosis, acanthosis with elongation of the rete ridges and a reduced or absent granular layer, often with collections of neutrophils in the epidermis, as well as papillary oedema and perivascular dermal inflammation.

The clinical differential diagnosis is mainly from seborrhoeic dermatitis, into which it may merge, eczema and a banal intertrigo; its sharp outline is fairly diagnostic.

Treatment initially can be with a strong topical corticosteroid but for maintenance hydrocortisone and bland preparations such as aqueous cream are preferable because of the risk of local side effects. Tar and dithranol should not be used in the flexures.

Reiter's syndrome

Cutaneous lesions in this condition may represent psoriasis precipitated by chlamydial infection or by other trigger factors, infective or otherwise. It is very rare in women. Thambar et al (1977) and Daunt et al (1982) have reported cases of vulval lesions equivalent to circinate balanitis. Kanerva et al (1982) showed, on electron microscopy, changes identical to those of pustular psoriasis in a patient with circinate balanitis.

ECZEMA

Atopic eczema

Atopic eczema rarely affects the vulva in adults even when it is severe and widespread.

Seborrhoeic dermatitis

This tends to occur in flexures; as well as in the genitocrural area (Fig. 6.32) and natal cleft, lesions

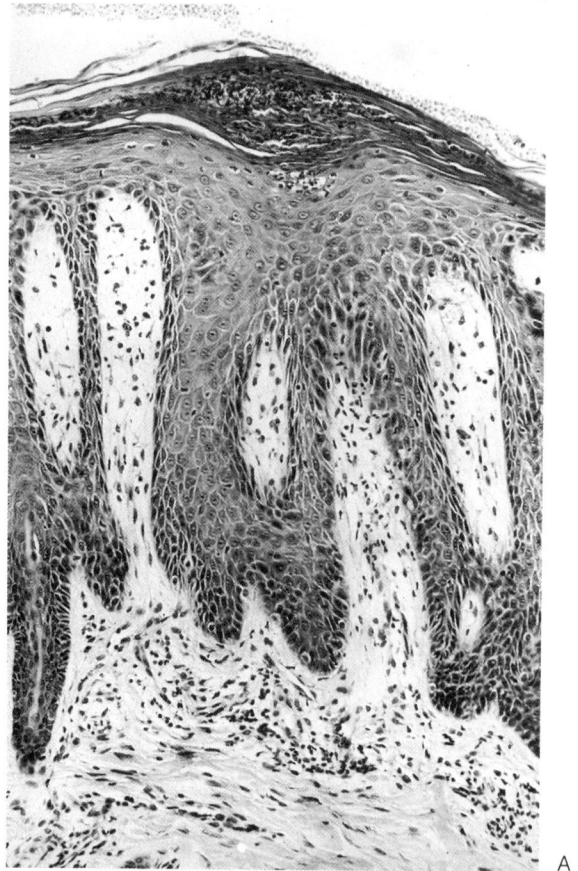

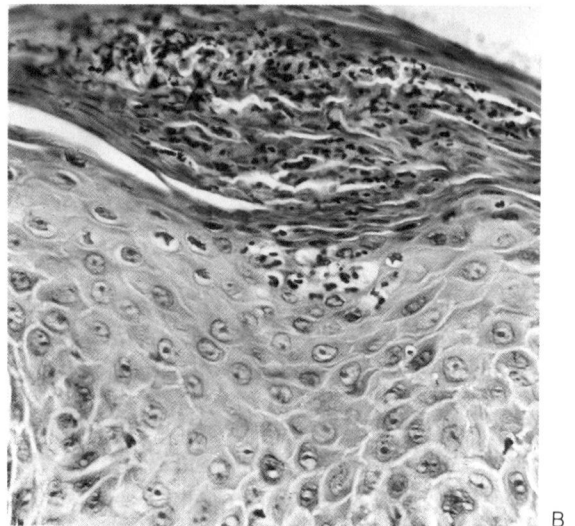

Fig. 6.31 (a and b) Psoriasis: parakeratosis, elongation of rete pegs, oedema of dermal papillae; a small Munro's abscess can be seen in the parakeratotic horny layer. (H & E × 135) (Reproduced from Beilby & Ridley (1987) by courtesy of the authors and publisher)

are likely to be found elsewhere, for example behind the ears and at the umbilicus. The lesions are orange-pink, slightly scaly, not well defined, and often secondarily infected.

Irritant and allergic reactions

The line between these two types is often difficult to draw where genital lesions are concerned.

Irritant (a direct effect on tissues without any allergic mechanism)

Bromination of swimming pools can cause genital burning (Rycroft & Penny 1983). Effects of bubble-baths are probably similar (Heller et al 1969). Douching is potentially harmful if toxic constituents are not well dissolved (and allergy to constituents e.g. scent is a possibility). However, Stock et al (1973) found no great ill to come of it in a US army population of 1600 women, 58% of whom used a douche. Deodorant sprays had a vogue a few years ago but now appear to be little used. They contained an emollient (a fatty ester), a fluorinated hydrocarbon as propellant and a scent, with or without an antiseptic. In 32 cases where allergy was suspected Fisher (1973) found only four confirmed by patch testing, the others presumably being irritant in nature and mainly due to the propellant when the spray was held too close to the skin.

Abortifacients may cause irritation on vulval contact. Podophyllum is an irritant. Maibach & Mathias (1985) described a case of severe dermatitis probably related to an irritant effect of a quaternary ammonium compound, methyl benzethonium chloride, and analogous to those cases of dequalinium necrosis described in the genital area of both sexes (Coles & Wilkinson 1965, Tilsley & Wilkinson 1965).

Allergic reactions (contact dermatitis)

This category is confined to cases where a true allergic response has arisen to a substance which is not an irritant.

Local antibiotic, anaesthetic and antihistamine preparations (as well as the preservatives they may contain) can all lead to sensitisation. Lignocaine is

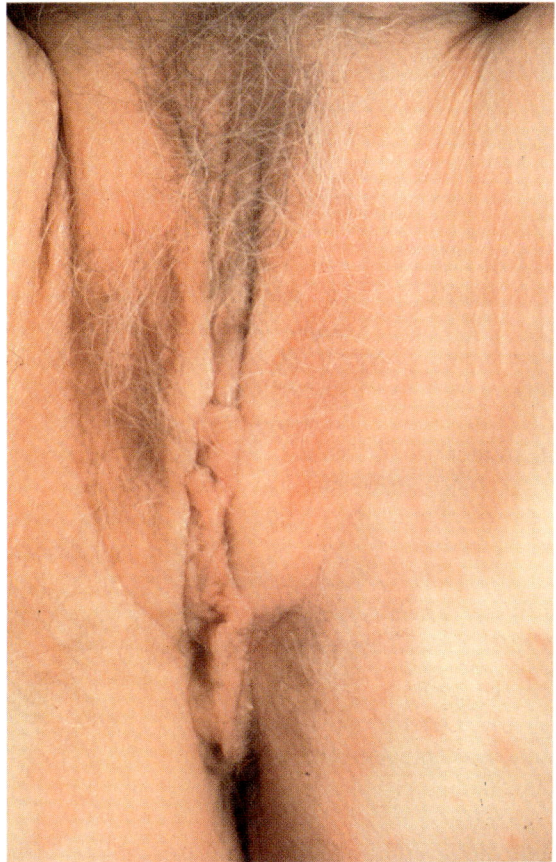

Fig. 6.32 Seborrhoeic dermatitis: diffuse erythematous lesions.

much less likely to do so than are other local anaesthetics.

Perfumes may also cause allergy; Larsen (1979) described its resulting from the incorporation of scent into a sanitary napkin. Sterry & Schmoll (1985) reported a patient with allergy to fragrance and to a disinfecting agent in self-adhesive pads. Guin & Haffley (1983) explored perfume allergy in one man and three women, all of the latter with vulval eczema. It seemed likely that allergy to perfume was responsible for the rash and that use of Mycolog®, a compound containing (as well as perfume) the preservative ethylenediamine, which is a strong sensitiser, had encouraged the development of allergy to the perfume compounds alpha-amylcinnammic aldehyde and alpha-amylcinnammic alcohol, which are weaker sensitisers. These latter substances may also be present in scented fabric softeners. Calnan (1978) reported a patient who developed an allergic reaction to oxypolyethoxy-dodecane anorectal ointment.

Allergic reactions have been reported to copper in the intra-uterine device (Romaguera & Grimalt 1981), and to vaginal applications (Robin 1978). The locally acting contraceptive preparations may induce allergy (Ridley 1981). Possible sources are chemical additives in sheaths and diaphragms (both affecting the male more commonly, since cutaneous surfaces are more susceptible than are mucosae), and active compounds or scents in spermicides, again more in the male. Patch testing is important and can be carried out in the ordinary way on the skin, since mucosal reactions do not seem to occur in the absence of positive cutaneous patch tests. Hindson (1966) recommended the list below, but new constituents of current substances under suspicion may have to be added.

Rubber condom (as is)
Chemical contraceptive used (as is)
Zinc mercaptobenzothiazole (1% in soft paraffin)
Dipentamethylthiuramdisulphide (1% in soft paraffin)
Zinc dithiocarbamate (1% in soft paraffin)
Zinc lupetimide (1% in soft paraffin)
Quinine hydrochloride (1% in water)
Phenyl mercuric acetate (0.01% in soft paraffin)
Hexyl resorcinol (1% in soft paraffin)
Oxyquinoline sulphate (1% in soft paraffin)
Phenoxypolyethoxy-ethanol (0.5% in soft paraffin)

As with any form of genital eczema where allergy is suspected, it is important to include the topical preparations used to treat the rash. Patch testing, of which details can be found in standard texts (Rook et al 1986) necessitates careful and experienced interpretation as well as access to a standard battery of commonly encountered allergens. It is therefore best carried out by the dermatologist, to whom patients not initially under his care should be referred.

Clinical and histological features

As regards appearances clinically, the end point of all these processes is diffuse oedematous erythe-

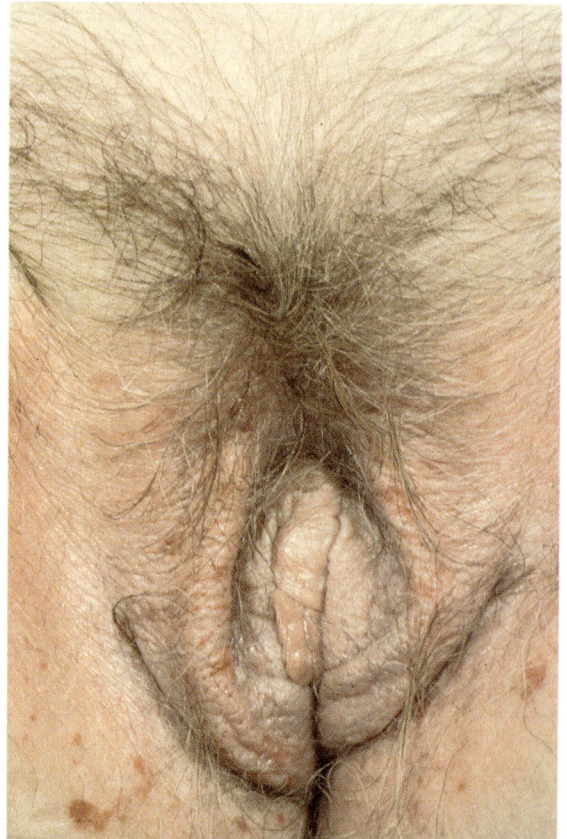

Fig. 6.33 Eczema with lichenification. (Reproduced from Beil-by & Ridley (1987) by courtesy of the authors and publisher)

ma; subsequent lichenification (p. 168) will render the area thick and pale (Fig. 6.33). Secondary infection will lead to soggy malodorous areas and acute soreness. The differential diagnosis may include an acute *Candida* vulvovaginitis (Figs. 6.34 a & b).

Histologically (Fig. 6.35), there is spongiosis, sometimes acanthosis and parakeratosis, and a mid-dermal infiltrate, with the changes of lichenification in chronic cases.

Management

Treatment of eczema calls for the removal of any known, or suspected, causative factor coupled with soothing applications such as potassium permanganate 1 in 10 000 or saline, as wet compresses or as simple bathing (a bidet can be useful here), a mild

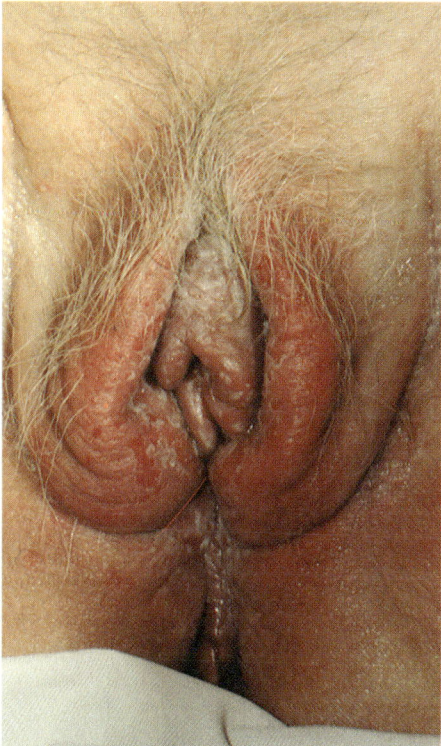

A

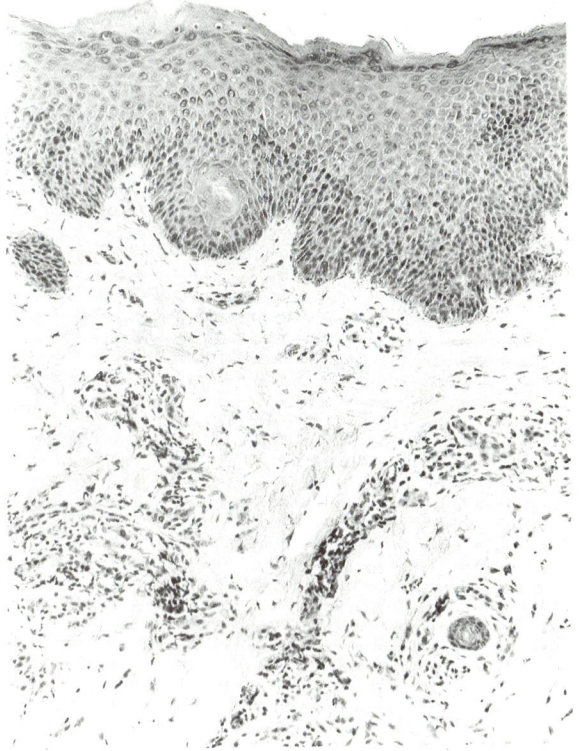

B

Fig. 6.34 (a) Candida vulvitis: redness and oedema in a diabetic patient. (b) Infection with *Candida* in a diabetic: hypae of *Candida* visible in stratum corneum. (PAS × 240) (By courtesy of Dr C H Buckley)

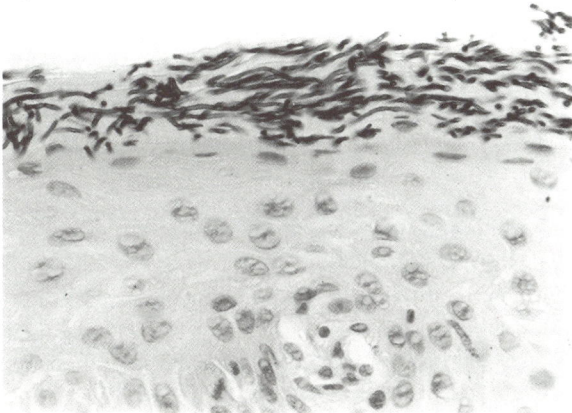

Fig. 6.35 Eczema: parakeratosis spongiosis, inflammatory infiltrate.

corticosteroid preparation, and treatment of any secondary infection. In very acute cases rest in bed with a hairdryer placed directing a current of cold air on the area is helpful.

When lesions are moist and painful, a cream or lotion is easier to apply than an ointment. Ointments in general, however, are safer to use because they do not contain preservatives and hence avoid the risk of sensitisation to these compounds.

As regards corticosteroids, hydrocortisone is safest for long term treatment but stronger preparations, for example beta methasone 17 valerate, may have to be used in the acute stage and, from time to time, in acute flares subsequently. Such flares are often precipitated by hot weather. Secondary infection may be by bacteria or *Candida* or both. If it is severe a systemic antibiotic should be given for a bacterial moiety; as regards *Candida*, however, ketoconazole is not now advisable because of its hepatoxic side effects, and nystatin is not absorbed.

Local antiCandida agents include nystatin, as well as clotrimazole and related compounds which have the advantage of some antibacterial activity. The choice of a more powerful antibacterial agent is more difficult; some antibiotics readily sensitise and the use of others may encourage resistant strains to develop. Mupirocin is a new agent which may be free of these hazards. Otherwise the tetracycline group, for example oxytetracyline, is reasonably safe and effective, or one may employ antiseptics such as chinoform (which, however, has the disadvantage of staining), or hydroxyquinoline. All these agents can be obtained in combinations with topical corticosteroids of various strengths.

A poor response should arouse suspicion of a local allergy, perhaps partly masked by a corticosteroid; appropriate measures, including patch testing at a time when the condition has settled, can then be taken.

Advice should be given on keeping weight down and on the avoidance of constrictive clothing which tends to press skin folds together; many of these patients will have chronic problems and can benefit from long term guidance and supervision.

LICHEN SIMPLEX: LICHENIFICATION

Definition

It cannot be denied that the terminology of the conditions now to be discussed gives non-dermatologists some difficulty. Nevertheless the conditions are of great importance and have held their names for some considerable time so the substance of their nomenclature should be mastered, and with it their essential morphology.

Lichen is a term used in describing many lesions which have an appearance of closely set papules as their main characteristic; hence lichen simplex and the closely related lichenification, lichen planus, lichen sclerosus et atrophicus. The derivation may be from a resemblance to the mossy surface of lichen on a tree. Some distinct conditions similarly named have no relevance when the vulva is under consideration, for example lichen amyloidosus. Moreover the terms 'lichenoid' as in many drug rashes and 'lichenoides' as in an entity such as pityriasis lichenoides chronica stem from lichen planus only and imply resemblance to the distinctive features of lichen planus, rather than to those of lichen simplex or lichenification, or of any other conditions which include the word 'lichen' in their names.

In lichen planus and lichen sclerosus et atrophicus closely set papules are indeed found, but in lichen simplex and lichenification the appearance is a similitude only; the normal rhomboidal pattern of the skin, magnified as the result of uniform thickening, gives the impression of papulation. In lichen simplex, the skin was apparently normal at the onset (i.e. the patient was suffering from pruritus vulvae (p. 217)), whereas in secondary lichenification the skin was the seat of some other condition which had become thickened in response to scratching and rubbing. Thus a lichenified vulva is one which has undergone the process of lichenification; the dermatologist's task is to determine if there was any underlying condition at the outset (as in lichenified eczema) or if the skin would have appeared normal (lichen simplex). The association of lichen simplex and lichenification with rubbing led to their being called neurodermatitis in the past, 'neuro' here being employed in the physical rather than the psychological sense (Whitlock 1976), but this is an outmoded term.

Clinical features

While many genital dermatoses readily lichenify, the area, particularly the clitoris and labia majora, is a common site too for lichen simplex. The same may be said of the scrotum, which is homologous with the labia majora. The peri-anal skin has a similar tendency.

Although in lichenification which is secondary to some pre-existing physical lesion there may be some signs of the underlying lesion, they are usually masked and one sees only, as in lichen simplex, thickened, slightly scaly, pale or earthy skin with accentuated markings and a diffuse outline (Fig. 6.36). Attacks of itching will make it red and swollen and perhaps excoriated; as they settle the area will become dry, thick scaly and perhaps pigmented. The thickened skin often fissures in the natal cleft. On the inner aspects of the labia majora the skin tends to look strikingly white. The findings are thus variable but usually easily recognisable.

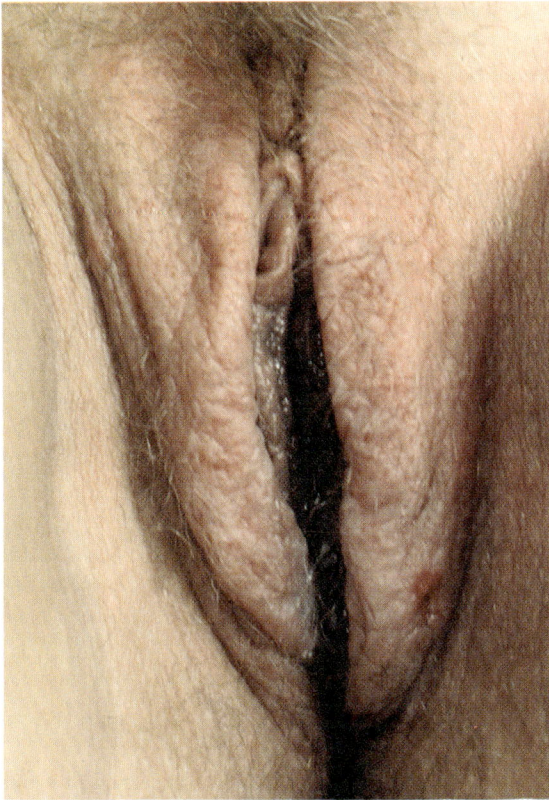

Fig. 6.36 Lichen simplex: dull earthy coloured thickening of labia majora. (Reproduced from Beilby & Ridley (1987) by courtesy of the authors and publisher)

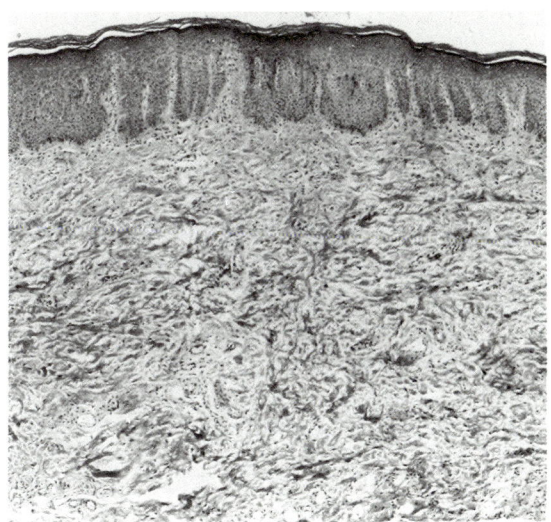

A

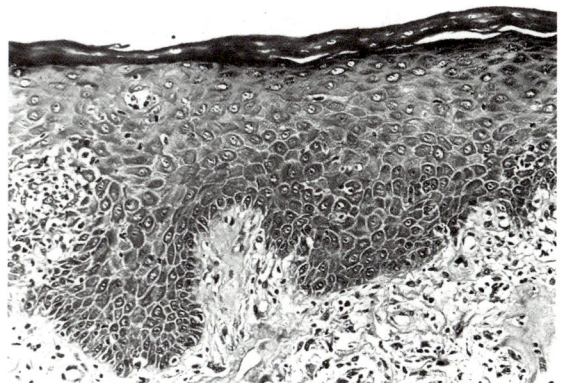

B

Fig. 6.37 (**a** and **b**) Lichen simplex: hyperkeratosis and parakeratosis, acanthosis, lengthened broad rete pegs, chronic inflammatory dermal infiltrate. (By courtesy of Dr C H Buckley and Dr D McGibbon)

Once attacks of itching have been triggered off by even mild physical factors or by emotional ones or those of unknown origin, the thickening, itching and further thickening tend to be self perpetuating.

The histology (Fig. 6.37) shows hyperkeratosis, occasional parakeratosis, marked acanthosis, lengthened rete ridges and an infiltrate of chronic inflammatory type in the dermis. In appropriate cases, traces of an underlying dermatosis may also be present.

Marks & Wells (1973 a & b) noted that in lichen simplex there was evidence of hyperplasia of all the cells in the epidermis, compared with the situation in psoriasis where it was only the keratinocytes which were so affected. The labelling index was increased as in psoriasis but the transit time was slower.

Management

Clinical and histological diagnosis is usually simple, but management carries the responsibility of ensuring that an underlying lesion is not missed. The patient should be reassured that there is no question of infection or malignancy (past views on a possible relation to malignancy are discussed on p. 191). A mild sedative at night is often helpful. The withdrawal of potential sensitisers and irritants is essential. Treatment with plenty of bland emollients and a topical corticosteroid is initiated. Since

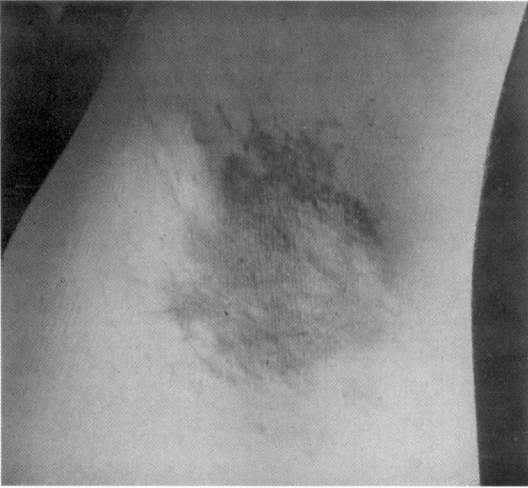

Fig. 6.38 Lichen planus: marked postinflammatory pigmentation in a flexural area.

the vulval skin is thin absorption of local preparations is good (while local side effects are more likely than in other areas because of this circumstance and because of the occlusion inevitable there). Normally therefore hydrocortisone is strong enough for symptomatic relief. However, where itching is severe and thickening considerable it is often reasonable to give a stronger preparation, for example betamethasone 17 valerate, at first to ensure rapid improvement. Such measures as alcohol injections (p. 218) are rarely, if ever, called for.

LICHEN PLANUS

This idiopathic (or sometimes drug-induced) condition may have an auto-immune background. Its association with other auto-immune diseases is probably significant, it is a well-recognised feature of graft-versus-host disease, and a significant association with HLA type HLA-DRI has now been demonstrated (Powell et al 1986).

The lesions occur on all areas of the skin and have a predilection for the oral mucosa. Vulval lesions, on keratinised or mucosal surfaces, are probably present more often than is recognised. They can be virtually confined to the vulva but more often appear as part of a widespread eruption. When they are on the keratinised skin lesions tend to disappear after weeks or months, often leaving

typical postinflammatory pigmentation (Fig. 6.38), but on the mucosal aspects, as in the mouth, they are more persistent.

Lesions on keratinised skin

Typical lesions on keratinised areas are purplish, flat-topped, polygonal shiny papules, sometimes slightly hyperkeratotic (Fig. 6.39).

The histology (Fig. 6.40) is that of lichen planus elsewhere: hyperkeratosis, acanthosis, an increased granular layer and a dense subepidermal band-like infiltrate, mainly composed of T cells, which extends up to the basal layer where there may be liquefaction degeneration and the formation of colloid bodies; the rete ridges become long and pointed.

The histological diagnosis is as a rule definite and may be required when, clinically, fairly pale isolated papules can resemble those of lichen sclerosus et atrophicus.

Management

The lesions often itch but symptomatic treatment with a topical corticosteroid or, occasionally, intralesional corticosteroid injections to a confluent area, is effective.

Mucosal and erosive lesions

On the mucosal aspect, however, diagnosis and management are less easy. Sometimes one sees a typical milk-white network on the inner aspects of the labia minora, resembling the buccal lesions. Here the histology is also likely to be reasonably helpful, although to achieve a biopsy is less simple. The presence of lesions elsewhere is obviously of assistance in such cases.

Problems arise when the only finding is an eroded, perhaps bullous and atrophic, painful area on the inner aspects of the labia minora, often with marked loss of substance (Fig. 6.41 a and b). Examination and biopsy are difficult and histology may in any case show only an atrophic ulcerated epithelium and a non-specific infiltrate; liquefaction degeneration of the basal layer is always a useful pointer to lichen planus. Again there is a parallel with eroded and atrophic oral lesions. The main

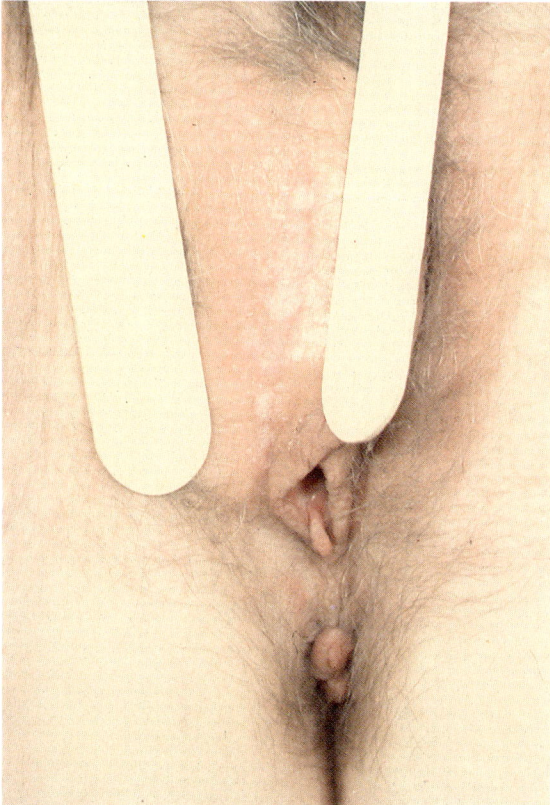

Fig. 6.39 Lichen planus: flat shiny polygonal papules. (Reproduced from Beilby & Ridley (1987) by courtesy of the authors and publisher)

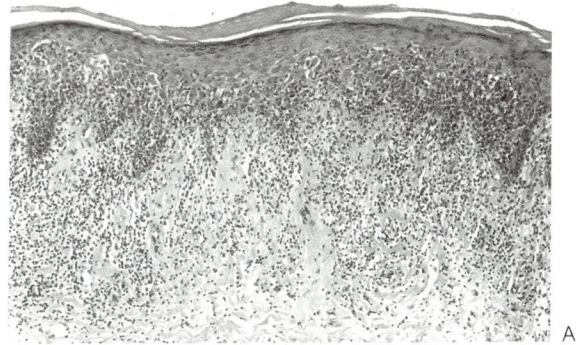

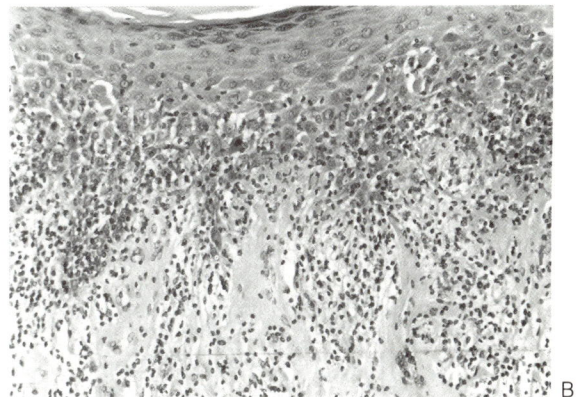

Fig. 6.40 Lichen planus: hyperkeratosis, prominent granular layer, irregular acanthosis and sawtooth pattern. Destruction of basal layer; band-like inflammatory infiltrate. (a) H & E × 75; (b) H & E × 165 (by courtesy of Dr C H Buckley)

problem in differential diagnosis is to distinguish it from cicatricial pemphigoid; if lesions elsewhere are not helpful the positive immunofluorescence (direct and also sometimes indirect) usually found in cicatricial pemphigoid is likely to be so.

Vaginal lesions

Vaginal lesions in lichen planus have been poorly documented in the past, largely because of the lack of clinical and histological specificity. Possible examples were reported by Weber (1927), Gougerot & Burnier (1937) and Crotty et al (1980). Pelisse et al (1982, 1983) and Hewitt et al (1985) have, however, reported cases with good evidence of lichen planus in the lesions themselves and/or in lesions elsewhere. These patients had desquamative gingivitis, erosive vulval lesions and a desquamative vaginitis, sometimes with synechiae, which may

cause stenosis. The author has seen several such patients all with good evidence of lichen planus elsewhere, past or present, and/or histological confirmation from genital lesions. The vaginal lesions are painful and haemorrhagic (Fig. 6.42 a). Some have the more usual oral lichen planus lesions rather than gingivitis (Fig. 6.42 b). One had undergone multiple attempts at surgery to relieve vaginal obstruction. It is tempting to think that cases reported as desquamative inflammatory vaginitis by Gray & Barnes (1965) and others, and discussed by Gardner & Kaufman (1981), may have been similar, though synechiae and lesions elsewhere were not described.

Management

Treatment of erosive lichen planus, vulval or vaginal, is difficult. Attempts can be made to introduce

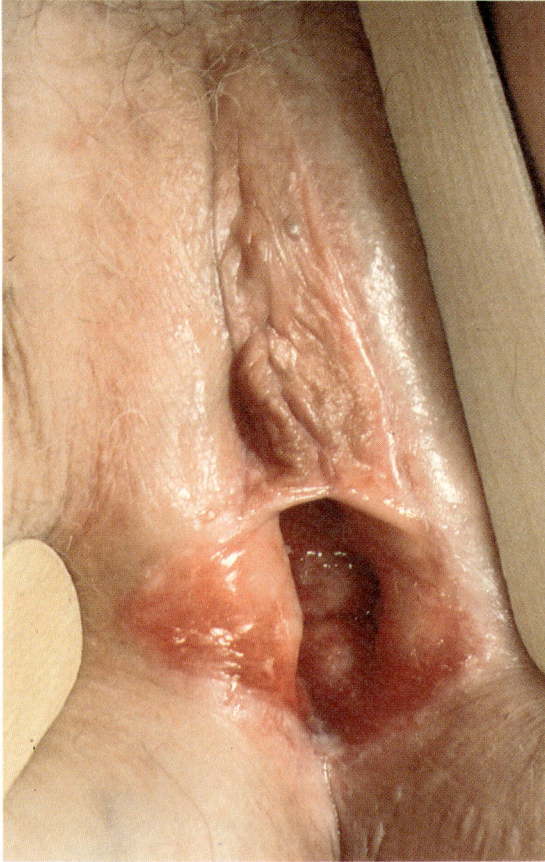
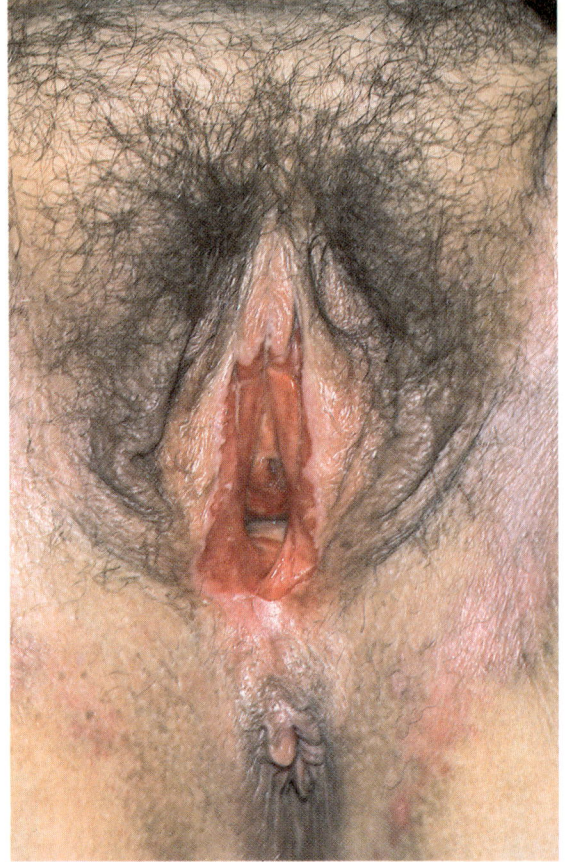

A   B

Fig. 6.41 Lichen planus (**a**) eroded areas in a patient with proven lichen planus elsewhere. (**b**) eroded areas in a patient with oral lichen planus. (Reproduced from Beilby & Ridley (1987) by courtesy of the authors and publisher)

corticosteroids into the vagina, for example with a foam preparation. Systemic steroids by and large seem to give the best results. After reports of the value of oral griseofulvin in severe oral lichen planus this drug is worth trying, but in the author's experience is of little help. Etretinate proved disappointing in the mouth (Hammersley et al 1984) and is equally without value at the vulva. Dapsone has been suggested (Falk et al 1985) at 50 mg a day for 3 months in eroded lesions of mouth, hands and feet, but has not proved helpful so far at the vulva.

The prognosis for healing is poor, lesions as far as one can tell persisting indefinitely. This is of concern not only because of the troublesome symptoms but because of the risk of malignancy. Oral lesions of this type are well known to be premalig-

nant. Wallace (1971) described one carcinoma in five patients with chronic vulval lichen planus. One wonders if in some cases excision and grafting would be justifiable, as has been found sometimes helpful in erosive lichen planus of palms and soles, or indeed if partial excision or a vulvectomy should be considered. Certainly follow-up should be assiduous.

LICHEN SCLEROSUS ET ATROPHICUS (LSA)

In the classification of the International Society for the Study of Vulvar Disease (p. 190) lichen sclerosus et atrophicus (LSA) is the only dermatosis de-

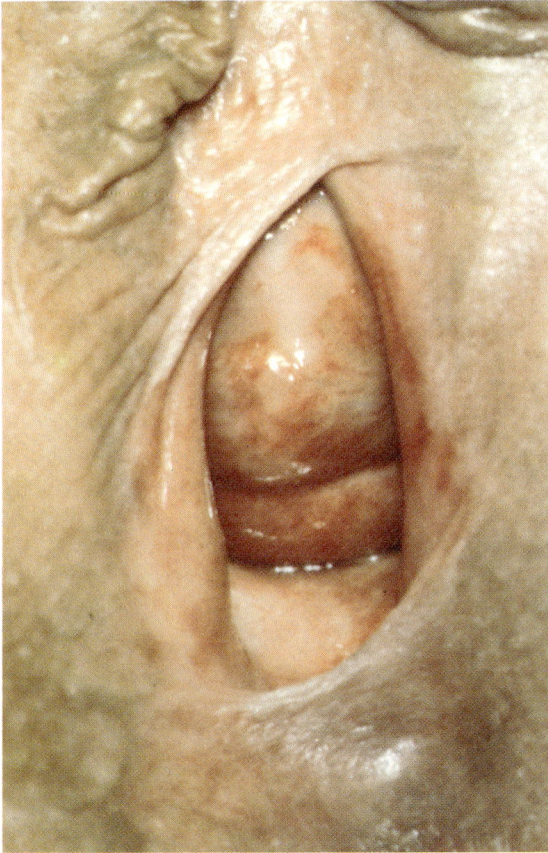

A

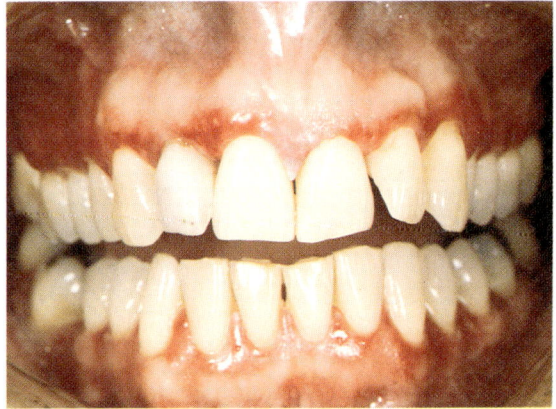

B

Fig. 6.42 Lichen planus (a) haemorrhagic areas on vaginal wall in a patient with erosive vulval and vaginal lesions and recurrent vaginal synechiae. (**b**) lichen planus gingivitis. (courtesy of Miss J Hughes)

fined with its name, yet even so it has been truncated to lichen sclerosus; this decision was because of evidence of 'metabolic activity in the epidermis', a suggestion that has not been followed up or enriched by later work. In any case there should be no difficulty in accepting something of this sort; to say it is atrophic is not to say that it is dead. Atrophic the clinical lesions very often are, so dermatologists tend to retain the adjective 'atrophicus'. However, all work on lichen sclerosus or lichen sclerosus et atrophicus is clearly referring to the same condition, and use of either form is not likely to cause problems.

The clinical findings are distinctive but variable and it is perhaps the latter feature which gives rise to the difficulty some non-dermatologists have in recognising the condition. The dermatologist, for his part, must adhere to fairly firm clinical and histological criteria and not make the diagnosis in their absence. The condition was described originally by Hallopeau (1889) as lichen plan scléraux and its histology by Darier (1892) and it was thought to be a variant of lichen planus. Others have considered it as a variant of morphoea (localised scleroderma). It is perhaps best to regard morphoea and LSA as extreme ends of a spectrum.

Lichen sclerosus et atrophicus is found in men, women and children and on all parts of the body. It may be commoner in white races but has been described in the negro and Bantu (Barclay et al 1966, Dogliotti et al 1974). In a current series (Meyrick Thomas et al 1987b), of 350 women and children with histologically confirmed LSA, only three (Asian) non-white patients were found, but although this figure seems a little low it has not been compared with the racial composition of the appropriate population.

Aetiology

Familial incidence though rare is well reported, for example by Hunt (1954), Barker & Gross (1962), Wallace (1971), Hofs (1978) and Friedrich & McLaren (1984), as well as Murphy et al (1982) who reported LSA in three sisters, one of whom had pernicious anaemia and vitiligo, and Meyrick Thomas & Kennedy (1986) reporting vulval LSA in identical twins.

As regards HLA types, Harrington & Gelsthorpe (1981) found the incidence of HLA-B40 increased in 50 women with LSA compared with controls, but the finding was not statistically significant. Holt & Darke (1983) added 23 women and controls to the total and found a significant link with HLA-AW30/31 and HLA-B4 in LSA. Meyrick Thomas et al (1984b), however, found no significant association with HLA types in 92 women and 28 men with LSA. Friedrich & McLaren (1984) studied two families with LSA (mother and two daughters in each) and proposed follow-up to see if certain HLA types were common to those affected.

Wallace (1971) had suspected a significant association with vitiligo. Later evidence (Goolamali et al 1974, Harrington & Dunsmore 1981, Meyrick Thomas et al 1982, 1987b) has demonstrated in women an association with auto-immunity in terms of increased auto-antibodies and auto-immune disease in the patient, and auto-immune disease in the patient's family; the same association in men has also now been shown (Meyrick Thomas et al 1983, 1984a). The conditons most often linked in affected women are thyroid disease and alopecia areata.

The link with auto-immune disease, though it certainly exists, is fairly weak, with about 21% of subjects having auto-immune disease and 22% a family history of auto-immune disease, while 44% have one or more auto-antibodies. Moreover it seems that the auto-immune diathesis stamps no particular character on the lesions; thus in 250 women there was no difference in duration, onset and relation to puberty or the menopause, sites of involvement or malignant change (Meyrick Thomas et al 1987b).

Achlorhydria has been noted in some cases of 'vulval dystrophy' of which many were probably LSA (23% of 269 'dystrophy' patients for example reported by Jeffcoate 1962) and perhaps this point should be examined again in proved cases, in view of the link with auto-immune diseases including pernicious anaemia noted above. Lavery (1984) found achlorhydria in 10 of 18 patients categorised as 'chronic vulval dystrophy' and has speculated, but so far without firm evidence, about a relationship between the effect of urogastrone (epidermal growth factor) on skin and on gastric acidity and an opposing effect of somatostatin. The role, in general, of epidermal growth factor is, however, uncertain (Lancet 1985b). Johansson and Nordlind (1986) noted, in two out of four patients with LSA, immunoreactivity within some cells of the epidermis to material like vasoactive intestinal polypeptide. This work must be regarded as a preliminary finding of uncertain significance.

Friedrich & Kalra (1984), noting the therapeutic effect of local testosterone, studied testosterone metabolism in 30 women with vulval LSA before the use of testosterone and subsequently in ten. They found that initially serum dihydrotestosterone and androstenedione levels were significantly decreased and free testosterone raised compared with controls. After treatment dihydrotestosterone and total testosterone levels rose. They suggested therefore that the enzyme 5α-reductase is involved in pathogenesis. The figures, while interesting, represent somewhat crude estimates of subtle local changes and their significance remains uncertain.

Cantwell (1984) who has over the years attributed scleroderma and morphoea to pleomorphic and variably acid-fast bacteria has now alleged the presence of similar organisms in four cases of LSA—three women and one man—but his findings must remain controversial; Aberer et al (1985) have suggested Borrelia burgdorferi as a cause of morphoea, but this has not been confirmed.

Barnes & Douglas (1985) have found an increase in a collagen inhibitor enzyme and an absence of collagenase in LSA compared with normal vulval tissue and that from other vulval conditions; they were using whole skin extracts, however, as cell cultures and the findings must be regarded with caution; the same authors (Douglas and Barnes 1986) have suggested that the activity of elastase is increased.

Whimster (1973) showed that a split skin graft taken from the thigh was transformed at the vulva into LSA, whereas a full thickness vulval LSA graft transferred to the thigh returned to normal, and the essential mystery of this remains unexplained. Foulds (1980) noted that LSA overtook a grafted area on the scalp and Ellis & Crow (1982) that LSA recurred in a full thickness peri-anal graft. Most striking of all, di Paola et al (1982) found that LSA (clinically and histologically confirmed) developed in a bilateral gracilis myocutaneous graft, which had its own blood supply and deep dermal tissue, when the graft had been used to repair a vulvec-

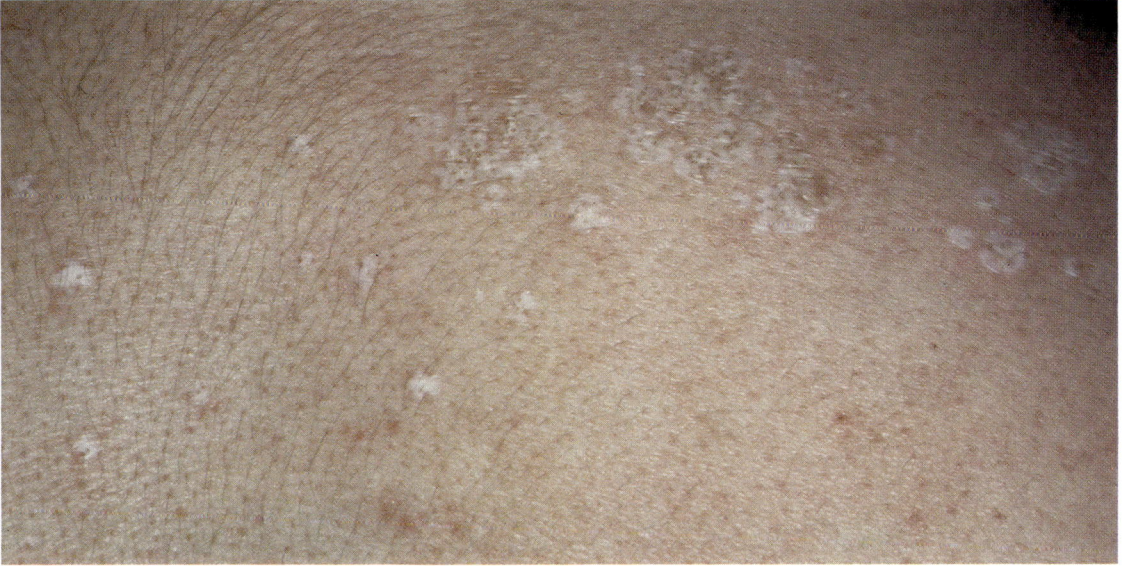

Fig. 6.43 Lichen sclerosus et atrophicus: typical lesions on back. (By courtesy of Dr M Moyal-Barracco)

tomy in a patient with a vulval carcinoma and LSA.

These findings must be accounted for by any aetiological theory. All that can be said is that the aetiology remains uncertain. Possible approaches include the study of skin 5α-reductase levels, of collagen subtypes (the latter may be of particular interest in connection with the suggested relation to morphoea to be discussed below) and of fibroblasts.

Clinical appearance and associated conditions

The morphology of LSA is distinctive. Firm flat polygonal ivory, or ivory-pink, often translucent papules, sometimes with a central plug, are seen singly or in confluent crinkly plaques (Fig. 6.43). Pallor of such areas is often striking. Purpura and telangiectasia are common (Fig. 6.44), and bullae may occur.

Plaques can be quite firm as well as white and have a confluent guttate pattern, in which case they merge clinically into morphoea, especially in its guttate form, with which it is generally considered to be significantly associated (13 cases in 380 of both sexes (Wallace 1971) 12 in the current 350 women in our own series (Meyrick Thomas et al 1987b)) (Fig. 6.45). Both conditions can become

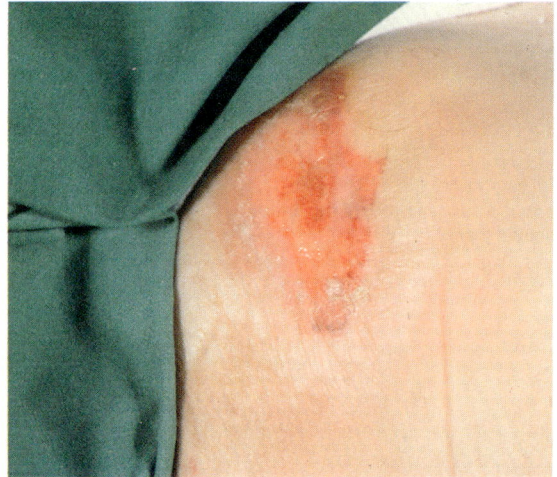

Fig. 6.44 Lichen sclerosus et atrophicus: crinkly atrophic plaque of upper inner thigh with marked central extravasation of blood. (Reproduced from Beilby & Ridley (1987) by courtesy of the authors and publisher)

bullous, morphoea more commonly, and it is possible that the diagnosis is often confused, or indeed that the conditions are part of a disease spectrum.

Lesions may occur anywhere on the trunk (Fig. 6.46), upper and lower limbs as well as the

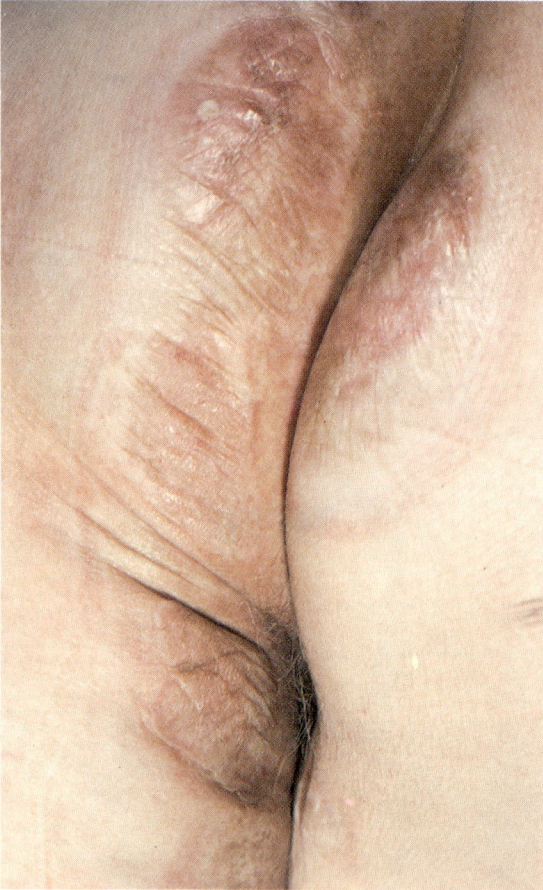

Fig. 6.45 Patient with lichen sclerosus et atrophicus, also showing plaques of morphoea with typical violaceous edge.

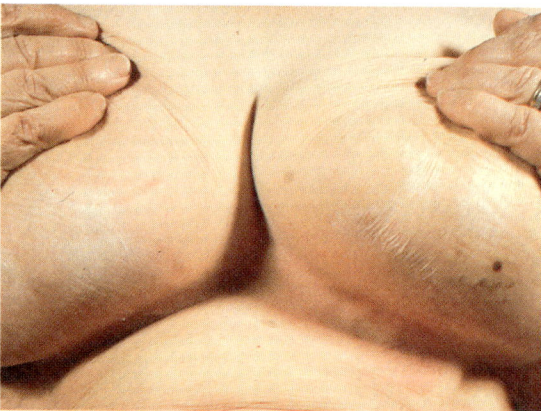

Fig. 6.47 Lichen sclerosus et atrophicus: typical lesions on wrists.

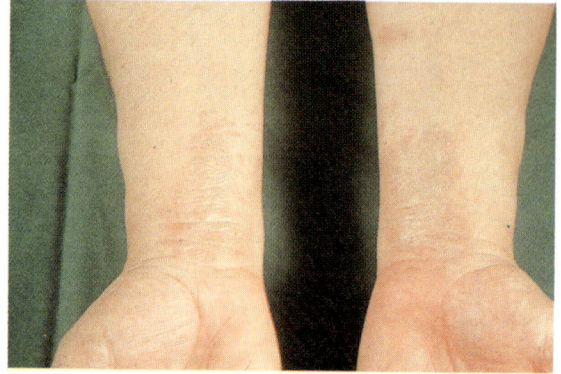

Fig. 6.46 Lichen sclerosus et atrophicus: flat ivory papules on the breast. (Reproduced from Beilby and Ridley 1987 by courtesy of the authors and publisher)

anogenital area. The front of the wrists (Fig. 6.47) is a common, and the scalp an uncommon, site. The Koebner phenomenon is often to be seen, for example at the site of a scratch, and Yates et al (1985) have described LSA at the site of radiotherapy for carcinoma of the breast in two women who had no lesions elsewhere.

The existence of oral lesions is disputable, and histological confirmation is rarely forthcoming. Ravits & Welsh (1957) reported mouth lesions in three men, two of whom had LSA elsewhere. Greyish-white and atrophic patches were noted, and the histology was suggestive of LSA. Miller (1957) reported a histologically compatible example, and one has been seen by Sarkany (1986 personal communication). Wallace (1971) noted no definite oral lesions in his series. Lichen planus is possibly significantly associated with LSA; Wallace had 6 cases in 380, although in our series (Meyrick Thomas et al 1987b) the incidence is now only 2 in 350 cases. It is possible that some examples of oral lesions in LSA may in fact be of lichen planus. It has already been noted that originally LSA was thought to be a variant of lichen planus. Miller (1957) comprehensively reviewed such lines of thought in earlier reports, including also those which illustrated overlap and confusion between morphoea and LSA as regards oral lesions.

Connelly & Winkelmann (1985) reported four patients, (two men and two women) who had LSA, morphoea and lichen planus and found eight other similar conjunctions in the literature. They suggested that a link is not unexpected in view of the

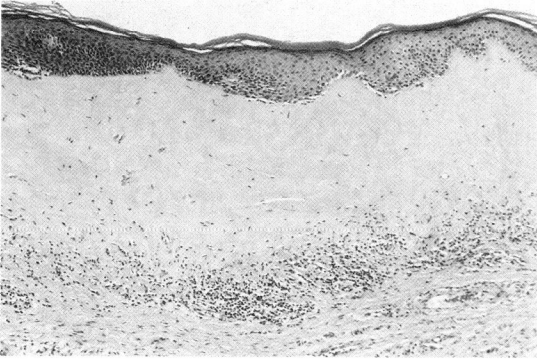

Fig. 6.48 Lichen sclerosus et atrophicus: atrophic epidermis, hyalinised dermis with lower band of inflammatory cells. (H & E × 60) (By courtesy of Dr C H Buckley)

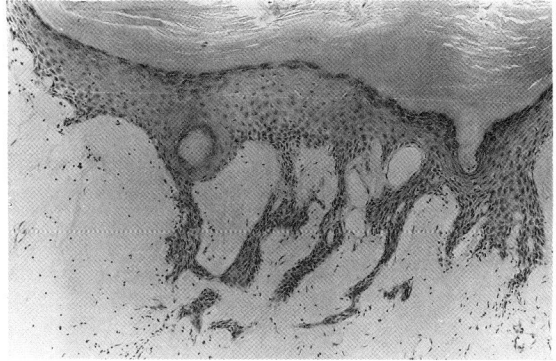

Fig. 6.49 Severe lichen sclerosus et atrophicus: hyperkeratosis, pointed rete ridges, hyalinisation. (H & E × 75) (Reproduced from Beilby & Ridley (1987) by courtesy of the authors and publisher)

co-existent lichenoid and sclerodermatous eruptions seen in graft-versus-host disease.

Histology

The histology is distinctive (Fig. 6.48). In early lesions there is hyperkeratosis, mild acanthosis and follicular plugging, but in later lesions the epidermis is atrophic. The dermis is initially oedematous and hyalinised, with a lower border of inflammatory cells disposed as a lichenoid band and in later lesions more condensed and with fewer cells. Extravasated red cells are a common feature. Electron microscopy (Mann & Cowan 1973) showed that melanocytes were absent in active lesions. Dermal material was seen in the epidermis. The dermal collagen was abnormal and the elastin appeared increased, contrary to studies with light microscopy and to other electron microscopic studies, for Kint & Geerts (1975) noted collagen fibrils between epidermal cells, an abnormal basement membrane, condensation and homogenisation of basal cell tonofibrils, and a reduced dermal elastin. Godeau et al (1982) demonstrated an elastase-type protease in vulval fibroblasts, and Frances et al (1983) changes in collagen subtypes using electron-microscopy and immunofluorescence.

Bushkell et al (1981) found fibrin at the dermo-epidermal junction in 7 of 24 vulval LSA biopsies by immunofluorescence, and Dickie et al (1982) found fibrin at the same site in 12 of 16 similar specimens with, in addition, C3 and IgM, each in four of the 12 positive specimens. Miller & Griffiths (1982) however showed that trauma in normal skin could give a somewhat similar finding, that is, fibrin and sometimes IgM along the basement membrane zone, in 7 of 10 cases, while complement was found in all, so the findings are probably essentially non-specific.

The changes described by Wallace & Whimster (1951) and Wallace (1971) as 'leukoplakia' (p. 189) probably represent the changes seen in severe LSA. There is epithelial hyperplasia, and a reversion to increased keratinisation, with or without mild atypia; the lower margin of the epidermis is irregular with pointed or forked rete ridges, and hyalinisation and loss of elastic tissue are noted in the dermis (Fig. 6.49).

The main differential diagnosis histologically is from morphoea. Patterson & Ackerman (1984) concluded in a study of 24 cases that the two conditions were distinct and favoured as criteria for the diagnosis of LSA a vacuolar change at the dermo-epidermal junction, and a lichenoid lymphocytic infiltration beneath the papillary dermis, whereas in morphoea the subcutis and reticular dermis show sclerosis and inflammatory infiltration.

In long-standing lesions of the LSA (and perhaps in early ones) both clinical and histological features become less distinctive, hence much uncertainty in diagnosis and in discussion.

LSA in males

In the male, LSA is now known to be one cause of phimosis in school-aged boys. Chalmers et al (1984) noted it in 14 (of whom 13 were aged 5 to 11 years) of 100 cases. Removal of the prepuce relieves symptoms in children. Follow-up has not so far determined whether when there were lesions on the glans they cleared, persisted or recurred developed in later life.

In adult men, a recent series of 25 patients with LSA revealed that 3 had only extragenital and 22 only penile lesions (Meyrick Thomas et al 1987a). The peri-anal area was not involved. It may be that some of these younger men had LSA dating back to childhood. The end result of untreated penile LSA in men is an atrophic and scarred lesion rather similar to that of cicatricial pemphigoid, though

histology and immunofluorescence will usually distinguish the two. The general term for such an appearance is 'balanitis xerotica obliterans' and most in cases this condition appears to have developed from LSA.

LSA in female children

In little girls the lesions may be genital, with or without extragenital involvement. Probably some have solely extragenital lesions but this has not been seen in our histologically confirmed series of 20 children; the youngest age at which lesions were seen is 6 months but it is conceivable that the true

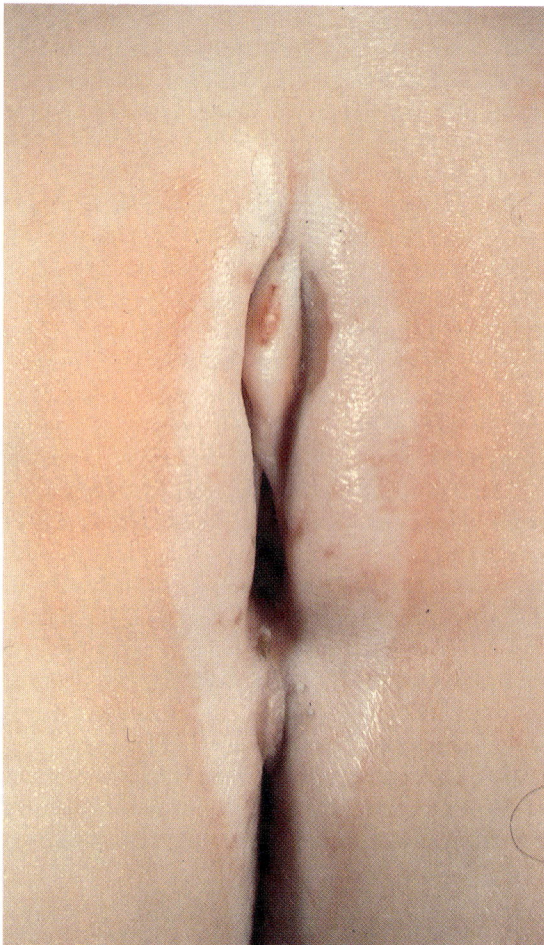
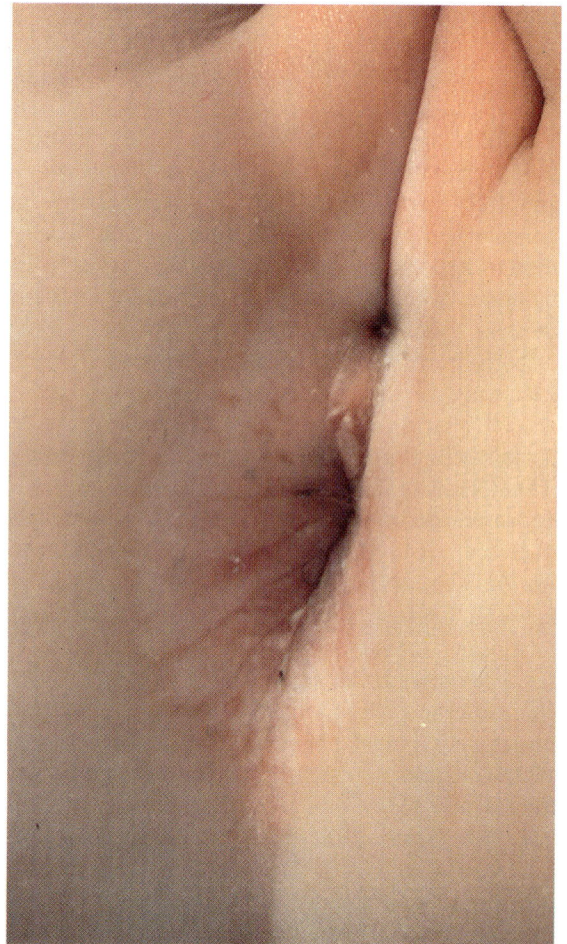

A   B

Fig. 6.50 Lichen sclerosus et atrophicus: typical pallor and speckling in a child (**a**) vulval; (**b**) peri-anal. (Reproduced from Beilby & Ridley (1987) by courtesy of the authors and publisher)

onset was earlier. In one of the patients of Clark & Muller (1967) the onset was at the age of 4 weeks, and the lesions in a case report by Cario et al (1984) were said to date from birth. The extragenital lesions are often profuse and the Koebner phenomenon is not unusual at the site of a scratch or injection. Clark & Muller (1967) commented on facial LSA in their patients, but it is hard to accept such findings which have not been noted in other reports in the literature and were not met with in our series.

The genital lesions may be obvious, and may or may not involve the peri-anal area. Sometimes however they are minute and evident only on close inspection when a child is brought along complaining of itching or soreness on defaecation or urination, for example a tiny whitish crimson-speckled frill around the clitoris. Equally, very widespread lesions may cause virtually no symptoms (Fig. 6.50). Rarely obliteration of contours is so extreme that a congenital abnormality is suspected and an examination under anaesthetic, to explore the area and taken a biopsy, may be necessary (Fig. 6.51).

The pallor may suggest vitiligo, but in that condition the texture of the skin is normal.

One child in our series with peri-anal LSA had intractable constipation which necessitated hospital admission and treatment with enemata before the diagnosis was made and the symptoms relieved by appropriate local treatment. Infection with staphylococci or streptococci may require systemic antibiotics (Fig. 6.52). Labial adhesions in small children attributable to LSA do not appear to have been reported but may have been missed. LSA may be mistaken for sexual abuse (p. 224); sexual abuse and LSA may of course co-exist.

Prognosis

As there is uncertainty as to age of onset, so there is doubt as to the clearance of anogenital LSA in little girls (it is agreed that extragenital lesions often remit). It has been generally thought (Wallace 1971) that in about two-thirds of patients the anogenital lesions will clear around puberty. Detailed follow-up has, however, not been available. Török et al (1975) could not comment on the postmenarchal course. Clark & Muller (1967) noted improvement in about half of their cases but relied in part on

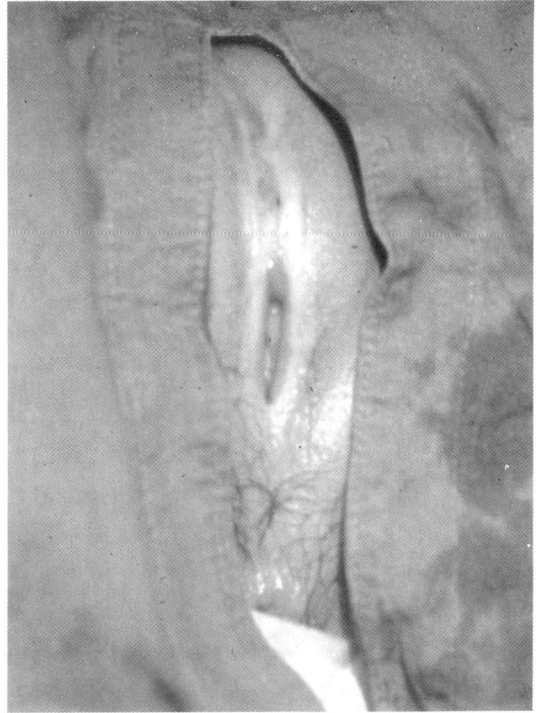

Fig. 6.51 Lichen sclerosus et atrophicus: extreme atrophy with no normal landmarks visible.

questionnaires for information. Kindler (1953) observed genital LSA in six girls and saw no improvement over a period of several years, in at least one case until after the menarche. It is interesting that in Wallace's account the regression is mainly of symptoms rather than of signs; he noted that in some 'apparent resolution' was followed by recurrence; and he commented that of 32 patients presenting between the ages of 15 and 30 years, 19 had had symptoms in childhood, as had 10 of 52 patients presenting between the ages of 30 and 45 years.

It is certainly the case that the condition often looks and feels better by the time of puberty, but proof that it really remits is as yet lacking. The author has seen one girl whose vulva looked virtually normal after puberty but whose biopsy still showed definite LSA.

As the condition seems not to remit in the middle aged and elderly (except at extra-genital sites), it is a tenable proposition that in fact it does not remit at

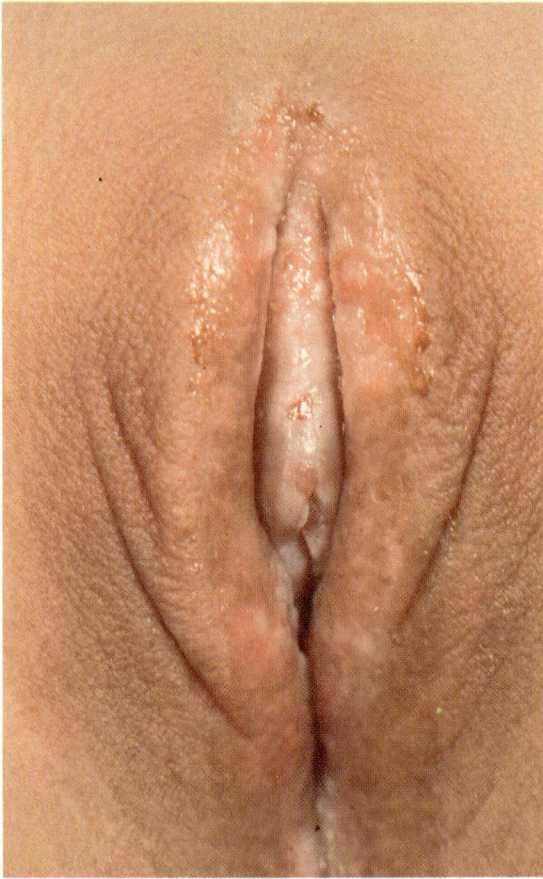

A

Fig. 6.52 (a and b) Lichen sclerosus et atrophicus: lesions in children with secondary infection.

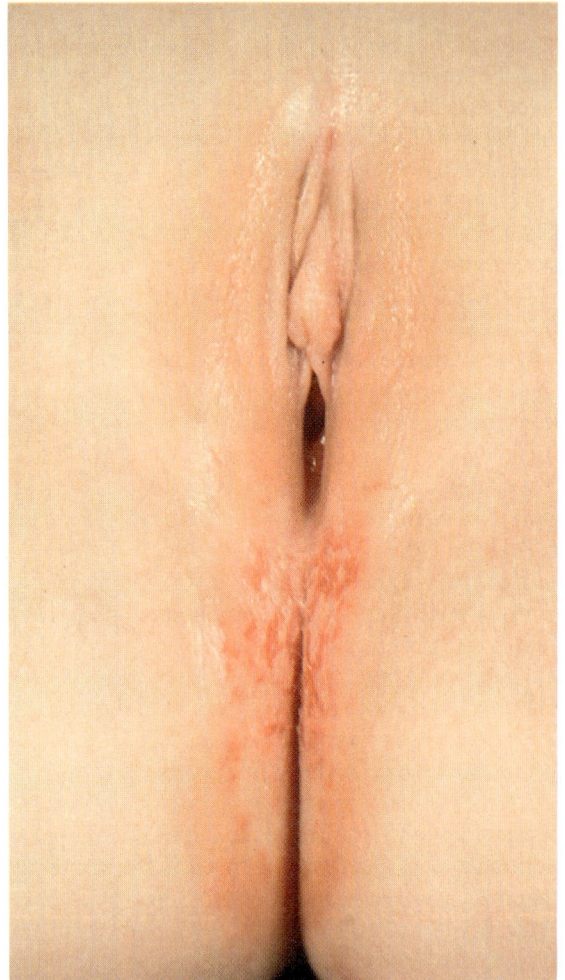

B

any stage, and this would be supported by the history of symptoms in childhood recollected by so many young women who appear with LSA.

In such young patients, dyspareunia may be a problem but pregnancy appears to be uneventful, however marked the stenosis and atrophy of the vestibule, and parents of children can be reassured accordingly.

Treatment

This is essentially as in adults but with even more reliance on bland preparations and the milder corticosteroids. Testosterone ointment is usually avoided. Systemic treatment is not indicated.

LSA in women

In women the lesions are most often anogenital. In our series, now of 350 women and children histologically confirmed as cases of LSA (Meyrick Thomas et al 1987b), 19% had trunk involvement. The vulva was involved in 98%, the anogenital area was affected in 54%, and the vulval without the anal area in 46%. The involvement of the peri-anal area (Fig. 6.53) usually completes with the vulva a figure-of-eight outline. The anal lesions may remit and recur, as may those on the trunk, but the vulval lesions appear to persist. The sites of election at the vulva are all aspects of the labia minora and the clitoris, as well as the inner aspects of the labia majora and the genitocrural folds (Fig. 6.54). Where the pallor is striking vitiligo may be suspected, but

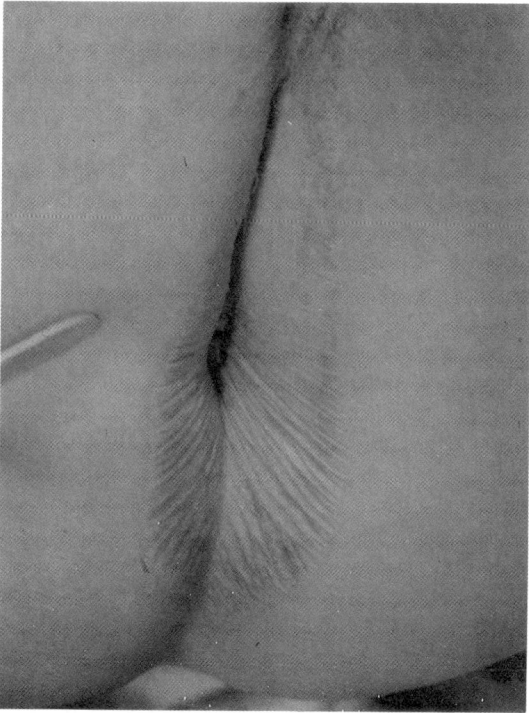

Fig. 6.53 Lichen sclerosus et atrophicus: crinkly atrophy of peri-anal area.

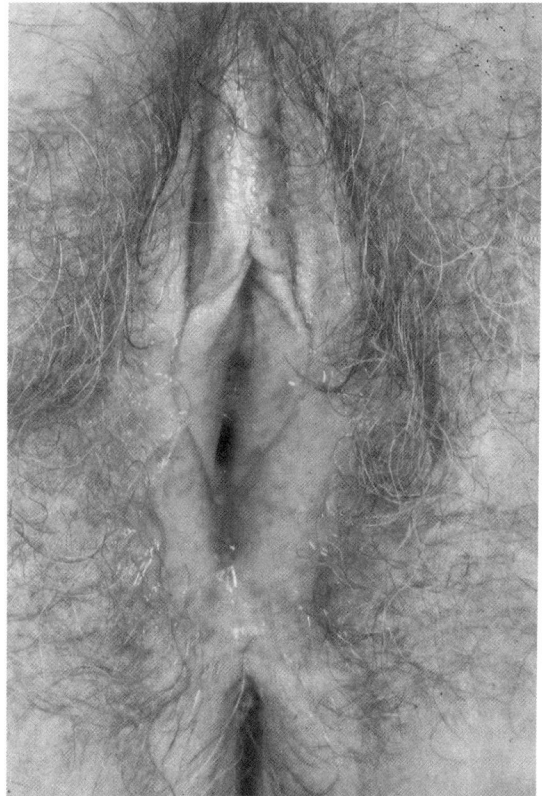

A

usually there is no difficulty in differentiation since the texture of the skin in vitiligo is normal. A few lesions are sometimes seen as atrophic papules on the outer aspect of the labia majora and on the mons pubis. Occasionally, as in children, lesions may be minimal, being seen as white patches on the inner labia minora (Fig. 6.55) or as tiny whitish speckled clitoral areas. In advanced cases contours are obliterated, the labia minora and majora disappear and loss of substance is marked (Fig. 6.56 a and b). The introitus is narrowed and the whole area is shiny, waxy and speckled. The vagina itself is not involved but stenosis of the orifice occurs.

Such severe lesions may ultimately leave only a pinhole meatus (p. 195); others may become thickened, eroded and fissured. A common appearance is of a honeycomb-like white plaque at the introitus, often with reddish fissuring and erosion (Fig. 6.57). It is such changes which correlate with the histological changes described by Wallace & Whimster over several years, and summarised by Wallace (1971), as leukoplakia. There is hyperkeratosis accompanied by irregular forked rete pegs, with or without atypia, and dermal hyalinisation.

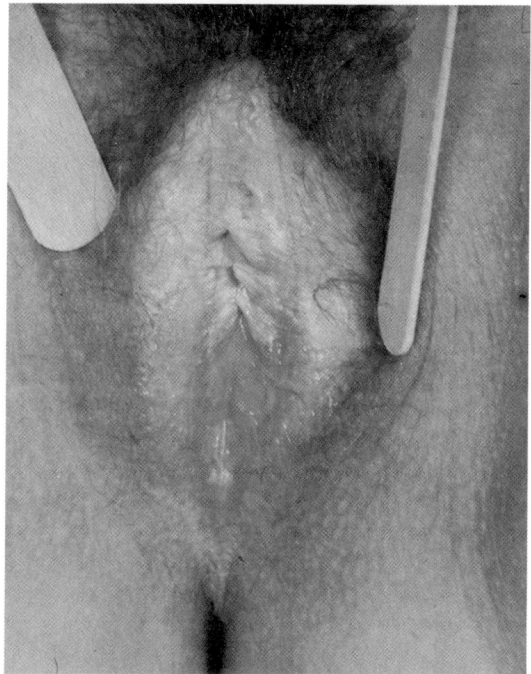

B

Fig. 6.54 (a and b) Lichen sclerosus et atrophicus: loss of contour, pallor and atrophy in young woman. (Reproduced from Beilby & Ridley (1987) by courtesy of the authors and publisher)

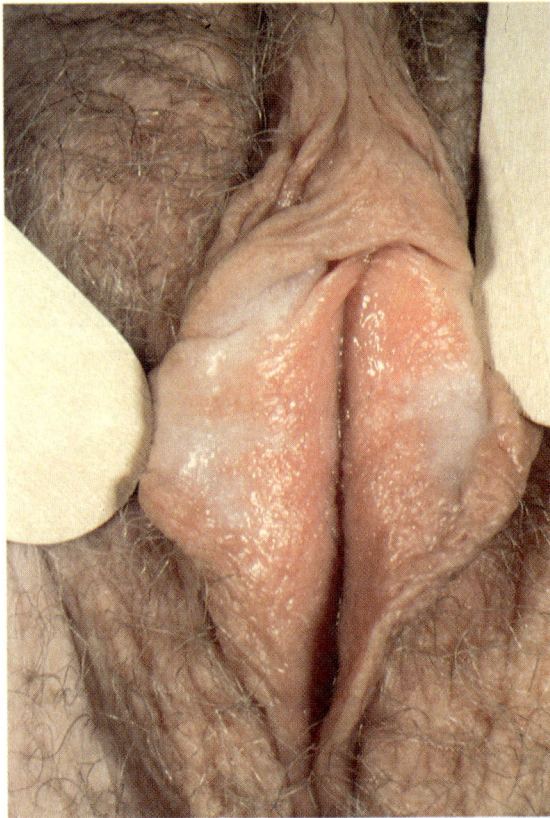

Fig. 6.55 Lichen sclerosus et atrophicus: small patches on labia minora.

Sometimes LSA of any degree of objective severity thickens in response to rubbing and scratching, and then it appears pale or earthy and puffy, the picture of lichenification (Fig. 6.58 a and b). The underlying condition may be masked completely and becomes apparent only when a topical corticosteroid has reversed the process by breaking the itch/scratch cycle. The histology (Fig. 6.59) in these cases shows a combination of features, lichenification per se and LSA.

Adhesions are a further potential complication, though except at the clitoris a rare one. In such cases separation of fused tissue is possible, but re-adhesion readily occurs. The labia minora or the clitoris, or both areas, may be affected. In one patient, seen a year or two after puberty, periclitoral adhesions resulted in a pseudocyst containing smegma, and the tissues rapidly resealed themselves even after careful dissection and removal of redundant skin (Fig. 6.60).

Management and Treatment

It is essential to reassure the patient that she has a well-recognised dermatological condition which, while it is unlikely to disappear, can be almost always satisfactorily controlled with simple local measures. Such reassurance is especially important in those who have been seen by gynaecologists speaking of 'leukoplakia' and who may even have been threatened with vulvectomy.

One should then establish whether or not the patient requires treatment at all. A few patients are entirely symptomless.

For the others, the next move is encouragement to use plenty of bland emollients of a nature that is tolerated. Some prefer thick greasy preparations and others thinner creams. The preparations should be used liberally, and particularly in relation to intercourse and after washing. If symptoms persist, hydrocortisone 2.5% is prescribed. If this helps, as it usually does, its use may be reduced in frequency or 1% prescribed instead. If it does not help a stronger corticosteroid is reasonable for a short period (or even a long one if use is intermittent and small amounts applied). Fissures and open areas may become infected and a local antiseptic or antibiotic will be called for.

If all these measures fail, testosterone propionate, as a 2% ointment in petrolatum or unguentum Merck, is often given, especially when there is little thickening clinically. This preparation was originally used empirically as a thickener of the skin and is widely employed in the United States. Friedrich (1971) showed its benefit with a controlled trial, but the subjects had various vulval dystrophies and one wonders if the effect is in some way nonspecific. The same applies to the benefits noted by Ambrosini et al (1984) in 75% of their 187 patients. Side effects may occur, both local (clitoral enlargement) and general (increased libido). A few patients like the ointment but many do not seem to be helped. If it is employed it should be used for several weeks. It is not usually given to children, though Gardner & Kaufman (1981) say that it is safe to use a 1% preparation for a short period. Progesterone cream (Jasionowski & Jasionowski 1979) is also thought to be of value. As regards systemic treatment Itala et al (1984) found benefit

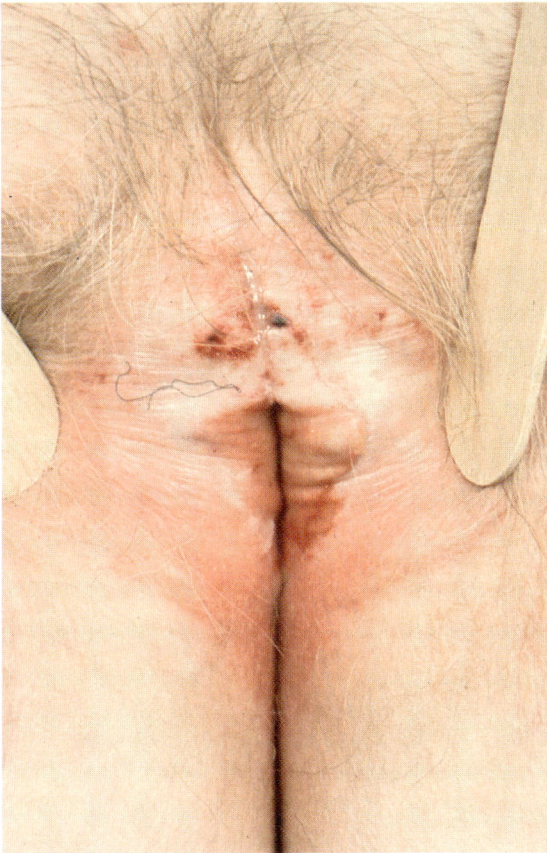

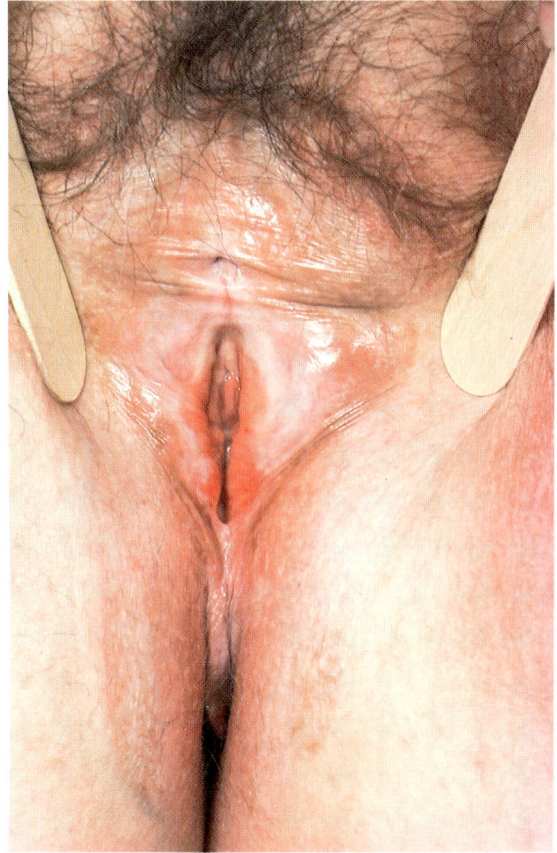

A

B

Fig. 6.56 Lichen sclerosus et atrophicus: extensive atrophy and loss of substance with erythema and telangiectasia. (Reproduced from Beilby & Ridley (1987) by courtesy of the authors and publisher)

from etretinate in five patients, as did Romppannen et al (1984) in 19 patients, though Neuhofer & Fritsch (1984) were not impressed with its effect in their eight patients. All these trials were uncontrolled. Penneys (1984) noted symptomatic improvement with potassium paraminobenzoate in an uncontrolled trial in five patients with LSA. The use of hydrochloric acid is without foundation, and for chloroquine, which has its advocates, there appears to be no firm evidence of benefit, although its potentiality for ocular side effects is well recognised.

August & Millard (1980) used a cryoprobe to remove localised troublesome areas. Simple excision, or the use of the carbon dioxide laser to remove a small area, is a similar approach. Surgery can be helpful in separating fused surfaces, for example in

uncovering a sealed-off clitoris, though the patient must then assiduously keep the surfaces separated to prevent re-attachment. Ratz (1984), using the laser, treated a patient with penile LSA, and Lobraico (1984) found the method helpful in 19 out of 28 women. Kaufman & Friedrich (1985) reported on ten patients with large areas so treated; five were followed up and three of them had a recurrence within 18 months and one patient later. The recurrent lesions may, it is thought, be 'newer' and more susceptible to local measures. It does not seem as if the laser has anything to offer, bearing in mind that the treatment requires a general anaesthetic and leaves considerable discomfort in its wake. Grafting is open to similar objections. The same may be said of alcohol injections. Local subcutaneous corticosteroids (triamcinolone) injections, however,

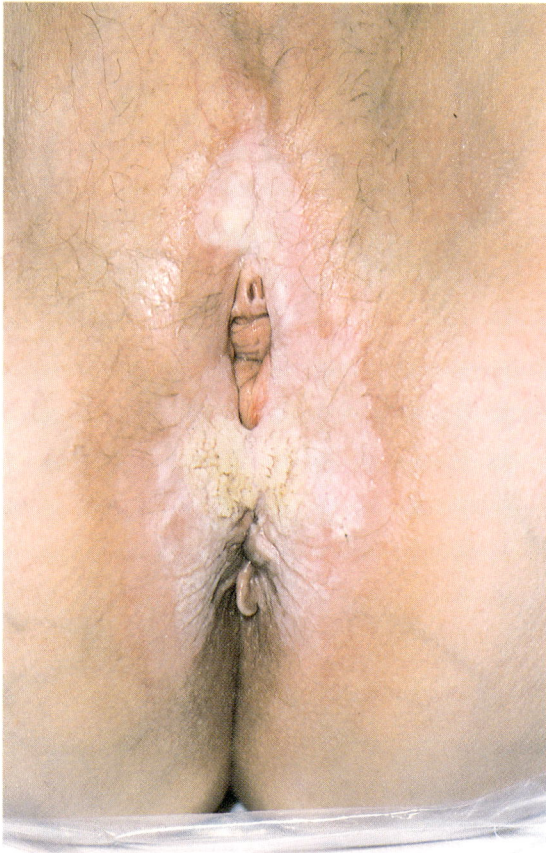

Fig. 6.57 Lichen sclerosus et atrophicus (vulvectomy); with thick white plaque formation.

are less traumatic, not requiring a general anaesthetic, and can be helpful.

In difficult cases where the introitus is particularly involved the perineoplasty technique of Paniel (Paniel et al 1984, Paniel 1986) may be applicable. Apparently the vaginal mucosa, when brought down on to the vestibule, does not become transformed into LSA.

Above all vulvectomy, with its mutilating results and morbidity, must be avoided unless there is unequivocal evidence of malignancy. Recurrence at the edges is prompt. Rettenmaier et al (1985) described the use of a skinning vulvectomy, with split skin grafting, and this is certainly a less mutilating approach; but two patients out of four showed recurrence after 4 and 8 years. Given current topical measures, circumstances justifying such intervention must surely be very rare.

LSA and malignancy

Lichen sclerosus et atrophicus at extragenital sites appears to have no potential for malignancy. Whether or not this is true in the genital or anogenital area is uncertain. Basal cell carcinoma in vulval LSA has been reported in two cases and the association may be fortuitous (McAdams & Kistner 1958, Meyrick Thomas et al 1985); the same may apply to the malignant melanoma reported by Friedman et al (1984). The frequency and significance of the association of vulval LSA with squamous cell carcinoma are hard to assess, not least because probably many women with LSA never see a dermatologist and because many vulvectomy specimens from patients with carcinoma are never adequately examined for LSA.

The incidence of LSA in squamous cell carcinoma of the vulva

McAdams & Kistner (1958) found LSA, carefully defined, in 16 of 400 cases of squamous cell carcinoma, and 'leukoplakia', presumably LSA, in 31; some examples noted as 'chronic dermatitis with sclerosis' may well have been LSA. Buscema et al (1980) studied 98 cases of squamous cell carcinoma and found 'dystrophies' in half of them. Mabuchi et al (1985) tried to establish precursors of cancer (presumably squamous cell carcinoma, but this is not stated) of the vulva, using a control series for comparison. 'Leukoplakia' and 'inflammation' of the vulva appeared to be significant; however, as this information was attained by a retrospective interview its value is clearly limited. Zaino et al (1982) examined squamous cell carcinoma in 60 women having a vulvectomy, and classified surrounding skin in terms of the International Society for the Study of Vulvar Disease nomenclature (p. 190). In only two patients was the surrounding skin normal. Thus 32 had 'atypical hyperplastic dystrophy', 15 lichen sclerosus, 14 hyperplastic dystrophy, 4 mixed dystrophy and 19 carcinoma in situ (some showed more than one abnormality). Using very subtle criteria (Hewitt 1986) for the histology of LSA, Hewitt (1984) cited his own earlier findings (Hewitt & Pelisse 1976) of LSA in 96% of

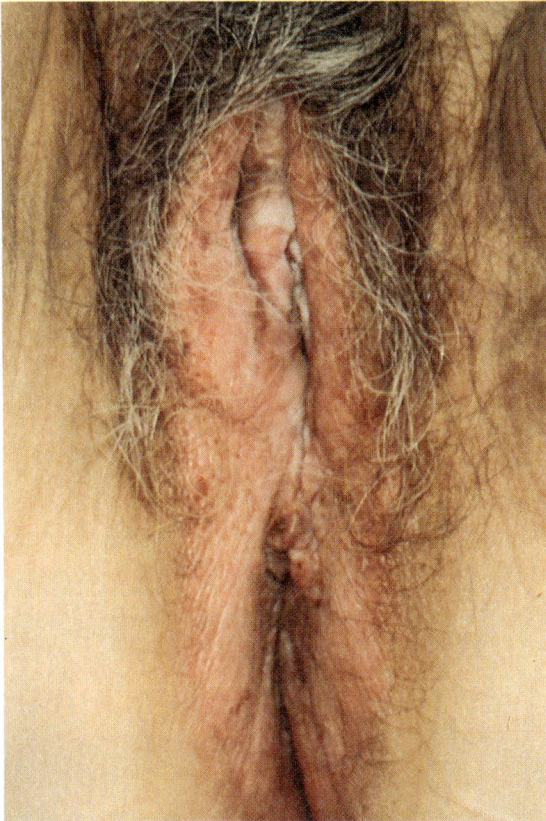

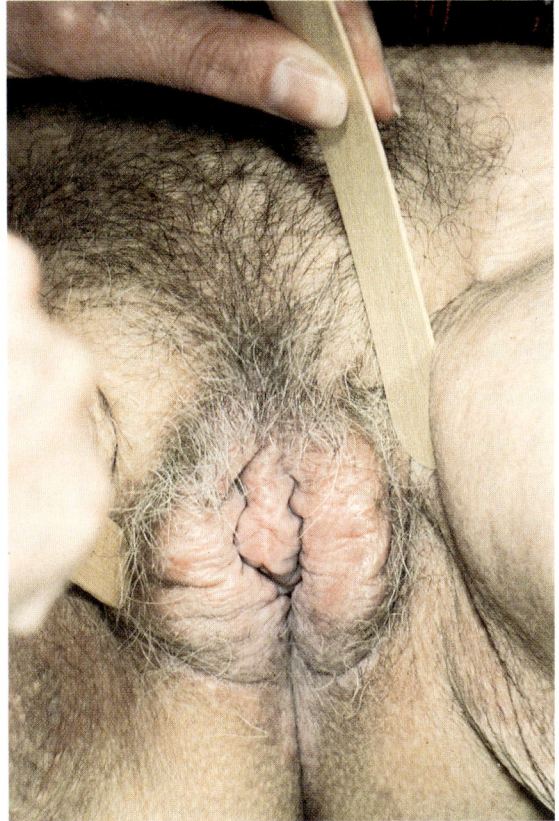

A

B

Fig. 6.58 (**a & b**) Lichen sclerosus et atrophicus: with lichenification especially of the clitoris.

104 cases of squamous cell carcinoma and those of Dottenwille (1982) of LSA in all of 40 cases of squamous cell carcinoma.

The incidence of squamous cell carcinoma in LSA of the vulva

Role of vulval intra-epithelial hyperplasia. Although Buckley et al (1984) considered that vulval intra-epithelial neoplasia (VIN) seems not to arise actually within the epidermis that is affected by LSA, these authors noted that VIN and LSA may co-exist and this may add to the score of malignancies found with LSA. An example (Fig. 6.61) is that of a woman 82 years of age who, while on immunosuppressive therapy for pemphigoid, developed a vast mass of genital warts, some areas of

which had progressed from VIN 3 to invasive carcinoma, and at the same time was found to have extensive vulval LSA which had been entirely symptomless. Another example (Fig. 6.62) is a woman with known LSA who developed recurrent large warty masses, showing VIN 3 with an area of invasive cancer in which HPV16 was found. These patients (Ridley 1986) appear akin to those males reported by Frances et al (1984) who had warty tumours arising on penile LSA (although in these cases the lesions were not thought to be malignant); and indeed to cases of verrucous carcinoma and squamous cell carcinoma arising on so-called pseudo-epitheliomatous micaceous balanitis (Lortat-Jacob & Civatte 1961, 1966), which may be a variant of LSA. Warts and LSA are indeed sometimes found together, and thus any squamous cell

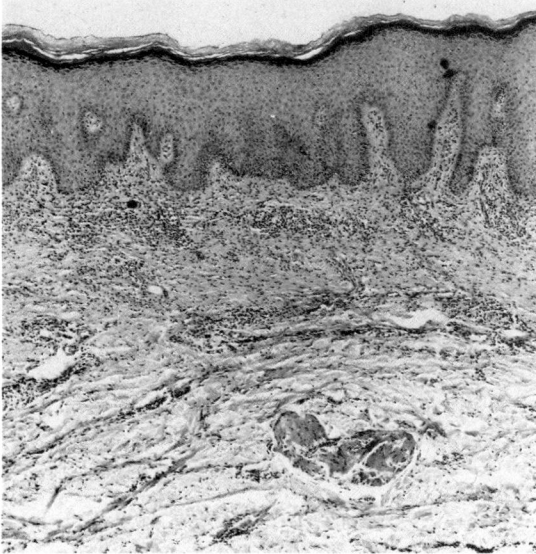

Fig. 6.59 Lichen sclerosus et atrophicus: features of lichenification superimposed on lichen sclerosus et atrophicus. (H & E × 13) (By courtesy of Dr D McGibbon)

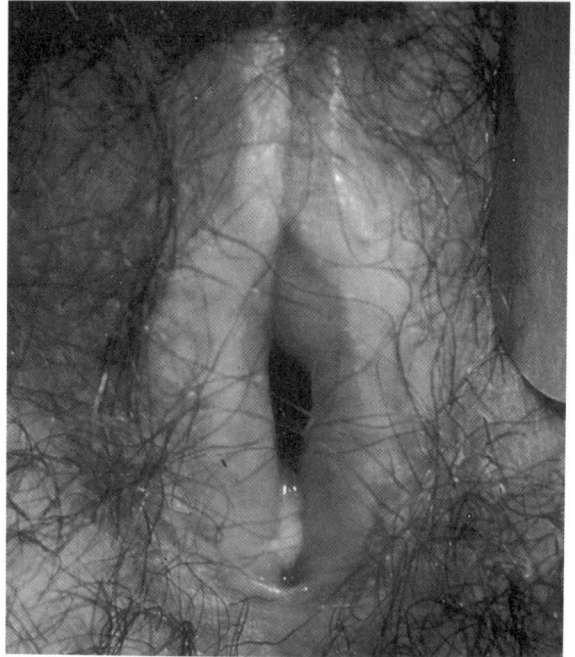

A

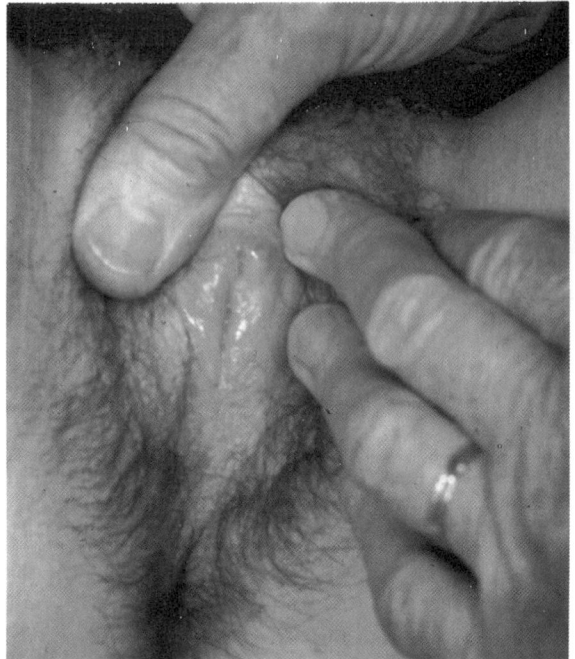

B

Fig. 6.60 Lichen sclerosus et atrophicus: lesions in a young girl: (a) at presentation; (b) with formation of clitoral 'pseudocyst'.

carcinoma which develops may be aetiologically related to the HPV and VIN rather than to the LSA per se. It may be relevant that Crum et al (1984), discussing VIN in general, noted that in younger patients there was strong evidence of HPV infection and low risk of progression to cancer, while older ones had less evidence of HPV infection and a greater risk of invasive cancer. However, these considerations can be no more than speculative when the role of the HPV in oncogenesis is still under investigation and while the incidence of subclinical HPV infection in LSA is unknown; HPV may act for example as a cofactor in inducing carcinoma and not necessarily by way of VIN.

Squamous cell carcinoma arising in the apparent absence of vulval intra-epithelial neoplasia. Wallace (1971) noted 12 women with squamous cell carcinoma of the vulva out of 290 with LSA; and Hart et al (1975) 5 out of 107, though these latter authors noted that in their patients the squamous cell carcinoma seemed to arise in areas uninvolved by LSA. In our current series of histologically proved LSA in 350 women (Meyrick Thomas et al 1987b), squamous cell carcinoma has been seen in 15 (not including the two associated with known HPV infection noted above). Common

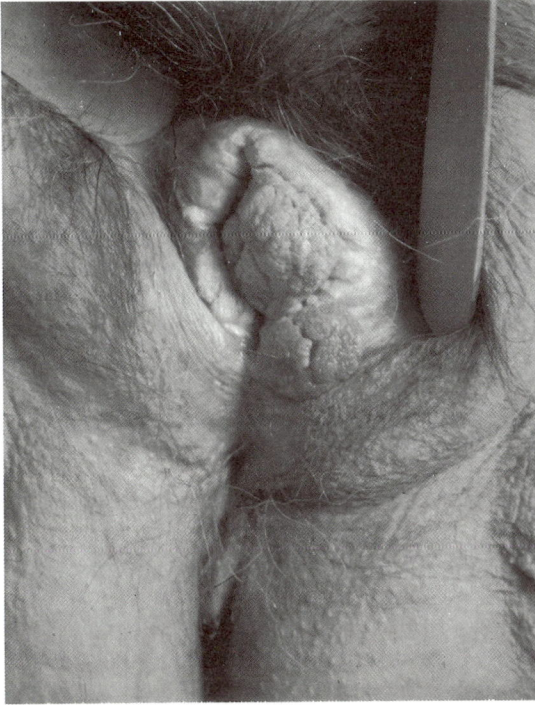

Fig. 6.61 Lichen sclerosus et atrophicus: genital warts and squamous carcinoma overlying lichen sclerosus et atrophicus. (By courtesy of C M Ridley 1975 The Vulva. Major Problems in Dermatology 5. Lloyd Luke)

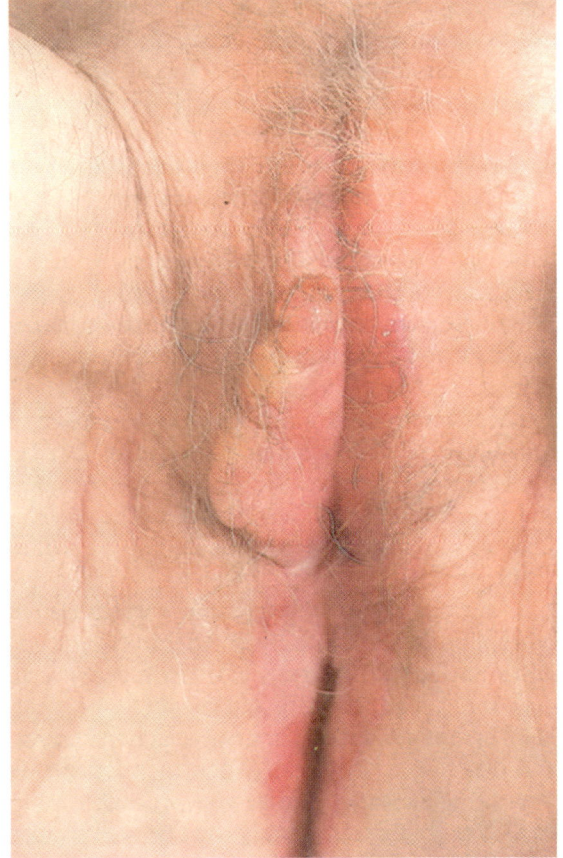

Fig. 6.62 Lichen sclerosus et atrophicus: warty lesions (HPV16) on underlying lichen sclerous et atrophicus.

sense suggests that this is a greater incidence than would be found in unaffected women. Moreover, in 20 cases of LSA Newton et al (1987) found that on flow cytometry 20% showed aneuploidy, a feature often denoting malignant potential.

The vulval lesions appear to arise mainly from thinly keratinised mucosal aspects. Recently, however, squamous cell carcinoma has been reported in peri-anal (i.e. keratinised) skin (Sloan & Goepel 1981, Ellis & Crow 1982).

The general assumption has been that while atrophy itself may be premalignant, superimposed irritation plays a part too and that the current, more effective, treatment has therefore cut down any risks there may have been. Two examples will show that this may be too facile an explanation. The first, personal, example is of two elderly women who had squamous cell carcinoma (without evidence of wart infection) and florid LSA. The LSA had been entirely symptomless. The second is

a case report from Cario et al (1984). They reported a West Indian girl 18 years of age with a squamous cell carcinoma (rare at that age) with surrounding changes of histologically proved LSA, said to have been present from birth (an unusual history and LSA are rare in the negro). The lesions were quite symptomless so chronic irritation would appear to have played no part.

Conclusion

The lack of resolution of the relationship between LSA and malignancy is a prime example of how much work is rendered without value because of difficulties in terminology, and also of the inherent problem of there not being a certain marker for the histological diagnosis of LSA. However, a careful study of squamous cell carcinoma now might yet yield unequivocal results, to confirm or refute Hewitt's assertion that all or almost all vulval squamous cell carcinomas have LSA as their background. It is particularly important that the whole of the vulva should be studied, since tissue immediately surrounding a carcinoma may be misleading. Much of the older work may be invalidated for this reason. The presence or absence of HPV infection should also be carefully noted. Where fresh tissue for DNA hybridisation is not available, new techniques will allow hybridisation to be carried out on fixed tissue (p. 73).

These interrelated questions—the incidence of squamous cell carcinoma in LSA and of LSA in squamous cell carcinoma—are of great importance, and highly relevant to them is that of the place of LSA in discussion of what is meant by vulval 'dystrophy'.

As regards clinical management, a watch should be kept on patients with LSA. After initial settling down on therapy, intervals of a few months seem reasonable. The patient should be told to come earlier if symptoms worsen, or if any area breaks down and does not readily heal. When such lesions are found, the patient should be seen at shorter intervals. Usually they are simply the result of friction with mild infection and they soon resolve. If not, the area should certainly be biopsied.

'DYSTROPHY'

Comments on historical terminology and current usage

In much of the literature on the vulva, particularly gynaecological and histopathological, one will meet the term vulval dystrophy. Dysplasia is sometimes used as a synonym for dystrophy but is better confined, if used at all, to conditions which are malignant for premalignant (as in the original terminology of the International Society for the Study of Vulvar Disease, where dysplasia corresponded to vulval intraepithelial neoplasia).

The term dystrophy is a vague one, implying 'defective nutrition'. It was introduced by Jeffcoate & Woodcock (1961) and its use consolidated over the years by Jeffcoate (1962) in his well-known

textbook of gynaecology. He considered chronic epithelial dystrophy to be a neutral descriptive term for any intractable vulval lesion not otherwise classified.

To realise why Jeffcoate felt impelled to choose this term one must look at the historical background, and as the subject is of prime importance from both practical and theoretical viewpoints some time spent on its unfolding is warranted. Such a survey will show what the term replaced and indicate that the time may have come for a further change.

Historical survey

A welter of terms has been applied from the end of the 19th century to describe those vulval lesions which were characterised by atrophy and shrinkage, which appeared to be associated with the development of carcinoma and which could not be clearly related to recognised skin conditions as seen elsewhere such as psoriasis or eczema. It is a reasonable contention that these were all in fact examples of LSA, defined by Hallopeau in 1889; and the arguments for this will be advanced later.

Thus one has the descriptions (cited by Ricci 1945) given by Weir in 1875 of 'ichthyosis' of the tongue and vulva, by Schwimmer (1877) of 'leukoplakia' (a term used to imply a potentially malignant change in mucosal or mucocutaneous tissue); and that by Breisky (1885) of vulval 'kraurosis' (which means brittle). Shelley & Crissey (1953) supplied a translation of this latter account:

the labia minora are apparently missing, in that they are plastered to the mucous surface of the labia majora, so that the edges alone remain indicated by shallow furrows. From the mons veneris to the urethral orifice the integument is drawn tight over the clitoris . . . . The general effect of this extensive shrivelling is a striking smallness and inflexibility of the vestibular portion of the vulva . . . which may indeed . . . offer abnormal resistance . . . in coitus . . . The skin . . . appears whitish and dry . . . while the adjacent skin parts involved are shiny and dry, pale reddish grey, covered also with faded whitish spots, and show ectatic vascular branching here and there.

Jayle (1906) considered that these changes could occur without leukoplakia. Berkeley & Bonney (1909) and Bonney (1938) thought the lesions should be subdivided into 'kraurosis' which was characterised by an inflammatory and benign condition of the vestibule and introitus, and (entirely separate and distinct) 'leukoplakic vulvitis' which was characterised by white areas and had a malignant potential.

The account by Berkeley & Bonney of leukoplakic vulvitis described vulval and peri-anal lesions and some on the thighs, appearing red, later very white (hence the name), cracked, smooth and atrophic; histologically there was at first a thickened epidermis, with a dermal infiltrate, a subepidermal homogenous zone and a loss of elastic tissue, culminating in a thin epidermis and dermal sclerosis with no inflammatory cells. The term 'leukoplakia' here was used in referring to changes in keratinised skin.

Kraurosis on the other hand they described as confined to the introitus, vestibule, urethral orifice, perhaps the clitoris. The tissue was red, shiny, later 'pale yellow and glistening'. There was vaginal stenosis, the labia minora and clitoris disappear. Histologically there was striking atrophy, much inflammation, and no oedematous homogeneous subepidermal zone.

The incidence of malignancy in kraurosis or leukoplakic vulvitis (in all, 19 cases in 10 years) was not stated, but, in every case of carcinoma of the vulva (58 in 10 years) these authors dealt with, leukoplakic vulvitis was present. It was correlated with 'maximum hypertrophy of the interpapillar epidermal process'.

As regards treatment of leukoplakic vulvitis they found X-rays helpful—could this have been a factor in their incidence of malignancy? They advised excision if this failed—wide excision because of recurrence. In kraurosis they also advocated surgical removal of affected tissue. Darier (1928) retained the original definition of kraurosis, with its lack of thigh and peri-anal lesions. In the USA, Taussig (1929) also contributed to this debate, describing a leukoplakic vulvitis, which began as a hypertrophic and ended as an atrophic condition with inflammatory infiltrate and a subepidermal 'collagenous' zone. He used the term kraurosis for the end stage of this leukoplakic vulvitis, whereas Berkeley & Bonney had totally separated the two.

Later correlations

Wallace and Whimster (1951), Wallace (1955) and Whimster (1959), in a series of accounts summarised by Wallace (1971), tried to overcome the confusion surrounding kraurosis, leukoplakic vulvitis and leukoplakia and their relation to LSA. They proposed that cases indisputably showing typical LSA, clinically and histologically, should be noted as such, that the terms kraurosis and leukoplakic vulvitis should be dropped, and that where the appearance originally described by Breisky as kraurosis was seen without clear evidence of LSA it should be termed 'primary atrophy'. Primary atrophy thus comprised cases with no extragenital LSA, no peri-anal LSA, and no vulval LSA papules; there was some potential for malignant change, and whereas Berkeley and Bonney had found no hyalinisation histologically, but much inflammation, the picture of primary atrophy was described by Wallace and Whimster as an atrophic epidermis, reduced elastic tissue, hyalinised collagen and some inflammatory cells—changes which would all be compatible with a late LSA. They wished to retain the term leukoplakia as a histological entity, characterised by marked dermal hyalinisation, sometimes a dermal infiltrate, and a hyperkeratotic epidermis with lengthened, irregular forked rete pegs with or without cellular atypia. It was distinguishable from lichenification by its lack of acanthosis, spongiosis and parakeratosis as well as by the irregularity of the epidermal downgrowths and the marked hyalinisation (Fig. 6.63) (some histopathologists believe that in simple lichenification one may see somewhat similar changes, though with hyalinisation that is mild and confined to the papillary dermis (McGibbon 1985—personal communication). They noted it in tissue adjacent to 20 squamous cell carcinomas, and regarded it as premalignant. In retrospect it seems as if they were describing something very similar to the 'maximum hypertrophy of the intrapapillar epidermal processes' of Berkeley & Bonney. They found this change as a sequel to rather than as a precursor of atrophy, thus differing from Taussig.

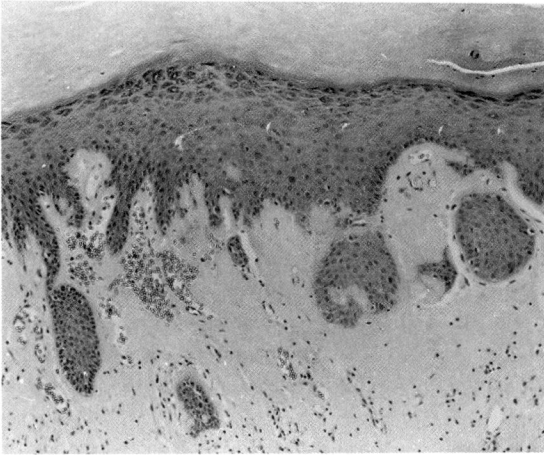

Fig. 6.63 'Leukoplakia' as described by Wallace & Whimster: hyperkeratosis with lengthened irregular and forked rete pegs, with or without atypia, marked dermal hyalinisation. (H & E × 15) (By courtesy of Dr D McGibbon)

Table 6.1 International Society for the Study of Vulvar Disease

Vulval dystrophies
The term 'dystrophy' characterises the many disorders of epithelial growth and nutrition which result in otherwise unclassified alterations of the surface architecture. Included within the general classification of the vulval dystrophies are those vulval changes variously described in the past as leukoplakia, kraurosis, atrophic dystrophy, hyperplastic vulvitis, leukoplakic vulvitis, neurodermatitis. The gross changes seen on the vulva may be diffuse or localised and may be seen as thickened or thinned. White or red colour changes may be evident. These lesions should be specifically classified according to their microscopic features as follows:

I.	Hyperplastic dystrophy	
	A. Without atypia	
	B. With atypia	
II.	Lichen sclerosus	
III.	Mixed dystrophy	(lichen sclerosus with foci of epithelial hyperplasia)
	A. Without atypia	
	B. With atypia	

Detailed histological definitions and descriptions were given of each condition noted above; atypia was classified as mild, moderate or severe, with or without dystrophy. (The histological minutiae have been discussed by Beilby & Ridley (1987).)

Although usually to be found arising on LSA or on primary atrophy, they believed that occasionally it developed on a vulva which was apparently normal or which showed simple lichenification.

It was at this stage that Jeffcoate & Woodcock (1961) tried to simplify that situation; beginning with an analysis of all putative causes of vulval malignancy (and noting with perspicacity the possibility of a 'field change') they went on to consider leukoplakia and leukoplakic vulvitis. They commented that, ironically, the clinician expected the pathologist to give him the diagnosis of leukoplakia, whereas the pathologist felt this was a clinical diagnosis and would have no part in it. The authors analysed too the confusion noted above between the writings of Berkeley & Bonney and those of Taussig, and then turned to LSA. Here they saw that between LSA and (clinical) leukoplakia and kraurosis there was no essential difference. Their conclusion was that the same end point might come from different aetiological factors and that 'the vulval and perianal regions are subject to chronic skin changes, the particular characteristics of which are probably conditioned by environment rather than causes', and '. . . irrespective of their appearances, all these intractable skin changes, for which a specific cause is not clear, are best given clinically an all-embracing and non-committal title such as "chronic epithelial dystrophy"'.

As a development of this concept Gardner & Kaufman (1969) suggested a histopathological classification with headings of hyperplastic dystrophy, atrophic dystrophy (LSA), and mixed dystrophies (LSA with adjacent areas of epithelial hyperplasia). In 1975 Gardner and Kaufman were closely associated with the proposal of the International Society for the Study of Vulvar Disease (ISSVD) (Friedrich 1976) to expand this scheme somewhat, and the resulting classification has been widely used since then (Table 6.1).

The classification is strictly histopathological, the concept and definition of atypia being developed in some detail, while the only concession to clinical background is to note that lesions may be diffuse or localised, thickened or thinned, red or white.

The current position

At this stage it is worth trying to extract the essentials which are still applicable from these older descriptions and classifications.

The kraurosis and leukoplakic vulvitis of Berkeley & Bonney were, judging from their accounts, essentially unitary and fully compatible with their being different patterns of LSA. The same applies to Taussig's kraurosis and leukoplakic vulvitis, which he indeed regarded as stages in one disease process, although it would be generally agreed that atrophy is the precursor rather than the end result.

Wallace & Whimster hoped by the term primary atrophy to avoid controversy when there was no indubitable evidence of LSA. However, on their histological and clinical findings, the fact that many developed unequivocal LSA (98 out of 120 of their cases were so categorised in the end) and everyday clinical experience of patients who may on one visit have obvious LSA papules and on another none, there seems little doubt that (with the possible exception of a few cases of lichen planus and perhaps plasma cell vulvitis of Zoon) all these patients could safely be reclassified as LSA and the term primary atrophy dropped.

What of the concept of leukoplakia by the same authors? Unfortunately the discrepancy between the clinical picture, implicit in its title, and its definition as a histological entity has given rise to some confusion. The findings however are vital; for such a histological appearance certainly corresponds to an active, painful fissured lesion of LSA (red or white); it is reversible with modern treatment but might perhaps have progressed to carcinoma in earlier days. The lesion should be recognised as almost if not quite invariably a severe phase of LSA. The occasional puzzling specimen of lichenification with minimal hyalinisation noted above is unlikely to offer much difficulty in practice; we should regard it, in these circumstances, as an essentially benign process. In the past, however, with little effective local treatment, it is conceivable that similar findings were indeed associated with malignancy, and this would correlate with the suspicion of Wallace & Whimster that these changes were sometimes seen on the lichenified vulva or even on an otherwise apparently normal one. As an alternative, one may surmise that all such examples are in fact found on an underlying LSA, perhaps masked by lichenification and patchy in character—both findings frequently encountered in practice.

The term leukoplakia remains in use for oral lesions, at the recommendation of the World Health Organisation (Kramer 1980), defined as a white patch or plaque that cannot be characterised clinically or pathologically as any other disease. This restores its original mucosal or mucocutaneous origin and its original domain. The definition is thus one of exclusion with no positive histopathological criteria. As regards the vulva, however, it should now no longer be employed.

As regards Jeffcoate's chronic epithelial dystrophy, and its incorporation in the ISSVD classification, this framework is somewhat oversimplified and artificial and would benefit from clinical enrichment. The original devisors of the schemes appreciated that well-defined entities, such as psoriasis or eczema, should be recognised separately, but to many others dystrophy appeared as an all-embracing term which tended to relieve one of any responsibility for further clinical delineation.

As a consequence the pathologist in effect takes on major responsibility in management which may not necessarily be on appropriate lines. Perhaps the most disturbing circumstance is that mention of atypia could spur a gynaecologist to vulvectomy, whereas if the naked-eye morphological findings were interpreted correctly the condition would be recognised as being amenable to treatment, for example an inflamed LSA. Equally, the lumping together of many diseases leads to some blurring of the issue as to whether or not cancer is significantly associated with vulval atrophies, especially LSA, for in many series other conditions—such as lichen simplex—would have been included in the total of chronic epithelial dystrophy.

The list of terms which in 1976 were recommended by the ISSVD for abolition is as follows:

Leukoplakia

Leukokeratosis

Leukoplakic vulvitis

Lichen sclerosus et atrophicus (retaining lichen sclerosus)

Hyperplastic vulvitis

Neurodermatitis

Kraurosis vulvae

Bowen's disease

Erythroplasia of Queyrat

Carcinoma simplex

Table 6.2

ISSVD (Friedrich 1976)	DERMATOLOGICAL CORRELATIONS
Hyperplastic dystrophy	
without atypia	Lichen simplex; and lichenification of an underlying dermatosis
with atypia	Mainly vulval intra-epithelial neoplasia; the overall architecture would have to be taken into account.
Lichen sclerosus (LSA was contracted to lichen sclerosus in the belief that it is 'metabolically active')	Lichen sclerosus et atrophicus
Mixed dystrophy (Lichen sclerosus with foci of epithelial dystrophy)	
without atypia	LSA and lichenification
with atypia	'Leukoplakia' (see text) ie severe LSA; LSA and VIN.

Neurodermatitis is an outmoded term for lichenification (p. 168). Bowen's disease is better termed carcinoma in situ or vulval intra-epithelial neoplasia (but Bowen lives on in the clinical variant of vulval intra-epithelial neoplasia termed 'bowenoid papulosis' (p. 271). Erythroplasia of Queyrat has always been mainly applied to penile lesions. Primary atrophy was not on the list but could also be removed from current terminology. Lichen sclerosus et atrophicus rather than lichen sclerosus remains the term preferred by dermatologists.

The ISSVD scheme has, however, the virtue of clarity, in spite of its oversimplification and clinical poverty, and meanwhile a scheme of dermatological correlations can be drawn up within the present classification (Table 6.2).

The future

The International Society of Gynecological Pathologists (ISGYP) recently proposed a new classification for consideration:

1. Non-neoplastic epithelial disorders of skin and mucosa

A. Lichen sclerosus (lichen sclerosus et atrophicus)
B. Squamous hyperplasia, not otherwise specified (NOS)
C. Other dermatoses
2. Mixed non-neoplastic and neoplastic epithelial disorders
When lichen sclerosus or squamous hyperplasia is associated with vulval intra-epithelial neoplasia (VIN) (see p. 267) both diagnoses should be reported, eg lichen sclerosus with VIN I, II or III.

At the 9th Congress of the ISSVD in 1987 a scheme essentially similar but with some modification was drawn up and ratified by the Congress:

Non-neoplastic epithelial disorders of vulval skin and mucosa
1. Lichen sclerosus
2. Squamous cell hyperplasia (formerly hyperplastic dystrophy)
3. Other dermatoses
Mixed epithelial disorders may occur. In such cases it is recommended that both conditions be reported. For example: lichen sclerosus with associated squamous cell hyperplasia (formerly classified as mixed dystrophy) should be reported as lichen sclerosus and squamous cell hyperplasia. Squamous cell hyperplasia with associated vulval intra-epithelial neoplasia (formerly hyperplastic dystrophy with atypia) should be diagnosed as vulval intraepithelial neoplasia. Squamous cell hyperplasia is used for those instances in which the hyperplasia is not attributable to another cause. Specific lesions or dermatoses involving the vulva (eg psoriasis, lichen planus, lichen simplex chronicus, Candida infection, condyloma acuminatum) may include squamous cell hyperplasia, but should be diagnosed specifically and excluded from this category.

The scheme will go forward to the ISGYP, and it is likely that this Society too will adopt it. The footnotes will, it is hoped, establish continuity for those used to the old terminology as well as offering further elucidation of the main categories. A new era of clarity and interdisciplinary cooperation has been ushered in.

Conclusions

The wheel which Jeffcoate began to turn in his scheme of rationalisation has now come full circle, for instead of using chronic epithelial dystrophy as a term for otherwise uncategorised lesions we can fairly confidently attribute all to LSA, with or without lichenification, while separating off such entities as eczema, lichen simplex, etc.

If this contention is untenable then there may indeed be entities peculiar to the vulva. If we think it is tenable, then the vulva is shown as an area where we can fully account for all its cutaneous lesions, where what to the non-dermatologist may appear an expanse featureless except for fissuring, atrophy and thickening can be satisfactorily scanned and interpreted by the clinician and pathologist in co-operation. The first view is typified by the statement of Douglas (1983) that the vulva should be considered 'as an organ and not as part of the integument . . . thus the erstwhile relationship of skin disease in general, which both dermatologists and gynaecologists were wont to assume is now less obvious—indeed almost non-existent'; while the second is represented by the comment of Weisfogel (1969) 'although the area involved is genital, the tissue concerned is skin'.

If we are to ascribe to LSA all cases of the appearance so well described by Breisky a century ago, and to sweep away much of the intervening controversy, we must be cautious and discriminating. Vulval LSA may have a less specific histology than that of LSA elsewhere; the same applies to lichen planus on non-keratinised surfaces. Difficulties of access in obtaining specimens, the different character of vulval skin as regards physiology and pathophysiology (Britz & Maibach 1979a and b, Britz et al 1980), and paucity of information on normal histological appearances (Harper & McNichol 1977 and Jones 1983 notwithstanding) amply account for this fact. Nevertheless we must beware of labelling cases as LSA without adequate evidence. Many problems will arise; a case may be clinically acceptable as LSA but histologically lack specific changes and require multiple biopsies to

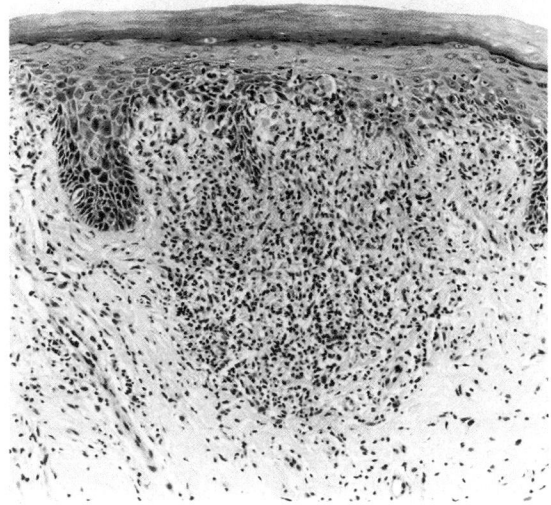

Fig. 6.64 Lichen sclerosus et atrophicus: the infiltrate at this stage has a somewhat lichenoid appearance. (H & E × 13) (By courtesy of Dr D McGibbon)

establish the diagnosis, or the histology may look lichenoid with a dense subepidermal band and many plasma cells (Fig. 6.64); there are patients with clinically and histologically borderline (in particular, women with doubtful pallor and atrophy whose main complaint is of recurrent splitting in the perineum) where perhaps only time will give a definite answer.

THE VULVA IN INFANCY AND CHILDHOOD

While, especially in later childhood, most of the lesions seen are best considered in the same way as their counterparts in adults, there are some general points to be considered and a few special lesions to note under this separate heading.

The anatomy of the vulva is somewhat different in children. The labia majora and pubic hair not having developed, the labia minora are relatively prominent, and the introitus is normally quite fiery in appearance. Congenital abnormalities are noted elsewhere (p. 25).

Examination can be difficult. Vaginal examination, if necessary, is best done by a gynaecologist, probably under general anaesthesia.

Urethral prolapse

This is noted on page 201.

Vulvovaginitis

Vulvovaginitis may result from poor hygiene, foreign bodies, infection with gonorrhoea or threadworms with or without anal symptoms. Reactions to bubble-baths are well recognised. Reactions to fabric softeners and washing powders are often mooted but most remain unproved. Vulvovaginitis may also occur in the prodromal state of acute fevers. Capraro et al (1974) reported it in patients with microperforate hymen, where the urine as in the normal child enters the vagina on micturition but then cannot escape. Contact allergic dermatitis is rare in childhood. Hypo-oestrogenism is sometimes held to account for a vulvovaginitis in children approaching puberty; this is probably true in the sense that it renders the mucosa susceptible to infection. Local oestrogen cream, used perhaps every night for a week or two, may help, though many gynaecologists are reluctant to use it in childhood.

Chronic bullous disease of childhood (linear IgA disease) is discussed elsewhere (p. 161).

Labial adhesions

These are fairly common in infancy (a 1.4% incidence according to Christensen & Øster 1971). The assumption has been that a lack of oestrogen is responsible for the adhesions, largely because of the age incidence.

Capraro & Greenberg (1972) found in 50 patients that children mainly presented before the age of 2 years. All were premenarchal, though seven showed evidence of sexual development and one-third were asymptomatic. Two patients had a renal abnormality and one a microperforate hymen. None was seen before the age of 2 months, but nevertheless the lesions can, when noticed, raise some anxiety as regards congenital vulval abnormality.

A pinhole meatus is present, usually just under the clitoris, but the labia minora are fused for all (in the majority of cases) or for most of their length. Urinary symptoms may follow. In some cases urinary infection has occurred, either primarily and perhaps causing fusion, or as a consequence of it.

Management

The labia can be separated surgically under anaesthesia, manually by the mother or by the use of bland or oestrogen-containing creams. Christensen & Øster (1971) favoured manual separation with a bland cream. Jenkinson & McKinnon (1984) followed 10 girls and found that all the adhesions separated spontaneously within 18 months. They strongly supported the awaiting of spontaneous resolution on the grounds of avoiding anaesthesia, with yet the possibility of occasional recurrence of the adhesions, and of the risk of local or systemic side effects from oestrogen cream.

Labial fusion may also rarely follow epidermolysis bullosa (p. 159) and LSA.

Napkin eruptions

Irritant rashes

Most of these rashes in infants (British Medical Journal 1981) are non-specific, and irritant, arising in relation to irritation from urine by wetting (and not by the effect of ammonia produced by urea-splitting organisms). Staphylococcal secondary infection is common and so is infection with *Candida*, whether primary or secondary. The mother may have a focus of *Candida* infection and the child may have a rectal reservoir. The role of detergents and fabric softeners is disputed.

Collipp et al (1985) have claimed that low zinc levels in hair, and sparse hair, are linked with napkin rashes in normal infants but confirmation is awaited.

There is a diffuse erythema with relative sparing of the folds.

Atopic eczema and seborrhoeic dermatitis

Atopic eczema and seborrhoeic dermatitis may also affect the napkin area and the two can be difficult to differentiate. Seborrhoeic dermatitis in infants is probably not identical to seborrhoeic dermatitis in adults.

Lesions in these cases will be more definite with redness and scaling and probably lesions elsewhere on the body, which may assist in the differential diagnosis. Yates et al (1983a and b) found initial clinical features unreliable in distinguishing between seborrhoeic dermatitis and atopic eczema in infancy; the blood IgE levels were of more value.

Napkin psoriasis

Here lesions in the napkin area and elsewhere look identical to those of adult psoriasis. *Candida* infection is common. The lesions remit spontaneously. Opinions vary as to whether or not psoriasis will develop later, but the likelihood is that napkin psoriasis does indicate a true psoriatic diathesis (Crow & Hargreaves 1968, Andersen & Thomsen 1971, Neville & Finn 1975).

Infantile gluteal granulomata

Cases of this unusual condition, commoner in the male, have been reported by Tappeiner & Pfleger (1971), Bonifazi et al (1981), Uyeda et al (1973), and Lovell & Atherton (1984). It appears to be a new eruption and, as well as *Candida* and occlusion, fluorinated corticosteroids are believed to be responsible.

There are oval, livid nodules with eroded surfaces, often appearing as a napkin rash is beginning to improve, and affecting the convexities of the napkin area. Eventually they regress and may leave scars.

Histology shows dermal oedema with a dense plasma cell and lymphocytic infiltrate together with vascular dilatation, fibrinoid necrosis and haemosiderin.

However, lesions essentially similar but where there was no use of topical corticosteroids have been reported in nine incontinent elderly women (Maekawa et al 1978), and here occlusion and irritation from excreta may have been the causative factors.

Management

Treatment in all these napkin rashes is mainly with mild topical corticosteroids and antiseptics and antibiotics, for example miconazole-hydrocortisone. No corticosteroid stronger than hydrocortisone should be used at this site in infancy, because of the risks of local atrophy and systemic absorption (and even of wasting—Johns & Bower 1970). If *Candida* infection is troublesome and a gut reser-

voir suspected or proved a course of oral nystatin is wise.

The area should be kept as dry and open as possible. Disposable napkins and one-way polypropylene napkin liners are helpful. When the condition improves bland preparations will suffice.

The differential diagnosis of lesions in the napkin area in infants must include such rarities as Letterer–Siwe disease (histiocytosis X), acrodermatitis enteropathica and congenital syphilis.

THE VULVA IN OLD AGE

Physiological atrophy of the vulva

Atrophy of the vulva as part of the normal ageing process is mild and symptomless.

Atrophic vaginitis

This is common in the postmenopausal woman. Except in as far as there may be a discharge which can cause vulval irritation it is irrelevant to vulval disease. In particular lichen sclerosus et atrophicus does not affect the vagina. Lichen planus may do so, but its desquamative telangiectatic appearance is unlikely to be confused with postmenopausal atrophy.

Similar changes in the oestrogen-responsive urethral epithelium may be responsible for some urinary symptoms.

Labial adhesions

Labial adhesions in the elderly are probably not analogous to the infantile condition, but raise the question of an underlying dermatological cause. Patients with this problem have been reported by Taylor (1941), Chuong & Hodgkinson (1984), Parkinson & Alderman (1984), and Savona Ventura (1985) and Kato et al (1986). All these patients were rendered incontinent because of accumulation of urine behind the fused tissue. In this older group, the pinhole meatus appears to be, in the main, posteriorly situated whereas in children it is anteriorly placed. In some of these cases oestrogen cream is said to have been effective but this might have been by virtue of its emollient qualities; others required surgical separation.

Cicatricial pemphigoid readily leads to adhesions

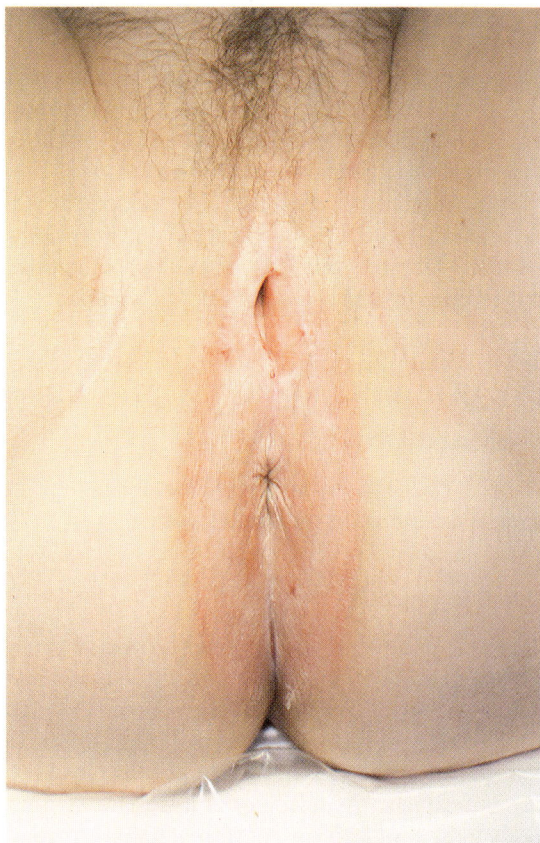

Fig. 6.65 Lichen sclerosus: only a small meatus is left.

(Damanski et al 1969 commented on by McCallum 1969), but it is rare and moreover lesions elsewhere tend to help towards a diagnosis.

Lichen planus would seem to be a possible candidate in view of the stenosis it may cause in the vagina, but vulval lesions are eroded and extensive without showing any tendency to fuse together.

Lichen sclerosus et atrophicus often leads to adhesions which seal off the clitoris, less often to labial adhesions as such; however, it can, by virtue of its destruction of the labia minora, lead (and not only in the elderly) to a fusion of tissue which obliterates the urethral and vaginal orifices (p. 181) (Fig. 6.65, 6.66 a and b); since the condition is relatively common it could well account for the majority of the cases.

A dermatologist should be asked to see any such case so that histological and, if necessary, immunofluorescence studies can be carried out.

Miscellaneous conditions

Angiomas and angiokeratomas are common in the elderly. Symptoms are, however, rare. Uncontrolled diabetes leads to a *Candida* vulvovaginitis, and incontinence and immobility to intertrigo with secondary infection. A condition analogous to infantile gluteal granuloma has been described in elderly incontinent women by Maekawa et al (1978).

MISCELLANEOUS LESIONS

Miscellaneous causes of vulvitis or vulvovaginitis

Some causes are noted in the section on infancy and childhood (p. 193) and old age (p. 195).

Vulvitis and vulvovaginitis, and often intertrigo, may be associated with incontinence, fistulae, retained tampons or other foreign bodies, neoplasia, vaginal adenosis (Blaikley et al 1971) or indeed any cause of vaginal discharge. Poor hygiene can be responsible. The causal role of tight occlusive clothing is problematical, but symptomatic improvement may follow its avoidance in vulvitis (or intertrigo) of any causation.

Davis (1971) reported six cases as salivary vulvitis following orogenital contact; the vulva was reddened; in two cases bacterial factors were probably relevant but this could not always be proved. He postulated saliva as a cause and suggested that one should suspect it if unusual pathogens, or no pathogens, were found in a case of vulvitis.

Drugs

Thomson (1986) has reported 2 cases of vulvitis in women taking the retinoid etretinate.

Hormonal factors

Hypo-oestrogenism may be concerned in vulvitis in children and possibly in labial adhesions in children. In adults, while it may certainly produce an atrophic vaginitis, the vulva is not likely to be involved except secondarily from the discharge. The redness and soreness of the vestibule tentatively attributed to involutional changes by Wallace (1971) may or may not be an entity.

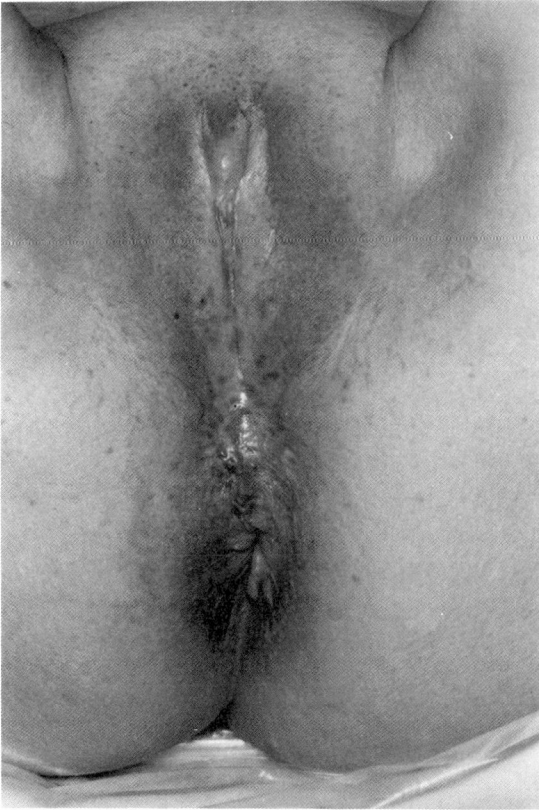

A

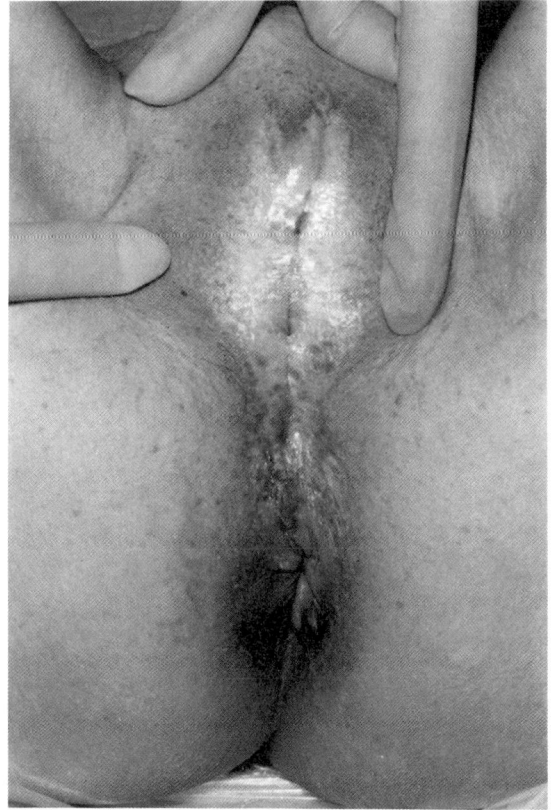

B

Fig. 6.66 (**a and b**) Lichen sclerosus in a woman aged 65, causing fusion of tissue to leave only a pinhole orifice.

Nutritional factors

Lack of riboflavine produces an eczematous genital rash and was described in male prisoners of war (Whitfield 1947). Lack of zinc is relevant in acrodermatitis enteropathica and related conditions.

Haemorrhagic lesions of the mucosae, including the vulva and vagina, may be found in scurvy. Parks & Martin (1948) thought vulvitis could be caused by blood dyscrasia and anaemia, and Hunt (1954) commented on a vulvitis in iron deficiency. Swift (1936) thought that hydrochloric acid and cod liver oil helped patients with pruritus to absorb Vitamin A while Gross (1941) used Vitamin B and liver in 'kraurosis', and Jeffcoate (1949) used hydrochloric acid and iron.

It is difficult to assess the findings in older papers in view of the very different general state of nutrition encountered at that time. There is no evidence that vulvitis in well-nourished subjects is related now to any such deficiency.

Lesions related to anogenital therapy

Contact dermatitis is noted elsewhere (p. 165). Preparations prescribed for vulval use are likely frequently to reach the vagina. Little harm appears to follow. However, substances can readily be absorbed through the vaginal mucosa, for example oestrogen cream (Rigg et al 1978). Donlan & Scutero (1975) reported a patient with an eosinophilic pneumonia and rash, which was probably related to the use of a vaginal cream which contained a sulphonamide, allantoin and aminacrine. Dutton et al (1983) thought that the liberal application of a corticosteroid cream to the vulva facilitated development of the tampon-associated toxic shock syndrome.

An aperient containing an anthraquinone (Dorbanex®) can result in discoloration of urine, vaginal secretions and skin (p. 150).

Long use of suppositories containing dextropropoxyphene have resulted in ulceration of the anus, rectum and vagina (Laplanche et al 1984), Fenzy & Bogomoletz (1986). Eigler et al (1986) described four patients in whom extensive chronic anorectal ulceration appeared to be caused by abuse of ergotamine–tartrate suppositories, clearing rapidly when the drug was withdrawn.

Cryotherapy of the cervix or vagina is followed by a discharge which may cause a vulvovaginitis.

Oedema

Urticaria or angio-oedema (including hereditary angio-oedema (Warin 1983)) may affect the vulva.

Cases of urticaria and pruritus, vulval or generalised, with nasal symptoms and sometimes anaphylaxis, have been reported in women after intercourse and attributed to an IgE-mediated allergy to seminal fluid (Chang 1976, Friedman et al 1984, Freeman 1986). Oral antihistamines or the use of a condom are advocated, and desensitisation may be successful (Friedman et al 1984, Frisch et al 1984).

Oedema is a common accompaniment of any vulval inflammation, for example eczema. Fluid will accumulate readily in the loose vulval tissue, and gross examples of this have been seen following peritoneal dialysis (Cooper et al 1983, Kopecky et al 1985), where the fluid was found to be an indication of a small inguinal hernia which was not necessarily clinically apparent, or of peritoneofascial defects.

Postpartum oedema following use of a 'birthing chair' was reported by Goodlin & Frederick (1983). Davenport & Richardson (1986) described 2 patients with a band uniting the labia minora following such oedema. The four cases with initially unilateral postpartum oedema reported by Ewing et al (1979), of whom three died despite antibiotics and steroids, were probably of infective (perhaps endotoxic) origin. Rainford (1970) noted gross vulval oedema in pre-eclampsia. Oedema may be a sign of Crohn's disease.

Lymphostatic disorders: lymphoedema

Lymphoedema may be primary, consequent upon congenital hypoplasia, or secondary.

Primary lymphoedema

Primary lymphoedema can sometimes be improved by surgery, and may be investigated by lymphangiography (Kinmonth 1982, Eichner et al 1983) either locally via vesicles or by way of the foot.

Large amounts of fluid may be discharged locally (Ma'Luf & Weed 1971). An immune deficit was associated, perhaps because of loss of lymphatic fluid into the gut, in the case of severe lymphoedema involving the genital area reported by Shelley & Wood (1981).

Secondary lymphoedema

Secondary lymphoedema may follow chronic infection, for example filariasis, obstruction by malignant deposits, surgery (especially if associated with lymphadenectomy) or radiotherapy given, for example, for cancer of the cervix or endometrium.

The lymphoedema may not always be clinically apparent but many cases are marked by chronic firm swelling which may in time show small vesicles or develop a verrucose surface (Fisher & Orkin 1970). True lymphangiomas are distinct.

Complications of lymphoedema

In both types of lymphoedema, the oedematous tissue is subject to recurrent streptococcal infection which, in turn, increases the obstruction. The attacks of cellulitis are associated with pain, tenderness, rigors and malaise. They are best treated with benzyl penicillin and penicillin V or with erythromycin if there is allergy to penicillin, and penicillin V can also be given with benefit on a long term basis as a prophylactic. Norburn & Coles (1960) reported a relevant case.

In primary or secondary lymphoedema a lymphangiosarcoma or angiosarcoma (p. 247) may occasionally develop (for example, the case reported by Huey et al 1985). Selective localisation of other malignancies to a lymphoedematous limb is discussed by Tatnall & Mann (1985). An immune deficit may be responsible.

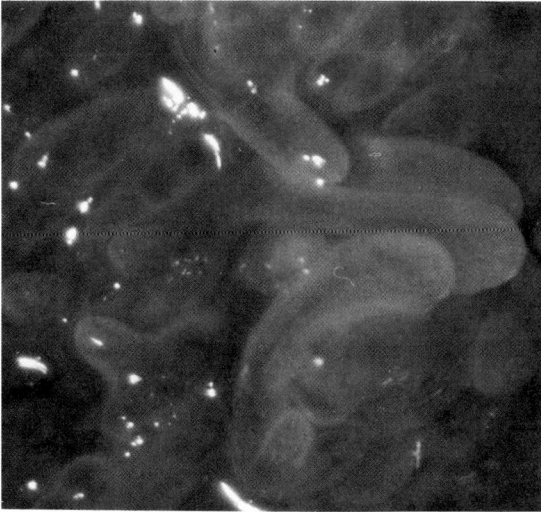

A

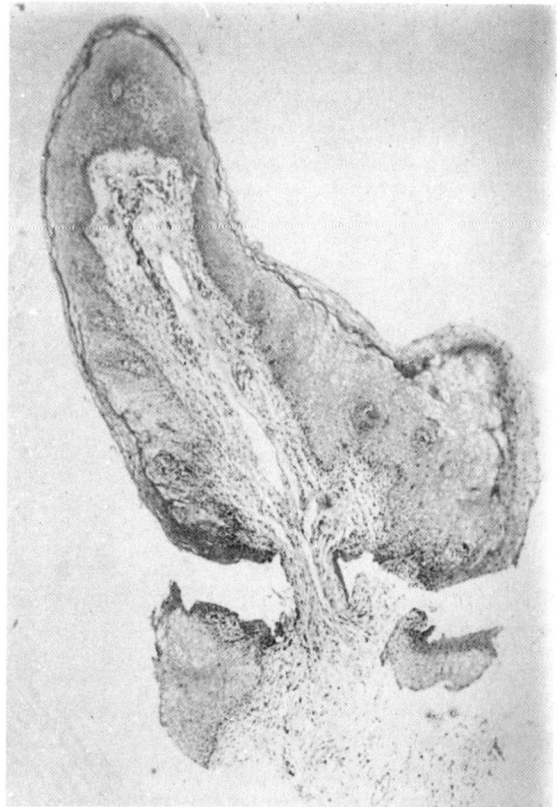

B

Fig. 6.67 (a) Vulval vestibular warts showing a papillary pattern. (By courtesy of Dr M Campion) (b) Vestibular papilla with evidence of HPV infection (koilocytosis) (H & E × 13)

Varicose veins of the vulva

Vulval varicosities, usually accompanied by similar lesions of the legs, are the consequence of chronic pelvic congestion, portal hypertension or obstructive pelvic lesions, and are common in pregnancy where, in addition, increased pelvic blood flow is relevant. A hormonal factor may be involved since pregnancy lesions often develop in the first trimester (Gallagher 1986).

After delivery, some lesions thrombose spontaneously. Where they do not do so, and where there are no leg varicosities, further investigation by venography and computerized tomography scan is indicated.

Where vulval varices are a problem, elevation of the foot of the bed during sleep and supporting pads are helpful. Active treatment includes ligation and sclerosing injections. The techniques are discussed by Gallagher (1986) in a review of vulval varicosities.

Hirsutes papillaris vulvae

Described by Altmeyer et al (1982) under this title, the papillomata were somewhat similar to pearly penile papules, a fairly common condition in the male (Neinstein & Goldenring 1984 found them in 23 out of 151 subjects studied). The pattern was of linear grouped frond-like or 'hairy' lesions on the inner aspects of the labia minora, and this area may be homologous with the tissue affected in the male. A few similar lesions are often seen at the vestibule and were described by Friedrich (1983b) as vestibular papillae.

The histology shows a core of connective tissue. They may be variants of normal but it is important to differentiate them from tiny genital warts. The difference is usually fairly marked with colposcopy and application of acetic acid, when warts are more keratinised and have branching stalks or appear sessile, with koilocytosis on histological examination. Nevertheless, recent descriptions of some types of subclinical wart infection (Growdon et al 1985, Campion et al 1986) raises the possibility that all these vulval lesions are in fact warty (Fig. 6.67)—or that human papilloma virus may be found in normal vestibular papillae and in hirsutes papillaris vulvae (see also p. 220).

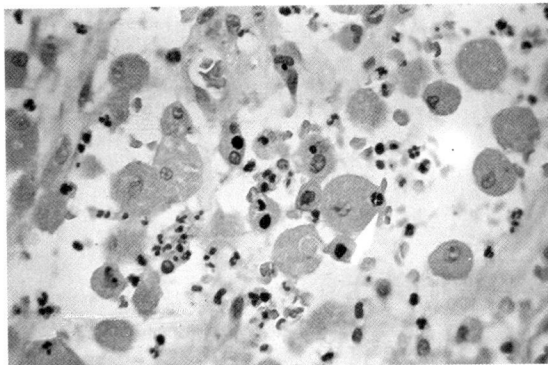

Fig. 6.68 Malakoplakia of the vulva: numerous large histiocytes are shown, some containing dense calcified Michaelis Guttman inclusions (arrow). (H & E × 300) (by courtesy of Dr R W Emmerson)

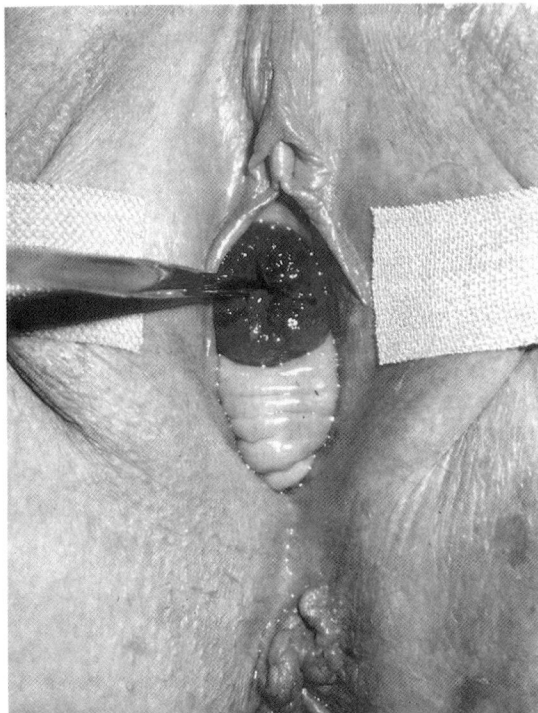

Fig. 6.69 Strangulated urethral prolapse

Malakoplakia

This unusual condition appears to be aetiologically related to bacteria but its presentation is not such as to suggest an infective origin.

The term means 'soft plaque'. The condition was described first by Michaelis & Guttman (1902) and given its name shortly afterwards.

Many of the patients are immunosuppressed and it is thought that inadequate clearance of a bacterial infection, often *E. coli* or an infection by an unusual strain, is responsible for the lesions. Arul & Emmerson (1977) described a vulval example and reviewed the literature which up to that time had featured cutaneous lesions only in two cases, one on the trunk and one (in a man) peri anal. Chalvardjian et al (1980) reported three examples involving the vagina, the cervix, and the ovary as part of a pelvic mass. Lin et al (1979) recorded a patient with vaginal lesions. Strate et al (1983) described a patient with vaginal polyps in which histology was granulomatous. Histiocyte-like cells with granular cytoplasm contained bacilliform bodies and cultures grew a mucoid form of *E. coli*. This lesion appeared to be similar to malakoplakia. Stanton & Maxted (1981) and Chen & Hendricks (1985) have reviewed the subject. The latter authors reported a woman with cervical and pelvic lesions and found no further vulval lesions in the literature. They quoted the successful treatment in a multifocal case

by using cholinergic agonists to raise the level of cyclic guanosine monophosphate in mononuclear cells.

The patient of Arul & Emmerson was an immunosuppressed woman 75 years of age with punched-out vulval lesions yielding *E. coli* on culture. The histology (Fig. 6.68) showed a granulomatous infiltrate of histiocytic cells rich in PAS positive granules. The cells contained Michaelis–Guttman bodies, thought to be encrustations of calcium phosphate round incompletely phagocytosed bacteria. There was a scanty connective tissue stroma containing lymphocytes and plasma cells.

The differential diagnosis of malakoplakia includes Crohn's disease and other granulomata unless typical Michaelis–Guttman bodies are seen.

URETHRAL LESIONS

Neoplasms are dealt with elsewhere (p. 314).

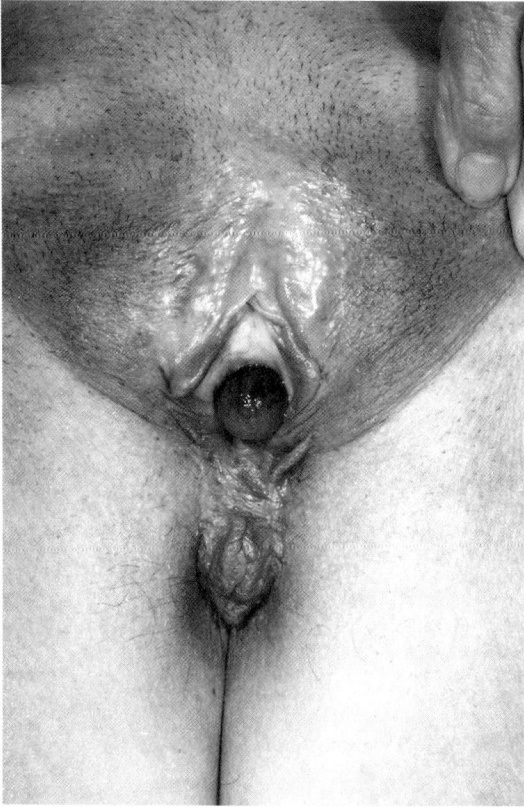

A

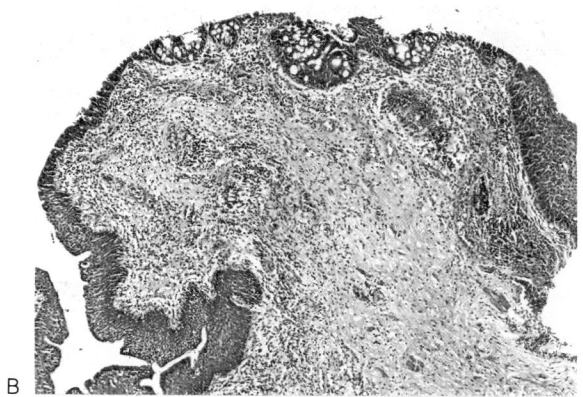

B

Fig. 6.70 (a) Urethral caruncle (b) urethral caruncle: the epithelium shows features of transitional and mucinous types, and the stroma is chronically inflammed (H & E × 20). (By courtesy of Dr C M Buckley)

Urethral prolapse

Unlike vaginal prolapse, which may make the anatomy of the vulva hard to interpret but which is unlikely to give rise to diagnostic difficulty, urethral prolapse can cause some confusion by resembling a neoplasm (Fig. 6.69). It may occur at any age, but is commonest in childhood and in the elderly.

The tissue is red and swollen. The histology shows vascular engorgement, thrombosis and dis-tension with a non-specific inflammatory infiltrate. Excision is usually carried out.

Urethral caruncle

A caruncle, usually found in middle-aged or elderly women, is a chronically inflamed and everted part of the mucosa (Fig. 6.70a). It appears as a bright-red nodule or polyp which may be painful and may bleed. The histology (Fig. 6.70b) is of a vascular inflammatory lesion but, in distinction to a pro-lapse, it also shows glandular structures or islands of epithelium in the stroma. The differential diagnosis is again from a neoplasm and this may not be easy clinically or indeed histologically since the islands of epithelium may be mistaken for in-vasive cells.

Treatment is by local destruction, for example with the cautery.

Urethral diverticula

Urethral diverticula occur in the upper portion of the posterior urethral wall. They have been attri-buted to congenital or infective changes; the latter is more likely, infection in one of the peri-urethral glands leading to a breakthrough into the urethral lumen (Beilby & Ridley 1987). The histology shows transitional columnar or squamous epithelium together with signs of non-specific inflammation.

REFERENCES

Aberer E, Neumann R, Stanek G 1985 Is localised scleroderma a Borrelia infection? Lancet ii: 278 (c)

Ackerman A B 1972 Focal acantholytic dyskeratosis. Archives of Dermatology 106: 702–706

Ackroyd J F 1985 Fixed drug eruptions. British Medical Journal 290: 1533–1534

Alexander A M 1974 Pseudofolliculitis diathesis. Archives of Dermatology 109: 729–730

Altmeyer P, Chilf G -N, Holzmann H 1982 Hirsuties papillaris vulvae (Pseudokondylome der vulva). Der Hautarzt 33: 281–283

Ambrosini A, Becagli L, Scrimin F, de Salvia D, Resta P, Gambato M 1984 Topical testosterone propionate in the therapy of vulvar dystrophies. European Journal of Gynecological Oncology 5: 58–63

Andersen S L C, Thomsen K 1971 Psoriasiform napkin dermatitis. British Journal of Dermatology 84: 316–319

Ansell I D, Hogbin B 1973 Crohn's disease of the vulva. Journal of Obstetrics and Gynaecology of the British Commonwealth 88: 376–378

Arul K J, Emmerson R W 1977 Malakoplakia of the skin. Clinical and Experimental Dermatology 2: 131–135

Atherton D J, Massam M, Wells R S, Harries J T, Pincott J R 1978 Genital Crohn's disease in a 6 year old boy. British Medical Journal i: 552

August P J, Milward T M 1980 Cryosurgery in the treatment of lichen sclerosus et atrophicus of the vulva. British Journal of Dermatology 103: 667–670

Baccaredda-Boy A, Crovato F 1970 Maladie de Crohn. Archives Belges de Dermatologie et Syphiligraphie 26: 125–128

Bandy L C, Addison A, Parker R T 1983 Surgical management of rectovaginal fistulas in Crohn's disease. American Journal of Obstetrics and Gynecology 147: 359–363

Barclay D L, Macey H B, Reed R J 1966 Lichen sclerosus et atrophicus of the vulva in children: A review and report of 5 cases. Obstetrics and Gynecology 27: 637–642

Barile M F, Graykowski E A, Driscoll E J, Riggs D B 1963 L form of bacteria isolated from recurrent aphthous stomatitis lesions. Oral Surgery, Oral Medicine and Oral Pathology 16: 1395–1402

Barker L P, Gross P 1962 Lichen sclerosus et atrophicus of the female genitalia. Archives of Dermatology 85: 362–371

Barnes C J, Douglas C P 1985 Preliminary findings on levels of collagenase and its tissue inhibitor in some vulval dystrophies. Journal of Obstetrics and Gynaecology 6: 55–56

Barth J H, Reshad H, Darley C R, Gibson J R 1984 A cutaneous complication of Dorbanex therapy. Clinical and Experimental Dermatology 9: 95–96

Bartholdson L, Hultborn A, Hulten L, Roos B, Rosencrantz M, Ahren C 1977 Lymph drainage from vulva and foot as demonstrated by 198Au. Acta Radiologica (Therapy) 16: 209–218

Beilby J O W, Ridley C M 1987 The pathology of the vulva. In: Fox H (ed) Haines and Taylor's Gynaecological and Obstetrical pathology Churchill Livingstone, Edinburgh

Berkeley C, Bonney V 1909 Leukoplakic vulvitis and its relation to kraurosis vulvae and carcinoma vulvae. Proceedings of the Royal Society of Medicine 3: (Part 2) 29–51

Betson J R, Chiffelle T Z, George R P 1962 Pilonidal sinuses involving the clitoris. American Journal of Obstetrics and Gynecology 84: 543–545

Bhatia N N, Bergman A, Broen E M 1984 Advanced hidradenitis suppurativa of the vulva. Journal of Reproductive Medicine 29: 436–440

Bitar A, Giroux J M 1970 Treatment of benign familial pemphigus (Hailey–Hailey) by skin grafting. British Journal of Dermatology 83: 402–404

Blaikley J B, Dewhurst C J, Ferreira A P, Lewis T L T 1971 Vaginal adenosis: clinical and pathological features with special reference to malignant change. Journal of Obstetrics and Gynaecology of the British Commonwealth 78: 1115–1122

Bloom S R, Polak J M 1983 Regulatory peptides and the skin. Clinical and Experimental Dermatology 8: 3–18

Bonifazi E, Garofalo L, Lospalluti M, Scarigno, A, Coviello C, Meneghini C L 1981 Granuloma gluteal infantum with atrophic scars. Clinical and histological observations in 11 cases. Clinical and Experimental Dermatology 6: 23–29

Bonney V 1938 Leukoplakic vulvitis and the conditions liable to be confused with it. Proceedings of the Royal Society of Medicine 31: 1057–1060

Borglin N E, Söderström J, Wehlin L 1966 Eosinophilic granuloma (histiocytosis X) of the vulva. Journal of Obstetrics and Gynaecology of the British Commonwealth 73: 478–486

Bowers P W, Powell R J 1983 Effect of thalidomide on orogenital ulceration. Lancet ii: 799–800

Boyce D C, Valpey J M 1971 Acute ulcerative vulvitis of obscure etiology. Obstetrics and Gynecology 38: 440–443

Breathnach S M 1985 The cutaneous amyloidoses. Archives of Dermatology 121: 470–475

Breisky D 1885 Über kraurosis Vulvae. Zeitschrift für Heilkunde 6: 69–80

British Medical Journal (leading article) 1981 Nappy rashes. British Medical Journal 282: 420–421

Britz M B, Maibach H I 1979a Human labia majora skin: transepidermal water loss in vivo. Acta Dermato-Venereologica 59: (Supplement 85) 23–25

Britz M B, Maibach H I 1979b Human cutaneous vulvar reactivity to irritants. Contact Dermatitis 5: 375–377

Britz M B, Maibach H I, Anjo D M 1980 Human percutaneous penetration of H C: the vulva. Archives of Dermatological Research 267: 313–316

Brodin M B 1980 Balanitis circumscripta plasmacellularis. Journal of the American Academy of Dermatology 2: 33–35

Brooke B N 1978 Dyspareunia: a significant symptom in Crohn's disease. British Medical Journal i: 1199 (correspondence)

Brown Z A, Stenchever M A 1977 Genital ulceration and infectious mononucleosis. Report of a case. American Journal of Obstetrics and Gynecology 127: 673–674

Brownstein M H, Mehregan A R, Bikowski B, Lupulescu A, Patterson J C 1979 The dermatopathology of Cowden's syndrome. British Journal of Dermatology 100: 667–673

Buchholz F, Schubert C, Lehmann-Willenbrock E 1985 White sponge nevus of the vulva. International Journal of Gynaecology and Obstetrics 23: 505–507

Buckley C H, Butler E B, Fox H 1984 Vulvar intraepithelial neoplasia and microinvasive carcinoma of the vulva. Journal of Clinical Pathology 37: 1201–1211

Bunney M H, Noble I M 1974 Red skin and Dorbanex British Medical Journal i: 731 (c)

Burgdorf W 1981 Cutaneous manifestations of Crohn's disease. Journal of the American Academy of Dermatology 5: 689–695

Burke D A, Adams R M, Arundell F D 1969 Febrile ulceronecrotic Mucha Habermann's disease. Archives of Dermatology 100: 200–206

Burnett J W, Goldner R, Calton G J 1975 Cowden's disease: Report of 2 additional cases. British Journal of Dermatology 93: 329–336

Burns R A, Reed W B, Swatek F E, Omieczynski D T 1967 Familial benign chronic pemphigus. Induction of lesions by Candida albicans. Archives of Dermatology 96: 254–258

Buscema J, Stern J, Woodruff J D 1980 The significance of the histologic alterations adjacent to invasive vulvar carcinoma. American Journal of Obstetrics and Gynecology 137: 902–909

Bushkell L L, Friedrich E G, Jordon R E 1981 An appraisal of routine direct immunofluorescence in vulvar disorders. Acta Dermato-Venereologica 61: 157–161

Calnan C D 1978 Oxypolyethoxydodecane in an ointment. Contact Dermatitis 4: 168–169

Cantwell A R 1984 Histologic observations of pleomorphic, variably acid-fast bacteria in scleroderma, morphoea, and lichen sclerosus et atrophicus. International Journal of Dermatology 23: 45–52

Capraro V J, Greenberg H 1972 Adhesions of the labia minora: a Study of 50 patients. Obstetrics and Gynecology 39: 65–69

Capraro V J, Dillon W P, Gallego M B 1974 Microperforate hymen. A distinct clinical entity. Obstetrics and Gynecology 44: 903–905

Cario G M, House M J, Paradinas F J 1984 Squamous cell carcinoma of the vulva in association with mixed vulvar dystrophy in an 18 year old girl. British Journal of Obstetrics and Gynaecology 91: 87–90

Carroll J M, Kuwabara T 1968 Ocular pemphigus. An electron microscopic study of the conjunctival and corneal epithelium. Archives of Ophthalmology 80: 683–695

Case Records of the Massachussetts General Hospital. Presentation of a Case. Castleman B, McNeely B U (eds). New England Journal of Medicine 282: 862–868

Caulfield J B, Wilgram G F 1963 An electron microscope study of dyskeratosis and acantholysis in Darier's disease. Journal of Investigative Dermatology 41: 57–65

Chalmers R J G, Burton P A, Bennett R F, Goring C C, Smith P J B 1984 Lichen sclerosus et atrophicus. A common and distinctive cause of phimosis in boys. Archives of Dermatology 120: 1025–1027

Chalvardjian A, Ricard L, Shaw R, Davey R, Cairns J D 1980 Malacoplakia of the female genital tract. American Journal of Obstetrics and Gynecology 138: 391–394

Chang T W 1976 Familial allergic seminal vulvovaginitis. American Journal of Obstetrics and Gynecology 126: 442–444

Chen K T K, Hendricks E J 1985 Malakoplakia of the female genital tract. Obstetrics and Gynecology 65: 84S–87S

Chernosky M E, Derbes V J, Burks J W 1957 Lichen sclerosus in children. Archives of Dermatology 75: 647–652

Chorzelski T P 1962 Experimentally induced acantholysis in Hailey's benign pemphigus. Dermatologica 124: 21–30

Chorzelski T P, Kudejko J, Jabloska S 1984 Is papular acantholytic dyskeratosis of the vulva a new entity? American Journal of Dermatopathology 6: 557–560

Chorzelski T P, Jablonska S 1986 Papular acantholytic dyskeratosis of vulva. American Journal of Dermatopathology 84: 363–365

Christensen E H, Øster J 1971 Adhesions of labia minora (synechia vulvae) in childhood. Acta Paediatrica Scandinavica 60: 709–714

Chuong C J, Hodgkinson C P 1984 Labial adhesions presenting as urinary incontinence in post-menopausal women. Obstetrics and Gynecology 64: 81S–84S

Clark J A, Muller S A 1967 Lichen sclerosus et atrophicus in children. A report of 24 cases. Archives of Dermatology 95: 476–482

Coles R B, Wilkinson D S 1965 Necrosis and dequalinium. I: balanitis. Transactions of the St John's Hospital Dermatological Society 51: 46–48

Collipp P J, Kuo B, Castro-Magana M, Chen S Y, Salvatore S 1985 Hair zinc, scalp hair quantity, and diaper rash in normal infants. Cutis 35: 66–70

Connelly M G, Winkelmann R K 1985 Coexistence of lichen sclerosus, morphea and lichen planus. Report of 4 cases and review of the literature. Journal of the American Academy of

Dermatology 12: 844–851

Cooke B E D 1979 Clinical and immunological features. In: Lehner T, Barnes C G (eds) Behcet's syndrome. Academic Press, London, p 143

Cooper J C, Nicholls A J, Simms J M, Platts M M, Brown C B, Johnson A G 1983 Genital oedema in patients treated by continuous ambulatory peritoneal dialysis. British Medical Journal 286: 1923–1924

Coppola G, Muscardin L M 1986 Papular acantholytic dyskeratosis. American Journal of Dermatopathology 84: 364

Crosti C, Riboldi A 1975 Eritoplasia plasmacellular benigna vulvare. Giornale Italiano di Dermatologia—Minerva Dermatologica: 110: 386–389

Crotty C P, Su W P D, Winkelmann R K 1980 Ulcerative lichen planus. Follow up of surgical excision and grafting. Archives of Dermatology 116: 1252–1256

Crow K D, Hargreaves G K 1968 Infantile pustular psoriasis. Transactions of the St John's Hospital Dermatological Society 54: 42–45

Crowe F W 1964 Axillary freckling as a diagnostic aid in neurofibromatosis. Annals of Internal Medicine 61: 1142–1143

Crum C P, Liskow A, Petras P, Keng W C, Frick H C 1984 Vulvar intraepithelial neoplasia (severe atypia and carcinoma in situ). A clinic-pathologic analysis of 41 cases. Cancer 54: 1429–1434

Damanski M, Barker M E, Sheehan J F 1969 Unusual cause of urinary obstruction. British Medical Journal ii: 385

Darier J 1892 Lichen plan scléreux. Annales de Dermatologie et de Syphiligraphie 3: 833–837

Darier J 1928 Kraurosis de la vulve. Précis de Dermatologie, 4th edn. Masson et Cie, Paris, p 465

Daunt S O'N, Kotowski K E, O'Reilly A P, Richardson A T 1982 Ulcerative vulvitis in Reiter's syndrome: a case report. British Journal of Venereal Diseases 58: 405–407

Davenport D M, Richardson D A 1986 Labial adhesions secondary to postpartum vulvar edema. Report of 2 cases. Journal of Reproductive Medicine 31: 523–527

Davis B A 1971 Salivary vulvitis. Obstetrics and Gynecology 37: 238–240

Davis J, Shapiro L, Baral J 1983 Vulvitis circumscripta plasmacellularis. Journal of the American Academy of Dermatology 8: 413–416

de Castro P, Jorizzo J L, Rajaraman S, Solomon A R, Briggaman R A, Raimer S S 1985 Localized vulvar pemphigoid in a child. Pediatric Dermatology 2: 302–307

Dégos R, Ébrard G 1958 Leukokératose papillomateuse buccogenitale familiale. Bulletin de la Société Française de Dermatologie et Syphiligraphie 65: 242

de Oliveira Neto M P 1972 Sarcoidose com lesoes da vulva. Revista Brasileira de Medicina 29: 134–139

de Saxe M, Kromberg J G R, Jenkins T 1984 The Aarskog (facio-digital-genital) syndrome in South Africa. South African Medical Journal 65: 299–303

Devroede G, Schlaeder G, Sanchez G. Haddad H 1975 Crohn's disease of the vulva. American Journal of Clinical Pathology 63: 348–358

Dicken C H, Powell S T, Spear K L 1984 Evaluation of isotretinoin treatment of hidradenitis suppurativa. Journal of the American Academy of Dermatology 11: 500–502

Dickie R J, Horne C H W, Sutherland H W, Bewsher P D, Stankler L 1982 Direct evidence of localised immunological damage in vulvar lichen sclerosus et atrophicus. Journal of Clinical Pathology 35: 1395–1397

di Paola G R, Rueda-Leverone N G, Becardi M G 1982 Lichen

sclerosus of the vulva recurrent after myocutaneous graft: a case report. Journal of Reproductive Medicine 27: 666–668

Dogliotti M, Bentley-Phillips C B, Schmann A 1974 Lichen sclerosus et atrophicus in the Bantu. British Journal of Dermatology 91: 81–85

Donatsky O 1976 Comparison of cellular and humoral immunity against streptococcal and adult human oral mucosa antigens in relation to exacerbation of recurrent aphthous stomatitis. Acta Pathologica et Microbiologica Scandinavica 84: 270–282

Donlan C J, Scutero J V 1975 Transient eosinophilic pneumonia secondary to use of a vaginal cream. Chest 67: 232–233

Donsky H J, Mendelson C G 1964 Squamous cell carcinoma as a complication of hidradenitis suppurativa. Archives of Dermatology 90: 488–491

Dottenwille M N 1982 Cancer invasif de la vulve et lichen scléreux vulvaire. Thèse, Paris. Cited by Hewitt 1984

Douglas C P 1983 Vulvar dystrophies. In: Studd J (ed) Progress in obstetrics and gynaecology, Vol. 3. Churchill Livingstone, Edinburgh

Douglas C P, Barnes C F J 1986 Proteolytic enzyme activity measured on extracellular matrix in vulval dystrodries. Journal of Obstetrics and Gynaecology 6: 193–195

Dupree E L, Lee R A 1973 Histiocytosis X in the female genital tract. Obstetrics and Gynecology 42: 201–204

Duray P H, Merino M J, Axiotis C 1983 Warty dyskeratoma of the vulva. International Journal of Gynecological Pathology 2: 286–293

Dutton A H, Hayes P C, Shepherd A N, Geirsson A 1983 Vulvo-vaginal steroid cream and toxic shock syndrome. Lancet i: 938 (c)

Ebling F J G 1986 Hidradenitis suppurativa: an androgen-dependent disorder. British Journal of Dermatology 115: 259–262

Eglin R P, Lehner T, Subak-Sharpe J H 1982 Detection of RNA complementary to herpes simplex virus in mononuclear cells from patients with Behcet's syndrome and recurrent oral ulcers. Lancet ii: 1356–1360

Eichner E, Danese C, Katz G 1983 Vulvar lymphatics as demonstrated by vital dyes and lymphangiography. International Surgery 68: 175–177

Eigler F W, Schaarschmidt K, Gross E, Richter H J 1986 Anorectal ulcers as a complication of migraine therapy. Journal of the Royal Society of Medicine 79: 424–426

Ellis J P, Crow K D 1982 A case of LSA of perineum with carcinomata of vulva and perianal area and recurrent lichen sclerosus in a full thickness skin graft. Case Presentation: XVI Congressus Internationalis Dermatologiae p 212

Evron S, Leviatan A, Okon E 1984 Familial benign chronic pemphigus appearing as leukoplakia of the vulva. International Journal of Dermatology 23: 556–557

Ewing T L, Smale L E, Elliott F A 1979 Maternal deaths associated with postpartum vulvar edema. American Journal of Obstetrics and Gynecology 134: 173–179

Falk D K, Latour D L, King L E 1985 Dapsone in the treatment of erosive lichen planus. Journal of the American Academy of Dermatology 12: 567–570

Fenzy A, Bogomoletz W V 1986 Anorectal ulceration due to abuse of dextropropozyphene and paracetamol suppositories. Journal of the Royal Society of Medicine 80: 62

Fisher A A 1973 Allergic reaction to feminine hygiene spray. Archives of Dermatology 108: 801–802

Fisher I, Orkin M 1970 Acquired lymphangioma. Archives of Dermatology 101: 230–234

Fitzsimmons J S, Guilbert P R, Fitzsimmons E M 1985 Evidence of genetic factors in hidradenitis suppurativa. British Journal of Dermatology 113: 1–8

Forman L 1966 The skin and the colon. Transactions of the St John's Hospital Dermatological Society 52: 139–154

Foulds I S 1980 Lichen sclerosus et atrophicus of the scalp. British Journal of Dermatology 103: 197–200

Frances C, Wechsler J, Meimon G, Labat-Robert J, Grimaud J A, Hewitt J 1983 Investigation of intercellular matrix macromolecules involved in lichen sclerosus. Acta Dermato-Venereologica (Stockholm) 63: 483–490

Frances C, Boisnic S, Lessana-Leibowitch M, Hewitt J 1984 Tumeur dyskératosique génitale masculine. Deux observations. Annales de Dermatologie et de Vénéreologie 111: 233–236

Freeman S 1986 Women allergic to husband's sweat and semen. Contact Dermatitis 14: 110–112

Friedman D, Haim S, Paldi E 1971 Refractory involvement of cervix uteri in a case of pemphigus vulgaris. American Journal of Obstetrics and Gynecology 110: 1023–1024

Friedman R J, Kopf A W J, Jones W B 1984 Malignant melanoma in association with lichen sclerosus on the vulva of a 14 year old. American Journal of Dermatopathology 6: (Supplement 1) 253–256

Friedman S A, Bernstein I L, Enrione M, Marcus Z H 1984 Successful long-term immunotherapy for human seminal plasma anaphylaxis. Journal of the American Medical Association 251: 2684–2687

Friedrich E G 1971 Topical testosterone for benign vulvar dystrophy. Obstetrics and Gynecology 37: 677–679

Friedrich E G 1976 New nomenclature for vulvar disease. Report of the Committee on terminology. Obstetrics and Gynecology 47: 122–124

Friedrich E G 1983a Vulvar disease. In: Saunders W B (ed) Major problems in obstetrics and gynecology 9, 2nd edn. W B Saunders, Philadelphia, ch 44, p 61

Friedrich E G 1983b The vulvar vestibule. Journal of Reproductive Medicine 28: 773–777

Friedrich E G, Kalra P S 1984 Serum levels of sex hormones in vulvar lichen sclerosus and the effect of topical testosterone. New England Journal of Medicine 310: 488–491

Friedrich E G, MacLaren N K 1984 Genetic aspects of lichen sclerosus. American Journal of Obstetrics and Gynecology 150: 161–166

Friedrich E G, Burch K, Bahr J P 1979 The vulvar clinic; an eight year appraisal. American Journal of Obstetrics and Gynecology 135: 1036–1040

Friedrich E G 1987 Vulvar vestibulitis syndrome. Journal of Reproductive medicine 82: 110–114

Frisch C, Pujade-Lauraine M D, Leynadier F, Dry J 1984 Rush hyposensitisation for allergy to seminal plasma. Lancet i: 1073

Gallagher P G 1986 Varicose veins of the vulva. British Journal of Sexual Medicine 13: 12–14

Gardner H L, Kaufman R H 1969 Benign diseases of the vulva and vagina. C V Mosby, St Louis

Gardner H L, Kaufman R H 1981 Benign diseases of the vulva and vagina, 2nd edn. G K Hall, Boston

Garnier G 1954 Vulvite érythématose circonscrite bénigne à type érythroplasique. Bulletin de la Société Française de Dermatologie et Syphiligraphie 61: 102–104

Garnier G 1957 Benign plasma cell erythroplasia. British Journal of Dermatology 69: 77–81

Gellert A, Green E S, Beck E R, Ridley C M 1983 Erythema nodosum progressing to pyoderma gangrenosum as a complication of Crohn's disease. Postgraduate Medical Journal 59: 791–793

Gianotti F, Caputo R 1985 Histiocytic syndromes: a review.

Journal of the American Academy of Dermatology 13: 383–404

Godeau G, Frances C, Hornebeck W, Brechemier D, Robert L 1982 Isolation and partial characterization of an elastase-type protease in human vulva fibroblasts: Its possible involvement in vulvar elastic tissue destruction of patients with lichen sclerosus et atrophicus. Journal of Investigative Dermatology 78: 270–275

Goodlin R C, Frederick I B 1983 Postpartum vulvar edema associated with the birthing chair. American Journal of Obstetrics and Gynecology 146: 334

Goodman R M, Smith E W, Paton D, Bergman R A et al 1963 Pseudoxanthoma elasticum: a clinical and histological study. Medicine 42: 297–334

Goolamali S K, Barnes E W, Irvine W J, Shuster S 1974 Organ-specific antibodies in patients with lichen sclerosus. British Medical Journal iv: 78–79

Gougerot H, Burnier R 1937 Lichen plan du col utérin, accompagnant un lichen plan jugal et un lichen plan stomacal. Lichen plurimuqueux sans lichen cutané. Bulletin de la Société Française de Dermatologie et Syphiligraphie 44: 637–640

Gray B K, Lockhart-Mummery H E, Morson B C 1965 Crohn's disease of the anal region. 6: 515–524

Gray L A, Barnes M L 1965 Vaginitis in women, diagnosis and treatment. American Journal of Obstetrics and Gynecology 92: 125–134

Greaves M W 1986 Histiocytic proliferative disorders. In: Rook A, Wilkinson D S, Ebling F J G, Champion R H, Burton J L (eds) Textbook of Dermatology 3rd edn. Blackwell Scientific, Oxford, ch 44

Greene S L, Muller S A 1985 Netherton's syndrome. Report of a case and review of the literature. Journal of the American Academy of Dermatology 13: 329–337

Greenspan A H, Shupack J L, Foo S H, Wise A C 1985 Acanthosis nigricans like eruption hyperpigmentation secondary to triazinate therapy. Archives of Dermatology 121: 232–235

Greer I A 1984 Orange periods. British Medical Journal 289: 323

Grimmer H 1968 Apokrine miliaria der vulva (subcorneale schweissdrüsen-retention). Zeitschrift für Haut und Geschlechts-Krankheiten 43: [123]–[132]

Gross P 1941 Non-pellagrous eruptions due to deficiency of Vitamin B complex. Archives of Dermatology 43: 504–531

Growdon W A, Fu Y S, Lebherz T B, Rapkin A, Mason G D, Parks G 1985 Pruritic vulvar squamous papillomatosis: evidence for human papillomavirus etiology. Obstetrics and Gynecology 66: 564–568

Guin J D, Haffley P 1983 Sensitivity to α-amylcinnamic aldehyde and α-amylcinnamic alcohol. Journal of the American Academy of Dermatology 8: 76–80

Hallopeau H 1889 Lichen plan scléreux. Annales de Dermatologie et de Syphiligraphie 2nd Series 10: 447–449

Hamilton P A, Brown P, Davies J D, Salmon P R 1977 Crohn's disease; an unusual cause of dyspareunia. British Medical Journal ii: 101

Hammersley N, Ferguson M M, Simpson N B 1984 Etretinate treatment in erosive lichen planus of the oral mucosa. In: Cunliffe W J, Miller A J (eds) Retinoid therapy. MTP, Lancaster

Harper W F, McNicol E M 1977 A histological study of normal vulval skin from infancy to old age. British Journal of Dermatology 96: 249–253

Harrington C I, Dunsmore I R 1981 An investigation into the incidence of autoimmune disorders in patients with lichen sclerosus et atrophicus. British Journal of Dermatology 104: 563–566

Harrington C I, Gelsthorpe K 1981 The association between LSA and HLA-B40. British Journal of Dermatology 104: 561–562

Hart W R, Norris H J, Helwig E B 1975 Relation of lichen sclerosus et atrophicus of the vulva to development of carcinoma. Obstetrics and Gynecology 45: 369–377

Hazelrigg D E, Stoller L J 1977 Isolated familial benign chronic pemphigus. Archives of Dermatology 113: 1302 (correspondence)

Heller R H, Joseph J M, Davis H J 1969 Vulvovaginitis in premenarcheal child. Journal of Pediatrics 74: 370

Hewitt J 1984 Conditions étiologiques du carcinome invasif d'emblée de la vulve. Possibilité d'un traitement proplylactique? Journal de Gynécologie, Obstetrique et Biologie de la Reproduction 13: 297–303

Hewitt J 1986 Histiologic criteria for lichen sclerosis of the vulva. Journal of Reproductive Medicine 31: 781–787

Hewitt J, Pelisse M 1976 Correlation between cancer and lichen sclerosis of the vulva: preliminary report. In: Friedrich E G, Gregori C A, Lynch P J (eds) Proceedings of the International Conference of the ISSVD

Hewitt J, Pelisse M, Lessana-Leibowitch M et al 1985 Le syndrome vulvovagino-gingival: nouveau groupement caractéristique du lichen plan érosif plurimuqueux. Revue de Stomatologie et de Chirurgie Maxillo-Faciale 86: 57–65

Highet A S, Warren R E, Staughton R C D, Roberts S O B 1980 Streptococcus milleri causing treatable infection in perineal hidradenitis suppurativa. British Journal of Dermatology 103: 375–382

Hindson T C 1966 Studies in contact dermatitis XVI—contraceptives. Transactions of the St John's Hospital Dermatological Society 52: 1–9

Hofs von W 1978 Familiiärer lichen sclerosus et atrophicans bei Vater, mutter und 9 jahriger Tochter. Dermatologische Monatsschrift 164: 633–639

Holland R M, Greiss F C 1983 Perineal Crohn's disease. Obstetrics and Gynecology 62: 527–529

Holt P J A, Darke C 1983 HLA antigens and Bf allotypes in lichen sclerosus et atrophicus. Tissue Antigens 22: 89–91

Hu C H, Michel B, Farber E M 1985 Transient acantholytic dermatosis (Grover's disease). Archives of Dermatology 121: 1439–1441

Huey G R, Stehman F B, Roth L M, Ehrlich C E 1985 Lymphangiosarcoma of the edematous thigh after radiation therapy for carcinoma of the vulva. Gynecologic Oncology 20: 394–401

Hughes B R, Holt P J A, Marks R 1987 Trimethoprim associated fixed drug eruption. British Journal of Dermatology 116: 241–242

Humphrey L J, Playforth H, Leavell U W 1969 Squamous cell carcinoma arising in hidradenitis suppurativa. Archives of Dermatology 100: 59–62

Hunt E 1954 Diseases affecting the vulva, 4th edn. Henry Kingston, London, ch 11, p 65

Hutchinson P E, Summerly R, Lawson R S 1976 Progressive postoperative gangrene: a reminder. British Journal of Dermatology 194: 89–95

Iglesias J, Almirall R, Puig Tintore L M 1984 Acne vulgaris of the vulva. Journal of Reproductive Medicine 29: 466–467

Itala J H, Allevato M A J, di Paola G R, Gomez Ruada N M 1984 Treatment of lichen sclerosus et atrophicus of the vulva with aromatic retinoid Ro 9359. Journal of Reproductive Medicine 29: 467

Izumi A K, Shmunes E, Wood M G 1971 Familial benign chronic pemphigus. The role of trauma including contact sensitivity. Archives of Dermatology 104: 177–181

Jackson R 1984 Melanosis of the vulva. Journal of Dermatologic Surgery and Oncology 10: 119–121

Janaki V R, Premalatha S, Raghuveera Rao N, Thambiah A S 1980 Lawrence-Seip syndrome. British Journal of Dermatology 103: 693–696

Jasionowski E A, Jasionowski P A 1979 Further observations on the effect of topical progesterone on vulvar disease. American Journal of Obstetrics and Gynecology 134: 565–567

Jayle F 1906 Le kraurosis vulvae. Revue de Gynécologie et de Chirurgie Abdominale 10: 633–668

Jeffcoate T N A, 1949 Pruritus vulvae. British Medical Journal ii: 1196–1200

Jeffcoate T N A 1962 Principles of gynaecology, 2nd edn. Butterworths, London

Jeffcoate T N A, Woodcock A S 1961 Premalignant conditions of the vulva, with particular reference to chronic epithelial dystrophies. British Medical Journal ii: 127–134

Jenkinson S D, Mackinnon A E 1984 Spontaneous separation of fused labia minora in prepubertal girls. British Medical Journal 289: 160–161

Johansson O, Nordlind K 1986 Immunoreactivity to material like vasoactive intestinal polypeptide in epidermal cells of lichen sclerosus et atrophicus. The American Journal of Dermatopathology 8: 105–108

Johns A M, Bower B D 1970 Wasting of napkin area after repeated use of fluorinated steroid. British Medical Journal i: 347–348

Jolliffe D S, Sim-Davis D 1977 Cicatricial pemphigoid in a young girl: report of a case. Clinical and Experimental Dermatology 2: 281–284

Jones I S C 1979 An assessment of vulval pigmentation. New Zealand Medical Journal 89: 348–350

Jones I S C 1983 A histological assessment of normal vulval skin. Clinical and Experimental Dermatology 8: 513–521

Jonquières E D L, de Lutzky F K 1980 Balanites et vulvites pseudo-érythroplasiques chroniques. Aspects histopathologiques. Annales de Dermatologie et de Vénérologie 107: 173–180

Joosef L A, Koudstaal J, Oswald F H 1964 Chromidrosis vulvae. Nederlandsch Tijdschrift voor Verloskunde und Gynaecologie 64: 179–187

Jorgenson R J, Levin L S 1981 White sponge nevus. Archives of Dermatology 117: 73–76

Jorizzo J L, Hudson R D, Schmalstieg F C et al 1984 Behçet's syndrome: Immune regulation, circulating immune complexes, neutrophil migration and colchicine therapy. Journal of the American Academy of Dermatology 10: 205–214

Jorizzo J L, Taylor R S, Schmalstieg F C et al 1985 Complex aphthosis: a forme fruste of Behçet's syndrome? Journal of the American Academy of Dermatology 13: 80–84

Joulia P, le Coulant P 1954 La maladie de Mucha, sa place actuelle dans la nosologie dermatologique. Minerva Dermatologica 29: 172–178

Kanerva L, Kousa M, Niemi K M, Lassus A, Juvakoski T, Lauharanta J 1982 Ultrahistopathology of balanitis circinata. British Journal of Venereal Diseases 58: 188–195

Kao M S, Paulson J D, Askin F B 1985 Crohn's disease of the vulva. Obstetrics and Gynecology 46: 329–333

Kato K, Kondo A, Takita T, Mitsuya H 1986 Labial adhesions in a diabetic woman. Urologia Internationalis 41: 455–456

Kaufman R H, Friedrich E G 1985 The carbon dioxide laser in the treatment of vulvar disease. Clinical Obstetrics and Gynecology 28: 220–229

Kauppinen K, Stubb S 1985 Fixed eruptions: causative drugs and challenge tests. British Journal of Dermatology 112: 575–578

Kennedy C, Hodge L, Sanderson K V 1978 Skin changes caused by D-penicillamine. Clinical and Experimental Dermatology 3: 107–116

Kierland R B, Epstein J G, Weber W E 1957 Eosinophilic granuloma of skin and mucous membrane. Association with diabetes insipidus. Archives of Dermatology 75: 45–54

Kindler T 1953 Lichen sclerosus et atrophicus in young subjects. British Journal of Dermatology 65: 269–297

King D T, Hirose F M, King L A 1978 Simultaneous occurrence of familial benign chronic pemphigus (Hailey–Hailey disease) and syringoma on the vulva. Archives of Dermatology 114: 801

Kinmonth J B 1982 The lymphatics: surgery, lymphography and diseases of the chyle and lymph systems, 2nd edn. Arnold, London

Kint A, Geerts M L 1975 Lichen sclerosus et atrophicus; an electron microscopic study. Journal of Cutaneous Pathology 2: 30–34

Kissmeyer A, With C 1922 Clinical and histological studies on the pathological changes in the elastic tissue of the skin. British Journal of Dermatology 34: 221–237

Klostermann G F 1972 Weibliche Gerschlechtsorgane. Vierter teil: vulva, vagina, urethra. In: Vehlinge E (ed) Handbuch der Speziellen Pathologischen Anatomie und Histologie. Springer-Verlag, Berlin, p 219

Kopecky R T, Funk M M, Kreitzer P R 1985 Localized genital edema in patients undergoing continuous ambulatory peritoneal dialysis. Journal of Urology 134: 880–884

Korting G W, Theisen H 1963 Circumscripte plasma cellulare Balanoposthitis und Conjunctivitis bei der selben person. Archive für Klinishe und Experimentelle Dermatologie 217: 495–504

Kramer I R H 1980 Oral leukoplakia. Journal of the Royal Society of Medicine 73: 765–767

Kremer M, Nussenson E, Steinfeld M, Zuckerman P 1984 Crohn's disease of the vulva. American Journal of Gastroenterology 79: 376–378

Lancet (editorial) 1982 Clinical stains for cancer. Lancet i: 320–321

Lancet (editorial) 1984 Management of toxic epidermal necrolysis. Lancet ii: 1250–1252

Lancet (editorial)1985a Thalidomide in dermatology and leprosy. Lancet ii: 80–81

Lancet (editorial) 1985b Polypeptide growth factors: a clinical perspective. Lancet ii: 251–253

Laplanche C, Grosshans E, Heid G 1984 Anorectal ulcerations after prolonged use of suppositories containing dextropropoxyphene. Annales de Dermatologie et de Vénéreologie 111: 347–355

Larsen W G 1979 Sanitary napkin dermatitis due to the perfume. Archives of Dermatology 115: 363

Larsson E, Westermark P 1978 Chronic hypertrophic vulvitis: a condition with similarities to cheilitis granulomatosa (Melkersson–Rosenthal syndrome). Acta Dermato-Venereologica 50: 92–93

Laugier M P, Hunziker N, Vidmar B 1971 L'oedeme isolé de la grand lèvre. Complication cutanée de la maladie de Crohn. Bulletin de la Société Française de Dermatologie et de Syphiligrahie 78: 98–100

Lavery H A 1984 Vulval dystrophies: new approaches. In: Fox H (ed) Clinics in obstetrics and gynaecology, 11, No. 1 p 155–169

Lawee D, Shafir M S 1983 Solitary penile ulcer associated with infective mononucleosis. Canadian Medical Association Journal 129: 146–147

Lehner T 1968 Autoimmunity in oral diseases, with special reference to recurrent oral ulceration. Proceedings of the Royal Society of Medicine 61: 515–524

Lehner T, Barnes C G 1979 Behcet's syndrome: clinical and immunological features. Academic Press, London

Leigh I M, Sanderson K V, Atherton D J, Wells R S 1979 Hypozincaemia in infancy. British Journal of Dermatology 101: (Supplement 17) 73–75

Leppard B, Delaney T J, Sanderson K V 1973 Chronic benign familial pemphigus. Induction of lesions by herpesvirus hominis. British Journal of Dermatology 88: 609–613

Levantine A V 1973 Vulval swelling in a patient with Crohn's disease. Proceedings of the Royal Society of Medicine 66: 48

Lever W L, Schaumburg-Lever G 1983 Histopathology of the skin, 6th edn. J B Lippincott, Philadelphia

Lin J A, Caraeta P F, Chang C H, Uchwat F, Tseng C H 1979 Malacoplakia of the vagina. Southern Medical Journal 72: 326–328

Lindskov R 1984 Acute febrile neutrophilic dermatosis with genital involvement. Acta Dermato-Venereologica 64: 559–561

Lipschutz B 1913 Über eine eigenartige Geschwürsform des weiblichen Genitales (ulcus vulvar acutum). Archiv für Dermatologie and Syphilis (Berlin) 114: 363–396

Lobraico R V 1984 A clinical review of lichen sclerosus treated with the CO_2 laser. Journal of Reproductive Medicine 29: 469–470

Lortat-Jacob E, Civatte J 1961 Balanite pseudo-epitheliomateuse, kératosique et micacée. Bulletin de la Société Française de Dermatologie et Syphiligraphie 68: 164–167

Lortat-Jacob E, Civatte J 1966 Balanite pseudo-epitheliomateuse, kératosique et micacée. Bulletin de la Société Française de Dermatologie et Syphiligraphie 73: 931–935

Lovell C R, Atherton D J 1984 Infantile gluteal granulomata: Case report. Clinical and Experimental Dermatology 9: 522–525

Lyles J W, Knox J M, Richardson J B 1958 Atypical features in familial benign chronic pemphigus. Archives of Dermatology 78: 446–453

Mabuchi K, Bross D S, Kessler I I 1985 Epidemiology of cancer of the vulva. A case-control study. Cancer 55: 1843–1848

McAdams A J, Kistner R W 1958 The relationship of chronic vulvar disease, leukoplakia and carcinoma in situ to carcinoma of the vulva. Cancer 11: 740–757

McCallum D I 1969 Unusual cause of urinary obstruction. British Medical Journal ii: 637

McCallum D I, Gray W M 1976 Metastatic Crohn's disease. British Journal of Dermatology 95: 551–554

McCallum D I, Kinmont P D 1968 Dermatological manifestations of Crohn's disease. British Journal of Dermatology 80: 1–8

Machnicki S 1953 Diphtheria of the vulva and of the vagina. Abstract from Polish. Zeitschrift für Haut-Und Geschlechtskrankenheiten 86: 368

McLintock D G 1985 Phimosis of the prepuce of the clitoris: indication for female circumcision. Journal of the Royal Society of Medicine 78: 257–258

Maekawa Y, Sakazaki Y, Hayashibara T 1978 Diaper area granuloma of the aged. Archives of Dermatology 114: 382–383

Maibach H I, Mathias C T 1985 Vulvar dermatosis and fissures—irritant dermatitis from methyl benzethonium chloride. Contact Dermatitis 13: 340

Mallinson C N, Bloom S R, Warin A P, Salmon P R, Cox B 1974 A glucagonoma syndrome. Lancet ii: 1–5

Ma'luf T J, Weed J C 1971 Chylous metrorrhea. A case report. Obstetrics and Gynecology 37: 277–281

Mann P R, Cowan M A 1973 Ultrastructural changes in four cases of lichen sclerosus et atrophicus. British Journal of Dermatology 89: 223–231

Mann P R, Haye K R 1970 An electron microscope study on the acantholytic and dyskeratotic processes in Darier's disease. British Journal of Dermatology 82: 561–566

Marks R, Wells G C 1973a Lichen simplex: morphodynamic correlates. British Journal of Dermatology 88: 249–256

Marks R, Wells G C 1973b A histochemical profile of lichen simplex. British Journal of Dermatology 88: 557–562

Marsden R A, McKee P H, Bhogal B, Black M M, Kennedy L A 1980 A study of benign chronic bullous dermatosis of childhood and comparison with dermatitis herpetiformis and bullous pemphigoid occurring in childhood. Clinical and Experimental Dermatology 5: 159–172

Mehregan A H 1986 Pinkus' Guide to Dermatohistopathology 4th edn. Appleton-Century-Crofts, East Norwalk, Connecticut

Mensing H, Janner M 1981 Vulvitis plasmacellularis Zoon. Zeitschrift für Hautkrankheiten 56: 728–732

Meyrick Thomas R H, Holmes R C, Rowland Payne C M E, Ridley C M, Sherwood F, Black M M 1982 The incidence of development of autoimmune diseases in women, after the diagnosis of lichen sclerosus et atrophicus. British Journal of Dermatology 104: (Supplement 22) 29

Meyrick Thomas R H, Kennedy C T C 1986 The development of lichen sclerosus et atrophicus in monozygotic twin girls. British Journal of Dermatology 114: 377–379

Meyrick Thomas R H, Ridley C M, Black M M 1983 The association of lichen sclerosus et atrophicus and autoimmune related disease in males. British Journal of Dermatology 109: 661–664

Meyrick Thomas R H, Ridley C M, Black M M 1984a The association of lichen sclerosus et atrophicus and autoimmune related disease in males—an addendum. British Journal of Dermatology 111: 371

Meyrick Thomas R H, Ridley C M, Sherwood F, Black M M 1984b The lack of association of lichen sclerosus et atrophicus with HLA-A and B tissue antigens. Clinical and Experimental Dermatology 9: 290–292

Meyrick Thomas R H, McGibbon D H, Munro D D 1985 Basal cell carcinoma of the vulva in association with vulval lichen sclerosus et atrophicus. Journal of the Royal Society of Medicine Supplement II 78: 16–18

Meyrick Thomas R H, Ridley C M, Black M M 1987a Clinical features and therapy of lichen sclerosus et atrophic affecting males. Clinical & Experimental Dermatology 12: 126–128

Meyrick Thomas R H, Ridley C M, MacGibbon D H, Black M M 1987b Lichen sclerosus and autoimmunity—a study of 350 women. British Journal of Dermatology (in press)

Michaelis L, Guttman C 1902 Ueber Einschlusse in Blasentumoren. Zeittschrift für Klinische Medizin (Berlin) 47: 208–215

Mikhail G R, Drukker B H, Chow C 1967 Pemphigus vulgaris

involving the cervix uteri. Archives of Dermatology 95: 496–498

Mikhail G R, Fachnie D'A M, Drukker B H, Farah R, Allen H M 1979 Generalised malignant acanthosis nigricans. Archives of Dermatology 115: 201–202

Miller R A W, Griffiths W A D 1982 Experimentally induced complement and immunoglobulin deposition along the basement membrane zone (BMZ) and in dermal blood vessels. British Journal of Dermatology 106: 275–279

Miller R F 1957 Lichen sclerosus et atrophicus with oral involvement. Archives of Dermatology 76: 43–55

Morgan W P, Leicester G 1982 The role of depilation and deodorants in hidradenitis suppurativa. Archives of Dermatology 118: 101

Mortimer P S, Dawber R P R, Gales M A, Moore R A 1986a A double-blind controlled cross-over trial of cyproterone acetate in females with hidradenitis suppurativa. British Journal of Deomatology 115: 263–268

Mortimer P S, Dawber R P R, Gales M A, Moore R A 1986b Mediation of hidradenitis suppurativa by androgens. British Medical Journal 292: 245–248

Moss T R, Stevenson C J 1981 Incidence of male genital vitiligo. Report of a screening programme. British Journal of Venereal Diseases 57: 145–146

Mountain J C 1970 Cutaneous ulceration in Crohn's disease. Gut 11: 18–26

Moynahan E J 1974 Acrodermatitis enteropathica: A lethal inherited human zinc deficiency disorder. Lancet ii: 399–400

Murphy F R, Lipa M, Haberman H F 1982 Familial vulvar dystrophy of lichen sclerosus type. Archives of Dermatology 118: 329–331

Neill S M, Smith N P, Eady R A J 1984 Ulcerative sarcoidosis: a rare manifestation of a common disease. Clinical and Experimental Dermatology 9: 277–279

Neinstein L S, Goldenring J 1984 Pink pearly papules: an epidemiologic study. Journal of Pediatrics 105: 594–595

Neuhofer J, Fritsch P 1984 Treatment of localised scleroderma and lichen sclerosus with etretinate. Acta Dermato-Venereologica 64: 171–174

Neville E A, Finn O A 1975 Psoriasiform napkin dermatitis—a follow-up study. British Journal of Dermatology 92: 279–285

Newton J A, Camplejohn R S, McGibbon D H 1987 A flow cytometric study of the significance of DNA anenploidy in cutaneous lesions. British Journal of Dermatology 117: 169–174

Norburn L M, Coles R B 1960 Recurrent erysipelas following vulvectomy. Journal of Obstetrics and Gynaecology of the British Commonwealth 67: 279–280

Norris J F B, Cunliffe W S 1986 Failure of treatment of familial widespread hidradenitis suppurativa with isoretinoin. Clinical and Experimental Dermatology 11: 579–583

Northcutt A D, Vanover M J 1985 Nodular cutaneous amyloidosis involving the vulva. Archives of Dermatology 121: 518–521

Nürnberger F, Müller G 1967 Elektronenmikroskopische Untersuchungen über die Akantholyse bei Pemphigus familiaris benignus. Archive für Klinische und Experimentelle Dermatologie 228: 208–219

O'Keefe R, Dagg J H, McKie R M 1987 The staphylococcal scalded skin syndrome in two elderly immunocompromised patients. British Medical Journal 295: 179–180

Orfanos C E, Schloesser E, Mahrle G 1971 Hair destroying growth of Corynebacterium tenuis in the so-called trichomycosis axillaris. Archives of Dermatology 103: 632–639

Paniel B J, Truc J B, de Margerie V, Chantraine J, Poitout P 1984 La vulvo-perineoplastie. Journal de Gynécologie, Obstetrique et Biologie de la Reproduction 13: 91–100

Paniel B J, Truc J B, Decroix Y, Poitout P 1986 Vulvoperineoplasty. Journal of Reproductive Medicine 31: 983–984

Parkinson D J, Alderman B 1984 Vulval adhesions causing urinary incontinence. Postgraduate Medical Journal 60: 634–635

Parks J 1941 Diphtheritic vaginitis in the adult. American Journal of Obstetrics and Gynecology 41: 714–715

Parks J, Martin S 1948 Reactions of the vulva to systemic diseases. American Journal of Obstetrics and Gynecology 55: 117–130

Patterson J A K, Ackerman A B 1984 Lichen sclerosus et atrophicus is not related to morphea. A clinical and histological study of 24 patients in whom both conditions were reputed to be present simultaneously. American Journal of Dermatopathology 6: 323–335

Peckham B M, Maki D G, Patterson J J, Hafez G -R 1986 Focal vulvitis: A characteristic syndrome and cause of dyspareunia. American Journal of Obstetrics and Gynecology 154: 855–864

Pelisse M, Hewitt J 1976 Erythematous vulvitis en plaques. Proceedings of the 3rd Congress of the International Society for the Study of Vulvar Disease, p 35–37

Pelisse M, Leibowitch M, Sedel D, Hewitt J 1982 Un nouveau syndrome vulvo-vagino-gingival. Lichen plan érosif plurimuqueux. Annales de Dermatologie et de Vénéreologie 109: 797–798

Pelisse M, Hewitt J, Leibowitch M et al. 1983. Le syndrome vulvo-vagino-gingival: groupement significatif du lichen plan érosif plurimuqueux. Annales de Dermatologie et de Vénéreologie 110: 953–956

Penneys N S 1984 Treatment of lichen sclerosus with potassium para-aminobenzoate. Journal of the American Academy of Dermatology 10: 1039–1042

Portnoy J, Ahronheim G A, Ghibu F, Clecner B, Joncas J H 1984 Recovery of Epstein Barr virus from genital ulcers. New England Journal of Medicine 311: 966–968

Powell F C, Rogers R S, Dickson E R, Moore S B 1986 An association between HLA DR1 and lichen planus. British Journal of Dermatology 114: 473–478

Prezyna A P, Kalyanaraman B 1977 Bowen's carcinoma in vulvo-vaginal Crohn's disease (regional enterocolitis): report of first case. American Journal of Obstetrics and Gynecology 128: 914–915

Radman H M, Bhagavan B S 1972 Pilonidal disease of the female genitals. American Journal of Obstetrics and Gynecology 114: 271–272

Rainford D J 1970 Southey's tubes and vulval oedema. British Medical Journal iv: 538

Ratz J L 1984 Carbon dioxide laser treatment of balanitis xerotica obliterans. Journal of the American Academy of Dermatology 10: 925–928

Ravits H G, Welsh A L 1957 Lichen sclerosus et atrophicus of the mouth. Archives of Dermatology 76: 56–58

Reed O M, Mellette J R, Fitzpatrick J E 1986 Cutaneous lentiginosis with atrial myxomas. Journal of the American Academy of Dermatology 15: 398–402

Rettenmaier M A, Braly P S, Roberts W S, Berman M L, Disaia P J 1985 Treatment of cutaneous vulvar lesions with skinning vulvectomy. Journal of Reproductive Medicine 30: 478–480

Reyman L, Milano A, Demopoulos R, Mayron J, Schuster S 1986 Metastatic vulvar ulceration in Crohn's disease. American Journal of Gastroenterology 81: 46–49

Rhodes A R, Silverman R A, Harrist T J, Perez-Atayde A R 1984 Mucocutaneous lentigines cardiomuco-cutaneous myxomas and multiple blue nevi: The LAMB syndrome. Journal of the American Academy of Dermatology 10: 72–82

Ricci J 1945 One hundred years of gynaecology 1800–1900. Blakiston, Philadelphia

Ridley C M 1975 The vulva. Major problems in dermatology 5. W B Saunders, London

Ridley C M 1977 Epidermolysis bullosa with unusual features: Inversa type. Proceedings of the Royal Society of Medicine 70: 576–577

Ridley C M 1981 Contraception and the skin. British Journal of Family Planning 7: 67–70

Ridley C M 1982 Zinc deficiency developing in treatment for thalassaemia. Journal of the Royal Society of Medicine 75: 38–39

Ridley C M 1983 Vulval dysplasia. British Journal of Hospital Medicine 32: 223

Ridley C M 1985 Cicatricial pemphigoid. American Journal of Obstetrics and Gynecology 152: 916 (letter)

Ridley C M 1986 Genital warts with malignant transformation and in association with lichen sclerosus et atrophicus (LSA) in elderly women: 2 cases. Journal of Reproductive Medicine 31: 984–985

Rigg L A, Hermann H, Yen S S C 1978 Absorption of estrogens from vaginal creams. New England Journal of Medicine 298: 195–197

Robboy S J, Ross J S, Prat J, Keh P C, Welch W R 1978 Urogenital sinus origin of mucinous and ciliated cysts of the vulva. Obstetrics and Gynecology 51: 347–351

Robin J 1978 Contact dermatitis to acetarsol. Contact Dermatitis 4: 309–310

Rocamora A, Santonja C, Vives R, Varona C 1986 Sebaceous gland hyperplasia of the vulva: a case report. Obstetrics and Gynecology 68: 63S–65S

Romaguera C, Grimalt F 1981 Contact dermatitis from a copper containing IUCD. Contact Dermatitis 7: 163–164

Romppanen U, Tuimala R, Ellmen J 1984 Etretinate (Tigason) in the treatment of dystrophic changes of the vulva—an open study. Dermatologica 169: 247

Rook A, Wilkinson D S, Ebling F J G, Campion R H, Burton J C, (eds) 1986 Textbook of dermatology, 4th edn. Blackwell Scientific, Oxford

Rose P G, Johnston G C, O'Toole R V 1984 Pure cutaneous histiocytosis X of the vulva. Obstetrics and Gynecology 64: 587–590

Roujeau J C, Rowland Payne C M E, Guillaume J C, Penso D, Saiag P, Revuz J, Touraine R 1986 Lyell's syndrome—Créteil's experience in 87 cases. British Journal of Dermatology 115 (Supplement 30): 25

Rowell N R 1984 Histocompatibility antigens (HLA) in dermatology. British Journal of Dermatology 111: 347–357

Rudd N L, Nimrod C, Holbrook K A, Byers P H 1983 Pregnancy complications in Type IV Ehlers-Danlos syndrome. Lancet i: 50–53

Rycroft R J G, Penney P T 1983 Dermatoses associated with brominated swimming pools. British Medical Journal 287: 462

Salem O S, Steck W D 1983 Cowden's disease (multiple hamartoma and neoplasia sydrome). A case report and review of the English literature. Journal of the American Academy of Dermatology 8: 686–696

Sarkany I 1959 Grenz ray treatment of familial benign chronic pemphigus. British Journal of Dermatology 71: 247–252

Sarona-Ventura C 1985 Labial adhesions in postmenopausal women with hip joint disease. Australian and New Zealand Journal of Obstetrics & Gynaecology 25: 303–304

Saylan T, Saltik I 1982 Thalidomide in the treatment of Behcet's syndrome. Archives of Dermatology 118: 536

Schuermann H 1960 Plasmocytosis circumorificialis. Deutsche Zahnarztliche Zeitschrift 15: 601

Sehgal V H, Gangwan O P 1986 Genital fixed drug eruptions. Genito-Urinary Medicine 62: 56–58

Shackelford G D, Bauer E A, Graviss E R, McAlister W H 1982 Upper airway and external genital involvement in epidermolysis bullosa dystrophica. Radiology 143: 429–432

Shaffer B, Copelan H W, Beerman H 1957 Pseudoxanthoma elasticum. A cutaneous manifestation of a systemic disease; report of a case of Paget's disease and a case of calcinosis with arteriosclerosis as manifestations of this syndrome. Archives of Dermatology 76: 622–630

Shelley W B 1972 Consultations in dermatology. W B Saunders, Philadelphia

Shelley W B 1974 Consultations in dermatology II. W B Saunders, Philadelphia

Shelley W B, Crissey J T 1953 Classics in clinical dermatology. C C Thomas, Springfield

Shelley W B, Miller M A 1984 Electron microscopy, histochemistry and microbiology of bacterial adhesion in trichomycosis axillaris. Journal of the American Academy of Dermatology 10: 1005–1014

Shelley W B, Wood M G 1981 Transformation of the common wart into squamous cell carcinoma in a patient with primary lymphoedema. Cancer 48: 820–824

Shuttleworth D, Graham-Brown R A C, Hutchinson P E, Joliffe D S 1985 Cicatricial pemphigoid in D-penicillamine treated patients with arthritis—a report of three cases. Clinical and Experimental Dermatology 10: 392–397

Shy K K, Eschenbach D A 1981 Fatal perineal cellulitis from an episiotomy site. Obstetrics and Gynecology 54: 292–298

Sinha M R 1982 Fixed genital drug eruption due to dapsone. A case report. Leprosy in India 54: 152–154

Singer A, Campion M S, Clarkson P K, Mc Cance D J 1986 Recognition of subclinical human papillomavirus infection of the vulva. Journal of Reproductive Medicine 31: 985–986

Sison-Torre E Q, Ackerman A B 1985 Melanosis of the vulva. A clinical simulator of malignant melanoma. American Journal of Dermatopathology 7: 51–60 (Supplement)

Sloan P J M, Goepel J 1981 Lichen sclerosus et atrophicus and perineal carcinoma: a case report. Clinical and Experimental Dermatology 6: 399–402

Souteyrand P, Wong E, MacDonald D M 1981 Zoon's balanitis (balanitis circumscripta plasmacellularis). British Journal of Dermatology 105: 195–199

Sparks M K, Kuhlman D S, Prieto A, Callen J P 1985 Hypercalcaemia association with cutaneous squamous cell carcinoma occurence as a late complication of hidradenitis suppurativa. Archives of Dermatology 121: 243–246

Stacy D, Burrell M O, Franklin E W 1986 Extramammary Paget's disease of the vulva and anus: use of intraoperative frozen-section margins. American Journal of Obstetrics and Gynecology 155: 519–532

Stage A H 1985 Cicatricial pemphigoid of the vulva. American Journal of Obstetrics and Gynecology 152: 916–917

Stage A H, Humeniuk J M, Easley W K 1984 Bullous pemphigoid of the vulva: a case report. American Journal of Obstetrics and Gynecology 150: 169–170

Stanton M J, Maxted W 1981 Malacoplakia: a study of the literature and current concepts of pathogenesis, diagnosis and treatment. Journal of Urology 125: 139–146

Starink T M, Hausman R 1984 The cutaneous pathology of facial lesions in Cowden's disease. Journal of Cutaneous Pathology 11: 331–337

Steinkampf M P, Reilly S D, Ackerman G E 1987 Vaginal agglutination and hematometra associated with epidermolysis bullosa. Obstetrics and Gynecology 69: 519–521

Stern J K, Rosen T 1982 Balanitis plasmacellularis circumscripta (Zoon's balanitis plasmacellularis). Cutis 25: 57–60

Sterry W, Schmoll M 1985 Contact urticaria and dermatitis from self-adhesive pads. Contact Dermatitis 13: 284–285

Stewart W D, Light M J 1984 Successful treatment of hidradenitis suppurativa with etretinate. Dermatologica 169: 258

Stock R J, Stock M E, Hutto J M 1973 Vaginal douching: Current concepts and practices. Obstetrics and Gynecology 42: 141–146

Strate S M, Taylor W E, Forney J P, Silva F G 1983 Xanthogranulomatous pseudotumor of the vagina: Evidence of a local response to an unusual bacterium (mucoid E.Coli). American Journal of Clinical Pathology 79: 637–743

Sumathipala A H T 1984 Penile ulcer in Crohn's disease. Journal of the Royal Society of Medicine 77: 966–967

Sutton R L 1935 In: Sutton R L (ed) Diseases of the skin, 9th ed, Vol. 2. C V Mosby, St Louis, p 1389

Swanson D L, Dahl M V 1981 Pemphigus vulgaris and plasma exchange: Clinical and serologic studies. Journal of the American Academy of Dermatology 4: 325–328

Sweet R D 1979 Acute febrile neutrophilic dermatosis—1978. British Journal of Dermatology 100: 93–99

Swift B H 1936 Achlorhydria as an aetiological factor in pruritus vulvae, associated with kraurosis or leukoplakia. Journal of Obstetrics and Gynaecology of the British Empire 43: 1053–1077

Szymanski F J, Caro M R 1955 Pseudoxanthoma elasticum. Review of its relationship to internal disease and report of an unusual case. Archives of Dermatology 71: 184–189

Tappeiner J, Pfleger L 1971 Granuloma glutaeale infantum. Hautarzt 22: 383–388

Tatnall F M, Mann B S 1985 Non-Hodgkin's lymphoma of the skin associated with chronic limb lymphoedema. British Journal of Dermatology 113: 751–756

Tatnall F M, Barnes H M, Sarkany I 1985 Sarcoidosis of the vulva. Clinical and Experimental Dermatology 10: 384–385

Taussig F J 1929 Leukoplakic vulvitis and cancer of the vulva (etiology, histopathology, treatment, five-year results). American Journal of Obstetrics and Gynecology 18: 472–503

Taylor W N 1941 Vulvar fusion: two cases with urological aspects. Journal of Urology 45: 710–714

Thambar I V, Dunlop R, Thin R N, Huskisson E C 1977 Circinate vulvitis in Reiter's syndrome. British Journal of Venereal Diseases 53: 260–262

Thiers H, Moulin G. Rochet Y, Lieux J 1968 Maladie de Hailey-Hailey à localisation vulvaire predominante. Étude génétique et ultra-structurale. Bulletin de la Société Française de Dermatologie et Syphiligraphie 75: 352–355

Thomas R, Barnhill D, Bibro M, Hoskins W, Hambridge W 1986 Histiocytosis X in gynecology: a case presentation and review of the literature. Obstetrics and Gynecology 67: 46S–49S

Thomson J 1986 Etretinate and vulvitis. Retinoids Today and Tomorrow 5: 49

Tilsley D A, Wilkinson D S 1965 Necrosis and dequalinium. II vulval and extra-genital ulceration. Transactions of the St John's Hospital Dermatological Society 51: 49–54

Török E, Orley J, Goracz G, Daroczy J 1975 Lichen sclerosus et atrophicus in children. Clinical and pathological analysis of 33 cases. Modern Problems in Paediatrics 17: 262–271

Toth F, Szeker V, Nemet J, Varga T 1969 Histochemische und elektronen mikroskopische Untersuchungen an einem pri-

maren eosinophilen Vulvagranulom. Strahlentherapie 138: 530

Troy J L, Silvers D N, Grossman M E, Jaffe I A 1981 Penicillamine–associated pemphigus: is it really pemphigus? Journal of the American Academy of Dermatology 4: 547–555

Uyeda K, Nakayasu K, Takaishi Y, Sotomatsu S 1973 Kaposi sarcoma-like granuloma on diaper dermatitis. Archives of Dermatology 107: 605–607

Vakilzadeh F, Kolde G 1985 Relapsing linear acantholytic dermatosis. British Journal of Dermatology 112: 349–355

Van der Putte S C J, Oly H B, Storm I 1986 Papular acantholytic dyskeratosis of the penis. American Journal of Dermatopathology 84: 365–366

van Joost T 1971 A rare case of vulvar ulcer of acute onset. Nederlands Tijdschrift voor Geneeskunde 115: 1080–1082

van Joost T, Faber W R, Manuel H R 1980 Drug induced anogenital cicatricial pemphigoid. British Journal of Dermatology 102: 715–718

Verbov J L 1973 The skin in patients with Crohn's disease and ulcerative colitis. Transactions of the St John's Hospital Dermatological Society 59: 30–36

Verburg D J, Burd L I, Hoxtell E O, Merrill L K 1974 Acrodermatitis enteropathica in pregnancy. Obstetrics and Gynecology 44: 233–237

Vermesh M, Deppe E, Zbella E 1984 Non-puerperal traumatic vulvar hematoma. International Journal of Gynaecology and Obstetrics 22: 217–219

Wagenberg H R, Downham T F 1981 Chronic edema of the vulva: a condition similar to cheilitis granulomatosa. Cutis 27: 526–527

Wallace H J 1955 Vulval atrophy and leukoplakia. In: Bowes R K (ed) Modern trends in obstetrics and gynaecology (second series). Butterworth, London, pp 386–394

Wallace H J 1971 Lichen sclerosus et atrophicus. Transactions of the St John's Hospital Dermatological Society 57: 9–30

Wallace H J, Whimster I W 1951 Vulval atrophy and leukoplakia. British Journal of Dermatology 63: 241–257

Warin R 1983 The role of trauma in the spreading weals of hereditary angio-oedema. British Journal of Dermatology 108: 189–194

Warkel R L, Jager R M Focal acantholytic dyskeratosis of the anal canal. American Journal of Dermatopathology 84: 362–363

Weber F R 1927 A note on lichen planus of the vulva. British Journal of Dermatology 39: 521–522

Weedon D Papular acantholytic dyskeratosis of vulva. American Journal of Dermatopathology 84: 363

Weisfogel E 1969 Aims of joint gynecologic, dermatologic and pathologic vulvar clinics. New York State Journal of Medicine 69: 1184–1186

Whimster I W 1959 The nature of leukoplakia. Nederlandsch Tijdschrift voor Geneeskunde 103: 2469–2471

Whitfield R G S 1947 Anomalous manifestations of malnutrition in Japanese prison camps. British Medical Journal ii: 164–168

Whitlock F A 1976 Psychophysiological aspects of skin diseases. Major problems in dermatology 8. W B Saunders, London, ch 7, pp 110–127

Woodruff J D, Babaknia A 1979 Local alchohol injection of the vulva: discussion of 35 cases. Obstetrics and Gynecology 54: 512–514

Woodruff J D, Parmley T H 1983 Infection of the minor vestibular gland. Obstetrics and Gynecology 62: 609–612

Work B A 1980 Pyoderma gangrenosum of the perineum. Obstetrics and Gynecology 55: 126–128

Yates V M, Kerr R E I, Mackie R M 1983a Early diagnosis of

infantile seborrhoeic dermatitis and atopic dermatitis—
clinical features. British Journal of Dermatology 108: 633–
638

Yates V M, Kerr R E I, Frier K, Cobb S J, Mackie R M 1983b
Early diagnosis of infantile seborrhoeic dermatitis and atopic
dermatitis—total and specific IgE levels. British Journal of
Dermatology 108: 639–645

Yates V M, King C M, Dave V K 1985 Lichen sclerosus et
atrophicus following radiation therapy. Archives of Dermatology 121: 1044–1047

Zaino R J, Husseinzadeh N, Nahhas W, Mortel R 1982 Epithelial alterations in proximity to invasive squamous carcinoma
of the vulva. International Journal of Gynecological Pathology
1: 173–184

Zoon J J 1952 Balanoposthite chronique circonscrite bénigne à
plasmacytes. Dermatologica 105: 1–7

Zoon J J 1955 Balanitis und vulvitis plasmacellularis. Dermatologica 111: 157

7

Historical and psychological considerations: subjective and traumatic conditions of the vulva
J J Bradley and C M Ridley

GENERAL ASPECTS

Historical aspects

Vulval lesions are not well described in early medical literature, though references are to be found in the Talmud, the Bible and Egyptian papyri of the second millenium BC; perhaps the first accurate descriptions were those of Avicenna in the 11th century and they were followed by those of Renaissance writers such as Severinus Pineus in the 16th century (Fig. 7.1 a and b) and Van den Spieghel in the 17th century. In 1857 the histology of the genitalia was described and dermatologists began to note and name vulval lesions such as 'leukoplakia' and 'kraurosis'.

Ricci (1943, 1945) is an authority on all historical aspects of gynaecological medicine and surgery; Leonardo (1944), Graham (1950) and Mettler (1947) are also rich sources; Ploss et al (1935) deals particularly with the anthropological significance of female anatomy and physiology.

Etymology

The vagina (sheath) and mons veneris (hill of Venus) are obvious appellations. Vulva is from the Latin for covering and was originally used for the uterus. Isidorus in 600 AD described the labia as being like doors (valvae) and Leonardo (1944) pointed out that in the fourth century Babylonian

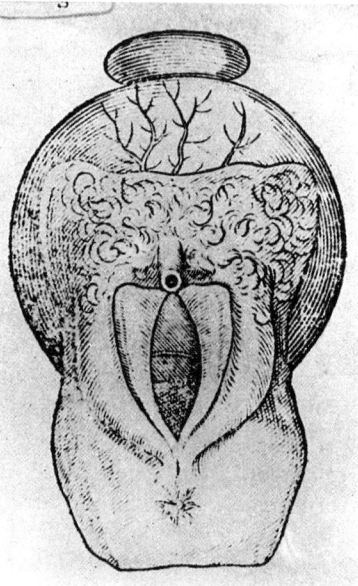

A

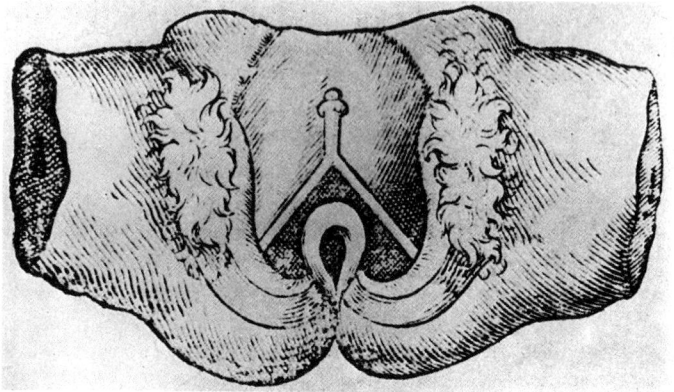

B

Fig. 7.1 (a and b) Earliest pictures of the external genitalia of the female: Severinus Pineus (1550–1619). Reproduced from the Genealogy of gynaecology, James V Ricci, Blakiston, Philadelphia 1943 (courtesy of McGraw Hill) Dr C M Ridley (1975) The vulva. Major problems in dermatology 5. Lloyd Luke.

Talmud the labia were described as hinges. Clitoris is usually thought to come from a Greek word meaning 'to close' and, some would say, 'key'.

'Hymen' obviously suggests a connection with the god of marriage. In ancient Greece, Hymen as a personal divinity was probably called into being to personify a cry 'Hymen' in the wedding song. The wedding song was known as a *Hymenaios* and the god himself was also entitled Hymenaios. The refrain of the wedding song thus became 'Hymen o Hymenaie'. Hymen is recorded as a word for any type of membrane from the fourth century BC and presumably existed before that. However, although in 16th century editions of fourth century commentaries on Terence and Virgil there are tales of a Hymen who rescued virgins and comments on a vaginal hymen which guarded virginity, the word was not apparently to be found as referring specifically to the vaginal membrane before the seventh century. Its use in this way was firmly established in the 16th century at the time of Vesalius. Conceivably the words for the god and for the membrane were simply homophones, an odd coincidence; alternatively, 'hymen' did indeed originally refer to the vaginal membrane and had lost this connotation by the time it first occurred in the literature as meaning a membrane in general.

The vulva in art and literature

One may contrast the somewhat crudely feminist viewpoint of Judy Chicago and her moulded ceramic 'vulval' plates (Fig. 7.2 a) with more subtle formalisations, for example on Greek pots, or even indeed the logo of the 'International Society for the Study of Vulvar Disease' (Fig. 7.2 b).

In literature the archetypal patterns so well delineated by Bodkin (1963) encompass many aspects of sexuality; the psychophysiological echoes of which she speaks reinforce and enrich intellectual appreciation.

Cultural and sociological factors

Attitudes to vulvovaginal disease will be affected by the social and cultural background. Trotula in the 11th century (Mason-Hohl 1940) said 'since these organs happen to be in a retired location, women on account of modesty and the fragility and deli-

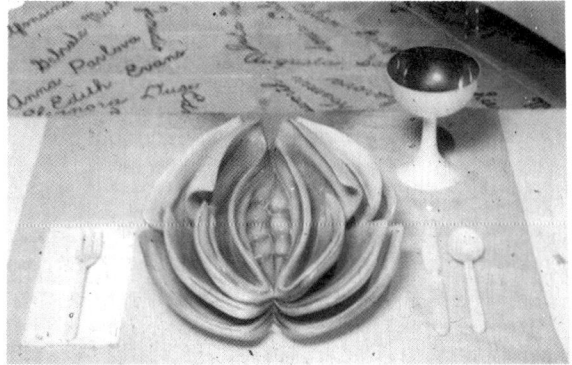

A

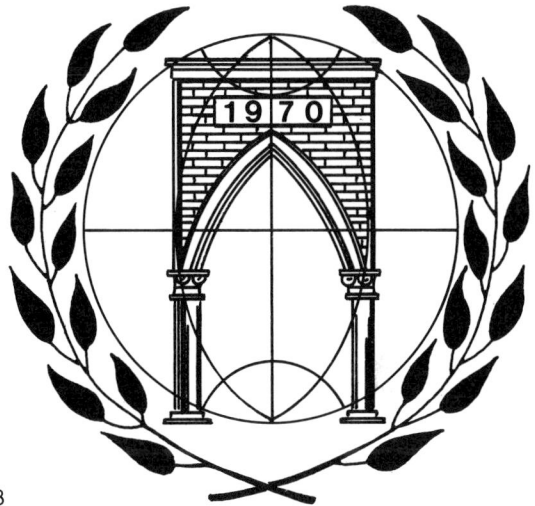

B

Fig. 7.2 (a) Moulded ceramic plate by Judy Chicago, American feminist (b) logo of the International Society for the Study of Vulvar Disease.

cacy of the state of these parts dare not reveal the difficulties of their sicknesses to a male doctor'. Some women still feel something of this, hence in part the popularity of such hospitals as there are which are staffed by women, and the tendency of women with vulval lesions to go to women dermatologists and gynaecologists. The women who have such views are a mixed group comprising the shy, those not wishing to be examined by a man for religious reasons, those who believe that men are often not sympathetic to women with these complaints, and some who simply seem to feel that they establish better rapport with a woman. Many doctors, male and female, will not be able to associate themselves with such views, but it is impossible to deny that they exist.

Sociological factors are also of importance in recognition, acceptance and treatment of sexually transmitted disease; the history of that subject and its interaction with society were intensively considered by Selvin (1985), Kampmeier (1985) and Reiss (1985).

PSYCHIATRIC DISORDERS AND THE VULVA

The genitalia and secondary sexual characteristics loom large in the body image of both sexes and it is hardly surprising that the vulva, representing an area of the body that is a source of pleasure, guilt, pride, embarrassment and procreation, should be a focus for anxieties, preoccupations, delusions and even hallucinations.

It follows that the physical examination of such a psychologically sensitive area should be conducted with gentleness, tact and perceptive awareness in a relaxed but thorough manner. Women frequently complain of feeling embarrassed, humiliated or demeaned by genital examination, but the presence of a chaperone (sometimes a sexual partner), explanation and reassurance will minimise the danger of distress and may be positively therapeutic. In spite of a climate of sexual liberation and what amounts to an information explosion on sexual matters in the popular press and women's magazines, a surprisingly large number of women are ignorant of their genital anatomy and many need gentle education with diagrams and encouragement to explore their own bodies.

Any vulval symptom, pain, irritation or observable lesion, is likely to give rise to anxiety, the degree of which will be dependent on the disability it causes, the patient's personality, the context in which it occurs and the reactions of the sexual partner. Relatively minor disorders may become a focus for displaced anxiety and guilt, particularly that relating to sexuality and sexual relationships. When taking a history it is important to allow a woman sufficient time and sympathetic interest to talk about personal problems, which will give the doctor an opportunity for further exploration of her lifestyle and relationships which might have a bearing on the presenting symptom. It is debatable whether any vulval symptoms (apart from some cases of pain and hallucinatory experiences) are purely psychogenic, though they may be perpetuated by psychological mechanisms (Whitlock 1976). On the other hand, the stress of adverse life events such as bereavement and divorce may induce white cell dysfunction, allowing the patient to be more prone to fungal or viral infection. Bartrop et al (1977) reported depression of the mitotic response of lymphocytes in 29 subjects whose spouses had died 6 weeks earlier, and similar results have been reported by other workers (Kronfol et al 1983, Schliefer et al 1983). A review of emotion and immunity (Lancet 1985) concluded that the relationship between them may prove to be another strong argument for a return towards 'whole person' medicine, but in a robust rejoinder (Hall 1985) it has been pointed out that there has been no evidence of any significant increase in illnesses that could be attributed to defects in immunity in air crews who survived the stresses of the 1939–45 war. However, the field of psychosomatic inter-relationships is fraught with difficulties, not least because of problems in communication between clinicians, psychologists and immunologists; it has been further reviewed recently (Lancet 1987).

Almost any genital symptom may be interpreted by a patient as being due to sexually transmitted disease and a high proportion of patients will be self-referred to sexually transmitted disease (STD) clinics. Some, of course, will indeed be suffering from such a disease and all will need an opportunity to ventilate their feelings (except perhaps some habitual attenders) and given appropriate reassurance, treatment, or referral to a gynaecologist, dermatologist or psychiatrist. Although it has been estimated that 30% of patients attending STD clinics are probable psychiatric cases based on the General Health Questionnaire (GHQ) (Pedder & Goldberg 1970), compared with 12% of the general population (Goldberg et al 1976), the patient's presenting symptoms may, of course, be due to organic disease, the psychiatric disorder being incidental. The psychiatric morbidity uncovered by the GHQ is generally anxiety or depression of mild to moderate severity, which would not warrant referral to a psychiatrist. Frost (1985) has shown that only 0.4% of new attenders in an STD clinic are thought to have overt psychiatric illness based on referral rates to psychiatrists from sexually transmitted disease clinics. Fitzpatrick et al (1986) in a study of 381 patients attending an STD clinic have found that while 43% had GHQ scores indicating that they were psychiatric cases, only 4% appeared to have an abnormal or unwarranted level of distress in relation to their presenting complaint.

The vast majority of emotional and psychiatric problems relating to the vulva are likely to be of relatively minor severity in psychiatric terms. Nevertheless, sensitive psychological management, which will include explanation, reassurance and above all time to listen to the patient, may ease or cut short unnecessary suffering. Misinterpretations of physical symptoms or signs by a patient may lead her to believe, for example, that a benign vulval wart is malignant, but she may be reluctant to express her anxiety. Anticipation of her fears and encouragement to express them followed by firm reassurance should give relief, whereas failure to do so may result in prolonged distress and rumination. Patients with serious vulval disease, such as carcinoma, have also been shown to benefit from imaginative pre- and postoperative counselling.

A woman with a fear or conviction of disease which is unresponsive to a simple psychotherapeutic approach, and which dominates her life and leads her from doctor to doctor, may justifiably be regarded as suffering from hypochondriasis (Barksy & Klerman 1983). This may be a symptom of an obsessional neurosis in which the patient may be able to accept reassurance for short periods, but then rapidly returns to her ruminations of serious disease and rejects any psychological interpretation of the symptom. There may be a degree of associated clinical depression which will respond to treatment with antidepressant drugs. Hypochondriasis may also be the presenting feature of severe depression, schizophrenia or monosymptomatic hypochondriasis, all of which may be grouped together as 'psychotic' disorders.

Psychotic disorders

The term 'psychosis' is applied to those illnesses in which patients suffer from delusions, hallucinations, or other disorders of the thought processes or mood which cause them to be out of touch with reality. The more florid forms of schizophrenia, mania or endogenous depression will be readily recognisable as frank mental illness and, although some patients may complain of vulval symptoms, they will be incidental to the overall picture. Apart from organic psychoses due to structural disease of the nervous system, metabolic disorders and drug intoxication or withdrawal (usually associated with disorientation and memory disturbance), categorisation as 'psychotic' is purely descriptive and does not have specific aetiological significance. However, the so called 'functional psychoses' (such as schizophrenia or endogenous depression) are syndromes which, once initiated, render the patient inaccessible to logical argument about certain ideas or symptoms, though insight may be retained in other respects. In practical terms, the patient is likely to be deeply distressed and bewildered by her symptoms, and may become suicidal or (more rarely) a danger to others.

A proportion of patients suffering from psychoses will present to general practitioners, physicians in genitourinary medicine, gynaecologists or dermatologists with vulval symptoms, without appearing to be obviously mentally ill. Superficially the presenting complaint may seem to be a straightforward one such as discomfort, irritation, anxiety about anatomical structure, fear of venereal disease, unpleasant discharges or odours. The doctor may initially be alerted to the possibility of psychosis by an unusual quality to the complaint. There may be a discrepancy between its apparent trivial nature and the emotional response (or vice versa) or a bizarre way of describing pain or sensations. After thorough physical examination the patient will be unable to accept assurances that no abnormality has been found. The more the woman is allowed to talk about her complaints, the more the diagnosis will become clear. It is important to encourage the patient to say what she believes to be the cause of her symptom and to express her ideas about its outcome and what she feels can be done to help her.

Recognition of the presence of major psychiatric illness rather than precise psychiatric diagnosis (if that is not a contradiction in terms) is required, and referral for appropriate psychiatric treatment. There is an understandable reluctance on the part of some physicians (Cotterill 1983) to alarm a patient who believes she has a physicial disorder by referring her to a psychiatrist and to risk the patient's refusing all medical care. Some doctors may feel confident in undertaking psychiatric management themselves, but in most cases it will be possible to persuade a patient to accept psychiatric consultation, at the same time offering a further appointment in the referring clinic.

Schizophrenia

Symptoms relating to the vulva are not common, though about one-fifth of schizophrenic patients do suffer from hypochondriacal delusions (Lucas et al 1962). The complaint is usually bizarre. The patient may feel that the appearance of her vulva has changed in a strange way, even to the extent that she fears she may be changing sex. Further questioning may reveal that she believes that it is due to some outside influence. Some schizophrenic patients experience tactile hallucinations in the genital area, or orgasmic sensations. Elaborate delusional explanations of these feelings may be elicited, such as the patient believing that she is being raped in her sleep.

A hyochondriacal preoccupation, short of frank delusions, may be a prodromal symptom of late onset schizophrenia (Kenyon 1976).

Endogenous depression

The well-recognised syndrome of gloom, early morning waking, weight loss, morning exacerbation of symptoms, loss of libido, self reproach and ideas of hopelessness and suicide may occur from adolescence to old age. A preoccupation with bodily health and functions is a frequent concomitant to the extent that it may be the leading symptom, and any mood changes noted may appear to be the effect rather than the cause of it.

The vulva may be the sole focus of symptoms from a vague feeling that 'something is wrong' to clearly defined localised persistent pain (Bradley (1963). The patient may have fears of often unspecified malignant or venereal disease, unrelieved by examination and negative laboratory tests, or a conviction that an unpleasant odour, which must be obvious to everyone around, emanates from the vulva. Soreness due to energetic use of deodorants

and disinfectants may be observed. She may admit to feelings of guilt about masturbation, or remote sexual indiscretions, when encouraged to speculate about the cause of her distress. Delusional ideas that the vulva has 'dried up' and that the vagina or urethra have been closed or obliterated may be encountered, and efforts to demonstrate that it is not so will be met with disbelief. Given adequate time, the patient will give a clear indication of the emotional loading of her symptoms. Fixed ideas of punishment, shame and the hopelessness of her case will emerge and the examining doctor should not shy from enquiring into whether she has considered suicide. Depressed patients are often relieved to be told that their illness is a well-recognised one and that it can be treated. Depressive illnesses may be self-limiting, but the judicious use of antidepressant drugs and/or electroconvulsive therapy, as an inpatient or outpatient (depending on the severity of illness and social circumstances) will cut short the period of suffering and perhaps prevent a suicide.

Monosymptomatic hypochondriacal psychosis

Hypochondriacal ideas of delusional intensity, unresponsive to repeated reassurance (often by a series of doctors unknown to each other) and without signs of schizophrenia or depression, may occur. The symptom may be centred on the vulva. It is generally a vague one, such as discomfort, or feeling 'not quite right' or dysmorphophobia, a disorder of perception of the body image in which the patient believes that the anatomical appearance is ugly or in some way abnormal. Such patients generally have a pre-existing personality disorder of obsessional or paranoid type. The symptom may persist for many years despite investigations, reassurance and even energetic psychiatric treatment. It does not usually progress to a full psychosis, but a significant number of patients ultimately commit suicide (Bebbington 1976, McKenna 1984).

Delusional parasitosis is an allied condition which is well known to dermatologists, though it is in fact relatively rare and an individual dermatologist may see only three or four cases in a professional lifetime (Lyell 1983). The syndrome occurs most commonly in middle-aged women who believe that they are infested with parasites, usually of the whole body, but sometimes confined to the perineum. The delusion will dominate the woman's life (and that of her family) and the secondary effects of repeated washing and use of strong antiseptics may be seen on examination. Psychiatric referral may be strongly resisted, but treatment with the neuroleptic drug pimozide 2–6 mg daily (therapy which is also effective in hypochondriacal psychosis and schizophrenia) can result in a dramatic remission within a few weeks (Monro 1980). The patient rarely develops full insight into the delusional nature of the symptoms, but is no longer preoccupied with them. Unfortunately, to avoid relapse long term treatment is usually necessary.

Epilepsy

Reports of vulval sensations or orgasm as part of an epileptic aura, or equivalent, are uncommon, though isolated cases are to be found (Scott 1978). A distinction must be made between the sexual aura, which may have temporal lobe origin, and ictal genital sensory phenomena, which may have parietal lobe origin (Spencer et al 1983).

PRURITUS VULVAE

The term 'pruritus vulvae' should be reserved for patients who complain of itching for which no cause is apparent. (Pruritis is an incorrect spelling, tempting to non-dermatologists because of the false analogy with dermatitis, etc.)

Diagnosis

A patient who complains of itching may be found to have any one of a variety of physical conditions: a neoplasm, pediculosis, a vaginal discharge whether normal or abnormal, any dermatosis including ill-defined allergic and irritant reactions, and many others. She may also have a vaginitis, proctitis or cervicitis without obvious discharge or cutaneous change; if these factors are dealt with the itching subsides. The same applies to children or young adults with a threadworm infestation. The engorgement and varicosities of pregnancy or the premenstrual state can occasionally produce symptoms, and prolapse may also be responsible.

A careful history and examination are therefore essential. If the area appears totally normal the diagnosis of pruritus vulvae is reasonable. Simple thickening is also consistent with that diagnosis; time will tell whether the thickening is secondary only to itching (lichen simplex) or to some underlying cutaneous lesion (lichenification). (These terms are discussed fully on p. 168). The other reservation as regards physical findings is that an eczema may have been set up as a result of irritant reactions or allergy to local applications used initially on a physically normal but itching vulva; the situation may then have been compounded by heat, obesity and friction.

In this situation, above all it is important to attempt to unravel causation and keep the patient under observation until she is completely symptom free and/or the train of events is clear. If this principle is not observed conditions which are important to treat will be missed.

After local factors have been excluded a systemic cause should be considered, although such a cause usually leads to generalised rather than localised pruritus. It is prudent to exclude iron deficiency and blood dyscrasias.

If these findings too are negative the patient may then be considered to have pruritus vulvae. A patient in this strictly defined category is relatively rare, less common for example than one with the burning vulva syndrome (with which cases may well have been confused in the past).

Aetiology

The pharmacological, physiological and psychological elements in itching were reviewed by Savin (1980). The uncertainties under these headings apply to itching of any area, but a further mystery is why some areas seem particularly prone to become itching and to be rubbed, thus setting off a self-perpetuating state; the anogenital area is commonly affected but the nape of the neck and sometimes the upper back are also sites with a similar tendency.

Whitlock (1976) critically surveyed the literature on pruritus, particularly in its psycho-physiological aspects. Some quotations will convey his views:

Minor physical factors often start a condition which is aggravated and potentiated by a variety of tensions and frustrations . . . Practically all writers agree that in any group of patients with generalised or local pruritus a large percentage will be suffering from a variety of skin diseases directly responsible for the initiation of the symptoms. However there will be a small number of patients whose symptoms cannot be explained in this manner and it would appear to be this group which is more likely to show psychological symptoms of an acute or chronic kind . . . there is very limited evidence for the occurrence of primary psychogenic itching affecting patients in the absence of some coexistent dermatosis as the cause of the itching in the first place.

Whitlock has pointed out that in the older literature such terms as 'neurodermatitis' did not necessarily imply a psychogenic origin but referred to the putative role of nerve fibres in sensation. Such views were reflected in the suggestion of Webster (1891) that fibrosis could cause itching, or that thinning of the skin left nerve endings vulnerable (Krantz 1970)—concepts that were, however, somewhat facile and in any case did not explain the itching which occurs in clinically normal skin.

Management

The patient is usually an adult with long-standing symptoms arising before or after the menopause. The itching may or may not be localised to one particular area of the vulva.

An attempt must be made to assess psychological factors in the individual case. Patients often welcome assurance that the complaint is common and not 'imaginary'. Often discussion will at least enable the patient to accept the symptoms and not worry about them so much. Rarely, there may be true depression, whether primary or secondary, in which case the help of the psychiatrist should be sought. A mild sedative (e.g. hydroxyzine) at night often helps to break a habit of itching and rubbing. Bland emollients (e.g. aqueous cream) are safe to use lavishly and can help to prevent soreness arising after micturition. It is worth establishing that hygiene is adequate, but in general more harm comes from overvigorous cleansing than from the reverse and patients should be advised to avoid bubble-baths, disinfectants, etc., although most

will already have done so. Agents which readily sensitise (e.g. topical antihistamines and most topical anaesthetic creams) should be withdrawn and patch tests arranged if allergy to any local application appears already to have taken place. Lignocaine is a safe local anaesthetic from the point of view of sensitisation but many patients find the feeling of numbness that it induces a poor exchange for itching. Topical corticosteroids can help, but mainly in the cases where there is much lichenification; in these circumstances indeed it is often wise to use a strong corticosteroid to aid rapid resolution for review. Such preparations are best applied at night during bad periods, and otherwise only occasionally as necessary. Crotamiton topically is quite safe but probably rarely helpful.

In the last century, removal of the clitoris or resection of the pudendal nerve was practised (Ricci 1945), and as recently as Mering (1952) advocated denervation. Woodruff & Thompson (1972), Ward & Sutherst (1975), Woodruff & Babaknia (1979), and Sutherst (1979)—the latter in a double blind study—have reported that local injections of alcohol, a procedure requiring a general anaesthetic, may be helpful in patients with assorted causes of itching; many probably had lichen simplex but many also lichen sclerosus et atrophicus and other conditions. It is sad to note that nine of the patients of Ward & Sutherst (1975) had had a simple vulvectomy without benefit. Hammond & Johnson (1984) have used the carbon dioxide laser with good results in five patients with pruritus, three of whom had 'hyperplasia' and so may have had lichen simplex. Here again the treatment is painful and requires general anaesthesia.

Care and continuity of supervision are important if symptoms are to be relieved and underlying conditions discovered.

In summary, we may consider pruritus vulvae as a condition now fairly rare where some trigger, perhaps emotional or perhaps a usually trivial physical factor, has initiated itching in a susceptible subject; the itching then leads to an itching-scratching self-perpetuating state, with or without overt lichenification. With time and simple remedies most patients will either lose their symptoms or be much less troubled by them. More drastic measures will rarely if ever be justified.

VULVODYNIA: THE BURNING VULVA SYNDROME

These terms have arisen in the last few years. Vulvodynia (McKay 1985) is used to describe the symptom of vulval soreness or burning, often with dyspareunia, sometimes also with vaginal or perineal involvement, but not itching. The topic first came to notice when Weisfogel (1976) discussed it at the Congress of the International Society for the Study of Vulvar Disease, and the name was devised by Tovell & Young (1978).

Patients with such a complaint seem to have increased in number although it is possible that in the past it was mistaken for pruritus vulvae, especially where the history taker was not meticulously careful and the patient not markedly articulate. A helpful point in differentiation is whether the patient has the urge to scratch, which is present in itching and absent in burning.

Equally patients complaining of pain are excluded from the definition. This is a difficult subgroup which may not in fact be truly separable. It encompasses patients with pain of frankly psychiatric origin and those with pain of neurological or uncertain origin (Neill & Swash 1982), where often the pain is worse on sitting or of a throbbing nature.

Vulvodynia may have several easily comprehensible sources, for example *Candida* infections or contact dermatitis. On occasion the physical factor may be subtle, as for example in Crohn's disease (p. 141) or the very rare case of lipodystrophia centrifugalis reported by Rowland Payne et al (1985), when dyspareunia was caused by loss of fat in the vulval area.

When no physical cause can be found or the symptoms persist after the physical findings have been treated the term 'burning vulva syndrome' (BVS) is used.

In practice an adequate explanation is currently rarely found for the chronic state so vulvodynia and BVS tend to be used synonymously. Some would indeed prefer vulvodynia as a term for the idiopathic state as being more acceptable to the patient. Although the terms are cumbersome they conduce to our keeping an open mind and are therefore preferable to the earlier title of 'psychosomatic vulvovaginitis' (Gardner & Kaufman 1981).

Vulvodynia and the BVS are the subject of study for a task force of the International Society for the Study of Vulvar Disease (Young 1984) and it is to be hoped that collation of case reports and questionnaires on an international basis will elucidate the problem.

Burning vulva syndrome (BVS)

The patients are usually young but sometimes middle aged. They have a long history of consultations with a variety of specialists, sometimes of multiple sexually transmitted diseases, often of intensive investigation. They tend to be demanding and emotionally labile and to engender frustration and even exasperation in the doctor. They usually have dyspareunia and physical examination, apart from the occasional underlying coincidental conditions such as lichen sclerosus et atrophicus, is normal to the naked eye except for mild or marked erythema, either patchy or confluent, in the posterior part of the vestibule. Wallace (1971) noted introital erythema in some of his patients; some of these may have had lichen sclerosus et atrophicus or lichen planus, but some may have been examples of the BVS.

Mechanisms of sensation

Studies of the neurophysiology of pain may help to clarify the mechanism of symptoms. Mediators such as peptides and prostaglandins, and nerve fibres (including those at a distance from the vulva, for example around sites of genital tract surgery or in the neighbourhood of spinal foramina, where referred pain may be relevant) as well as the subject's level of perception may all be important. The consensus of opinion at present, and the subject was discussed in detail at the 1985 Congress of the International Society for the Study of Vulvar Disease, is that there is probably a spectrum of causation with some patients having exclusively psychogenic and some exclusively physical trigger factors; whereas most will be in between, with a physical trigger which has set off a self-maintaining complaint.

Such triggers may be surgical, and perhaps varicosities secondary to surgery such as were blamed by Beard et al (1984) for some cases of pelvic pain. Other factors readily come to mind such as *Candida* infections, intertrigo, etc. More subtle causes are now being explored, namely an inflammation of minor vestibular glands or the vestibule in general, and subclinical vulval warts.

Minor vestibular glands: 'focal vulvitis': vulval vestibulitis

Minor vestibular glands are found mainly in the posterior part of the vulva and are essentially normal. Robboy et al (1978) found them in 9 out of 19 autopsy specimens ranging in number from 2 to 10 around the hymeneal ring. The orifices are just visible to the naked eye. Woodruff & Parmley (1983) and Friedrich (1983) attributed symptoms to their inflammation, describing punctate erythema and tenderness relieved by a perineoplasty or laser treatment. Laser treatment seemed the more valuable since it can deal with glands in all parts of the vestibule more easily (Kaufman & Friedrich 1985). Follow up after treatment is as yet short. Recently Peckham et al (1986) have suggested that such inflammatory changes, while punctate, do not correspond well to the vestibular glands, and have suggested 'focal vulvitis' as an alternative name for the syndrome. Friedrich (1987) and Pyka et al (1987) in further clinical and histological studies however prefer the term vulval vestibulitis, and this seems more specific and accurate (see also p. 162).

Wart infection

Sometimes in BVS the introitus looks velvety and on colposcopy and after application of 5% acetic acid the typical appearance of 'microwarts' can be seen. Although it may be that some stalk-like lesions are non-infective, simple vestibular papillae (Friedrich 1983), many such lesions are probably undoubtedly warty in as far as human papillomavirus has been demonstrated in them (see p. 199) (Fig. 7.3). The difficulty is to assign significance to these findings. Such warts are common in the clitoral and urethral area where symptoms are rare; many patients have such warty changes at the posterior vestibule but are symptomless; warts visible to the naked eye do not give rise to burning sensation. Rigorous follow-up of patients whose symptoms have been relieved by laser treatment of the warts is necessary, as is study of a control series.

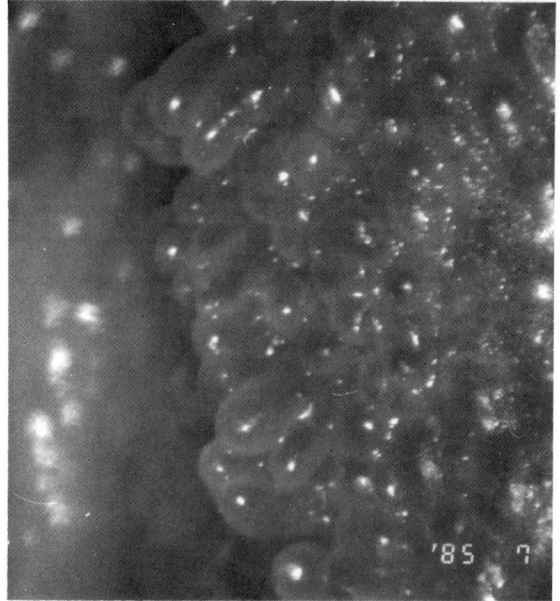

Fig. 7.3 Vulval vestibular microwarts showing a papillary pattern. (By courtesy of Dr M Campion)

Management

Reassurance and support may help to some extent and many patients do tend to improve slowly. On the assumption that the symptoms may be caused by 'occult' *Candida*, for example infection in the minor vestibular glands or in warty tissue, or elsewhere, long term anti-*Candida* therapy is often given with doubtful effect. The same applies to the short term use of strong topical corticosteroids, either frankly empirically or in the hope of dealing with '*Candida* hypersensitivity' (burning has been attributed to withdrawal of topical corticocosteroids but this must explain at most a very few cases). Local injections of alcohol, such as may help in pruritus, do not help patients with BVS but subcutaneous injections of triamcinolone into the affected areas may do so. A local anaesthetic preparation of low sensitising potential (lignocaine) may have some symptomatic value. Laser treatment is as yet of unproved efficacy; symptomatic improvement is common but recurrence of the complaint in a few months is a well-recognized sequel.

Psychogenic factors are generally agreed to be important but much morbidity of this type may be secondary rather than primary; in either case patients may fall into the 'chronic pain syndrome' category. Psychotropic drugs will help where there is true depression and may in other cases be used to alter the patient's perception of pain and burning; the dermatologist may prefer to enlist the help of an interested psychiatrist in such management.

MUTILATION

Mutilation is an emotive term. Self-induced trauma as for abortion or emotional reasons tends to arouse disapproval and even rejection in health care professionals, while necessary surgery for malignant disease and episiotomy may be perceived by the patient, if not by the surgeon, as mutilation.

Mutilation may be accidental, or as a result of sexual violence, and elicit appropriate concern and action. Sexual re-assignment surgery is condemned by those who see it as tampering with nature, but is sought eagerly by those who feel it will offer them greater fulfilment.

Cultural pressures force millions of children and young women to submit to traditional rituals such as infibulation, which may be life threatening or disabling. Those involved usually accept these practices as an inevitable part of their lives, even though those outside these cultures regard them with horror.

Ritual and cultural mutilation

Mutilation for cultural, religious or aesthetic reasons is unusual in Western society, though the current 'punk' fashion for adornment with metal rings has spread from the ears to other parts of the body, including the vulva (Healey 1978). There are reports of African tribes who measure female sexuality in terms of clitoral length and labial hypertrophy and whose girls are deliberately manipulated to stimulate enlargement of the clitoris and labia minora (Gelfand 1973).

The practice of what has been loosely termed 'female circumcision' has been carried on for many generations in more than 20 countries in Africa, from Nigeria in the West to Somalia and the Sudan in the East. It is also practised in Oman, South Yemen and the United Arab Emirates and among the Muslim population of Indonesia and Malaysia. It is estimated that as many as 74 000 000 women are involved (Hosken 1979). Christian missionaries have strongly deplored the practice over the last hundred years, but it is only in the last decade that concern has been expressed by the international community and by outspoken women in those countries affected, who see these mutilations as a way of maintaining female subjugation. There is a widespread belief that female circumcision is a requirement of the Islamic faith, though this has been repudiated by Muslim theologians; it is apparently viewed as an 'embellishment' rather than an ordinance like male circumcision (Shandall 1967). It is not practised in a number of Muslim countries, including Saudi Arabia. The custom is perpetuated by other religious groups, including Catholics, Protestants, Copts and Animists, and seems to be related more to cultural tradition than to religion.

The various types of operation subsumed under the description 'circumcision' (apart from removal of the prepuce of the clitoris) are illegal in the Sudan, though they are still practised (Fig. 7.4). Following newspaper reports that about six such operations are carried out annually in private hospitals in London (Observer 1982) women's rights groups have been campaigning for legislation to make such practices illegal in the United Kingdom. A Prohibition of Female Circumcision Act (1985) has now been passed.

Three types of operation are carried out:

1. Circumcision which involves the removal of the prepuce of the clitoris (Sunna circumcision).
2. Excision—clitoridectomy and excision of the labia minora.
3. Infibulation—which involves clitoridectomy, excision of the labia minora and of the anterior two-thirds or the whole of the medial part of the labia majora. The vaginal introitus is obliterated by sutures, apart from a very small opening for menstrual blood and urine. After this operation the girl's legs are bound together for up to 40 days to allow formation of scar tissue.

The type of operation and ritual surrounding it vary according to the country and culture. The operation is usually performed by older women, in some places with elaborate ceremony and in others without. No form of anaesthetic is used except

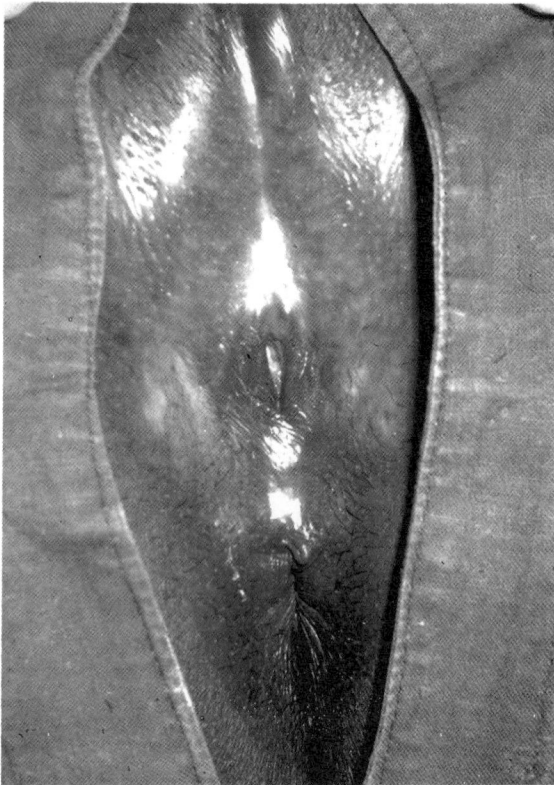

Fig. 7.4 Female circumcision.

when the operation is performed in hospital. The age at which it occurs varies from a few days old to late adolescence, or just before marriage.

The ritual is usually carried out in unhygienic surroundings and it is not surprising that there is a significant mortality from haemorrhage and infection, though accurate statistics are not available. Damage is often sustained to the urethra, bladder and vagina as the girl struggles to free herself. Haematocolpos and urinary problems occur as a result of obliteration of the vaginal introitus, and keloidal scars and calculi (Onuigbo 1976, Aziz 1980, Junaid & Thomas 1981) are also reported. Other than in the most minor operations sexual enjoyment is lost, and in infibulated women intercourse is impossible until the husband opens the vagina, often with a knife. Because of the fibrosis, dilatation of the vulva may be impossible in labour, with the result that the head tears the perineum.

Despite the obvious psychological trauma of the operation and its sequelae, the social pressures are so great that a girl and her parents will conform because of the danger of rejection, ridicule or unmarriageability (McLean 1980).

What possible motives can there be for what to Western eyes must be a wholly repugnant custom? Initiation into adulthood, preservation of virginity, hygiene and aesthetic reasons have all been advanced. By its apologists it is seen as a way of maintaining tribal cohesion, and by its critics as a means by which men subjugate women, perpetuated out of spite by women who have undergone mutilation themselves. Anthropologists have suggested that female circumcision may be partly the result of male ambivalence towards female sexuality, and partly a reaction of women to male circumcision (Bettelheim 1954). Myths current in some cultures are that the masculine element of a woman is her clitoris and a man's femininity is represented by his foreskin. It is believed that in order to avoid sexual ambiguity both must be removed.

Interference by well-meaning Westerners is resented, but in some countries there has been a growing desire to eradicate the customs of circumcision, excision and infibulation, and there does seem to be a slow decline in the practice. However, a tradition known to have existed for over 2000 years is likely to be eroded only extremely slowly.

Self mutilation

Mentally handicapped and psychotic patients may injure the vulva with their fingernails or with various foreign bodies, as part of a masturbatory act or as a response to delusions or hallucinations. The mental disorder in such cases is usually obvious. Injuries are sometimes caused by clumsy attempts to procure abortion. It will be the apparently 'normal' young woman who presents with atypical excoriation, ulcers or even haematuria who will be a diagnostic problem when investigations all prove negative. Reports of self mutilation of the female genitalia are uncommon in the literature, although relatively common among males, which may be surprising as self mutilation, in general, is much commoner in women than in men (French & Nelson 1972).

Such a patient will often give an irritatingly vague account of how and when the lesion began and, although consulting a doctor about it, she may seem inappropriately composed and phlegmatic. In fact, the lesion will have been caused by the patient herself using her nails, a needle, or by cigarette burns, though this may be very hard to demonstrate. Straightforward conscious malingering is relatively unusual, though it is possible, for instance, in a young woman held on remand in prison as a means of obtaining sympathy or hospital admission. The majority of patients producing artefacts fall into a category that is neither truly malingering, nor truly unconscious behaviour. Lyell (1979) sums it up neatly, 'it is done consciously perhaps, but with a consciousness that is made to act in that way by forces that are outside the patient's control'.

When suspicion has been aroused, a closer look at the patient's personality and current life situation is indicated. Such women are emotionally immature and not necessarily young. There may be a history of early emotional deprivation, due to parental loss or discord, or an overdependence on parents. The patient may admit to sexual frigidity and yet present in a flirtatious way, or like a coy child. She may express disappointment with a sexual partner and an inability to form stable relationships. A history of overdoses, cut wrists or drug abuse may be obtained and she may have been in trouble with the law. 'Blackouts', amnesias, or illnesses suggestive of hysterical conversion may be elicited during the course of taking her history.

A proportion of patients who produce self-inflicted lesions may appear to be superficially stable: a student nurse devoted to her profession, a devout religious postulant, or a middle-aged spinster caring for a cantankerous elderly mother, but under the apparent stability is a bewildered child reacting to some intolerable situation by a need to be 'ill'. Gentle enquiry into current tensions, frustrations or disappointments may be very revealing. Confrontation with the suspicion that she is causing the lesion herself will get nowhere, and the temptation to view the encounter in an adversarial way, by trying to 'catch the patient out' should be resisted. Judging the point at which to refer the patient to a psychiatrist can be difficult. If a good rapport has been established it may be possible to suggest that the lesion may be the effect of emotional problems (without accusing her of self mutilation) and subsequently share her care with a social worker. It is

important that the two therapists should maintain good communication with each other, as there may well be a tendency for the patient to play one off against the other.

Sexual violence

Rape

The Sexual Offences Act 1956 and 1976 Sexual Offences (Amendment) Act define rape as 'unlawful sexual intercourse with a woman without her consent and at that time the man knows that she does not consent to intercourse, or is reckless as to whether or not she consents to it'. It is further defined as sexual intercourse by fraud, threats, or if a woman is asleep, unconscious or mentally handicapped, or so young (under 16) as to be unable to understand the nature of the act. No age group from childhood to extreme old age is exempt. In practice, at least in the United Kingdom, probably most cases of rape go unreported because of fear of further distress caused by questioning, court appearances and reactions of relatives.

Injuries to the vulva may include bruising, fingernail scratches on the labia, dilatation of the introitus and sometimes rupture of the fourchette and perineum in young girls. Genital examination must be conducted with particular care because of the medicolegal implications (Knight 1976).

Trauma to the genitalia and other parts of the body, sexually transmitted disease and pregnancy will be anticipated complications, but the psychological trauma engendered by the experience of rape will, for most women, be the most serious effect, which can affect their lives for many years. At the time of the attack a woman may be literally paralysed by terror, fearing for her life. Others may resist violently (and perhaps suffer more physical injury thereby). The state of shock following the event may be shown by an immediate emotional response with a need to talk about it, while others will feel emotionally numb and be unable to communicate their distress. Surprisingly, some women carry on a normal life without telling anyone of their terrifying experience, but most will suffer nightmares, depression, feelings of unjustified guilt and shame, humiliation and anger. Reactions of relatives and friends, police and courts, and sometimes even doctors, may reinforce such feelings. The experience may lead to a temporary or long-lasting revulsion towards intercourse or any form of physical intimacy.

Many large towns in the United Kingdom now have rape crisis centres with a 24-hour emergency service. They offer invaluable advice to both women and the doctors treating them at the time of crisis, and also provide continuing psychological support (London Rape Crisis Centre 1984).

Sexual abuse in children

The current view is that this may be under-reported. Anal rather than, or as well as, vulval signs may be prominent and diagnostic (Hobbs and Wynne 1986). The question of abuse will arise when anogenital warts and mollusca (pp. 109, 125) are found, though in many cases there is probably no sexual connotation. Moreover, sexual factors may be wrongly invoked when some naturally occurring vulval condition is not recognised or is misinterpreted—for example lichen sclerosus et atrophicus (Handfield-Jones et al 1987) or (Hey et al 1986) Crohn's disease.

Accidental injury: haematomas

While similar lesions (Fig. 7.5) may follow rape, coital injury, non-accidental injury in children and indeed any form of trauma, many such cases are the result of falls on to sharp objects, damage from in-rush of water in water skiing and similar episodes.

Principles of treatment are noted on page 351.

Sexual re-assignment surgery

Female to male transexualism is rare. It has been estimated that of about 10 000 transexuals in the United States of America 4000 are female to male. About 400 female to male re-assignment operations were performed in 1980 in the United States (Lothstein 1982). Hoenig & Kenna (1974) have estimated from a survey in the Manchester region that the incidence of transexualism in England and Wales is 1 in 34 000 for males and 1 in 108 000 for females, suggesting that there are 181 female to male transexuals in this population.

Inevitably such cases attract publicity out of

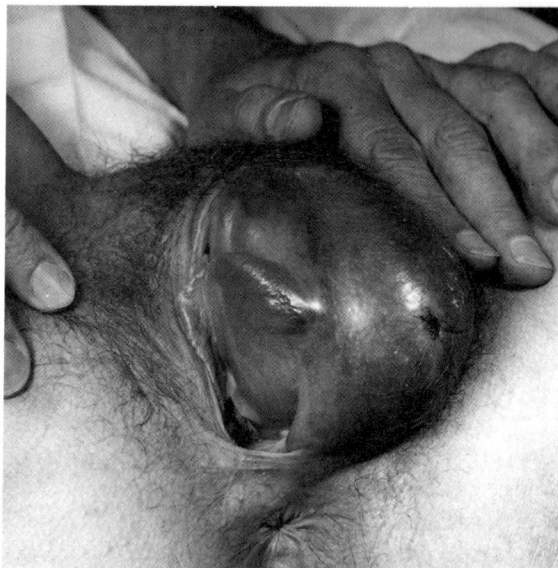

Fig. 7.5 Vulval haematoma (traumatic).

proportion to the incidence of the condition and complex social, psychological, ethical and legal issues are involved. It is controversial whether surgical attempts at constructing something approaching male genitalia are in the patient's interest though, in spite of the dearth of adequate follow-up studies, it might be justified in a small number of cases.

The typical patient has a conviction, from childhood, that she is psychologically a male trapped in a female body. She will be erotically attracted to women and will have the ambition to be a faithful husband. Masturbation is rarely practised because of a feeling of revulsion towards her genitalia, which are a constant reminder of femininity. Many such patients will live as men without resorting to surgery. Some will feel more relaxed by regular use of androgens which will suppress menses, cause deepening of the voice and growth of facial hair. Marked enlargement of the clitoris occurs and its erotic sensitivity increases. It is generally recommended (Money & Ambinder 1978) that no surgical intervention is made until the subject has undergone regular psychotherapy and lived as a male for 2 years. Some patients will be content with mastectomy, hysterectomy and oophorectomy; others will wish to proceed, in spite of the hazards of multiple operations, to the construction of an artificial phallus from skin grafts with a urinary tube. The clitoris is retained to allow orgasm (Money & Ambinder 1978). Davies (1985) has described these procedures.

Episiotomy

Between 1965 and 1973 the incidence of the use of episiotomy was found to have doubled from 24.4% to 46.7% in a study of obstetric practice in residents of Wales (Chalmers et al 1976), and episiotomy was performed in 62.5% of vaginal deliveries in the United States in 1979 (National Center of Health Statistics 1981). Thaker & Banta (1983) have summarised both the benefits and risks of episiotomy in a comprehensive review of the literature. Despite undeniable benefit in ease of delivery in a proportion of cases, the risk of infection, blood loss, poor anatomical results, postpartum pain and dyspareunia may well outweigh the benefits, and the authors concluded that arguments for the widespread use of episiotomy do not withstand scientific scrutiny.

Uncomplicated pregnancy entails many psychological adjustments to change of body image and episiotomy is seen as a further (and in many cases unnecessary) insult which leaves the woman feeling scarred both physically and psychologically. However small the actual cut may be, delays in suturing can interfere with the mother's first interaction with her baby, and pain and discomfort in the puerperium may disturb the establishment of breastfeeding. Dyspareunia shortly after delivery may cause a woman to lose confidence in her ability to have satisfying intercourse, which may persist long after any physical cause can be found for discomfort, which in turn may lead to marital disharmony and depression (Kitzinger 1981). However, antenatal and postpartum counselling about episiotomy may facilitate psychological adjustment (Reading et al 1983).

Vulvectomy

There have been very few studies of the psychosocial and sexual adjustment of patients who have undergone this severely disfiguring surgery. Di Saia et al (1979) reported on 18 patients treated with wide local excision rather than radical vulvectomy and found that all the patients maintained sexual responsiveness. A more detailed study has been made by Andersen & Hacker (1983) of 15 patients, aged between 50 and 70 years, who had undergone either total or partial vulvectomy. Psychological testing showed scores of depression comparable with other patients who had any form of cancer. Physical disabilities caused by leg oedema and urinary problems curtailed some social activities and there was a reduction of sexual activity and arousal. Numbness of the perineum and a loss of or failure to maintain orgasm (both with and without clitoral excision) contributed to this, leading, in some cases, to marital distress, disruption of body image and sexual anxiety.

A study by Moth et al (1983) of 14 women (aged between 32 and 60 years) who had undergone vulvectomy, and of nine of their sexual partners, revealed that although all the patients had had satisfactory sexual relationships before the operation about two-thirds reported dyspareunia and almost all some form of sexual dysfunction after the operation. The women disliked the appearance of the operation area and half of the men felt differently towards their wives' bodies. The women experienced reduced libido, depression and loss of self-confidence. The authors underlined the need for pre- and postoperative counselling for the patient and her partner to prepare them for the sexual problems likely to be encountered.

These points have been further stressed in a report by the same authors (Andreasson et al 1986) on a larger group; 25 women and 15 partners have now been studied following vulvectomy. More than half the women had both sexual dysfunction and psychological problems, while almost half the men had psychological problems.

The assumption that patients in the older age group will not wish to remain sexually active has been shown to be untrue, and it is noteworthy that many patients in these studies attempted to maintain a sexual life despite physical loss and emotional disruption.

Radiodermatitis

Radiation vaginitis may follow radiotherapy or radium therapy for the uterus, cervix or vagina, but radiotherapy is rarely used in the treatment of vulval malignancy, for vulval tissue is sensitive to X-rays and necrotic ulcers may result. Radiotherapy has in the recent past, however, been used to treat benign cutaneous vulval conditions such as lichen sclerosus et atrophicus, and the typical telangiectasia, atrophy and pigmentation can be recognised. Such tissue is recognised to be prone to the development of carcinoma.

REFERENCES

Andersen B L, Hacker N F 1983 Psychosexual adjustment after vulval surgery. Obstetrics and Gynecology 62: 457–62

Andreasson B, Moth I, Jensen S B, Bock J E 1986 Sexual function partners. Acta Obstetrica et Gynecologica Scandinavica 65: 7–10

Aziz F A 1980 Gynecologic and obstetric complications of female circumcision. International Journal of Gynaecology and Obstetrics 17: 560–563

Barksy A J, Klerman G L 1983 Overview: Hypochondriasis, bodily complaints and somatic styles. American Journal of Psychiatry 140: 273

Bartrop R W, Lazarus L, Luckhurst E, Kilah L G, Penny R 1977 Depressed lymphocyte function after bereavement. Lancet i: 834–836

Beard R W, Highman J A, Pearce S, Reginald P W 1984 Diagnosis of pelvic varicosities in women with chronic pelvic pain. Lancet ii: 946–949

Bebbington P E 1976 Monosymptomatic hypochondriasis, abnormal illness behaviour and suicide. British Journal of Psychiatry 128: 475–478

Bettelheim B 1954 Meaning of initiation, symbolic wounds: puberty rites and the envious male. Free Press, Glencoe Illinois, p 104–127

Bodkin M 1963 Archetypal patterns in poetry. Psychological Studies of Imagination. Oxford University Press

Bradley J J 1963 Severe localised pain associated with the depressive syndrome. British Journal of Psychiatry 109: 741–745

Chalmers I, Zlosnik J E, Johns K A et al 1976 Obstetric practice and outcome of pregnancy in Cardiff residents. British Medical Journal 1: 735

Cotterill J A 1983 Psychiatry and skin diseases. In: Rook A J, Maibach H I (eds) Recent advances in dermatology, No. 6. Churchill Livingstone, Edinburgh

Davies D M 1985 Plastic and reconstructive surgery: cosmetic surgery II. British Medical Journal 290: 1499–1501

Di Saia P J, Cressman W T, Rich W M 1979 An alternative approach to early cancer of the vulva. American Journal of Obstetrics and Gynecology 133: 825

Fitzpatrick R, Frost D, Ikkos C 1986 Survey of psychological disturbance in patients attending a sexually transmitted diseases clinic. Genitourinary Medicine 62: 111–115

French A P, Nelson H L 1972 Genital self-mutilation in women. Archives of General Psychiatry 27: 618–621

Friedrich E G 1983 The vulvar vestibule. Journal of Reproductive Medicine 28: 773–777

Friedrich E G 1987 Vulvar vestibulitis syndrome. Journal of Reproductive Medicine 82: 110–114

Frost D P 1985 Recognition of hypochondriasis in a clinic for sexually transmitted disease. Genitourinary Medicine 61: 133–137

Gardner H L, Kaufman R H 1981 Benign diseases of the vulva and vagina, 2nd edn. G K Hall, Boston, Massachusetts

Gelfand M 1973 Gross enlargement of the labia minora in an African female. Central African Journal of Medicine 19: (5) 101

Goldberg D P, Kay C, Thompson L 1976 Psychiatric morbidity in general practice and in the community. Psychological Medicine 656: 5–9

Graham H 1950 Eternal Eve. Heinemann London

Hall J G 1985 Emotion and immunity (correspondence). Lancet ii: 326–327

Hammond R, Johnson A 1984 Use of the carbon dioxide laser for relief of pruritus in vulval dystrophies. Journal of Obstetrics and Gynaecology 5: 125–126

Handfield-Jones S E, Hinde F J R, Kennedy C T C 1987 Lichen Sclerosus et atrophicus in children misdiagnosed as sexual abuse. British Medical Journal 294: 1404–1405

Healy T 1978 Those little perforations. World Medicine 14: 99–102

Hey F, Bucham P C, Littlewood J M, Hall R I 1986 Differential diagnosis in child sexual abuse. Lancet i: 283

Hobbs C J, Wynne J M 1986 Buggery in Childhood—common syndrome of child abuse. Lancet ii: 792–796

Hoenig J, Kenna J C 1974 The prevalence of transsexualism in England and Wales. British Journal of Psychiatry 124: 181–190

Hosken F 1979 The Hosken report: genital and sexual mutilation of females. Womens International Network News, Lexington, Mass

Junaid T A, Thomas S M 1981 Cysts of the vulva and vagina: a comparative study. International Journal of Gynaecology and Obstetrics 19: 239–243

Kampmeier R H 1984 Early development of knowledge of sexually transmitted disease. In: Holmes K K, Mårdh P-A, Sparling P F, Wiesner P G (eds) Sexually Transmitted Diseases. McGraw-Hill, New York, Ch 2, p 19

Kaufman R H, Friedrich E G 1985 The carbon dioxide laser in the treatment of vulvar disease. Clinical Obstetrics and Gynecology 28: 220–229

Kenyon F E 1976 Hypochondriacal states. British Journal of Psychiatry 129: 1–14

Kitzinger S 1981 Emotional aspects of episiotomy and postnatal sexual adjustment. In: Kitzinger S (ed) Episiotomy, physical and emotional aspects. National Childbirth Trust, London p 45–53

Knight B 1976 Sexual offences in legal aspects of medical practice, 2nd edn. Churchill Livingstone, London, ch 19, p 160–168

Krantz K E 1970 The anatomy and physiology of the vulva and vagina and the anatomy of the urethra and bladder. In: Philipp E E, Barnes J, Newton M (eds) Scientific foundations of obstetrics and gynaecology. Heinemann, London, section II, p 47

Kronfol Z, Silva J, Greden J, Dembinski S, Gardner R, Carroll B 1983 Impaired lymphocyte function in depressive illness. Life Science 33: 241–247

Lancet (editorial) 1985 Emotion and immunity. Lancet ii: 133–134

Lancet (editorial) 1987 Depression, stress and immunity. Lancet i: 1467–1468

Leonardo R A 1944 History of gynecology. Froben Press, New York

London Rape Crisis Centre 1984 Sexual violence. Women's Press Handbook Series, London

Lothstein L M 1982 Sex reassignment surgery: Historical, bioethical and theoretical issues. American Journal of Psychiatry 139: 417–426

Lucas C J, Sainsbury P, Collins J G 1962 A social and clinical study of delusions in schizophrenia. Journal of Mental Science 108: 747–758

Lyell A 1979 Cutaneous artefactual disease. A review, amplified by personal experience. Journal of the American Academy of Dermatology 1: 391–407

Lyell A 1983 The Michelson lecture: delusions of parasitosis. British Journal of Dermatology 108: 485–499

McKay M 1985 Vulvodynia versus pruritus vulvae. Clinical Obstetrics and Gynecology 28: 123–133

McKenna P J 1984 Disorders with overvalued ideas. British Journal of Psychiatry 145: 579–585

McLean S 1980 Female circumcision, excision and infibulation: The facts and proposals for change. Minority Rights Group Report No. 47, London

Mason-Hohl E 1940 The diseases of women, by Trotula of Salerno. Ward Ritchie, Los Angeles

Mering J H 1952 A surgical approach to intractable pruritus vulvae. American Journal of Obstetrics and Gynecology 64: 619

Mettler C C 1947 In: Mettler F A (ed) History of medicine Blakiston, Philadelphia, Toronto, ch 13 Obstetrics and gynecology, p 931, ch 10 Dermatology, p 661, ch 9 Venerology, p 601

Money J, Ambinder R 1978 Two year, real life diagnostic test rehabilitation versus cure. In: Brady J P, Brodie H K H (eds) Controversy in Psychiatry. W B Saunders, Philadelphia, p 833–845

Monro A 1980 Monosymptomatic hypochondriacal psychosis. British Journal of Hospital Medicine 24: 34–38

Moth I, Andreasson B, Jensen S B, Bock J E 1983 Sexual function and somato-psychic reactions after vulvectomy: a preliminary report. Danish Medical Bulletin 30: 27–30

National Centre for Health Statistics 1981 Data from the hospital discharge survey. (Furnished by Eileen McCarthy) Hyattsville, Maryland

Neill M E, Swash M 1982 Chronic perianal pain: an unsolved problem. Journal of the Royal Society of Medicine 75: 96–101

Observer 9 October 1982. Feature

Onuigbo W I B 1976 Vulval epidermoid cysts in the Igbos of Nigeria. Archives of Dermatology 112: 1405–1406

Peckham B M, Maki D G, Patterson J J, Hafez G-R 1986 Focal vulvitis: a characteristic syndrome and cause of dyspareunia. American Journal of Obstetrics and Gynecology 154: 855–864

Pedder J R, Goldberg D P 1970 A survey by questionnaire of psychiatric disturbance in patients attending a venereal disease clinic. British Journal of Venereal Diseases 46: 58–61

Ploss H H, Bartels M, Bartels P 1935 An historical gynaecological and anthropological compendium. Heinemann, London, ch VI The female genitalia: racial and ethnographical characteristics, p 276, anthropological, p 300

Pyka R E, Wilkinson E J, Friedrich E G, Crocker B P 1987 The histopathology of vulvar vestibulitis syndrome (in press)

Reading A E, Sledmere C M, Cox D N, Campbell S 1983 How women view post-episiotomy pain. British Medical Journal 284: 243–246

Reiss I L 1984 Human sexuality in sociological perspective. In: Holmes K K, Mårdh P-A, Sparling P F, Wiesner P G (eds) Sexually transmitted diseases. McGraw-Hill, New York, ch 4, p 39

Ricci J 1943 The genealogy of gynaecology 2000 BC–1800 AD. Blakiston, Philadelphia

Ricci J 1945 One hundred years of gynaecology 1800–1900. Blakiston, Philadelphia

Robboy S J, Ross J S, Prat J, Keh P C, Welch W R 1978 Urogenital sinus origin of mucinous and ciliated cysts of the vulva. Obstetrics and Gynecology 51: 347–351

Rowland Payne C M E, Harper J I, Farthing C E, Branfoot A C, Staughton R E 1985 Lipodystrophia centrifugalis. British Journal of Dermatology 113: Supplement 29 100–101

Savin J 1980 Itching. In: Rook A, Savin J (eds) Recent advances in dermatology 5. Churchill Livingstone, Edinburgh, p 221

Schliefer S J, Keller S E, Camerino M, Thornton J C, Stein M 1983 Suppression of lymphocyte stimulation following bereavement. Journal of American Medical Association 250: 374–377

Scott D 1978 Psychiatric aspects of sexual medicine. From Epilepsy 1978: Perspectives on epilepsy. Compiled by the British Epilepsy Association, Woking, pp 89–97

Selvin M 1984 Changing medical and societal attitudes toward sexually transmitted diseases: a historical overview. In: Holmes K K, Mårdh P-A, Sparling P F, Wiesner P G (eds) Sexually transmitted diseases. McGraw-Hill, New York, ch 1, p 3

Shandall A A 1967 Circumcision and infibulation of females. A general consideration of the problem and a clinical study of the complications in Sudanese women. Sudan Medical Journal 5: 178–212

Spencer S S, Spencer D D, Williamson P D, Mattson R H 1983 Sexual automatisms in complex partial seizures. Neurology 33: 527–533

Sutherst J R 1979 Treatment of pruritus vulvae by multiple intradermal injections on alcohol. A double-blind study. British Journal of Obstetrics and Gynaecology 86: 371–373

Thaker S B, Banta H D 1983 Benefits and risks of episiotomy: an interpretative review of the English language literature 1860–1980. Obstetrical and Gynecological Survey 38: (6) 322–338

Tovell H M M, Young A W 1978 Classification of vulvar diseases. Clinical Obstetrics and Gynecology 21: 955–961

Wallace H J 1971 Lichen sclerosus et atrophicus. Transactions of the St John's Hospital Dermatological Society 57: 9–30

Ward G D, Sutherst J R 1975 Pruritus vulvae: treatment by multiple intradermal alcohol injections. British Journal of Dermatology 93: 201–204

Webster J C Cited by Ricci 1945 q.v. p 419

Weisfogel E 1976 Battle with a unicorn. The burning vulva. Proceedings 3rd Congress International Society for the Study of Vulvar Disease

Whitlock F A 1976 Psychophysiological aspects of skin diseases. Major problems in dermatology, Vol. 8. W B Saunders, London, ch 7, p 110–127

Woodruff J D, Babaknia A 1979 Local alcohol injections of the vulva: discussion of 35 cases. Obstetrics and Gynecology 54: 512–514

Woodruff J D, Parmley T H 1983 Infection of the minor vestibular gland. Obstetrics and Gynecology 62: 609–612

Woodruff J D, Thompson B 1972 Local alcohol injections in the treatment of vulvar pruritus. Obstetrics and Gynecology 40: 18–20

Young A W 1984 Burning vulva syndrome: report of the ISSVD task force. Journal of Reproductive Medicine 29: 457

8

Tumour-like lesions and cysts of the vulva
H Fox and C H Buckley

TUMOUR-LIKE LESIONS

Ectopic tissues

Ectopic tissues in the vulva may not only mimic a true neoplasm by presenting as a localised mass but can themselves undergo neoplastic change.

Breast tissue

The presence of mammary tissue in the vulva, though rare, is the most frequently reported example of vulval ectopia, though strictly speaking the breast tissue is accessory rather than ectopic in nature. During the early stages of embryogenesis mammary tissue first appears as bilateral strap-like thickening of the epidermis (the 'mammary ridges') which extends from forelimb to hindlimb: this anlage usually persists to give rise to true breast tissue only in the thoracic region, the remainder of the ridge regressing by a process of atresia. Occasionally, however, atresia is incomplete and remnants of the mammary ridges persist away from the thoracic area and give rise to accessory breast tissue which is invariably situated along the so-called 'milk lines'. Accessory breast tissue may be associated with a nipple in the overlying skin.

Approximately 30 examples of vulval accessory breast tissue have been reported (Foushee & Pruitt 1967, Garcia et al 1978, Gugliotta et al 1983); the breast tissue is almost invariably situated in the labia majora, only one instance of localisation to the labia minora having been recorded (Mengert 1935), and has been associated with an overlying nipple in only two patients (Green 1936); the mammary tissue has been bilateral in 55% of cases.

Accessory vulval breast tissue may, occasionally, become clinically overt in young non-pregnant women who complain of cyclical swelling of, or discomfort in, the vulval area during the luteal phase of the menstrual cycle. Such cases are, however, exceptional and the vast majority of patients present with a vulval swelling during the later months of pregnancy; the masses may be firm or apparently cystic, are freely mobile, are not tethered to the overlying skin and can measure anything from 1 to 8 cm in diameter. Curiously, breast tissue does not usually present clinically during a first pregnancy, swelling commonly only occurring in later gestations.

A history of localised vulval swelling during late pregnancy should clearly arouse a clinical suspicion of accessory breast tissue, but nevertheless this condition is so rare that most vulval swellings in the pregnant woman will be due to other causes. The diagnosis is confirmed only by histological examination, which will reveal typical breast tissue showing physiological hyperplasia; some degree of secretory activity is usually apparent and in cases biopsied during the puerperium the mammary tissue characteristically shows well-marked lactationary change. It would be expected that a swelling due to pregnancy changes in accessory breast tissue would spontaneously regress after gestation and lactation, but in fact this is far from being inevitable and several patients have required extirpation of a persistent vulval mass many months after completion of their pregnancy and lactational period.

Accessory breast tissue in the vulva may present in non-pregnant women, largely because a pathological process has developed in the mammary tissue. Several examples of 'fibrocystic disease' in vulval breast tissue have been documented (Bell 1926, Dubrauzky 1960), this diagnosis being based largely upon the development of cystic change in the

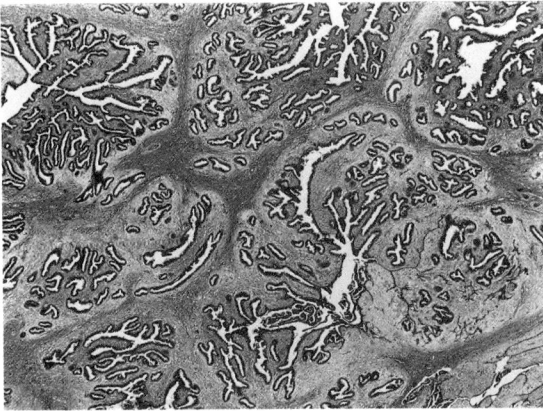

Fig. 8.1 A fibroadenoma developing in accessory vulval breast tissue. (H & E ×12)

mammary tissue. A number of fibro-adenomas arising in vulval breast tissue have also been described (Friedel 1932, Roth 1936, Fisher 1947, Siegler & Gordon 1951, Burger & Marcuse 1954, Foushee & Pruitt 1967, Hassim 1969); these vulval fibroadenomas were histologically identical with, or very similar to, those which commonly occur in normally sited breast tissue, but in very few, if any, of these cases had a definite origin from breast tissue been demonstrated. The presence of a fibroadenoma in the vulva does not necessarily mean that it has arisen from ectopic breast tissue for neoplasms of similar type can be derived from apocrine sweat glands. Hence a mammary origin in this site can be accepted only if there is clear evidence of derivation from non-neoplastic mammary tissue (Fig. 8.1); none of the reported cases fully meets this far from stringent criterion.

An intraductal papilloma developing in supernumerary vulval breast tissue has been described (Rickert 1980); this clearly arose within mammary lobules but the tumour closely resembled a papillary hidradenoma; this raises the possibility that some vulval lesions classed as papillary hidradenomas may in reality be papillomas of mammary origin. A number of mammary-type adenocarcinomas of the vulva, thought to have originated in accessory breast tissue, have also been documented (Green 1936, Hendrix & Behrman 1956: Guerry & Pratt-Thomas 1976, Guercio et al 1984, Cho et al 1985). In only one of these cases, however, was a definite derivation of the neoplasm from breast tissue established (Hendrix & Behrman 1956), the origin in the other cases being presumptive rather than proved. It has to be borne in mind that an adenocarcinoma derived from skin appendages may resemble a breast neoplasm and that, admittedly rarely, a carcinoma of the breast can metastasise to the vulva; the patient described by Guerry & Pratt-Thomas (1985) was suffering from bilateral carcinoma of the breast as well as having a vulvar adenocarcinoma and, as all three tumours were histologically identical, the decision that the vulval tumour was primary rather than metastatic appears to have been totally arbitrary. The tumour reported by Cho et al (1985) contained oestrogen receptors and stained positively for milk fat globulin protein; neither of these features, either singly or in combination, are, however, specific for tumours of mammary origin.

Salivary tissues

One example of salivary glandular tissue presenting as a vulval mass has been described (Marwah & Berman 1980). The salivary tissue was regarded as being ectopic in nature but, as it was associated with respiratory-type epithelium and cartilage, the true nature of this lesion is uncertain.

Nodular fasciitis

This is a benign proliferation of fibroblasts which is often mistaken for a sarcoma. It occurs most commonly in young adults and has a particular propensity for the upper limbs and trunk. The presenting complaint is usually of a rapidly growing nodule or mass which is often painful or tender, the history commonly being measured in weeks rather than months. The lesions are generally well circumscribed and measure less than 3 cm in diameter; the cut surface may be firm or gelatinous. Histologically the lesions consist predominantly of plump fibroblasts which resemble closely those seen in granulation tissue (Fig. 8.2); these cells are arranged in bundles and fascicles which are separated from each other by a myxoid stroma. There is often a mild or moderate lymphocytic infiltrate, and intercellular clefts, occasional cyst-like spaces, numerous small blood vessels and a generous sprinkling of mitotic figures are all characteristic

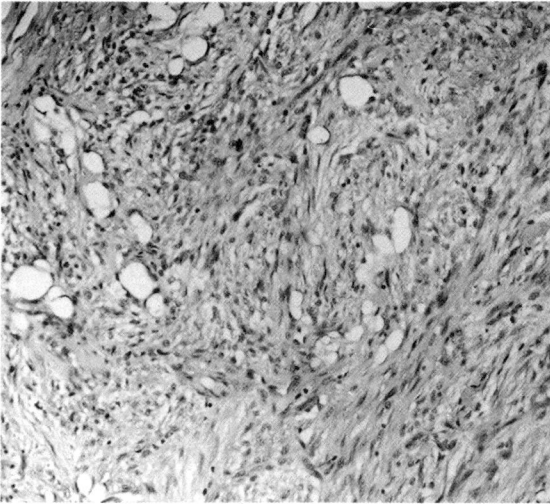

Fig. 8.2 Nodular fasciitis. Fibrocystic cells are arranged in fascicles and are infiltrating fat. (H & E ×70)

features. The cause of nodular fasciitis is unknown, though a widely held hypothesis is that the fibro-blastic proliferation represents a reaction to either injury or an inflammatory process. Nodular fasciitis is benign and almost invariably cured by local excision; incomplete removal may be followed, though rarely, by recurrence within a short time (Enzinger & Weiss 1983).

Only four cases of nodular fasciitis of the vulva have been fully documented (Roberts & Daly 1981, Gaffney et al 1982, Li Volsi & Brooks 1987), whilst one further example has been briefly alluded to in a large series of patients with this lesion (Allen 1972).

All the fully reported patients presented with a short history of a labial mass; they had mobile subcutaneous nodules, one being slightly tender, which measured 2 to 3 cm in diameter. In each case treatment was by wide local excision and the women were alive and well with no evidence of local recurrence, at intervals varying from 6 months to 2 years after treatment.

Desmoid tumour

This term is applied to a form of localised fibromatosis, which, though histologically bland, can attain a large size, tends to infiltrate neighbouring tissues and frequently recurs. The lesion tends to present as a deep-seated, firm, rapidly growing, non-tender subcutaneous mass and occurs most frequently in patients aged between 25 and 35 years. On section the mass is firm and white, often resembling scar tissue. It is poorly circumscribed and is formed of sweeping bundles of elongated, slender, spindle-shaped cells showing no atypia or mitotic activity which are separated from each other by abundant collagen. The infiltrative nature of this lesion often results in inadequate local excision and hence recurrence is common.

Only a single example of a desmoid tumour of the vulva has been described (Kfuri et al 1981). This arose in the right labium majus of a 19-year-old woman as an indurated mass measuring 7 × 2 cm; somewhat unusually for a lesion of this type the lesion was both painful and tender. The desmoid tumour described in this case developed at the site of a previous surgical exploration when what appeared to be inflammatory and scar tissue was removed; the true nature of the original lesion was therefore in some doubt but the vulval mass present 3 years later was clearly a desmoid tumour and hence was possibly a recurrence. The patient was treated, apparently successfully, by wide local excision.

Verruciform xanthoma

This epithelial lesion, which can mimic a squamous cell carcinoma, presents as a cauliflower-like, verrucous or papillomatous nodule. It is characterised histologically by uniform acanthosis without atypia, parakeratosis and an accumulation of foamy xanthomatous cells within the papillary dermis between, but not deep to, the acanthotic rete ridges. This benign lesion, which is of unknown aetiology and pathogenesis, is found most commonly in the oral cavity, but two examples have been reported as occurring in the vulval skin (Santa Cruz & Martin 1979). The first of these patients, aged 29 years, had noticed multiple warty lesions of the vulva for 17 years and was diagnosed clinically as suffering from multiple condylomata acuminata. The second patient, aged 43 years, presented with a polypoid sessile mass measuring 1.5 cm in diameter, near to the clitoris; this lesion was diagnosed clinically as a squamous cell carcinoma. In both these cases the correct diagnosis only became apparent on histological examination.

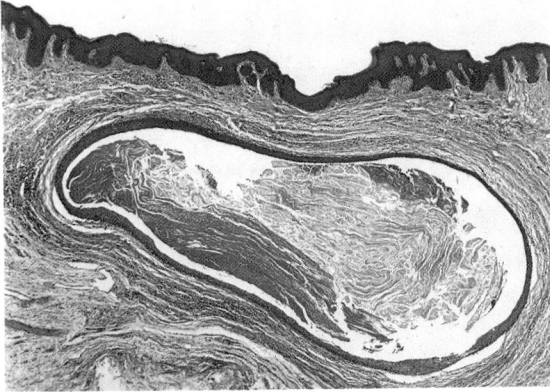

Fig. 8.3 Histological appearances of an epidermoid cyst of the vulva. The cyst is lined by squamous epithelium and contains keratinous material. (H & E ×25)

'Endometrioma'

This rather unsatisfactory term, implying as it does a neoplastic process, is used to describe the presence in the vulva of functional endometriosis. Vulval endometriosis has been reported following episiotomy and has occurred following implantation of menstrual fragments into a vulval surgical wound (Catherwood & Cohen 1951, Duson & Zelenik 1954). When it is found in the labia majora it is thought perhaps that endometrial metaplasia has occurred in the canal of Nuck or that menstrual fragments may have migrated along the canal (Janovski & Douglas 1972).

The lesion may be blue/purple and cystic or form a deep-seated, ill-defined firm or fluctuant mass, usually in the area of Bartholin's gland or the posterior fourchette. Cyclical swelling and discomfort have been reported in some cases and histological examination reveals the typical appearance of endometrial tissue with an associated fibrous response and accumulation of haemosiderin-laden macrophages (Novak & Woodruff 1979). Occasionally the covering skin may become ulcerated.

NON-NEOPLASTIC CYSTS OF THE VULVA

Cysts of the vulva may arise in developmental remnants, can form following blockage of gland ducts or may be the result of epithelial inclusions. They

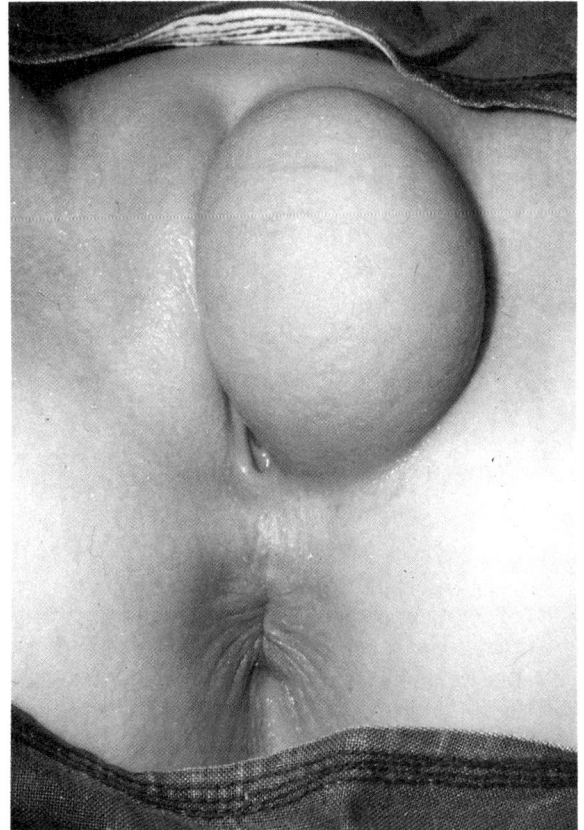

Fig. 8.4 An epidermoid cyst of the vulva. (By courtesy of Professor Sir John Dewhurst).

may also develop in endometriotic foci (Fox & Buckley 1982).

Epidermoid cysts

Cysts lined by stratified squamous epithelium and containing yellowish, grey-white, flaky or greasy, laminated keratinous debris occur most frequently in the labia majora (Fig. 8.3). In this site it is uncertain whether they are primary keratinous cysts or whether they have developed from ducts of sebaceous glands which have undergone squamous metaplasia. In the perineal area, they are most commonly the result of epithelial inclusions in obstetric scars.

Epidermoid cysts form discrete, often multiple, firm intradermal nodules which are usually tethered to the covering epithelium (Fig. 8.4). The cysts are benign, but on rare occasions squamous

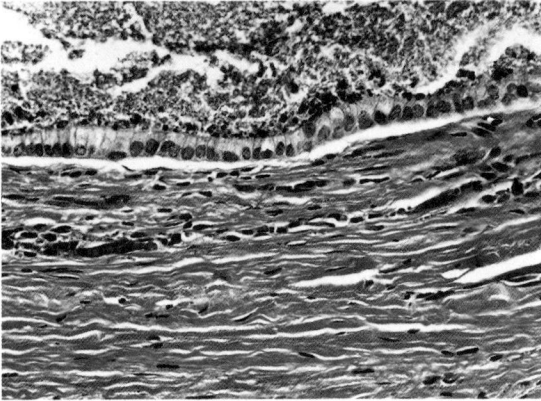

Fig. 8.5 A mucinous cyst of the vulva. The cyst is lined by columnar mucus-secreting cells and the cyst cavity (above) contains mucinous material. (H & E ×20)

carcinoma may develop within them (Novak & Woodruff 1979) and, not uncommonly, the cysts may leak, their contents eliciting a foreign-body inflammatory response in the adjacent stroma. The latter may result in partial or complete loss of the epithelial lining of the cyst, complete or partial disruption of the cyst and local scarring of the skin.

Cysts resulting from sebaceous gland blockage

These cysts, as distinct from epidermoid cysts with which they are commonly confused because of the similarity of their clinical appearance and distribution, result from the blockage of one or more of the numerous sebaceous glands of the labia majora and minora (Fig. 6.16 a and b). Unlike epidermoid cysts, they are commonly surmounted by a punctum through which the cyst contents may leak leading to crusting. The cysts are lined by squamous epithelium showing sebaceous differentiation and contain greasy yellow material. It is not unusual for these cysts to become infected and the resulting inflammation may result in loss of the lining epithelium and a foreign body response in the adjacent stroma as it does with the epidermoid cysts.

Mucinous cysts

Mucinous cysts are lined by a mucus-secreting columnar epithelium which may show focal squamous metaplasia (Fig. 8.5). They are not uncommon in

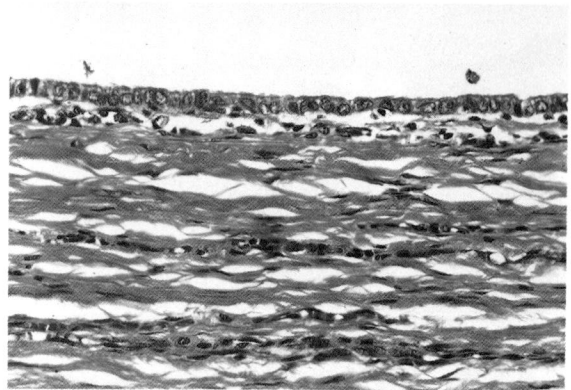

A

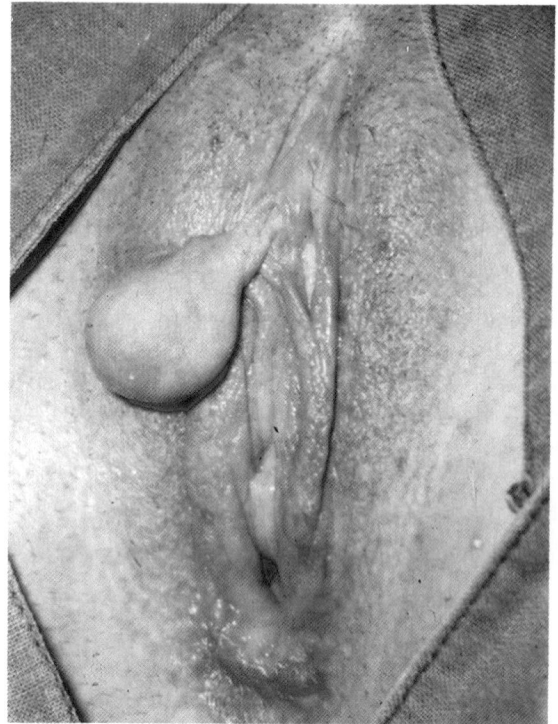

B

Fig. 8.6 (a) A mesonephric (Gartner's duct) cyst. The cyst is lined by a tall cuboidal epithelium and smooth muscle is present in the cyst wall (H & E ×240). (b) A developmental cyst.

the vestibule where they develop secondary to obstruction of the duct of one of the many minor mucus-secreting glands or from dysontogenetic urogenital sinus epithelium. The characteristics of the mucin are consistent with such an origin and are at variance with the older concept that the cysts are of Müllerian origin.

Mesonephric (Gärtner's duct) cysts

Cysts which develop from the remnants of the mesonephric duct arise in the lateral parts of the vulva. They are thin walled, contain clear colourless fluid and are lined by a cuboidal or low columnar epithelium; smooth muscle can be identified within their walls (Fig. 8.6 a and b).

Cysts of the canal of Nuck

These cysts develop from a peritoneal fragment or remnant which is carried into the labium majus by the round ligament as it passes from the abdominal cavity through the inguinal canal. The cysts occur in the upper part of the labium major and are lined by a single layer of flattened mesothelium.

Local excision of the cystic lesions described above is appropriate and adequate treatment. Some, however, are multiple and repeat excision may be necessary in some cases.

Bartholin's gland cyst

These cysts develop as a consequence of obstruction to the main duct of Bartholin's gland, which results in retention of secretion (Friedrich & Wikinson 1982). The cysts may measure anything from 1 to 10 cm in diameter and are found in the posterior part of the labium major. They contain clear, watery mucoid material and are lined by

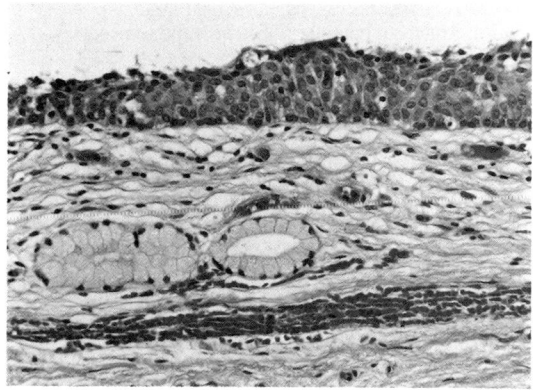

Fig. 8.7 A cyst of Bartholin's gland duct. The cyst is lined by transitional epithelium. (H & E ×195)

transitional epithelium which frequently undergoes partial or complete squamous metaplasia; compressed mucus-secreting glandular acini may be found in the cyst wall (Fig. 8.7).

Cysts of this type are prone to repeated infection and this may result in the formation of a Bartholin's gland abscess. Marsupialisation of the cyst will usually permit complete resolution of the infection but it must be remembered, although it is an uncommon happening, that carcinoma of Bartholin's gland may first present as a Bartholin's gland cyst due to ductal obstruction or abscess formation, and excision of the entire infected or cystic gland is to be recommended, particularly in the older patient.

REFERENCES

Allen P W 1972 Nodular fasciitis. Pathology 4: 9–26
Bell J W 1926 Supernumerary breast near labium. American Journal of Obstetrics and Gynecology 11: 507–509
Burger R A, Marcuse P M 1954 Fibroadenoma of vulva. American Journal of Clinical Pathology 24: 965–968
Catherwood A E, Cohen E S 1951 Endometriosis with decidual reaction in episiotomy scar. American Journal of Obstetrics and Gynecology 62: 1364–1366
Cho D, Buscema J, Rosenhein N B, Woodruff J D 1985 Primary breast cancer of the vulva. Obstetrics and Gynecology 66: 765–815
Dubrauzky V 1960 Gestielte Zystenmamma auf der Basis einer Brusedrusen anlage in der recuten Schamlippe. Zentralblatt für Gynakologie 82: 558–563
Duson C K, Zelenik J S 1954 Vulvar endometriosis apparently produced by menstrual blood. Obstetrics and Gynecology 3: 76–79
Enzinger F M, Weiss S W 1983 Soft tissue tumors. C V Mosby, St Louis

Fisher J H 1947 Fibroadenoma of supernumerary mammary gland tissue in vulva. American Journal of Obstetrics and Gynecology 53: 335–337
Foushee J H S, Pruitt A B 1967 Vulvar fibroadenoma from aberrant breast tissue. Obstetrics and Gynecology 29: 819–823
Fox H, Buckley C H 1982 Pathology for gynaecologists. Edward Arnold, London
Friedel R 1932 Ein Fibroadenom einer Nebenbrustdruse im rechten Labium Majus. Virchows Archiv 286: 62–69
Friedrich E G Jr, WIlkinson E J 1982 The vulva. In: Blaustein A (ed) Pathology of the female genital tract. Springer-Verlag, Berlin
Gaffney E F, Majmudar B, Bryan J A 1982 Nodular (pseudo-sarcomatous) fasciitis of the vulva. International Journal of Gynecological Pathology 1: 307–312
Garcia J J, Verkauf B S, Hochberg C J, Ingram J M 1978 Aberrant breast tissue of the vulva: a case report and review of the literature. Obstetrics and Gynecology 52: 225–228
Green H J 1936 Adenocarcinoma of supernumerary breasts of

the labia majora in a case of epidermoid carcinoma of the vulva. American Journal of Obstetrics and Gynecology 31: 660–663

Guercio F, Cesone P, Saracino A, Gatti M, Arisio R, Oberto F 1984 Adenocarcinoma in soto su ghandola mammaria aberrente in sede vulvare. Minerva Ginecologica 36: 315–319

Guerry R L, Pratt-Thomas H R 1976 Carcinoma of supernumerary breast of vulva with bilateral mammary cancer. Cancer 38: 2570–2574

Gugliotta P, Fibbi M, Fessia L, Canevini P, Bussolati G 1983 Lactating supernumerary mammary gland tissue in the vulva. Applied Pathology 1: 61–65

Hassim A M 1969 Bilateral fibroadenoma in supernumerary breasts of the vulva. Journal of Obstetrics and Gynaecology of the British Commonwealth 76: 275–277

Hendrix R C, Behrman S J 1956 Adenocarcinoma arising in a supernumerary mammary gland in the vulva. Obstetrics and Gynecology 8: 238–241

Janovski N A, Douglas C P 1972 Diseases of the vulva. Harper & Row, Maryland

Kfuri A, Rosenhein N, Durfman H, Goldstein P 1981 Desmoid tumor of the vulva. Journal of Reproductive Medicine 26: 272–273

Li Volsi VA, Brooks J J 1987 Nodular fasciitis of the vulva: a report of two cases. Obstetrics and Gynecology 69: 513–516

Marwah S, Berman M L 1980 Ectopic salivary gland in the vulva (choristoma): report of a case and review of the literature. Obstetrics and Gynecology 56: 389–391

Mengert W F 1935 Supernumerary mammary gland tissue on labia minora. American Journal of Obstetrics and Gynecology 29: 891–892

Novak E R, Woodruff J D 1979 Gynecologic and obstetric pathology, 8th edn. W B Saunders, Philadelphia, p 1–58

Rickert R R 1980 Intraductal papilloma arising in supernumerary vulvar breast tissue. Obstetrics and Gynecology 55: 84S–85S

Roberts W, Daly J W 1981 Pseudosarcomatous fasciitis of the vulva. Gynecologic Oncology 11: 383–386

Roth V 1936 Zystischen Adenofibrom auf der Basis einer persistierenden Brustdrusenanlage in der linken grossen Schamlippe. Zeitschrift für Geburstshilfe 112: 245–251

Santa Cruz D J, Martin S A 1979 Verruciform xanthoma of the vulva. American Journal of Clinical Pathology 71: 224–228

Siegler A M, Gordon R 1951 Fibroadenoma in a supernumerary breast of the vulva. American Journal of Obstetrics and Gynecology 62: 1367–1369

9

Non-epithelial and mixed tumours of the vulva
H Fox and C H Buckley

NON-EPITHELIAL TUMOURS

Mesenchymal neoplasms

All mesenchymal neoplasms of the vulva are either rare or extremely uncommon and for only a few tumours have sufficient cases been described to allow for any rational consideration of their natural history and prognosis when occurring at this site. Virtually all mesenchymal tumours, whether benign or malignant, present as enlarging, but otherwise asymptomatic, vulval masses which usually defy specific clinical diagnosis. Indeed, the clinical picture of these tumours may be extremely misleading for benign mesenchymal tumours, which are not uncommonly pedunculated because of the effects of gravity, may become ulcerated and secondarily infected, a not unexpected outcome in view of the effects of local moisture and warmth together with friction from tight underclothes. A benign tumour with an ulcerated surface and secondary infection producing reactive enlargement of regional lymph nodes can clearly impart a false impression of malignancy.

In general terms, vulval sarcomas occur principally in the labia majora, span a very wide age range from infancy to old age and do not show specific or diagnostic gross features. Haematogenous metastasis to the lungs is a common feature but spread to the regional lymph nodes is very variable.

In virtually all mesenchymal tumours diagnosis is dependent upon the histopathological findings. Unfortunately, accurate identification of many sarcomas by morphological critera alone can be difficult or even impossible, whilst electron microscopy is of only limited value in many of these neoplasms. Fortunately, greater accuracy is now attainable by immunohistochemical techniques using a range of antisera directed against soft-tissue marker antigens. The range and specificity of this technique are rapidly expanding and the topic has been the subject of a recent comprehensive review (Du Boulay 1985).

Tumours of smooth muscle

Leiomyoma. Benign smooth muscle neoplasms can arise in the vulva and are generally similar to their more commonly occurring counterparts in the uterine body; histologically, they are composed of smooth muscle fibres forming bundles and whorls; and there is often a pallisading arrangement with some interdigitating in a 'herring bone' fashion. The tumour cells are elongated with spindle-shaped nuclei and, by definition, have well-circumscribed, non-infiltrating margins, show little or no pleomorphism or atypia and contain less than two mitotic figures per ten high power fields (Tavassoli & Norris 1979).

Several histological variants of the conventional leiomyoma occur in the vulva and merit special attention. Cellular leiomyomas (Fig. 9.1) contain densely-packed spindle cells with elongated nuclei whilst epithelioid leiomyomas are formed of polygonal cells which have a centrally placed nucleus and clear, slightly vacuolated, cytoplasm (Fig. 9.2); neurolemmoma-like leiomyomas and symplastic leiomyomas, which contain large, bizarre, multinucleated cells, are now well recognised and can occur in the vulva.

Vulval leiomyomas are relatively uncommon and only about 70 examples have been recorded (Lovelady et al 1941, Palermino, 1964, Riedel 1964, Tavassoli & Norris 1979, Smit et al 1984), although

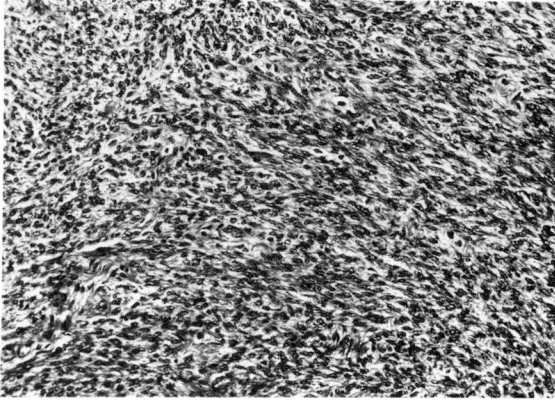

Fig. 9.1 A cellular leiomyoma. The neoplasm shows a much greater degree of cellularity than that encounted in a conventional leiomyoma but there is no pleomorphism or excess mitotic activity. These tumours are benign. (H & E ×120)

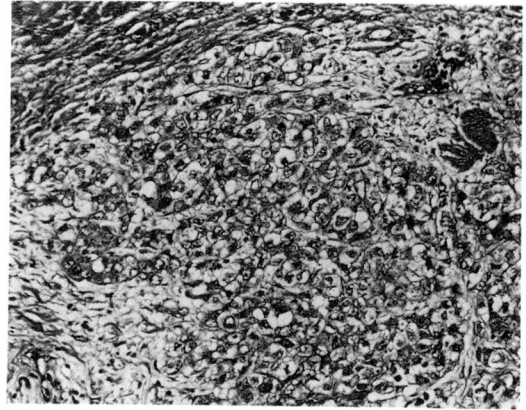

Fig. 9.2 An epithelioid leiomyoma. Many of the smooth muscle cells are polygonal and have abundant cytoplasm. (H & E ×120)

it is certain that many, if not most, such neoplasms now pass without specific comment. There is no known association with uterine leiomyomas and it is far from clear whether these tumours originate from the smooth muscle of the vulval erectile tissue, from the muscular elements of the round ligament or from the myo-epithelial cells of Bartholin's gland; most arise, however, in the labia majora and leiomyomas limited to the clitoris (Stenchever et al 1973) or Bartholin's gland (Tavassoli & Norris 1979, Katenkamp & Stiller 1980) are distinctly rare.

Vulval leiomyomas appear during the reproductive years and usually present as well-circumscribed, painless, non-tender nodules or swellings in the labia; they have a tendency to enlarge during pregnancy and are formed of firm, white whorled tissue. The absence of pain is a notable feature in view of the fact that cutaneous leiomyomas elsewhere are often exquisitely painful (Thompson 1985). The histological criteria, discussed below, for recognizing those vulval smooth muscle tumours which are likely to behave as low grade leiomyosarcomas are far from absolute (Tavassoli & Norris 1979) and hence all vulval leiomyomas should be treated by wide local excision.

Two cellular leiomyomas of the vulva have been described (Kaufman & Gardner 1965), one in a girl of 13 years of age and the other in a 35-year-old woman; neither neoplasm showed any cellular atypia or excess mitotic activity and both patients were apparently permanently cured by wide local excision. Two instances of an epithelioid leiomyoma of the vulva have been reported (Tavassoli & Norris 1979, Aneiros et al 1982); one arose in a 26-year-old woman who was well and tumour free one year after surgical excision, whilst the other, in a 25-year-old patient, recurred despite an absence of atypia or any excess of mitotic figures. Epithelioid leiomyomas, just as is the case with uterine smooth muscle tumours of similar type, should therefore be regarded as being more aggressive than conventional leiomyomas.

Leiomyosarcoma. Malignant smooth muscle neoplasms of the vulva take two forms. One is that of a clearly sarcomatous tumour with considerable pleomorphism and mitotic activity which may or may not be easily recognised as being of smooth muscle origin, whilst the other resembles closely a leiomyoma but nevertheless behaves in a malignant fashion (Fig. 9.3).

Easily recognisable leiomyosarcomas of the vulva, showing unmistakable histological evidence of malignancy, are rare, only 14 examples having been reported (DiSaia et al 1971, Davos & Abell 1976, Verhaegh et al 1977, Audet-Lapointe et al 1980, Smit et al 1984). These tumours have occurred in women aged from 35 to 84 years though the mean age at initial presentation was 51.6 years. Patients with a neoplasm of this type generally present with a progressively enlarging mass or nodule in the vulval

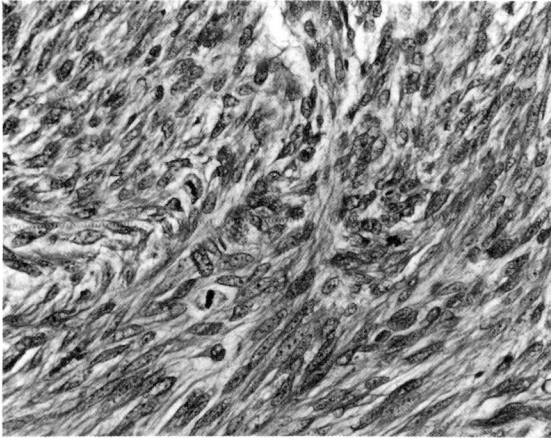

Fig. 9.3 A leiomyosarcoma in which many mitotic figures are present. There is, however, relatively little pleomorphism. (H & E ×240)

area and the length of the history is usually less than 12 months. Most leiomyosarcomas arise in the labia though some have been localised to the posterior fourchette or to the area of Bartholin's gland. In most of the reported cases initial treatment was by local excision and the true diagnosis was only recognised on histological examination. Only one of the 14 reported patients did not suffer tumour recurrence after initial local excision, this woman being alive and well 2½ years later. Six other patients were subjected to multiple local excisions for recurrent tumour or to radical surgery supplemented, in one instance, by radiotherapy, and were alive at intervals ranging from 2 to 6 years after initial treatment (though one of these women was known to have pulmonary metastases). Seven patients succumbed to their tumour, the length of survival ranging from 6 months to 16 years and death being usually due to pulmonary, hepatic or skeletal metastases. In most of these fatal cases initial local excision had been followed by radical vulvectomy supplemented, in many instances, by either radiotherapy, chemotherapy or by both modes of therapy. In some of these fatal cases radical surgery had been undertaken immediately after histological recognition of the true nature of the neoplasm, whilst in others this more aggressive approach had been delayed until tumour recurrence was apparent.

Clearly, the management of overtly malignant smooth muscle neoplasms of the vulva is somewhat unsatisfactory for it appears that the eventual outcome is related more to the inherent biological malignancy of the individual tumour than to the results obtained by any specific form of therapy. Quite obviously, however, local excision, even with wide margins, is an inadequate form of therapy and definitive treatment should almost certainly be by radical vulvectomy, probably with bilateral groin lymph node dissection. There is no clear-cut evidence that either radiotherapy or chemotherapy has any significant effect either in reducing the risk of recurrence or in the treatment of recurrent disease.

All the tumours discussed so far were overtly malignant and can be regarded as leiomyosarcomas of high grade malignancy. Tavassoli & Norris (1979) looked at the question of malignancy in smooth muscle neoplasms of the vulva from a quite different viewpoint. These workers studied 32 vulval neoplasms which were quite clearly of smooth muscle nature and attempted to define criteria for the recognition of those neoplasms which, whilst not having any obvious potentiality for metastatic spread, would nevertheless tend to behave as low grade leiomyosarcomas and recur locally after initial excision. They concluded that those neoplasms measuring more than 5 cm in diameter, having infiltrating margins and containing more than five mitotic figures per ten high power fields are very likely to recur and that tumours showing all these three features should be regarded as leiomyosarcomas and treated as such, this diagnosis being made irrespective of the degree, if any, of cellular atypia. Neoplasms showing two of these three features should be regarded as low grade leiomyosarcomas. Tavassoli & Norris point out, however, that smooth muscle tumours of the vulva can recur despite the absence of all three of these morphological indications of aggressive behaviour and that all leiomyomatous neoplasms should therefore be treated by wide local excision rather than by enucleation. Those neoplasms meriting a diagnosis of low grade leiomyosarcoma will tend to show a pattern of repetitive local recurrence and it is a moot point whether they should be treated by repeated local excisions or by radical vulvectomy.

A particular variant of malignant smooth muscle neoplasms of the vulva deserves specific mention,

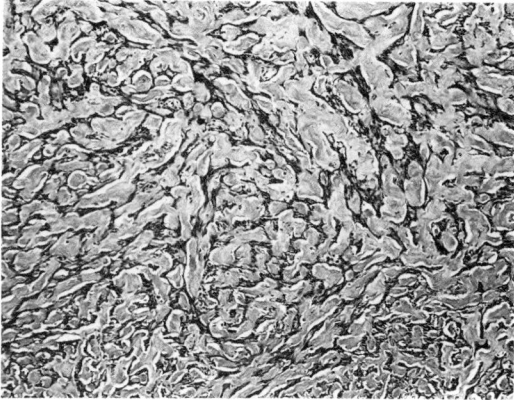

Fig. 9.4 A myxoid leiomyosarcoma. The tumour cells are separated by abundant myxoid tissue. Despite their lack of pleomorphism and mitotic activity these neoplasms behave in a malignant fashion. (H & E ×230)

this being the myxoid leiomyosarcoma (Fig. 9.4), two examples of which have been reported as occurring in the vulva (Salm & Evans 1985). These neoplasms differ from leiomyomas with myxoid change only in their relatively large size and their infiltrating margins for they do not commonly show any excess of mitotic figures. Of the two examples reported in the vulva, one was in an 88-year-old woman who died from unrelated causes 1 year after excision of the tumour without any evidence of local recurrence. The other was in a patient aged 57 years and recurred 1 year after local excision. These neoplasms have, in general terms, a high incidence of recurrence and a potentiality for distant metastasis; they should probably be treated as high grade leiomyosarcomas.

Tumours of striated muscle

Rhabdomyomas. Benign tumours of striated muscle are extremely uncommon. Two main types are recognised, the adult rhabdomyoma, formed of large round or polygonal cells with abundant granular cytoplasm, and the fetal rhabdomyoma, formed of elongated spindle cells which recapitulate the developmental stages of striated muscle. Some fetal rhabdomyomas have an abundant myxoid stroma whilst others are formed of densely packed interlacing fascicles of cells. The adult rhabdomyoma occurs almost exclusively in the head and neck area of adult men (usually over 40

years of age) whilst the fetal rhabdomyosarcoma develops principally in the head and neck area of males aged less than 3 years.

In recent years it has, however, become apparent that a significant proportion of rhabdomyomas occur in the vulvovaginal region in women aged between 20 and 50 years; there is some dispute as to whether these vulvovaginal rhabdomyomas are myxoid fetal rhabdomyomas, as suggested by Di Sant Agnese & Knowles (1980), or represent a specific type of rhabdomyoma, this latter view being espoused by Enzinger & Weiss (1983). These vulvovaginal tumours do appear to have distinctive clinical and histological features, and the delineation of a specific entity of 'genital rhabdomyoma' has considerable merit. These neoplasms, if indeed they are neoplasms rather than hamartomas or examples of reactive hyperplasia, usually present as asymptomatic nodules, rarely measure more than 3 cm in diameter and form a polypoid mass covered by epithelium. Histologically they are formed of relatively mature striated muscle fibres with distinct cross-striations; these fibres are separated by varying amounts of myxoid stroma and collagen.

Only two of the reported genital rhabdomyomas have arisen in the vulva rather than in the vagina (Di Sant Agnese & Knowles 1980). One was an asymptomatic nodule present for 1 year in a 24-year-old woman and the other presented as a nodule of 3 years duration in an episiotomy scar. In both cases local excision was curative.

Rhabdomyosarcoma. Rhabdomyosarcomas are highly malignant, rapidly growing neoplasms which not only spread at an early stage via the blood stream but also commonly metastasise to lymph nodes. Three histological types have been recognised: embryonic, alveolar and pleomorphic, the first two occurring principally in children and young adults and the last having a rather wider age range. The embryonal rhabdomyosarcoma tends to form oedematous, polypoid masses and usually has a myxoid stroma in which tumour cells may be sparse and widely scattered or abundant and closely packed. The tumour cells may be round or spindle shaped and show considerable pleomorphism (Fig. 9.5). Alveolar rhabdomyosarcomas are formed principally of round cells with scanty cytoplasm which are separated off into lobules by fibrous septa; central necrosis within these lobules imparts an

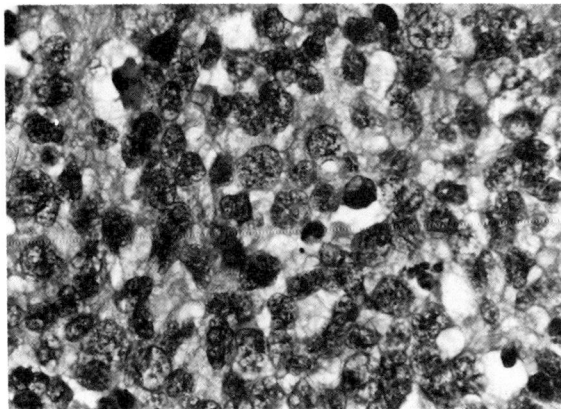

Fig. 9.5 Closely packed small round cells in an embryonal rhabdomyosarcoma. (H & E ×490)

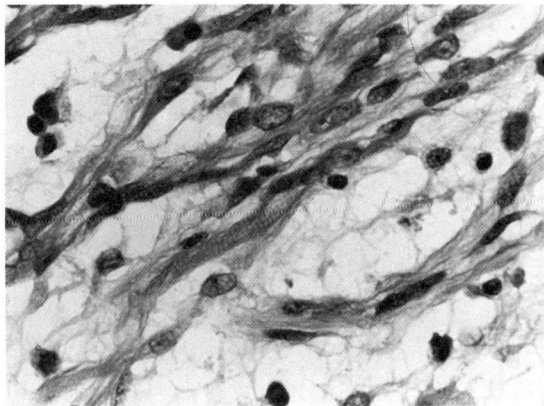

Fig. 9.6 Clearly visible cross-striations in a cell in a rhabdomyosarcoma. (H & E ×50)

alveolar pattern to the tumour. The pleomorphic rhabdomyosarcomas are, as their name suggests, pleomorphic sarcomas composed largely of spindle-shaped cells but with an admixture of larger cells which are often multinucleated and have abundant eosinophilic cytoplasm; it is possible, however, that many tumours placed into this diagnostic category are not actually of striated muscle origin (Enzinger & Weiss 1983).

The histological diagnosis of a rhabdomyosarcoma is dependent upon recognition of tumour cells which recapitulate embryonic stages in the development and differentiation of striated muscle cells. In only a minority of cases are cells with definite cross-striations present (Fig. 9.6) but large plump cells with abundant, eosinophilic, fibrillary or granular cytoplasm can often be presumed to be rhabdomyoblasts in those tumours with a typical embryonal or alveolar pattern. A definitive diagnosis of a rhabdomyosarcoma is commonly dependent upon the use of either electron microscopy or immunocytochemistry.

The literature on vulval rhabdomyosarcomas, though both sparse and unsatisfactory, leaves little doubt that neoplasms of this type are very uncommon at this site. DiSaia et al (1971) reported three rhabdomyosarcomas of the vulva, these occurring in women aged 18, 28 and 88 years respectively. The tumours were all in the labia majora and ranged in size from 1 to 10 cm in diameter; unfortunately, no histological details of these neoplasms were given and the criteria for their recognition as

rhabdomyosarcomas were not detailed. The two younger patients died, one 5 months and the other 9 months after initial presentation, this fatal outcome not being averted by local excision, radiotherapy and chemotherapy. One patient, aged 88 years, was alive and free of tumour 44 months after radical vulvectomy and bilateral groin node dissection; the small size of this neoplasm (1 cm in diameter), allied with the advanced age of the patient, prompts doubts about the rhabdomyosarcomatous nature of this tumour, doubts which the lack of histological detail can only reinforce.

Two examples of embryonal rhabdomyosarcoma of the vulva in young children have been described (James et al 1969, Talerman 1973). Both presented as rapidly growing vulval masses in 6-month-old girls; one patient was treated only by local excision and was alive and well 9 months later, whilst the other succumbed to local recurrence of her tumour 16 months after hemivulvectomy and radiotherapy. In neither of these cases was the rhabdomyosarcomatous nature of the tumour proved, the diagnosis in both being largely a matter of presumption.

Tumours of fibrous tissue

Fibroma. Vulval fibromas are relatively, but not absolutely, common (Lovelady et al 1941, Kaufman & Gardner 1965) and probably arise not primarily in the vulva itself but from the deeper connective tissues surrounding the introitus and the perineal body. Fibromas usually occur in the

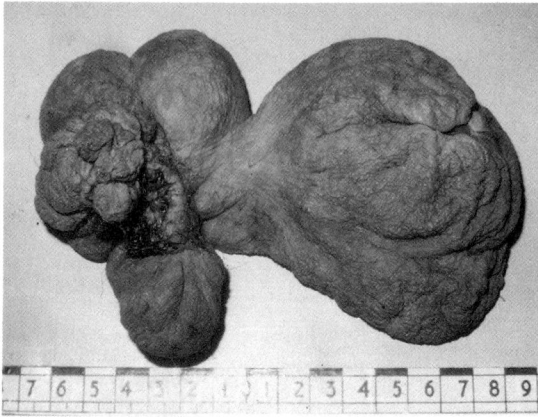

Fig. 9.7 An extirpated 'soft' fibroma of the vulva. (By courtesy of Professor Sir John Dewhurst)

labium majus and, although commonly measuring between 2 and 8 cm in diameter, can, on occasion, attain a huge size; they appear either as subcutaneous nodules or as pedunculated, pendulous, sometimes superficially ulcerated masses (Fig. 9.7). Fibromas are well circumscribed and formed of whitish-grey, firm tissue; histologically, parallel and interlacing bundles of fibrous tissue are seen.

The only complaint of women with a vulval fibroma is the presence of a nodule or mass; local excision is curative and there is no evidence that benign fibromas ever undergo malignant change.

Fibrosarcoma. Fibrosarcomas were, until quite recently, thought to be relatively common, largely because any highly cellular collagen-forming tumour or tumour-like lesion was indiscriminately placed into this category. The application of more stringent diagnostic criteria and the clearer recognition of such neoplasms as the malignant fibrous histiocytoma and of the various forms of fibromatosis have led to the current belief that fibrosarcomas are distinctly uncommon (Enzinger & Weiss 1983).

Fibrosarcomas can occur at any age and tend to form fleshy, rounded or lobulated masses; small tumours often appear deceptively well circumscribed whilst the larger neoplasms clearly have infiltrating margins. Histologically, fibrosarcomas tend to have a rather uniform pattern of spindle-shaped cells, with scanty cytoplasm and indistinct borders, arranged in bundles which are separated from each other by collagen fibres. Mitotic figures

are often a conspicuous feature but marked pleomorphism is not a characteristic of even the poorly differentiated fibrosarcomas.

Fibrosarcomas recur, invariably because of incomplete initial removal, in 50% of cases and metastasise principally by the haematogenous route to the lungs and skeleton, spread to lymph nodes being uncommon. Despite the propensity for recurrence and metastasis the overall 5-year survival rate is in the region of 60%, prognosis being directly related to the degree of differentiation of the tumour and, most importantly, to the number of mitotic figures.

Fewer than ten fibrosarcomas of the vulva have been described (Keller 1951, Woodruff & Brack 1958, DiSaia et al 1971, Davos & Abell 1976, Hall & Amin 1981), though it is far from certain that all these would currently be acceptable as true fibrosarcomas. These tumours have occurred in women aged between 30 and 67 years, with a mean age of 44 years, and most were in the labium majus, though one was confined to the clitoris and two involved the entire vulval area. The presenting complaint was usually that of an otherwise asymptomatic vulval mass and the length of history varied from 1 month to 2 years. Most of the tumours ranged from 6 to 8 cm in diameter but one was described as being 'as large as a grapefruit' and one was a huge mass measuring 25 cm in diameter and weighing 2.4 kg.

Of the eight patients for whom follow-up details were available, four were alive and well at intervals ranging from 4 to 9 years after initial treatment and four had died, all in less than 2 years of presentation, death being due in most instances to a combination of local recurrence and pulmonary metastases. All the patients who survived had been treated by radical vulvectomy together with either pelvic lymphadenectomy or bilateral inguinal node dissection. Of the four patients who died, one was terminally ill on admission and received no therapy, two were treated by simple vulvectomy and radiotherapy and one by wide local excision with bilateral inguinal lymphadenectomy.

It is clearly difficult to generalise about optimal therapy of vulval fibrosarcomas from such a limited number of cases but it does appear that radical surgery is the treatment of choice; radiotherapy appears to be of very limited value.

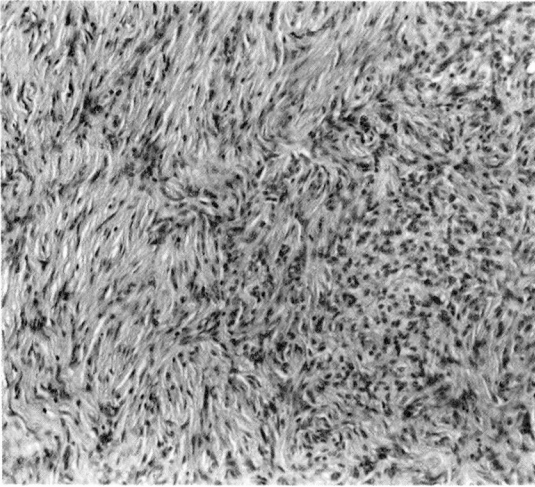

Fig. 9.8 A benign fibrous histiocytoma: the typical storiform pattern is not marked in this example. (H & E ×25)

Tumours of fibrohistiocytic origin

Benign fibrous histiocytoma. Tumours of this type are thought to arise from primitive mesenchymal cells which can differentiate into both fibroblastic and histiocytic cells; they are formed of a mixture of fibroblastic and histiocytic cells (Fig. 9.8) that are often arranged in a cartwheel (or 'storiform') pattern and are admixed with a variable number of lymphocytes, foam cells, multinucleated giant cells of foreign body type and siderophages (Enzinger & Weiss 1983). Pleomorphism and mitotic figures are notably absent and the lack of these features distinguishes the neoplasm from the malignant fibrous histiocytoma.

The benign fibrous histiocytoma occurs most commonly in the dermis or subcutis (where it is often referred to as a 'dermatofibroma') and although the extremities are the most frequent site of occurrence the lesion can also rarely involve the vulval skin (Beilby & Ridley 1987). The tumour presents as a slowly growing, hard, elevated or pedunculated lesion measuring, at most, a few centimetres in diameter. The overlying skin is reddened or reddish brown but is sometimes, if the tumour contains an abundance of siderophages, blackened. The tumours have poorly defined margins and on section are formed of moderately firm, yellow-brown or reddish tissue.

Between 5 and 10% of histologically benign

fibrous histiocytomas recur; there are no histological features which permit a forecast of possible recurrence and it is probable that in most cases tumour resurgence simply reflects inadequate local excision.

Dermatofibrosarcoma protuberans. This neoplasm, which develops most commonly on the trunk, is a nodular cutaneous tumour which is characterised histologically by a markedly storiform arrangement of its constituent cells. There has been much debate about the histogenesis of this tumour but the striking histological similarity of the dermatofibrosarcoma protuberans to a benign fibrous histiocytoma has led to its being identified as a fibrohistiocytic neoplasm. The neoplasm is, however, more infiltrative than a benign fibrous histiocytoma and has a greater tendency to recurrence, though on the other hand distant metastases occur much less commonly and after a considerably greater time interval than is the case with malignant fibrous histiocytomas; hence the current tendency is to classify the dermatofibrosarcoma protuberans as a fibrohistiocytic tumour of intermediate malignancy (Enzinger & Weiss 1983).

Dermatofibrosarcoma protuberans occurs as a slowly growing plaque within the dermis which has an eventual tendency to become nodular; the overlying skin may be ulcerated. On section, the tumour is firm and greyish white; the appearances may be altered by myxoid and, occasionally, cystic change but haemorrhage and necrosis are rare. Histologically, the tumour is locally infiltrative and formed of plump fibroblastic cells arranged in a distinctly storiform pattern. Vessels are not conspicuous, there is little pleomorphism and mitotic figures are not numerous; giant cells, xanthomatous cells and infiltrating inflammatory cells are sparse. Myxoid change occurs in some neoplasms and this tends to be accompanied by some loss of the characteristic storiform appearance. The tumour recurs in approximately 50% of cases (Taylor & Helwig 1962) whilst metastases, most commonly to the lung, occur in less than 1% of patients, almost invariably after several local recurrences.

Four cases of dermatofibrosarcoma protuberans of the vulva have been recorded (Davos & Abell 1976, Soltan 1981, Agress et al 1983, Bock et al 1985). Patients with these neoplasms have ranged

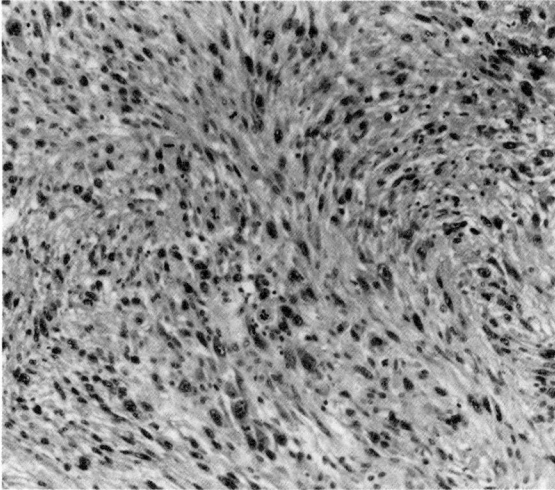

Fig. 9.9 A malignant fibrous histiocytoma. A whorled storiform pattern is clearly apparent but there is considerable pleomorphism and mitotic activity. (H & E ×45)

in age from 38 to 83 years and all presented with a slowly growing, painless, non-tender lump in the vulva, the length of the history varying from 10 months to 10 years. Three of the tumours were situated in the labium majus whilst one was near the mons pubis; the smallest was just over 4 cm in its longest diameter and two of the tumours measured 8 cm across. The masses were all mobile but the overlying skin was ulcerated in two cases. The neoplasms were all treated by wide local excision and three of the patients were alive and remained tumour free after surgery, two for 6 months at the time of reporting and one for 20 years. Local recurrence developed in one patient 5 years after local excision; she was treated by radical vulvectomy and was alive with disseminated breast cancer, but without further reappearance of her vulval tumour, 6 months later. There seems little doubt that wide local resection is the treatment of choice for this neoplasm and there does not appear to be any compelling necessity for lymph node dissection.

Malignant fibrous histiocytoma. Malignant fibrous histiocytomas appear most commonly during the seventh decade and occur most frequently in the muscles of the extremities and in the retroperitioneal space, where they present as multinodular, fleshy, whitish-grey masses that often appear deceptively well circumscribed. Histologi-

cally (Fig. 9.9) the most typical pattern is of plump spindle cells arranged in short fascicles in a storiform (cartwheel) fashion around slit-like vascular spaces. These are admixed with stout histiocytic cells which usually show considerable pleomorphism and with larger, relatively pleomorphic, fibroblastic cells arranged in a haphazard fashion. Xanthomatous cells and multinucleated giant cells are commonly present whilst mitotic figures, both normal and abnormal, are often a conspicuous feature. The overall recurrence rate following surgical extirpation of a malignant fibrous histiocytoma is 44% and 42% of such tumours give rise to metastases, usually in the lungs, lymph nodes and liver (Enzinger & Weiss 1983).

A small minority of malignant fibrous histiocytomas occur in the skin and subcutaneous tissues and here the incidence of metastatic spread is related to the depth of involvement, those tumours limited to the subcutaneous tissue having a metastatic rate of only 10% and those involving deeper structures, such as fascia, having a metastasis rate of 27%. Very superficial malignant fibrous histiocytomas, which are limited to the dermis, are often classed as 'atypical fibroxanthomas' and follow a generally benign course, only 10% recurring after surgical excision and metastases being very exceptional (Enzinger & Weiss 1983).

Only five malignant fibrous histiocytomas of the vulva have been reported, four as such (Davos & Abell 1976, Taylor et al 1985, Santala et al 1987) and one as a 'malignant fibroxanthoma' (Hensley & Friedrich 1973). These neoplasms arose in women aged between 38 and 79 years who presented with a history, varying in length from 2 to 12 months, of an enlarging vulval mass, this being painful in two cases; all the tumours were in the labia majora, two being ulcerated, and they ranged from 2.5 to 6 cm in diameter.

One patient was alive and tumour free 19 months after local excision of the tumour whilst two others, managed by radical vulvectomy and, in one case, bilateral groin node dissection, were also alive and well 5 months later; a fourth woman was treated by hemivulvectomy and unilateral groin node dissection and was tumour free at the time of reporting. The less fortunate fifth patient was subjected to radical vulvectomy together with pelvic and groin node dissection but developed a recurrence after

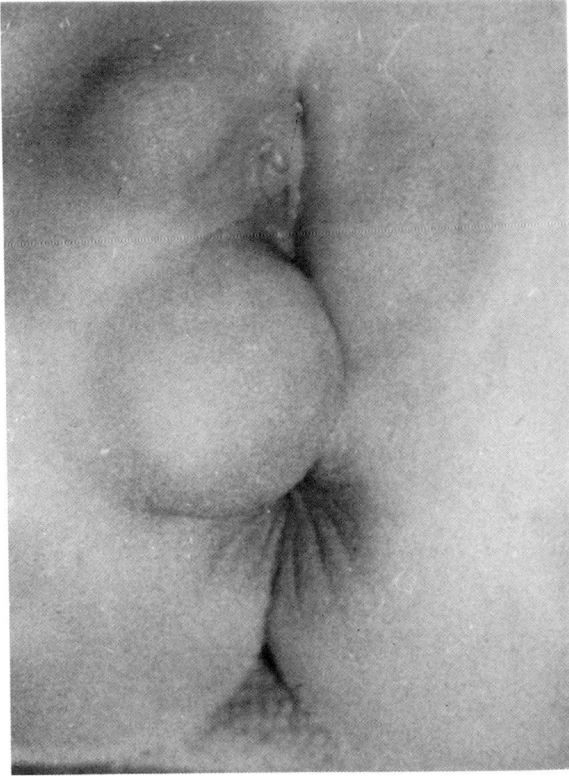

Fig. 9.10 A lipoma of the vulva. (By courtesy of Professor Sir John Dewhurst)

3 months; despite radiotherapy she died of pulmonary metastases 2 months later.

Tumours of fat

Lipoma. Benign lipomatous neoplasms of the vulva are relatively common and present either as soft, rounded, lobulated masses (Fig. 9.10) or as soft, pedunculated tumours (Lovelady et al 1941, Kaufman & Gardner 1965); they can, on occasion, be extremely large and attain a diameter as great as 17 cm. Most vulval lipomas develop from the fatty tissue of the labia majora but examples have been noted of clitoral localisation (Haddad & Jones 1960). Vulval lipomas can occur at any age and one has been described in a neonate (Fukaminzu et al 1982). Histologically these neoplasms are formed of mature fat cells which are often admixed with strands of fibrous tissue.

A number of histological variants of the typical lipoma have been described such as the pleomorphic lipoma, the spindle cell lipoma, the angiolipoma, the benign lipoblastoma and the myolipoma but these variants, with the single exception of a tumour of rather dubious nature classed as a 'haemangiofibrolipoma' (Tsoutsoplides 1980), have not been described in the vulva whilst there is no record of vulval involvement in any of the syndromes of diffuse lipomatosis.

Liposarcoma. Liposarcomas are the most common soft tissue sarcomas of adult life and ocur most frequently in the thigh, retroperitoneum, chest wall, breast, mediastinum and omentum; a number of histological types are recognised, such as the well-differentiated liposarcoma, the myxoid liposarcoma, the round cell liposarcoma and the pleomorphic liposarcoma. Reports of vulval liposarcoma are, however, extraordinarily rare, with only two reasonably persuasive accounts of such a neoplasm. One such tumour (Taussig 1937) developed in the labium majus of a 29-year-old woman; hemivulvectomy with superficial inguinal and femoral lymph node dissection was performed but the patient died 5 months later with metastases in the lung and skeleton. Brooks and LiVolsi (1987) described a large liposarcoma in a fifteen-year-old girl which involved the vulva and perineum; following excision the tumour recurred twenty months later, the patient dying from local disease thirty-one months after initial presentation.

Gondos and Casey (1982) reported a liposarcoma of the perineal body which presented as a hard lump of 2 months duration in a 38-year-old woman. The patient was subjected to posterior exenteration but developed a nodule of recurrent liposarcoma in the vagina 8 months later; this was treated by local excision followed by chemotherapy with Adriamycin and the patient was alive and tumour free 6 months later.

Tumours of vascular origin

Haemangioma. There is still some dispute as to whether haemangiomas are hamartomas or true neoplasms and a point in favour of the former view is they occur primarily in infancy and childhood. The lesion may be of the capillary type with easily recognisable small blood vessels of capillary calibre lined by a single layer of endothelial cells or of the

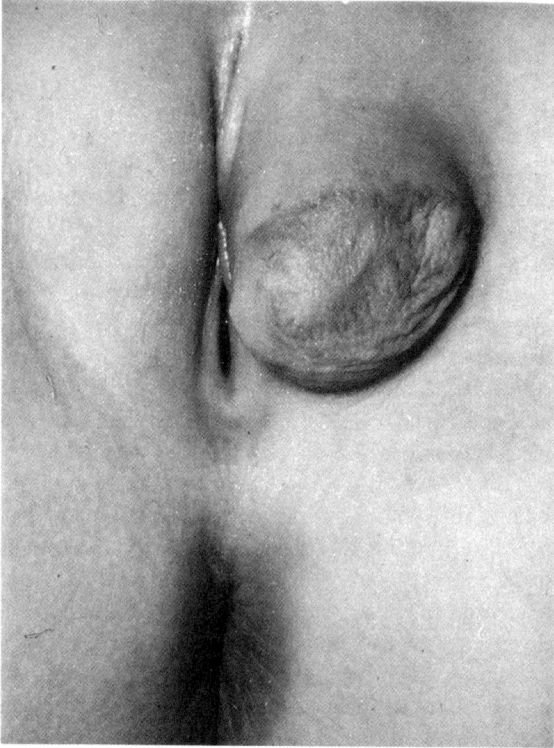

Fig. 9.11 A haemangioma of the vulva in a young child. (By courtesy of Professor Sir John Dewhurst)

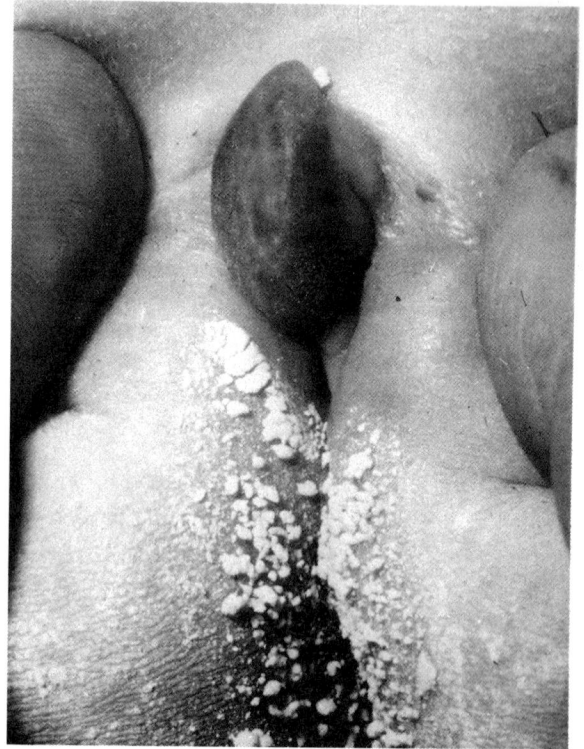

Fig. 9.12 A haemangioma of the clitoris in a neonate. (By courtesy of Professor Sir John Dewhurst)

cavernous variety with large vascular channels, again lined by a single layer of endothelial cells. Some capillary haemangiomas consist largely or partly of more solidly packed endothelial cells with only tentative blood vessel formation; such lesions are sometimes designated as benign haemangio-endotheliomas.

Clinically significant haemangiomas of the vulva are far from common but about 35 cases have been recorded (Lovelady et al 1941, Gerbie et al 1955, Darnalt-Restrepo 1957, Guilientetti 1959, Giannone & Avezzi 1969, Mobius & Krause 1974); such cases are usually reported because the haemangioma is large and unsightly (Fig. 9.11) and there can be little doubt that many cases of vulvar haemangioma either pass unrecorded or are insufficiently large for the parents of the child to seek medical aid. Those which have been described have commonly been of the cavernous type and have involved the labia, usually unilaterally but sometimes bilaterally.

Some examples of a cavernous haemangioma localised to the clitoris (Fig. 9.12) have been documented (Lovelady et al 1941, Haddad & Jones 1960, Kauffman-Friedman 1978); haemangiomas in this site produce clitoromegaly and this may lead to the patient being investigated for an intersex state or for congenital adrenal hyperplasia.

Only very large unsightly haemangiomas require treatment either by laser therapy or by plastic surgery. The 'strawberry' type of cavernous haemangioma usually remits spontaneously and hence does not require treatment; exceptionally oral steroids are required to control rapid enlargement and/or thrombocytopenia (Kasabach–Merritt syndrome).

Angiokeratoma. An angiokeratoma is often regarded as a variant of a haemangioma though its true nature is debatable; the consideration of this entity in this section is largely a matter of convenience and should not be regarded as indicating an adherence to the neoplastic concept of the angiokeratoma.

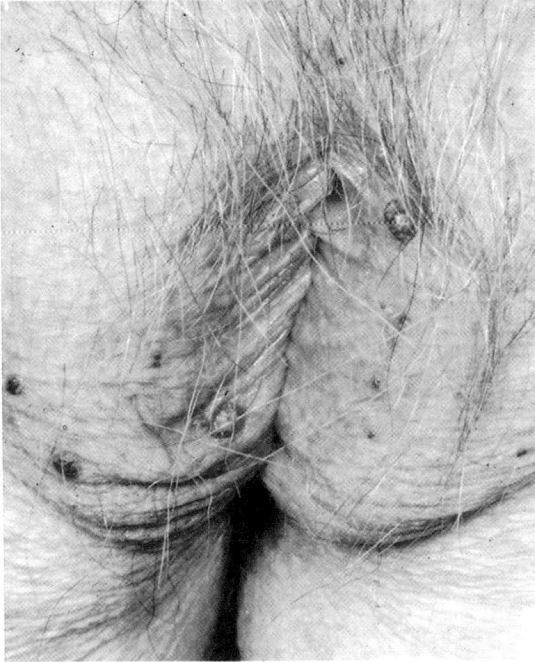

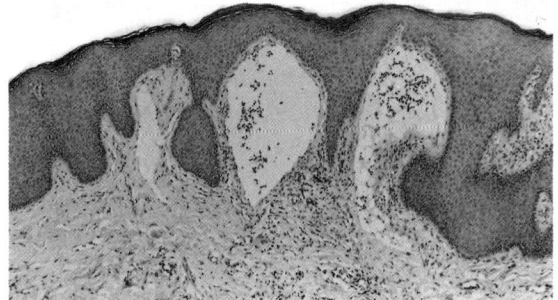

Fig. 9.14 An angiokeratoma of the vulva. Sinusoidally dilated vascular channels are present in the papillary dermis: they are surrounded by elongated rete ridges. (H & E ×15)

Fig. 9.13 Angiokeratoma—hyperkeratotic red lesions on labia majora

Vulval angiokeratomas are more common than their rather sparse coverage in the literature would suggest (Imperial & Helwig 1967, Blair 1970; Verbov & Manglabruks 1978, Uhlin 1980, Novick 1985, Dotters et al 1986); for though the vulva is by no means the only area in which these lesions develop it is certainly a site of predilection. Vulval angiokeratomas develop principally in women aged between 20 and 40 years and the vast majority arise in the labium majus. The lesions may be single but are, in 50% of cases, multiple, as many as 24 separate angiokeratomas having been noted in the vulva of one woman (Uhlin 1980). The lesions usually measure between 2 and 10 mm in diameter and may assume a papular, globular or warty appearance. In the early stages of their development angiokeratomas are commonly cherry red in colour but as they age their tint darkens to brown or black (Fig. 9.13).

Histologically, enormously dilated capillary vessels, often converted into a solitary, sinusoidal, vascular channel, are present in the papillary dermis (Fig. 9.14): the overlying epidermis shows a variable degree of hyperkeratosis and acanthosis with elongated rete ridges growing down to surround, and appearing almost to embrace, the dilated vascular channels in the dermis.

Angiokeratomas are often asymptomatic but may cause pruritus whilst bleeding from the lesion is not uncommon; the bleeding is usually of a relatively trivial degree, manifest only by spotting of the underclothes, but can occasionally be quite severe. The presence of a black, warty, bleeding lesion can arouse suspicions of a malignant melanoma which are, however, rapidly dispelled by histological examination of the locally resected lesion, a procedure which is curative.

Glomus tumour. The glomus tumour is a neoplasm which is thought to arise from the glomus body, a specialized form of arteriovenous anastomosis that serves in thermal regulation and is located in the dermis. The tumours occur most commonly in the subungual region, the digits and the palm but can occur in any site. They present, usually in adult life, as small blue-red tender nodules and histologically they consist of clusters of capillary-type vessels surrounded by cuffs of glomus cells set in hyalinised or myxoid stroma. The tumours are benign and are cured by simple excision.

Rare examples of glomus tumours at the vulva have been described. Kohorn et al (1986) reported a histologically confirmed lesion on the left labium minus causing dyspareunia and pain in a woman aged 45 years, and Katz et al (1986) a similar lesion at the same site in a woman aged 29 years.

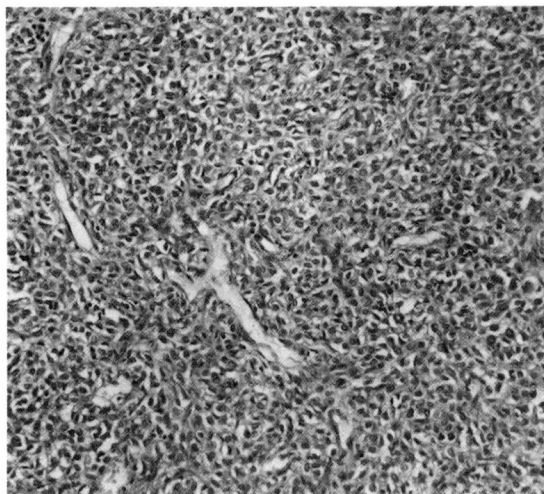

Fig. 9.15 A haemangiopericytoma. Tightly packed cells surround multiple vascular channels. A branching vessel in the centre of the field has a characteristic 'stag-horn' appearance.

Haemangiopericytoma. This uncommon, though not rare, neoplasm was first described by Stout & Murray (1942) who thought that it was derived from pericytic cells, a view which is generally, but not universally, accepted. The tumour occurs predominantly in young adults and has a propensity for the thigh, retroperitoneum and pelvic fossa. The characteristic histological picture (Fig. 9.15) is one of multiple vascular channels set amidst, and surrounded by, tightly packed cells which may be arranged in trabeculae, clumps or sheets: sometimes the tumour cells are disposed concentrically around the vascular channels in an 'onion-skin' pattern. The tumour cells are rounded, polygonal or spindle shaped and have round or ovoid nuclei, a moderate amount of cytoplasm and ill-defined borders. The vascular channels range in size from small vessels of capillary calibre to wide sinusoids and form a ramifying network within the tumour; very typically the dividing sinusoidal channels tend to have a 'stag-horn' appearance. The vessels are lined by a single layer of endothelial cells which is often markedly attenuated. A reticulin stain shows that the vessels within the neoplasm are supported by a well-defined basal lamina and that reticulin fibres enmesh individual tumour cells.

Many haemangiopericytomas appear to be benign but a proportion, variously estimated as between 11 and 56%, pursue a malignant course, recurring after initial excision and subsequently metastasising via the bloodstream to the lungs and skeleton. Some of the tumours which behave in a malignant fashion cause death within a few months but others run a more indolent course with metastases appearing between 5 and 15 years after initial excision and with patients living for prolonged periods with metastatic disease. The microscopic findings are not always clearly related to the malignancy or otherwise of the neoplasm and it has often been denied that there are any histological criteria for the recognition of malignancy in these tumours. In several large series it has, however, been found that cellular pleomorphism, foci of necrosis and the presence of more than four mitotic figures per ten high power fields all suggest that a particular haemangiopericytoma will behave in a malignant fashion (McMaster et al 1975, Enzinger & Weiss 1983).

Only seven instances of a haemangiopericytoma of the vulva have been adequately reported (De Sousa & Lash 1959, Reymond et al 1972, Davos & Abell 1976, Ambrosini et al 1980, Guercio et al 1982, Zakut et al 1985). The ages of the patients ranged from 15 to 60 years though four patients were aged less than 25 years at the time of initial diagnosis. The affected women all complained of an enlarging vulval mass, the length of history varying from 2 to 15 months but being usually less than 6 months; in two cases the patients also complained of pain in the region of the vulval mass. The tumour was in the labium majus in all except one of the patients in whom the neoplasm predominantly involved the clitoris. Four of the vulval haemangiopericytomas were treated by wide local excision, one by local excision and subsequent radiotherapy, one by hemivulvectomy and one by radical vulvectomy. Five of the patients were alive and well at the time of reporting, with follow-up periods ranging from 2 months to 19 years. Two of the neoplasms behaved, however, in a malignant fashion. One, in a 15 year-old girl, recurred within 2 months of local excision and led to the patient's death 5 months later with widespread metastases, neither radiotherapy or chemotherapy having any inhibitory effect on the relentless growth or spread of the tumour. The other malignant haemangiopericytoma was treated by radical vulvectomy, after which the patient was well for 14 years, only then to suffer a metastasis in the shaft of the femur; this appeared to respond reasonably well to radiotherapy. It should be noted that in neither of these two malignant haemangiopericytomas was there any overt histological evidence of malignancy.

There are no clear-cut guidelines for the management of a haemangiopericytoma of the vulva, though it is probable that wide local excision is the initial treatment of choice. If the histological appearances appear to be fully benign it would be reasonable not to pursue further treatment, though the possibility of recurrence or metastasis cannot be totally discounted. If the morphological features suggest that the neoplasm is malignant it is possible that adjuvant radiotherapy would be advisable. Certainly, all cases should be subjected to lengthy follow-up.

Aggressive angiomyxoma. These neoplasms present as large gelatinous masses which infiltrate the soft tissues of the female pelvis and perineum. They have a bland histological appearance with many blood vessels set in an abundant myxoid stroma which contains scattered stellate and spindle-shaped cells. These tumours, possibly because their infiltrative nature makes complete removal difficult, tend to recur locally in a repetitive and relentless fashion. There have been nine reported cases of aggressive angiomyxoma of the vulva (Steeper and Rosai 1983, Begin et al 1985, Hilgers et al 1986). All presented as a painless expanding vulval mass in women aged between 21 and 38 years. All but one of the tumours recurred locally after excision, some repeatedly.

Kaposi's sarcoma. This is now generally recognised as a neoplasm of vascular tissue though the exact cell of origin is uncertain (Enzinger & Weiss 1983). The tumour shows striking geographical variations, is circumstantially linked with cytomegalovirus infection and tends to occur particularly in immunocompromised individuals, having achieved considerable recent notoriety as a complication of the acquired immunodeficiency syndrome (AIDS).

The initial lesion is a blue-red nodule in the skin; usually the nodules are mutiple and gradually increase in both size and number, eventually to coalesce into plaques of polypoid growths; in about 15% of cases the initial lesion is, and remains, soli-

tary. Histologically the early lesions resemble granulation tissue with proliferating capillaries lined by plump endothelial cells and a surrounding scanty proliferation of immature spindle cells together with a marked infiltrate of mixed non-specific inflammatory cells. As the lesion ages it tends to lose its inflammatory component and become more cellular, commonly resembling a well-differentiated fibrosarcoma but differing from such a lesion by the presence of slit-like vascular spaces and the relative absence of mitotic activity.

The disease usually progresses in an indolent fashion with a course of 8 to 10 years and with only about 20% of afflicted individuals succumbing to the neoplasm; Kaposi's sarcoma developing in sufferers from AIDS appears, however, to follow a much more aggressive and rapidly fatal pathway.

Only two cases of Kaposi's sarcoma of the vulva have been noted. One (Hall et al 1979) arose in a 64-year-old woman who gave a 1-year history of vulval itching, and pain for the previous 2 months. She was found to have a large, raised, indurated, scaling lesion involving the entire right labium majus; multiple satellite nodules were present in the skin of the groin, buttock and thigh. A diagnosis of Kaposi's sarcoma was made after biopsy of the lesion and the patient treated with chemotherapy. The vulvar lesion responded well but the patient died of renal disease 1 month later; no residual tumour was found at autopsy. LiVolsi and Brooks (1987) refer briefly to a multifocal Kaposi's sarcoma of the vulva and perineum in an elderly woman; following radiotherapy she survived for 15 years.

The optimal treatment for Kaposi's sarcoma is yet to be defined, although both radiotherapy and chemotherapy have their advocates.

Angiosarcomas. Angiosarcomas are malignant neoplasms the cells of which manifest many of the functional and morphological characteristics of normal endothelium (Enzinger & Weiss 1983). The tumours may be sufficiently well differentiated as to bear a considerable resemblance to a benign haemangioma or so poorly differentiated that they mimic a carcinoma or a malignant melanoma.

Angiosarcomas are rare but most commonly arise in the skin and superficial soft tissues. The cutaneous angiosarcomas present as blue or red nodules which become multiple and tend gradually to convert into large ulcerated tumour masses; most are moderately differentiated and contain distinct vascular channels, albeit of irregular size and shape, which communicate with each other to create an anastomosing vascular network. About 40% of patients with an angiosarcoma succumb to their disease because of either distant metastases or extensive local recurrence.

Reports of vulval angiosarcomas have been sparse and rather unsatisfactory. Davos & Abell (1976) described an 83-year-old woman who presented with a 3-year history of an enlarging mass in the left labium majus; this was treated by local excision and was shown histologically to be a typical angiosarcoma, consisting in part of irregular vascular spaces containing erythrocytes and lined by large, atypical endothelial cells and partly of solid sheets of neoplastic cells. Unfortunately, no follow-up information was available for this patient. Bo et al (1976) reported a 49-year-old patient who presented with a 10-year history of a nodule in the left labium majus which had recently increased rapidly in size. The tumour, which was the 'size of a mandarin orange', formed an ulcerated mass which was treated by local excision. A diagnosis was made histologically of angiosarcoma, a diagnosis which is not convincingly supported by the histological illustrations, and the patient was alive and well 5 years later.

It is clearly impossible to make any generalisations about the management or prognosis of vulval angiosarcomas from these two cases but, in general terms, angiosarcomas are relatively resistant to radiation and are best treated by very wide excision.

Tumours of lymphatic origin

Lymphangioma. It is doubtful if lymphangiomas are true neoplasms, it being more probable that they arise from sequestrations of lymphatic tissue that fail to communicate normally with the lymphatic tree; these remnants may have some proliferative capacity but tend to enlarge principally by accumulation of fluid (Enzinger & Weiss 1983). Histologically the lesion consists of lymphatic spaces of variable size which are lined by thinned endothelial cells; these spaces are filled with proteinaceous fluid containing lymphocytes and, occasionally, a few erythrocytes.

Lymphangiomas of the vulva are uncommon and present as soft compressible masses, usually in the labia majora (Loveday et al 1941, Kaufman & Gardner 1965); they vary considerably in size but can attain a considerable bulk. Lymphangiomas usually occur in childhood; occasionally examples arise in adults but these probably represent an acquired lymphangectasia rather than a true lymphangioma. One example of a vulval lymphangioma occurring in a patient with congenital dysplastic angiopathy (Klippel–Trerauny–Weber syndrome) has been reported (Krebs et al 1984). The lesions of lymphangioma circumscriptum are small and have a typical frog-spawn-like appearance. They may communicate with deep lymphatic cisterns (Whimster 1974).

Local excision of a lymphangioma is curative; complete removal is, however, not always easy to achieve and recurrence can occur from residual tissue.

Lymphangiosarcoma. It is now recognised that malignant neoplasms of lymphatic vessels either do not occur or, if they do, are indistinguishable from an angiosarcoma (Enzinger & Weiss 1983).

Tumours of neural origin

Neurolemmoma. Neurolemmomas are slowly growing tumours which arise from the Schwann cells of nerve sheaths, hence their alternative name of 'Schwannomas'. They are encapsulated by the epineurium, but often eclipse the nerve from which they have arisen. Histologically, these neoplasms have two components, a highly ordered cellular component (Antoni A areas) and a loose myxoid component (Antoni B areas). The relative contributions of these two patterns varies and there may be an almost imperceptible blending or an abrupt transition from one to the other. Antoni A areas are formed of compact spindle cells arranged in short bundles or interlacing fascicles; nuclear palisading and a whorled pattern are characteristic features. In Antoni B areas spindled or ovoid cells are arranged haphazardly in a loose myxoid stroma. Neurolemmomas occur principally between the ages of 20 and 50 years and are usually solitary; they are occasionally multiple and have a more than fortuitous association with von Recklinghausens's disease (neurofibromatosis).

A few neurolemmomas of the vulva have been

described, most arising in the labia (Bryan 1955, Bianco & Samuel 1958, Dini 1959) but one being localised to the clitoris (Migliorini & Amato 1978). In all these cases the tumour presented as an indolently enlarging mass without any associated pain or tenderness. Diagnosis of such a lesion is, of course, not possible clinically and rests solely upon histological examination. It is important, however, that a clear distinction is drawn between a neurolemmoma and a neurofibroma (see below) in so far as whilst the latter has a definite potential for malignant change this possibility is so remote in neurolemmomas that it can be ignored; in this respect it should be noted that the presence of mitotic figures in an otherwise typical neurolemmoma is not an indication of malignancy (Enzinger & Weiss 1983). Surgical removal of a neurolemmoma is curative.

A variant of the conventional neurolemmoma is the multinodular or plexiform Schwannoma, which closely resembles a plexiform neurofibroma. An example of such a neoplasm occurring in the vulva was reported by Woodruff et al (1983). This tumour presented as a large mass in the labium majus of a 26-year-old woman; following surgical removal recurrences subsequently appeared first at 18 months and later at 22 months after original extirpation but the patient was alive and well 3½ years after initial diagnosis.

Some neurolemmomas consist largely of Antoni A areas without any significant admixture with Antoni B areas and these are classed as 'cellular neurolemmomas'. One such neoplasm has been described as occurring in the vulva, though it was inaccurately reported as a malignant Schwannoma (Lawrence & Shingleton 1978). This tumour arose in a 44-year-old woman and was recognised as malignant largely because of its high content of mitotic figures; as already remarked a plethora of mitoses is not necessarily indicative of malignancy in neurolemmomas and this patient was alive and well 1 year later.

Benign granular cell tumour. This neoplasm, previously known as a granular cell myoblastoma because of a now untenable view that it was of muscular origin, is currently thought, on the basis of morphological, ultrastructural and histochemical studies, to be derived from Schwann cells (Enzinger & Weiss 1983). The tumour usually arises in the dermal or immediately subcutaneous tissues, is poorly circumscribed and characteristically yellow or yellowish-grey on cutting. Histologically (Fig. 9.16 a, b) the lesion is formed of rounded or polygonal cells with indistinct margins, central vesicular nuclei and abundant, coarsely granular, eosinophilic cytoplasm; there is usually little pleomorphism and mitotic figures are either absent or extremely sparse. The tumour cells stain positively, though weakly, with PAS both before and after diastase and are usually arranged in ribbons or clumps which are separated from each other by fibrous septa. Sometimes a desmoplasmic reaction can largely engulf the tumour cells which then appear as scattered nests set in a dense fibrous stroma. In the case of those granular cell tumours situated in the dermis the overlying squamous epithelium commonly shows a pronounced pseudo-epitheliomatous hyperplasia which is not infrequently misdiagnosed as a squamous cell carcinoma. The neoplastic cells usually stain stongly positive for carcinogenic embryonic antigen (CEA) using the immunoperoxidase technique (Shousha & Lyssiotis 1979).

Ultrastructurally, these neoplasms have a very distinctive, virtually diagnostic, appearance, the cytoplasmic granules consisting of autophagic vacuoles which contain cellular debris such as mitochondria, myelin figures, fragments of rough endoplasmic reticulum and axon-like structures (Fisher & Wechsler 1962, Aparicio & Lumsden 1969, Carstens 1970, Sobel et al 1973, Weiser 1978).

Over 60 cases of benign granular cell tumour of the vulva have been reported (Birch & Sondag 1961, Radman & Bhagavan 1969, Coates & Hales 1973, Dgani et al 1978, Chambers 1979, King et al 1979, Lieb et al 1979, Zenetta et al 1981, Morris 1982, Lesoin et al 1983, Vold & Jerve 1984, Altaras et al 1985) though it is certain that many such neoplasms now pass unrecorded. In most instances the vulval lesion has been an isolated occurrence but occasionally a vulval tumour has formed one component of a syndrome in which multiple granular cell tumours arise, either synchronously or sequentially, in various parts of the body (Powell 1946, Gifford & Birch 1973). The vulval neoplasms can occur at any age and usually arise in the labia, though there have been two instances of the lesion being confined to the clitoris (Doyle & Hutchinson 1968, Degefu et al 1984). The patients invariably

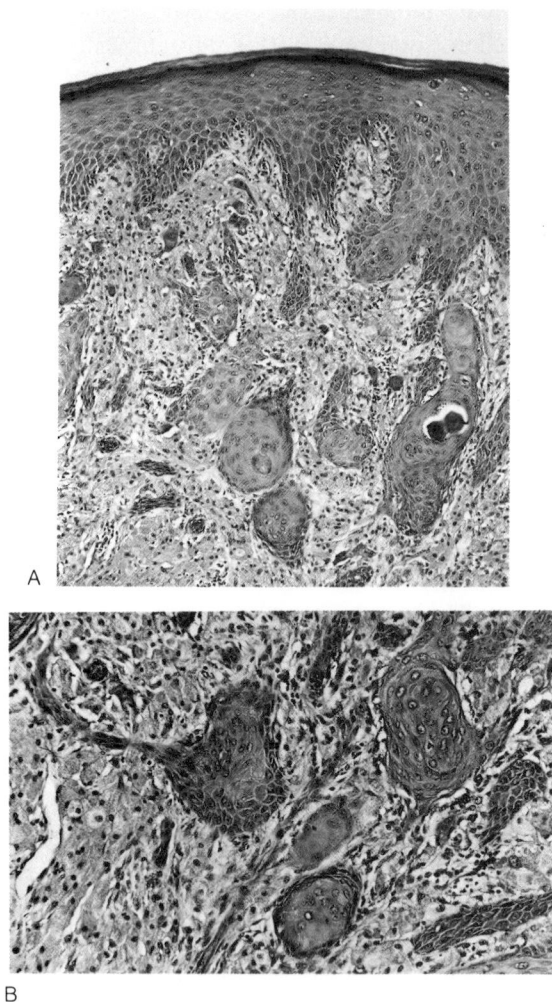

Fig. 9.16 (a) A benign granular cell tumour of the vulva. Rounded and polygonal cells with abundant granular cytoplasm occupy the debris. The overlying squamous epithelium shows a marked pseudo-epitheliomatous hyperplasm. (H & E ×70); (b) A higher power view of the tumour shown in (a). (H & E ×110) (c) A benign granular cell tumour. This lesion was yellowish and clinically was thought to be of sebaceous origin.

complain of a slowly growing, painless and non-tender lump or nodule; the history usually extends over months or years and the tumour rarely exceeds a diameter of 4 cm. The lump is commonly mobile but some cases of granular cell tumour situated in the upper dermis show skin tethering; the elevated overlying skin may be depigmented and occasionally ulcerated (Fig. 9.16 c). In the case of the more superficially situated tumours a diagnosis of a sebaceous cyst is often entertained whilst the more

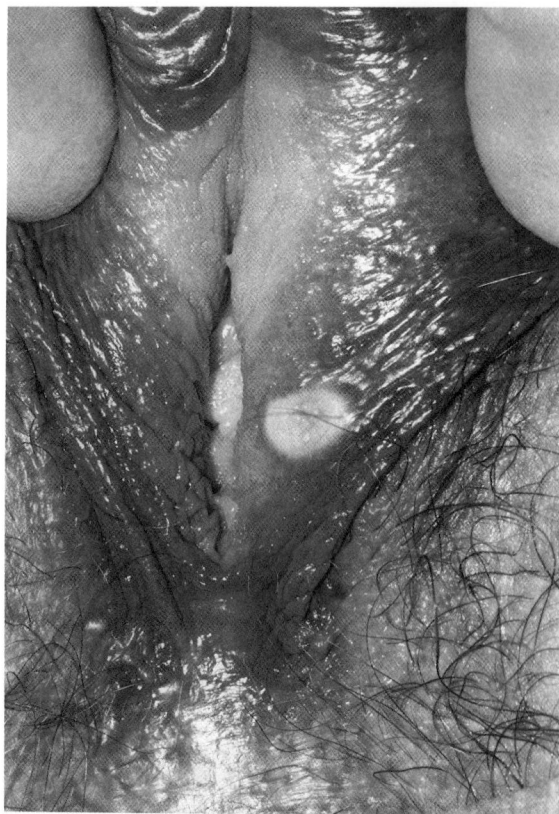

deeply located neoplasms may simulate a Bartholin's duct cyst, a Bartholin's gland adenoma or a fibroma. The tumour is thus rarely correctly diagnosed prior to operation and as it can appear deceptively well delineated, often with a well marked pseudocapsule, it may simply be enucleated. In fact, however, these neoplasms are not well circumscribed and groups of tumour cells are usually present beyond the apparent macroscopic limits of growth; hence in order to prevent recurrence wide local excision is required.

Ninety-eight per cent of granular cell tumours are benign and the patient is cured by simple surgical extirpation; the rare exceptions are considered below.

Malignant granular cell tumour. Malignant granular cell tumours are extremely uncommon and fall into two categories (Gamboa 1955); first are those which appear histologically benign but nevertheless behave in a malignant fashion, and second are others which not only behave biologically as a malignant tumour but which show, in some areas at least, considerable pleomorphism and mitotic activity. Only two examples of a malignant granular cell tumour of the vulva have been fully documented and in each case the tumour was recognised to be malignant only after it had given rise to metastases. The patient described by Mágori & Szegvári (1973) was aged 49 years when a histologically benign granular cell tumour was removed from her vulva; 16 months later she returned with a local recurrence which was extirpated only for her to present 4 months later with an inguinal lymph node metastasis. Following surgical removal of the inguinal lymph node the patient was well and without evidence of tumour at the time of reporting. Robertson et al (1981) reported a 33-year-old woman who presented with a mobile mass, measuring 3 cm in diameter, in her right labium majus which had been present for no less than 18 years. A histologically benign granular cell tumour was removed but the patient developed right inguinal lymph node metastases 5 years later; following block dissection of the right groin the patient was well and tumour free 6 months later.

Although both the women with vulval malignant granular cell tumours appear to have survived the overall survival for patients with neoplasms of this type is only about 40% (Cadotte 1974, Robertson et al 1981), the remainder dying with widely disseminated metastases, particularly to the lungs. Neither radical surgery nor radiotherapy appears to have any significant influence on the eventual prognosis (Enzinger & Weiss 1983).

Neurofibroma. Neoplasms of this type take several forms and are thought to be derived from Schwann cells, which have the facultative ability to synthesise not only myelin but also collagen (Lott & Richardson 1981, Enzinger & Weiss 1983).

The solitary neurofibroma occurs, by definition, in patients not suffering from von Recklinghausen's neurofibromatosis. Such neoplasms most commonly present as slowly growing, painless, often rather flabby nodules in the dermis or subcutis and are well circumscribed but not encapsulated. Histologically (Fig. 9.17) their most typical pattern is one of elongated Schwann cells with long, wavy nuclei which are separated from thick crenated bundles of collagen by a small or moderate amount of mucoid substance. Variation in the proportion of these

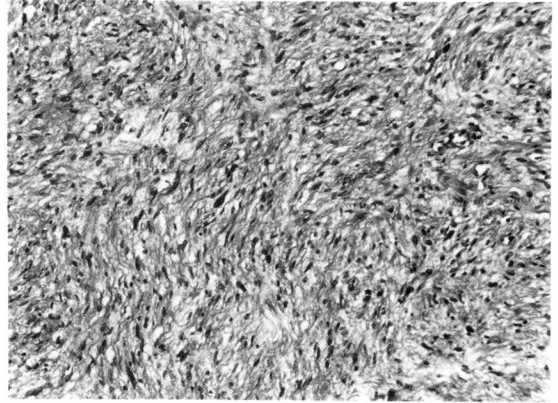

Fig. 9.17 A solitary neurofibroma in a patient without the stigmata of von Recklinghausen's disease. (H & E ×100)

different components can give rise to cellular, hyaline and myxoid variants.

In individuals with von Recklinghausen's disease, neurofibromas usually appear during childhood or adolescence. Some of these tumours do not differ in any respect from the solitary neurofibroma but others have a plexiform pattern with masses of expanded nerve branches which become broken up by proliferating Schwann cells and thick bundles of collagen. A diffuse form of neurofibroma also occurs in patients with von Recklinghausen's disease; this type forms an ill-defined plaque which spreads along connective tissue septa and between fat cells and consists predominantly of fibrillary collagen with an admixture of stubby Schwann cells.

The risk of malignant change in a solitary neurofibroma is extremely low but the risk for neurofibromas associated with von Recklinghausen's disease is estimated to be between 2 and 13% (Enzinger & Weiss 1983).

Over 20 cases of neurofibroma of the vulva have been reported. Two were solitary neurofibromas occurring in women with no evidence of von Recklinghausen's disease (Venter et al 1981); these two neoplasms, one in a woman of 19 years and the other in one aged 36 years, were exceptional in that they grew rapidly and attained hugh proportions (more than 25 cm in diameter). Both were successfully treated by local surgery. Lovelady et al (1941) briefly reported two small vulval neurofibromas (measuring 1 and 2 cm in diameter respectively) but did not comment on whether the patients were or were not suffering from von Recklinghausen's disease.

Most vulval neurofibromas have occurred in patients with clear-cut evidence of neurofibromatosis. In some instances the tumours have been confined to the labia (Miller 1979, Friedrich & Wilkinson 1985) but in others the clitoris has been the site of a plexiform neurofibroma, the resulting clitoromegaly in some instances being an isolated phenomenon and in others being associated with labial tumours (Petsche & Radinger 1954, Haddad & Jones 1960, Hoffmann 1963, Kenny et al 1966, Labardini et al 1968, Messina & Strauss 1976, Schepel & Tolhurst 1981, Greer & Pederson 1981, Milia et al 1982, Craven & Bresnahan 1983, Ravikumar & Lakshmanan 1983). Not surprisingly patients, usually children or adolescents, with clitoral enlargement due to a plexiform neurofibroma tend to be initially diagnosed as cases of intersex, this being particularly the case if accompanying labial tumours are incorrectly taken to be testes. It is highly probable that such cases tend to be selectively reported and thus place undue emphasis on neurofibromas involving the clitoris. It is equally probable that many examples of vulval neurofibromas in women with von Recklinghausen's disease pass unrecorded and these two factors make it difficult to assess the true incidence of vulval tumours in this disease, a difficulty accentuated by the inadequate recording of pathological findings and a manifest lack of understanding of the protean manifestations of von Recklinghausen's disease in many reports of cases. These difficulties are emphasised in the study by Schreiber (1963) of 33 female patients with neurofibromatosis; amongst these, ten had vulval abnormalities, none of which was subjected to pathological assessment. Schreiber regarded the vulval abnormalities as being due to 'elephantiasis nervosum', which he described as an 'overgrowth of skin and subcutaneous tissue which may or may not contain neurofibromas'. The exact nature of these lesions is a matter for debate but this report has, on the one hand, been interpreted as indicating that vulval neurofibromas are very uncommon in patients with von Recklinghausen's disease and, on the other hand, been taken to show that vulval neurofibromas occur frequently in this disorder. There is clearly a need for better clinical and pathological documentation of vulval abnormalities in cases of neurofibromatosis.

A solitary neurofibroma is usually adequately treated by local excision. In many cases of neurofibromatosis, however, the large number of tumours limits surgical therapy to those lesions which are large, painful or located in strategic areas where continued growth would impair organ function. Unfortunately the poorly delineated nature of many of these neoplasms means that surgical removal is often incomplete and that subsequent recurrences develop.

Malignant change occurs in a significant proportion of neurofibromas in patients with von Recklinghausen's disease and is usually manifest by rapid enlargement of, and pain in, a pre-existing lesion. Once malignant change has occurred radical surgery is indicated though even with such therapy less than 20% of patients survive for 5 years.

Malignant Schwannoma (synonyms: neurogenic sarcoma, neurofibrosarcoma). It is generally agreed that if a sarcomatous neoplasm arises in a peripheral nerve or in a pre-existing neurofibroma it can be regarded as a malignant Schwannoma; there is considerable controversy, however, about the recognition of a malignant Schwannoma outside these two settings, some claiming that they are common tumours of soft tissues and others that they rarely, if ever, occur in patients lacking the stigmata of neurofibromatosis. The malignant Schwannoma certainly closely resembles a fibrosarcoma and even when the neoplasm clearly arises from a nerve it cannot always be distinguished from such a tumour. Enzinger & Weiss (1983) maintain, however, that the presence of certain rather subtle histological features, such as peculiarities of nuclear shape, a tendency towards nuclear palisading and evidence of rudimentary tactoid differentiation, allow for the recognition of most, though probably not all, malignant Schwannomas.

Because the histological diagnosis of a malignant Schwannoma is fraught with both problems and controversy, it has proved difficult to define the prognosis of these neoplasms, but in Enzinger & Weiss's (1983) series the 5-year survival rate for patients with a malignant Schwannoma developing in the setting or von Recklinghausen's disease was only 15% whilst the equivalent survival rate for

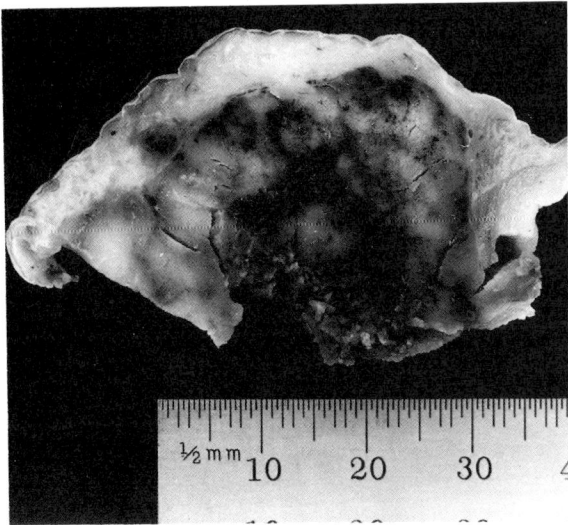

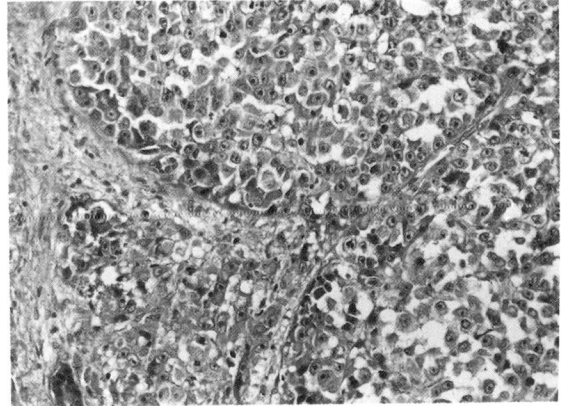

Fig. 9.19 Histological appearance of an epithelioid sarcoma of the vulva. The tumour characteristically grows in a multinodular fashion. (H & E ×40) (Reproduced from Ulbright et al 1983, with kind permission of the authors and the Editor of *Cancer*).

Fig. 9.18 An epithelioid sarcoma of the vulva. In this section of the right labium majus numerous white or haemorrhagic nodules of tumour are seen spreading below the skin surface. (Reproduced from Ulbright et al 1983, by kind permission of the authors and the Editor of *Cancer*).

patients with a malignant Schwannoma but without neurofibromatosis was 47%. There seems little doubt that the treatment of choice for these neoplasms is radical surgery; information about the value of radiotherapy or chemotherapy in the management of these tumours is too limited to permit any assessment of their therapeutic role.

Malignant Schwannomas of the vulva have been only rarely reported and their paucity is compounded by the high probability, as previously noted, that one of the vulval tumours described as a malignant Schwannoma (Lawrence & Shingleton 1978) should be more correctly regarded as a cellular neurolemmoma. DiSaia et al (1971) described two cases of malignant Schwannoma of the vulva; the tumours arose in women aged 25 and 42 years (neither of whom were apparently sufferers from neurofibromatosis), were small (2.5 cm in diameter) and situated in the labia majora; the patients were treated by radical vulvectomy and were alive and well at 18 months and 9 years respectively after initial diagnosis. These authors also described a third case in which the neoplasm arose in a predominantly peri-anal site but their report is flawed by the complete absence of any histological information and by the authors' failure to state their

criteria for the recognition of a malignant Schwannoma.

The only fully acceptable example of a malignant Schwannoma of the vulva was reported by Davos & Abell (1976); the patient, aged 40 years, presented with a 5-year history of a vulval nodule which had recently increased in size and become painful. The patient had no stigmata of von Recklinghausen's disease and the vulval mass, which was in the labium majus, measured 3 cm in diameter. The patient was treated by hemivulvectomy and was alive and well 2 years later. This neoplasm was shown histologically to be a sarcoma arising in a solitary neurofibroma and therefore fully merited the diagnosis of a malignant Schwannoma.

Mesenchymal tumours of uncertain origin

Epithelioid sarcoma. The epithelioid sarcoma, first described by Enzinger in 1970, is a rare but morphologically distinct soft tissue neoplasm which occurs most commonly in the extremities of adolescents and young adults. Its histogenesis is uncertain, for whilst some ultrastructural studies have suggested a possible origin from synovium many of the clinical and pathological characteristics of the tumour are more akin to those of a malignant fibrous histiocytoma.

Epithelioid sarcomas grow slowly but in a relentless fashion (Fig. 9.18); inadequate excision is inevitably followed by recurrence and, in many cases, by lymphatic and, later, vascular spread. The histological features (Fig. 9.19) are characteristic but nevertheless confusing and these neoplasms are often initially diagnosed as carcinomas or as necrotizing granulomatous inflammatory lesions. The tumour cells are grouped into nodules which commonly show central necrosis or hyalinisation; the cells are polygonal or fusiform with abundant strongly acidophilic cytoplasm which may show fine vacuolation or hyaline change. Spindle-shaped cells are often present and tend to aggregate at the periphery of the nodules; occasional multinucleated giant cells may be seen. In some cases an alveolar pattern is present whilst sometimes the tumour cells form nests or cords which are set in a densely fibrous stroma. Clefts have been noted in some tumours but these are possibly a fixation artefact. Pleomorphism is not usually a conspicuous feature whilst mitotic figures may be either sparse or fairly numerous. At the ultrastructural level the tumour cells are characterised by intercellular cytoplasmic interdigitations, an abundance of rough endoplasmic reticulum, many Golgi complexes and conspicuous intermediate-sized cytoplasmic filaments; there has been some dispute as to whether intercellular membrane junctions are present or not (Gabbiani et al 1972, Frable et al 1973, Blousten et al 1976, Patchefsky et al 1977, Mills et al 1981).

Five cases of epithelioid sarcoma of the vulva have been reported (Piver et al 1972, Gallup et al 1976, Hall et al 1980, Ulbright et al 1983). One of these tumours occurred in a 55-year-old woman but all the other patients were aged between 27 and 31 years. The patients presented with a history, varying in length from 8 weeks to 2 years, of a slowly enlarging, painless, nodular mass most commonly situated in the labium majus; ulceration occurred in only one case and in several of these patients the initial clinical diagnosis was that of a Bartholin's duct cyst. Three of the patients were treated by wide local excision whilst two were subjected to radical vulvectomy and bilateral groin lymph node dissection. Recurrences, at intervals varying from 6 weeks to 5 years after initial therapy, occurred in four patients, usually as multiple nodules in the vulva, groin, upper thigh or lower anterior abdominal wall, and all these women died with lung metastases, three within 2 years but one surviving for 11 years before succumbing to the neoplasm.

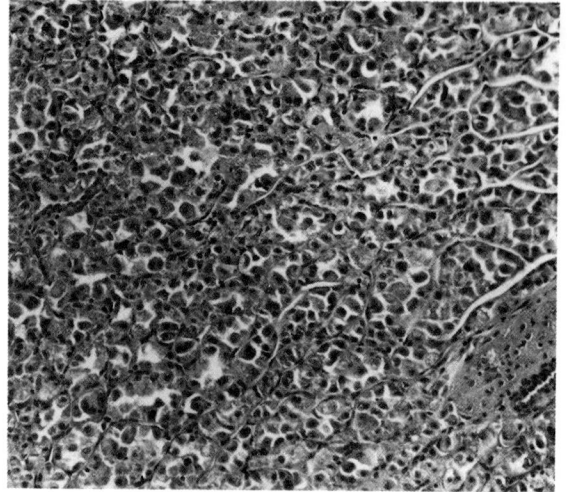

Fig. 9.20 An alveolar soft part sarcoma: the tumour cells are separated into islands by fibrous septae. (H & E ×80)

Only one patient, treated by wide local excision, did not suffer tumour recurrence, and she was alive and well 9 years later. These gloomy figures emphasize the point made by Ulbright et al (1983) that epithelioid sarcomas of the vulva appear to behave more aggressively than do similar neoplasms in extragenital sites and indicate the difficulties encountered in treatment. Radiotherapy appears to be ineffective against these tumours and Hall et al (1980) suggest that early surgical management, consisting of either very wide en bloc removal or radical vulvectomy with bilateral groin lymph node dissection, is the treatment of choice. Chemotherapy has been used to treat recurrences but without any great success and the role, if any, of this form of therapy is currently undetermined.

Alveolar soft part sarcoma. This is a rare soft tissue neoplasm which occurs most commonly in adolescents and young adults; the site of predilection in adult patients is the lower limb, particularly the thigh, whilst in children the tumour arises most commonly in the head and neck region. The alveolar soft part sarcoma is a slowly growing neoplasm which is nevertheless ultimately fatal in 50% of cases, metastasis occurring at a relatively early stage via the bloodstream to the lungs.

The tumour is usually poorly circumscribed, soft and friable. Histologically, fibrous septa compartment the tumour cells into sharply defined islands

(Fig. 9.20); within the cellular aggregates central degeneration and loss of cellular cohesion result in a pseudo-alveolar pattern. The tumour cells are large, rounded or polygonal, have central vesicular nuclei and abundant granular eosinophilic cytoplasm; there is little pleomorphism and mitotic figures are sparse (Enzinger & Weiss 1983). PAS staining shows a variable amount of intracellular glycogen and, in most but not all cases, PAS positive, diastase resistant crystals, the nature of which is unknown.

The histogenesis of the alveolar soft part sarcoma is obscure though it is possible that it is a neoplasm of specific nerve endings or chemoreceptors. The view, based largely on electronmicroscopic observations, that the neoplasm is a form of paraganglioneuroma has won wide support (Smetana & Scott 1951, Marshall & Horn 1961, Welsh et al 1972, Unni & Soule 1975), though many still have reservations about this concept (Enzinger & Weiss 1983).

There have been only two reports of an alveolar soft tissue sarcoma of the vulva. Shen et al (1982) described a 62-year-old woman in whom an asymptomatic mobile mass in the labium minus, measuring 4 cm in its largest diameter, was an incidental finding during a routine examination. The tumour was excised and, after a definitive pathological diagnosis of alveolar soft part sarcoma was attained, the patient was subjected to radical vulvectomy with bilateral groin node dissection; no further treatment was given and the patient was alive and tumour free 2 years later. Kondratiev & Kurillov (1971) had previously reported a vulval alveolar soft part sarcoma which arose in a 28-year-old woman and recurred 15 months after initial excision; the illustrations of this neoplasm are largely, but not entirely, convincing.

Two cases give little indication as to how vulval alveolar soft part sarcomas should be treated though there can be little doubt that wide local excision, probably with regional node dissection, is the initial treatment of choice. Theoretically, adjuvant therapy should also be given though postoperative radiation, whilst tending to reduce the incidence of local recurrence of these tumours, does not prevent distant metastases or prolong survival (Shen et al 1982); chemotherapy does not appear to have any significant effect on this neoplasm.

Germ cell tumours

Endodermal sinus tumour

The endodermal, or yolk sac, tumour is derived from germ cells and predominantly occurs in the gonads; it is well recognised, however, that neoplasms of this type can also develop in those extragonadal sites which traditionally harbour germ cell neoplasms, such as the pineal gland, the sacrococcygeal area or the mediastinum. The occurrence of endodermal sinus tumours in the lower female genital tract is less widely known though over 40 such neoplasms have been reported as arising in the vagina (Young & Scully 1984) and four endodermal sinus tumours of the vulva have been fully documented (Ungerleider et al 1978, Castaldo et al 1980, Krishnamurphy & Sampat 1981, Dudley et al 1983). It is assumed, but certainly not proved, that endodermal sinus tumours arising in this unusual site originate from germ cells which, during embryogenesis, have gone astray during their migration from the yolk sac to the developing gonad, but it is extraordinary that other types of germ cell tumour, such as dysgerminoma, have not been described as occurring in the vagina and vulva.

The endodermal sinus tumour is a highly aggressive, extremely malignant neoplasm which invades locally, spreads at an early stage to regional lymph nodes and disseminates widely within a short time of initial diagnosis. It has a complex histological character with a number of different microscopic patterns which can occur singly or in any combination or permutation. These include a loose, vacuolated network within which microcystic spaces form a honeycomb pattern, perivascular formations (Fig. 9.21) which mimic the endodermal sinus of the rat placenta (Schiller–Duval bodies), sheets or aggregates of small polygonal epithelial-like cells with clear cytoplasm and gland-like spaces lined by flat or cuboidal cells (Talerman 1982). A relatively constant feature is the presence, either within or outside of tumour cells, of small eosinophilic PAS positive, diastase resistant globules.

Patients with an endodermal sinus tumour have elevated plasma levels of alpha fetoprotein, this substance serving as an excellent marker to facilitate pre-operative diagnosis, to monitor the re-

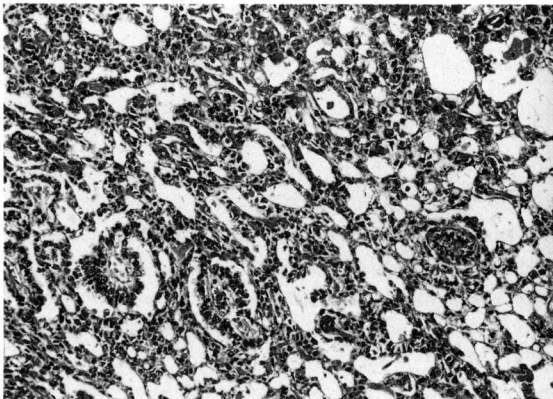

Fig. 9.21 An endodermal sinus tumour. Several typical Schiller–Duval bodies are seen. (H & E ×60)

sponse of the tumour to therapy and to indicate, at an early stage, tumour recurrence. The PAS positive globules within the tumour can be shown by immunocytochemical techniques to contain alpha fetoprotein.

The endodermal sinus tumour of the ovary is a neoplasm of infancy, adolescence and early adulthood and those occurring in the vulva follow this same pattern, the ages of the four patients with endodermal sinus tumours at this site being 22 months, 2 years, 14 years and 26 years; this last patient, unusually but not exceptionally old to be suffering a neoplasm of this type, was pregnant at the time of initial diagnosis. All the patients presented with a short history, measured in months rather than years, of a painless enlarging mass in the vulva, the tumour being in the labium majus in three cases and confined to the clitoris in one; the masses ranged in size from 1.5 to 12 cm in diameter.

One child, with tumour limited to the clitoris, was treated solely by wide excision and was well and tumour free 42 months after surgery. The course pursued by the tumour in the other three patients was less encouraging for all died, at periods varying from 6 to 23 months, with lymph node metastases followed by disseminated disease; one of these patients was treated by wide local excision and subsequent chemotherapy whilst the other two were subjected to a radical vulvectomy followed by chemotherapy and radiotherapy. Depression about the outlook for young patients with

a vulval endodermal sinus tumour should, however, be tempered by the fact that only one of the reported patients received what would currently be regarded as fully effective chemotherapy for a tumour of this type, namely triple combination therapy with vincristine, actinomycin D and cyclophosphamide (VAC) and it is of interest to note that six patients with vaginal endodermal sinus tumours were alive and free from disease at intervals varying from 2 to 9 years after treatment by surgery and VAC (Young & Scully 1984). The optimal management of a vulval endodermal sinus tumour would therefore appear to be initial control of the local disease by radical vulvectomy with groin and pelvic node dissection followed by a full course of chemotherapy with VAC (Dudley et al 1983). Such a therapeutic regime holds hope for considerable improvement of the prognosis for children and young women with an endodermal sinus tumour of the vulva.

Teratoma

There have been no detailed accounts of a vulval teratoma but Huffman et al (1981) briefly mention two tumours apparently of this type occurring in this anatomical region in children. One presented as a mass lateral to the fourchette in a 14-month-old infant and, being formed solely of rectal-type tissue, may well have been a developmental abnormality of the lower intestinal tract rather than a true teratoma. The second case, histological details of which were not given, arose from the perineum immediately adjacent to the anus rather than from the vulva.

Malignant lymphoma and leukaemia

Very few lymphomatous or leukaemic lesions of the vulva have been recorded and, unfortunately, many of the descriptions of such cases have been characterised by skimpiness of clinical detail, poor documentation of the histological findings and an inadequate period of follow-up. Furthermore most of the reports predate the currently used systems of nomenclature, and terms such as 'reticulum cell sarcoma' and 'lymphosarcoma' abound; as the true nature of these lymphomas can rarely be identified in contemporary terms they will, in this account, all be classed together as examples of non-Hodgkin's lymphoma.

Vulval involvement in lymphoma or leukaemia can, as with other sites in the female genital tract, be grouped under four headings:

1. Known cases of lymphoma or leukaemia with occult involvement of the vulva which is detectable only on autopsy examination.
2. Known cases of lymphoma or leukaemia in which clinically detectable lesions develop in the vulva.
3. Cases of disseminated lymphoma or leukaemia in which a vulval lesion is the presenting feature or part of the presenting clinical picture.
4. Initial localisation of a lymphoma to the vulva, this being the apparent site of a primary extranodal lymphoma.

The existence of primary extranodal lymphomas is not universally accepted, it being argued that such cases represent only an apparently primary localisation of what is always a multifocal disease. Occasional patients with vulval lymphoma have, however, survived for a significant number of years after only local treatment and this does suggest that primary lymphomas of the vulva may exist. Such a lesion should ideally, however, only be diagnosed if it fulfils the following criteria:

1. At the time of diagnosis the disease is clinically confined to the vulva and full investigation fails to reveal evidence of lymphoma elsewhere. A tumour can still be accepted as probably primary in the vulva if spread has occurred to local lymph nodes.
2. The peripheral blood and bone marrow do not contain any abnormal cells.
3. If further lymphomatous lesions appear at sites remote from the vulva, then at least several months should have elapsed between the appearance of the primary and secondary lesions.

None of the reported cases of vulval lymphoma meet these criteria to their full extent but, nevertheless, there have been seven cases which probably fall into this category, one of Hodgkin's disease (Hahn 1958) and six of non-Hodgkin's lymphoma (Taussig 1937, Ramioul 1952, Buckingham & McClure 1955, Iliya et al 1968, Wishart 1973,

Verhaegh et al 1977). The woman with Hodgkin's disease was 56 years old and presented with an indurated swelling in the region of Bartholin's gland that had been present for 1 year. Following local excision this patient was alive and well 5 years later. The ages of the patients with apparently primary non-Hodgkin's lymphoma of the vulva varied from 33 to 77 years; all presented with a vulval nodule, mass or ulcer and the length of the history ranged from 2 to 8 months. Most of the lesions were in the labia but one was principally localised to the clitoris. In one case the lymphoma developed in a woman who was immunosuppressed (Wishart 1973). All the patients received local treatment, either simple excision, radical vulvectomy or radical vulvectomy and radiotherapy. One woman was alive and well 5 years later, one alive and well 15 months later, one was alive but with local recurrence 6 months after surgery and one patient succumbed to inguinal node metastases and local recurrence after 3 years. One patient died of a pulmonary embolism 2 weeks after treatment whilst no follow-up details were provided for the remaining patient. It can be seen therefore that local therapy of an apparently primary lymphoma of the vulva can be successful in some cases, though many would consider that chemotherapy is also indicated.

Presentation of a disseminated or multifocal lymphoma as a vulval lesion is very rare. Schiller & Madge (1970) reported a patient in whom a vulval mass was the presenting clinical sign of a widespread non-Hodgkin's lymphoma whilst Eguwatu et al (1980) described a 13-year-old Nigerian girl who, although found to have an ovarian Burkitt's tumour, presented clinically with a rapidly enlarging vulval mass, biopsy of which showed the typical features of this form of lymphoma. The patient with a vulval extramedullary plasmacytoma reported by Doss (1978) also probably falls into this group for she died rapidly of widespread myelomatosis. A particular form of local presentation of a disseminated disease is the granulocytic sarcoma, which though appearing as a localised tumour is the harbinger of, and evolves into, a myeloid leukaemia; the vulval lesions reported by Joswig & Joswig-Priewe (1974), Gardaise et al (1974) and Laricchia et al (1977) all appear to fall into this category. Clearly a leukaemic process or a multi-

258 THE VULVA

focal lymphoma presenting with a vulvar lesion should be treated systemically.

Involvement of the vulva in patients with known lymphoma or leukaemia is also rare. Kulka (1932) described an example of clitoral priapism due to leukaemic infiltration in a patient known to be suffering from this disease whilst Plouffie et al (1984) reported an example of lymphomatous infiltration of Bartholin's gland in a patient with known non-Hodgkin's lymphoma.

Finally, there have been a few reports of vulval lymphoma in which too few clinical or pathological details have been given to allow for any comment as to their relationship or otherwise with multifocal or disseminated disease (Kelly 1972).

MIXED TUMOURS

Benign mixed tumours

Benign mixed tumours, or pleomorphic adenomas, occur most commonly in the salivary gland and are characterised by having both epithelial and mesenchymal components. They are traditionally thought to be derived from pluripotential myo-epithelial cells, though recent studies suggest that mixed tumours contain a spectrum of cell types, with epithelial cells at one end of the range and myoepithelial cells at the other; in between are relatively undifferentiated cells, some of which have characteristics of both epithelial and myo-epithelial cells, this indicating that a single progenitor cell gives rise to all the cell types seen in mixed tumours (Batsakis et al 1979).

The neoplasms are solitary and, although not encapsulated, well delineated; they usually have a lobulated or bosselated surface and on section may be firm, hard, cartilaginous or mucoid. Histologically the epithelial component forms tubules, small cysts, cords, nests and sheets. The epithelial cells are regular with rounded, often inconspicuous, nuclei and eosinophilic cytoplasm and are set in a chondromyxoid stroma in which mature cartilage is commonly present. Bone is sometimes seen and this appears to be a consequence of osseous metaplasia. Pleomorphism, cellular atypia and mitotic activity are not features of these neoplasms.

Five cases of benign mixed tumour of the vulva have been reported (Janovski & Douglas 1972, Wilson & Woodger 1974, Ordonez et al 1981, Rorat & Wallach 1984), all of which had the typical appearances of a pleomorphic adenoma as seen in salivary glands. The origin of such tumours in the vulva is obscure but it is probable that they arise either from Bartholin's gland or from vulval sweat glands; a theoretical possibility is that they originate from either accessory breast or ectopic salivary tissue in the vulva.

The age of patients with a benign mixed tumour of the vulva has ranged from 44 to 66 years with most women being over 60 years at the time of diagnosis. The invariable complaint has been of a painless lump which has usually been apparent for years rather than months, a mass having been present in one patient for 29 years before clinical presentation. All except one of the tumours arose in the left labium majus, the sole exception being sited adjacent to the clitoris. All the tumours measured less than 2.5 cm. in diameter and were mobile. The neoplasms were all treated by wide local excision and, at the time of reporting, none had recurred at follow-up intervals ranging from 4 months to 5 years. It is worth noting that 50% of parotid gland pleomorphic adenomas recur, almost certainly because of incomplete initial excision. There are no grounds for believing that pleomorphic adenomas in the vulva behave differently from their more common counterparts in the salivary gland and hence benign mixed tumours should be treated by generous local excision with a wide margin of adjacent normal tissue.

Malignant mixed tumour

If one excludes carcinosarcomas the term 'malignant mixed tumour' encompasses two quite distinct entities. The first is a pleomorphic adenoma which, although histologically benign, pursues a malignant course and metastasises and the other is a true carcinoma arising in an otherwise unremarkable pleomorphic adenoma (carcinoma ex mixed tumour).

Only one malignant mixed tumour of the vulva has been documented (Ordonez et al 1981), this being a typical carcinoma ex mixed tumour. The neoplasm presented, in a 69-year-old woman, as a polypoid tumour mass involving the left labium majus, the left lateral wall of the vagina, the peri-urethral area and the rectovaginal septum. A pelvic exenteration was performed and the tumour, which measured 7 cm in diameter, showed in some areas the typical appearances of a pleomorphic adenoma and in others the equally typical pattern of an adenoid cystic carcinoma. Local recurrence did not occur but 1 year later the patient, though still alive, had multiple pulmonary metastases.

REFERENCES

Agress R, Figge D C, Tamimi H, Greer B 1983 Dermatofibrosarcoma protuberans of the vulva. Gynecologic Oncology 16: 288–291

Altaras M, Jaffe R, Bernheim J, Ben Aderet N 1985 Granular cell myoblastoma of the vulva. Gynecologic Oncology 22: 352–355

Ambrosini A, Becagli L, de Bastiani B M 1980 Hemangiopericytoma of the vulva: a study of two cases. European Journal of Gynaecological Oncology 1: 198–200

Aneiros J, Garcia del Moral R, Beltran E, Nogales F F 1982 Epithelioid leiomyoma of the vulva. Diagnostic Gynecology and Obstetrics 4: 351–355

Aparicio S R, Lumsden C E 1969 Light and electron-microscopic studies on the granular cell myoblastoma of the tongue. Journal of Pathology 97: 339–355

Audet-Lapointe P, Paquin F, Guerard M J, Charbonneau A, Methot F, Morano G 1980 Leiomyosarcoma of the vulva. Gynecologic Oncology 10: 350–355

Batsakis J G, Regezi J A, Bloch D 1979 The pathology of head and neck tumors: salivary glands. Part 3. Head and Neck Surgery 1: 260–273

Begin L R, Clement P B, Kirk M E, Jothy S, McCaughey, Ferenczy A 1985 Aggressive angiomyxoma of pelvic soft parts: a clinicopathological study of nine cases. Human Pathology 16: 621–628

Beilby J O W, Ridley C M 1987 Pathology of the vulva. In: Fox H (ed) Haines and Taylors textbook of obstetrical and gynaecological pathology, 3rd edn. Churchill Livingstone, Edinburgh, pp 64–145

Bianco R, Samuel S 1958 Neurilemmoma della vulva. Tumori 44: 326–336

Birch H W, Sondag D R 1961 Granular cell myoblastoma of the vulva: report of five cases with special tissue stains in one. Obstetrics and Gynecology 18: 443–454

Blair C 1970 Angiokeratoma of the vulva. British Journal of Dermatology 83: 409–411

Blousten P A, Silverberg S G, Waddell W R 1976 Epithelioid sarcoma: case report with ultrastructural review, histogenetic discussion and chemotherapeutic data. Cancer 38: 2390–2400

Bo A V, Bianchi G, Kron G B, Miglioli P 1976 Si du un caso ad eccezionale sopravvenza di sarcoma della vulva. Minerva Ginecologica 28: 145–149

Bock J E, Andreasson B, Thorn A, Holck S 1985 Dermatofibrosarcoma protuberans of the vulva. Gynecologic Oncology 20: 129–135

Brooks J J, LiVolsi V A 1987 Liposarcoma presenting on the vulva. American Journal of Obstetrics and Gynecology 156: 73–75

Bryan W E 1955. Neurilemmoma of the vulva. Journal of Obstetrics and Gynaecology of the British Empire 62: 949–950

Buckingham J C McClure H J 1955 Reticulum cell sarcoma of the vulva: report of a case. Obstetrics and Gynecology 6: 138–143

Cadotte M 1974 Malignant granular cell myoblastoma. Cancer 33: 1417–1422

Carstens P H 1970 Ultrastructure of granular cell myoblastoma. Acta Pathologica et Microbiologica Scandinavica 78: 685–694

Castaldo T W, Petrilli E S, Ballon S C, Voet R L, Lagasse L D, Lubens R 1980 Endodermal sinus tumor of the clitoris. Gynecologic Oncology 9: 376–380

Chambers D C 1979 Granular cell myoblastoma of the vulva. Journal of the National Medical Association 71: 1071–1073

Coates J B, Hales J S 1973 Granular cell myoblastoma of the vulva. Obstetrics and Gynecology 41: 796–799

Craven E M, Bresnahan K 1983 Neuroma of the clitoris. Delaware Medical Journal 55: 341–342

Darnalt-Restrepo E 1957 Hemangiomas de la vulva et de la vagina. Rivista Colombiana de Obstetricia 8: 272–276

Davos I, Abell M R 1976 Soft tissue sarcomas of vulva. Gynecologic Oncology 4: 70–86

Degefu S, Dhurandhar H N, O'Quinn A G, Fuller P N 1984 Granular cell tumor of the clitoris in pregnancy. Gynecologic Oncology 19: 246–251

Dgani R, Czernobilsky B, Borenstein R, Lancet M 1978 Granular cell myoblastoma of the vulva: report of 4 cases. Acta Obstetricia et Gynecologica Scandinavica 57: 385–387

Dini S 1959 Rara isservazione di neurinoma del piccolo labbro vulvare. Archivo de Becchi 29: 867–875

De Sousa L M, Lash A F 1959 Hemangiopericytoma of the vulva. American Journal of Obstetrics and Gynecology 78: 295–298

DiSaia P J, Rutledge F, Smith J P 1971 Sarcoma of the vulva: a report of 12 patients. Obstetrics and Gynecology 38: 180–184

Di Sant Agnese P A, Knowles D M 1980 Extracardiac rhabdomyoma: a clinicopathological study and review of the literature. Cancer 46: 780–789

Doss L L 1978 Simultaneous extramedullary plasmacytomas of the vagina and vulva: a case report and review of the literature. Cancer 41: 2468–2471

Dotters D J, Fowler W C, Powers J K, McKune B K 1986 Argon laser therapy of vulvar angiokeratoma. Obstetrics and Gynecology 68: 56s–59s

Doyle W F, Hutchinson J R 1968 Granular cell myoblastoma of the clitoris. American Journal of Obstetrics and Gynecology 100: 589–590

Drescher H, Herzog W 1961 Über Neurofibromatose der Vulva und der Vagina. Zentralblatt für Gynäkologie 83: 743–750

Du Boulay C E H 1985 Immunohistochemistry of soft tissue tumours: a review. Journal of Pathology 146: 77–94

Dudley A G, Young R H, Lawrence W D, Scully R E 1983 Endodermal sinus tumor of the vulva in an infant. Obstetrics and Gynecology 61: 76S–79S

Eguwatu V E, Ejeckam G C, Okaro J M 1980 Burkitt's lymphoma of the vulva: case report. British Journal of Obstetrics and Gynaecology 87: 827–830

Enzinger F M 1970 Epithelioid sarcoma: a sarcoma simulating a granuloma or a carcinoma. Cancer 26: 1029–1041

Enzinger F M, Weiss S W 1983 Soft tissue tumors. C V Mosby, St Louis

Fisher E R, Wechsler H 1962 Granular cell myoblastoma—a misnomer: E M and histochemical evidence concerning its Schwann cell derivation and nature (granular cell Schwannoma). Cancer 15: 936–954

Frable W F, Kay S, Lawrence W, Schatzki P F 1973 Epithelioid sarcoma: an electron microscopic study. Archives of Pathology 95: 8–12

Friedrich E G, Wilkinson E J 1985 Vulvar surgery for neurofibromatosis. Obstetrics and Gynecology 65: 135–138

Fukaminzu H, Matsumoto K, Inoue K, Moriguchi T 1982 Large vulva lipoma. Archives of Dermatology 118: 447

Gabbiani G, Fu Y S, Kaye G I, Lattes R, Majno G 1972 Epithelioid sarcoma: a light and electron microscopic study suggesting a synovial origin. Cancer 30: 486–499

Gallup D G, Abel M R, Morley G W 1976 Epithelioid sarcoma of the vulva. Obstetrics and Gynecology 48 (Supplement 1): 14S–17S

Gamboa L G 1955 Malignant granular-cell myoblastoma. Archives of Pathology 60: 663–668

Gardaise J, Marie M, Bertrand G 1974 Chlorome a localizations génitales multiples. Semaine des Hôpitaux de Paris 51: 609–616

Gerbie A B, Hirsch M R, Greene R R 1955 Vascular tumors of the female genital tract. Obstetrics and Gynecology 6: 499–507

Giannone R, Avezzi G 1969 Emangioma cavernose della vulva. Revista Italiana de Ginecologia 53: 471–479

Gifford R, Birch H W 1973 Granular cell myoblastoma of multicentric origin involving the vulva: a case report. American Journal of Obstetrics and Gynecology 117: 184–187

Gondos B, Casey M J 1982 Liposarcoma of the perineum. Gynecologic Oncology 14: 133–140

Greer D M, Pederson W C 1981 Pseudo-masculinization of the clitoris. Plastic and Reconstructive Surgery 68: 787–788

Guercio E, Siliquini G P, Aimone V, Chiringhello B, Mutti F, Rolfo A 1982 Emangiopericitoma della vulva. Minerva Ginecologica 34: 451–460

Gulienetti R 1959 Haemangiomata of the external genitals. British Journal of Plastic Surgery 12: 228–233

Haddad H M, Jones H W 1960 Clitoral enlargement simulating pseudohermaphroditism. American Journal of Diseases of Children 99: 282–287

Hahn G A 1958 Gynecologic considerations in malignant lymphoma. American Journal of Obstetrics and Gynecology 75: 673–683

Hall D J, Burns J C, Goplerud D R 1979 Kaposi's sarcoma of the vulva: a case report and brief review. Obstetrics and Gynecology 54: 478–483

Hall D J, Grimes M H, Goplerud D R 1980 Epithelioid sarcoma of the vulva. Gynecologic Oncology 9: 237–246

Hall J S E, Amin U F 1981 Fibrosarcoma of the vulva: case reports and discussion. International Surgery 86: 185–187

Hensley G T, Friedrich E G 1973 Malignant fibroxanthoma: a sarcoma of the vulva. American Journal of Obstetrics and Gynecology 116: 289–291

Hilgers R D, Pai R, Barton S A, Aisenbrey G, Bowling M C 1986 Aggressive angiomyxoma of the vulva. Obstetrics and Gynecology 68: 605–625

Hoffman J 1962 Die Neurofibromatose der Vulva unter dem Erscheinungsbild eines Pseudohermaphroditismus. Zentralblatt für Gynäkologie 84: 961–966

Huffman J W, Dewhurst C J, Capraro V J 1981 The gynecology of childhood and adolescence, 2nd Edn. W B Saunders, Philadelphia

Iliya F A, Muggia F M, O'Leary J A, King T M 1968 Gynecologic manifestations of reticulum cell sarcoma. Obstetrics and Gynecology 31: 266–269

Imperial R, Helwig E B 1967 Angiokeratoma of the vulva. Obstetrics and Gynecology 29: 307–312

James G B, Guthrie W, Buchan A 1969 Embryonic sarcoma of the vulva in an infant. Journal of Obstetrics and Gynaecology of the British Commonwealth 76: 458–461

Janovski N A, Douglas C P 1972 Diseases of the vulva. Harper and Row, Hagerstown, Maryland

Joswig E H, Joswig-Priewe H 1974 Retikulumzellsarkom in Bereich der Vulva und Vagina. Zentralblatt für Gynäkologie 96: 1040–1043

Katenkamp D, Stiller D 1980 Unusual leiomyoma of the vulva with fibroma-like pattern and pseudoelastin formation. Virchows Archiv. A. Pathological Anatomy and Histology 388: 361–368

Katz V L, Askin F B, Bosch B D 1986 Glomus tumor of the vulva: a case report. Obstetrics and Gynecology 67: 43S–45S

Kauffman-Friedman K 1978 Hemangioma of clitoris-confused with adreno-genital syndrome: case report. Plastic and Reconstructive Surgery 62: 452–454

Kaufman R H, Gardner H L 1965 Benign mesodermal tumors. Clinical Obstetrics and Gynecology 8: 953–981

Keller J 1951 Fibrosarcoma of labium vulvae. Canadian Medical Association Journal 64: 574–576

Kelly J 1972 Malignant disease of the vulva. Journal of Obstetrics and Gynaecology of the British Commonwealth 79: 265–272

Kenny F M, Fetterman G H, Preeyasombat C 1966 Neurofibromata simulating a penis and labioscrotal gonads in a girl with von Recklinghausen's disease. Pediatrics 37: 956–959

King D F, Bustillo M, Broen E N, Hirose F M 1979 Granular cell tumors of the vulva: a report of three cases. Journal of Dermatologic Surgery and Oncology 5: 794–797

Kohorn E I, Merino M J, Goldenhersh M 1986 Vulvar pain and dyspareunia due to glomus tumor. Obstetrics and Gynecology 67: 41S–42S

Kondratiev L N, Kurillov A L 1971 Soft tissue alveolar sarcoma of the vulva. Arkhiv Patologii (Moscow) 33: 80–82

Krebs H B, Schneider V, Radford W L 1984 Congenital dysplastic angiopathy (Kleppel–Trenaunay–Webber syndrome) with vulvar involvement: a case report. Journal of Reproductive Medicine 29: 215–218

Krishnamurphy S C, Sampat M B 1981 Endodermal sinus (yolk sac) tumor of the vulva in a pregnant female. Gynecologic Oncology 11: 379–382

Kulka H 1932 Leukanischer Priapismus der Klitoris unter den Bilde eines Carcinoms. Archiv für Gynakologie 149: 450–461

Labardini M M, Kallet H A, Cerny J C 1968 Urogenital neurofibromatosis simulating an intersex problem. Journal of Urology 98: 627–632

Laricchia R, Wierdis T, Loiudice L, Trisolini A, Riezzo A 1977 Neoformazione vulvare (mieloblastoma) come prima manifestazione di una leucemia acuta mieloblastica. Minerva Ginecologica 29: 957–961

Lawrence W D, Shingleton H M 1978 Malignant Schwannoma of the vulva: a light and electron microscopic study. Gynecologic Oncology 6: 527–537

Lesoin A, Destée A, Lafitte J J, Jomin M 1983 Myoblastome à cellules granuleuses: revue de la littérature à propos 3 observations. Larc Medicale 3: 232–235

Lieb S M, Gallousis S, Freedman H 1979 Granular cell

myoblastoma of the vulva. Gynecologic Oncology 8: 12–20

Li Volsi V A, Brooks J J 1987 Soft tissue tumours of the vulva. In: Wilkinson E J (ed) Pathology of the vulva and vagina. Churchill Livingstone, New York, p 209–238

Lott I T, Richardson E P 1981 Neuropathological findings and the biology of neurofibromatosis. In: Riccardi V M, Mulvihill J J (eds) Neurofibromatosis (Von Recklinghausen's disease). Raven, New York, p 23–32

Lovelady S B, McDonald J R, Waugh J M 1941 Benign tumors of vulva. American Journal of Obstetrics and Gynecology 42: 309–313

McMaster M J, Soule E H, Ivins J C 1975 Hemangiopericytoma: a clinicopathologic study and long term follow-up of 60 patients. Cancer 36: 2232–2244

Mágori A, Szegvari M 1973 Rezidiverender und metastasierender Abrikossoff-Tumor de Vulva. Zentralblatt für Allgemeine Pathologie und Patholgischen Anatomie 117: 265–273

Marshall R B, Horn R C 1961 Nonchromaffin paraganglioma. Cancer 14: 779–787

Messina A M, Strauss R G 1976 Pelvic neurofibromatosis. Obstetrics and Gynecology 47: 63S–66S

Migliorini A, Amato A 1978 In tema de patologia neoplastica della vulva: raro caso di neurinoma del clitoride. Minerva Ginecologica 30: 543–545

Milia S, Firinh C, Pirisi G 1982 Neurofibrotomatosi con lacalizzazione vulvare: a proposito di un caso. Minerva Ginecologica 34: 1055–1058

Miller G C 1979 Neurofibromatosis affecting the vulva: case report. Military Medicine 144: 542–543

Mills S E, Fechner R E, Bruns D E, Brus M E, O'Hara M F 1981 Intermediate filaments in eosinophilic cells of epithelioid sarcoma: a light microscopic, ultrastructural and electrophoretic study. American Journal of Surgical Pathology 5: 195–202

Mobius W, Krause W 1974 Das Vulvahänabguin beim Säugling und Kleinkind und seine Behandlung. Zentralblatt für Gynäkologie 96: 280–286

Morris P G 1982 Granular cell myoblastoma of the vulva: report of two cases and review of the literature. Journal of Obstetrics and Gynaecology 2: 178–180

Novick N L 1985 Angiokeratoma vulvae. Journal of the American Academy of Dermatology 12: 561–563

Ordonez N G, Manning J T, Luna M A 1981 Mixed tumors of the vulva: a report of two cases probably arising in Bartholin's gland. Cancer 48: 181–185

Palermino D A 1964 Leiomyoma of the vulva: report of a case. Obstetrics and Gynecology 24: 301–302

Patchefsky A S, Soriano R, Kostianousky M 1977 Epithelioid sarcoma: ultrastructural similarity to nodular synovitis. Cancer 39: 143–152

Petsche H, Radinger C 1954 Ein Fall von Morbus Recklinghausen mit Ovarialaplasie und Pseudohermaphroditismus masculinus externus. Weiner Zeitschrift für Nervenhelkunde und deren Grenzgebiete 10: 252–259

Piver M S, Tsukada Y, Barlow J 1972 Epithelioid sarcoma of the vulva. Obstetrics and Gynecology 40: 839–842

Plouffie C, Tagandi T, Rosenberg A, Ferenczy A 1984 Non-Hodgkin's lymphoma in Bartholin's gland: case report and review of the literature. American Journal of Obstetrics and Gynecology 148: 608–609

Powell E B 1946 Granuloma cell myoblastoma. Archives of Pathology 42: 517–524

Radman H M, Bhagavan B S 1969 Granular cell myoblastoma of the vulva. Obstetrics and Gynecology 33: 501–505

Ramioul H 1952 Un nouveau cas de sarcome vulvaire (reticulo-

endothéliome malin) Gynaecologia 133: 74–81

Ravikumar V R, Lakshmanan D 1983 A solitary neurofibroma of the clitoris masquerading as an intersex. Journal of Pediatric Surgery 18: 617

Reymond R D, Hazra T A, Edlow D W Bawab M S 1972 Haemangiopericytoma of the vulva with metastasis to bone 14 years later. British Journal of Radiology 45: 765–768

Riedel H 1964 Zysten und Geschwülste des auseren Genitale und der Vagina. Zentralblatt für Gynäkologie 86: 1497–1508

Robertson A J McIntosh W, Lamont P, Guthrie W 1981 Malignant granular cell tumour (myoblastoma) of the vulva: a report of a case and review of the literature. Histopathology 5: 69–79

Rorat E, Wallach R E 1984 Mixed tumors of the vulva: clinical outcome and pathology. International Journal of Gynecological Pathology 3: 323–328

Salm R, Evans D J 1985 Myxoid leiomyosarcoma. Histopathology 9: 159–169

Santala M, Suonio S, Syrjänen K, Uronen M T, Saarikoski S 1987 Malignant fibrous histiocytoma of the vulva. Gynecologic Oncology 27: 121–126

Schepel S J, Tolhurst D E 1981 Neurofibromata of clitoris and labium majus simulating a penis and testicle. British Journal of Plastic Surgery 34: 221–223

Schiller H M, Madge G E 1970 Reticulum cell sarcoma presenting as a vulvar lesion. Southern Medical Journal 63: 471–472

Schreiber M M 1963 Vulvar von Recklinghausen's disease. Archives of Dermatology 88: 136–137

Shen T-J, D'Ablaing G, Morrow C P 1982 Alveolar soft part sarcoma of the vulva: report of first case and review of literature. Gynecologic Oncology 13: 120–128

Shousha S, Lyssiotis T 1979 Granular cell myoblastoma: positive staining for carcinoembryonic antigen. Journal of Clinical Pathology 30: 219–224

Smetana H F, Scott W F 1951 Malignant tumors of nonchromaffin paraganglia. Military Surgery 109: 330–349

Smit W L R, Knobel J, van der Merwe J V 1984 Leiomioom en leiomiosarcoom van die vulva: gevalbeskrywings. South African Medical Journal 66: 961–962

Sobel H J, Schwarz, R, Marquet E 1973 Light and electron microscopic study of the origin of granular cell myoblastoma. Journal of Pathology 109: 101–111

Soltan M H 1981 Dermatofibrosarcoma protuberans of the vulva. British Journal of Obstetrics and Gynaecology 88: 203–205

Steeper T, Rosai J 1983 Aggressive angiomyxoma of the female pelvis and perineum. American Journal of Surgical Pathology 7: 463–476

Stenchever M A, McDivett R W, Fisher J A 1973 Leiomyoma of the clitoris. Journal of Reproductive Medicine 2: 75–76

Stout A P, Murray W R 1942 Hemangiopericytoma: a vascular tumor featuring Zimmerman's pericytes. Annals of Surgery 116: 26–33

Talerman A 1973 Sarcoma botyroides presenting as a polyp on the labium majus. Cancer 32: 994–999

Talerman A 1982 Germ cell tumors of the ovary. In: Blaustein A (ed) Pathology of the female genital tract, 2nd edn. Springer-Verlag, New York, ch 24, p 602

Taussig F J 1937 Sarcoma of the vulva. American Journal of Obstetrics and Gynecology 33: 1017–1026

Tavassoli F A, Norris H J 1979 Smooth muscle tumors of the vulva. Obstetrics and Gynecology 53: 213–217

Taylor H T, Helwig E 1962 Dermatofibrosarcoma protuberans: a study of 115 cases. Cancer 15: 717–725

Taylor R N, Bottles K, Miller T R 1985 Malignant fibrous histiocytoma of the vulva. Obstetrics and Gynecology 66: 145–148

Thompson J A 1985 Therapy for painful cutaneous leiomyomas. Journal of the American Academy of Dermatology 13: 865–867

Tsoutsoplides G C 1980 Surgical management of extensive hemangiofibrolipoma of the vulva in an infant. American Journal of Obstetrics and Gynecology 136: 260–261

Uhlin S R 1980 Angiokeratoma of the vulva. Archives of Dermatology 116: 112–113

Ulbright T M, Brokaw S A, Stehman F B, Roth L M 1983 Epithelioid sarcoma of the vulva: evidence suggesting a more aggressive behaviour than extra-genital epithelioid sarcoma. Cancer 52: 1462–1469

Ungerleider R S, Donaldson S S, Warnke R A, Wilbur J R 1978 Endodermal sinus tumor: the Stanford experience and the first reported case arising in the vulva. Cancer 41: 1627–1634

Unni K K, Soule E H 1975 Alveolar soft part sarcoma, an electron microscopic study. Mayo Clinic Proceedings 50: 591–598

Venter P F, Rohm G F, Slabber C F 1981 Giant neurofibromas of the labia. Obstetrics and Gynecology 57: 128–130

Verbov H L, Manglabruks K 1978 Angiokeratoma of vulva. Dermatologica 156: 296–298

Verhaegh M, Clay A, Demaille M C, Caty A 1977 Les sarcomes vulvaires (à propos de 3 observations). Lille Médicale 22: 675–677

Vold I N, Jerve F 1984 Granular cell myoblastoma of the vulva: a report of three cases. Annales Chirurgiae et Gynaecologicae Fenniae 17: 281–283

Weiser G 1978 Granularzelltumor (Granulares Neurom Feyrter) und Schwannsche Phagen. Elektronenoptische Untersuchung von 3 faellen. Virchows Archiv A. Pathological Anatomy and Histology 380: 49–57

Welsh R A, Bray D M, Shipley F H, Meyer A T 1972 Histogenesis of alveolar soft part sarcoma. Cancer 29: 191–204

Whimster I W 1974 The pathology of lymphangioma circumscriptum (summary). British Journal of Dermatology 91: (Supplement 10) 35–36

Wilson D, Woodger B A 1974 Pleomorphic adenoma of the vulva. Journal of Obstetrics and Gynaecology of the British Commonwealth 81: 1000–1002

Wishart J 1973 Reticulosarcoma of the vulva complicating azathioprine-treated dermatomyositis. Archives of Dermatology 108: 563–564

Woodruff J D, Brack C B 1958 Unusual malignancies of the vulvo-urethral region: report of twelve cases. Obstetrics and Gynecology 12: 677–686

Woodruff J M, Marshall M L, Godwin T A, Funkhouser J W, Thompson N J, Erlandson R A 1983 Plexiform (multinodular) Schwannoma: a tumor simulating the plexiform neurofibroma. American Journal of Surgical Pathology 7: 691–697

Young R H, Scully R E 1984 Endodermal sinus tumor of the vagina: a report of nine cases and review of the literature. Gynecologic Oncology 18: 380–392

Zakut H, Lotan M, Lipnitzsky M 1985 Vulval haemangiopericytoma: a case report. Acta Obstetrica et Gynecologica Scandinavica 64: 619–621

Zenetta G, Bellorini R, Berra G 1981 Il mioblastoma a cellule granulose della vulva: presentazione di un caso. Chirurgia Italiana 33: 616–619

10

Epithelial tumours of the vulva
C H Buckley and H Fox

EPITHELIAL NEOPLASMS

Benign epithelial tumours

Benign epithelial tumours of the vulva are relatively common and may develop from the epidermis, the skin appendages or accessory breast tissue. The majority are of unknown aetiology.

Squamous papilloma

These are solitary lesions of the middle aged and elderly and resemble a skin tag (see below): they are of unknown aetiology.

They consist of a local, papillomatous overgrowth of the epidermis which is focally acanthotic and variably hyperkeratotic. There is no cellular atypia and the lesion is not regarded as having any malignant potential. The underlying stroma is fibrovascular connective tissue (Novak & Woodruff 1979).

Skin tag (fibro-epitheliomatous polyp, achrocordon)

These common lesions of the vulva (Friedrich et al 1979) are usually solitary, and appear as soft, sometimes wrinkled, polypoidal nodules of a similar colour to, or darker than, the surrounding skin. Though usually small, they may attain a striking size and appear pendulous (Fig. 10.1 a).

The tags have a fibrovascular connective tissue core covered by squamous epithelium which may be atrophic, or more commonly, mildly acanthotic and hyperkeratotic (Fig. 10.1 b).

Basal cell papilloma (seborrhoeic keratosis)

These lesions, which can develop in any part of the body, occur most commonly after middle age and may appear singly or in crops (Murphy et al 1984a); they show no particular predilection for the vulva. The lesions frequently cause irritation and occasionally pain but may be asymptomatic.

Basal cell papillomas appear as pale brown to black, soft, friable, greasy, granular, velvety or verrucous, flattened, rather irregular, 'stuck-on' plaques, which vary in size from a few millimetres to several centimetres. In some instances their heavy pigmentation may result in clinical confusion with melanoma. Morphologically the lesion is exophytic and somewhat papillary and lies superficial to the basal layer of the surrounding epidermis (Fig. 10.2a). It is composed of variably pigmented sheets and cords of cells which are similar throughout the lesion; they are small and regular and resemble those of the normal basal layer of the epidermis. Within the lesion there are keratin-containing cysts, so-called horn cysts, which may communicate with the skin surface (Fig. 10.2b). Small groups of the cells may show evidence of keratinisation; this is usually the result of irritation (Connors and Ackerman, 1976).

Keratoacanthoma

This is a rapidly growing, self-limiting neoplasm, for which a viral aetiology has been postulated. It is a rare finding on the vulva (Friedrich & Wilkinson 1982a) where it is most likely to be located on the external surface of the labia majora (Janovski & Douglas 1972, Rhatigan & Nuss 1985).

A keratoacanthoma appears firm, round, flesh coloured or red and in the course of a few weeks can develop into a well-demarcated hemispherical nodule with a central keratin-plugged crater 1 to 2 cm in diameter. Typically the lesion continues to grow for up to 6 months and then involutes leaving

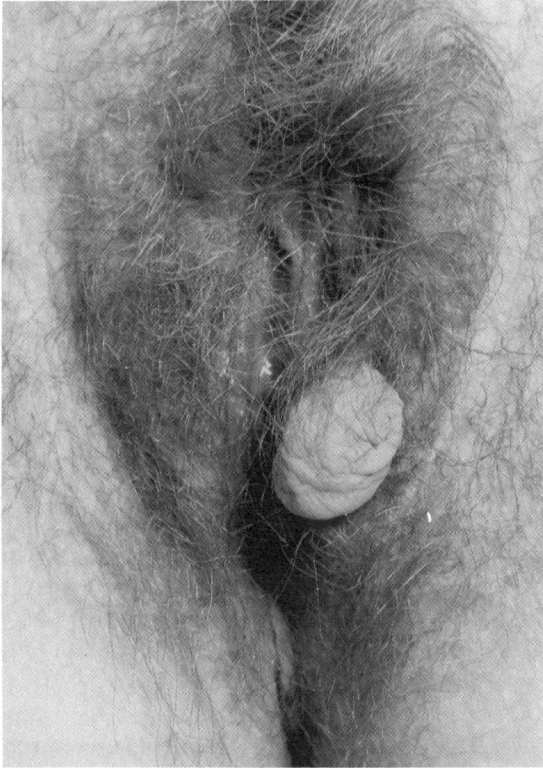

A

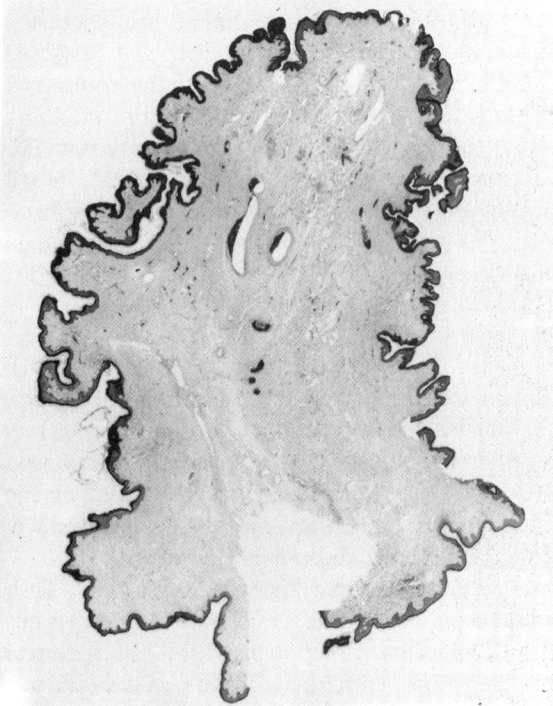

B

Fig. 10.1(a) Large fibro-epitheliomatous polyp; (b) histology.

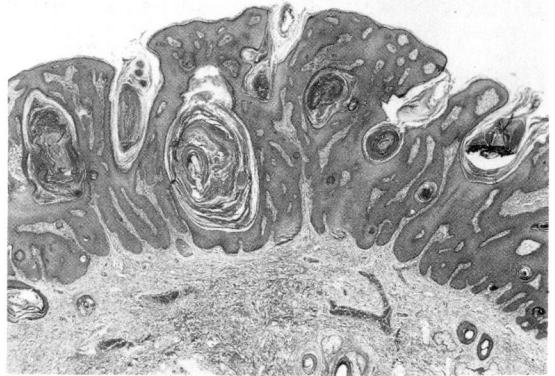

A

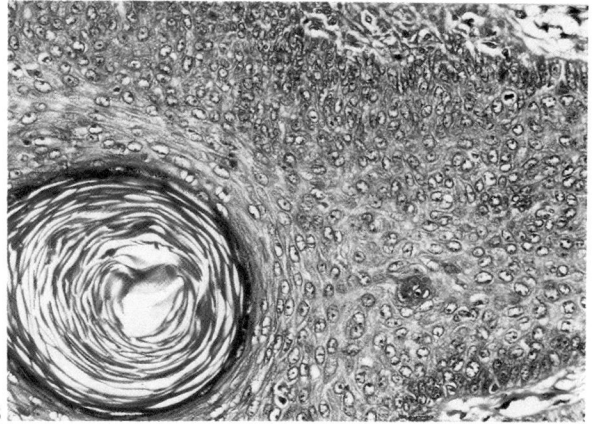

B

Fig. 10.2(a) Basal cell papilloma. The papillary epithelium encloses prominent keratin-containing cysts (H & E × 12) (b) Basal cell papilloma. The cells resemble those of the normal basal layer of the epidermis and are similar throughout; the cyst, to the left, contains laminated keratin. (H & E × 195)

a small depressed scar. Histologically (Fig. 10.3a) the papule is cup shaped, the centre being keratin filled and the margins formed by lobulated squamous cell masses and tongues. Each lobule is composed centrally of squamous cells with pale eosinophilic glassy cytoplasm and peripherally of a layer of small, darkly staining basal-like cells (Fig. 10.3b). The latter feature is helpful in differentiating the lesion from very well-differentiated squamous carcinoma, but distinguishing the two remains a problem both clinically and histologically. There is little cellular pleomorphism in the keratoacanthoma but mitoses, of normal form, may be numerous in the rapidly growing stage. Intracytoplasmic aggregates of desmosomes are a unique,

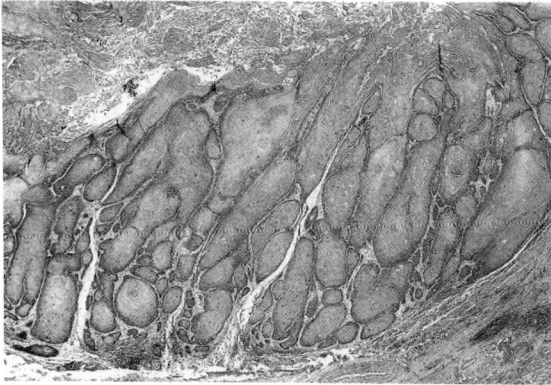

A

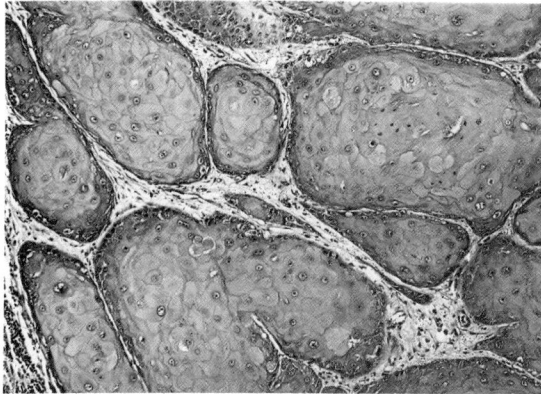

B

Fig. 10.3 Keratoacanthoma. (**a**) The wall of the lesion is formed by lobulated tongues of squamous epithelium; the keratin plug, within the crater, lies to the upper left. (H & E × 12) (**b**) The lobules of squamous cells with large pale cells centrally and small, darkly staining, basal-like cells at their periphery. (H & E × 60)

but not constant, feature of these tumours (Fisher et al 1972).

Persistent lesions may require excision and careful histological examination as opposed to curettage or biopsy. Indeed, it may be difficult for the pathologist to make the correct diagnosis without the opportunity to examine the lesion in its entirety.

Condylomata acuminata (genital warts)

Condylomata acuminata (see also p. 107) differ from the benign neoplasms described so far, in that a viral aetiology has been clearly demonstrated. They are the result of infection by human papillomavirus (HPV) (Gissmann et al 1982, Jablonska & Orth 1983) which is transmitted by sexual contact. They

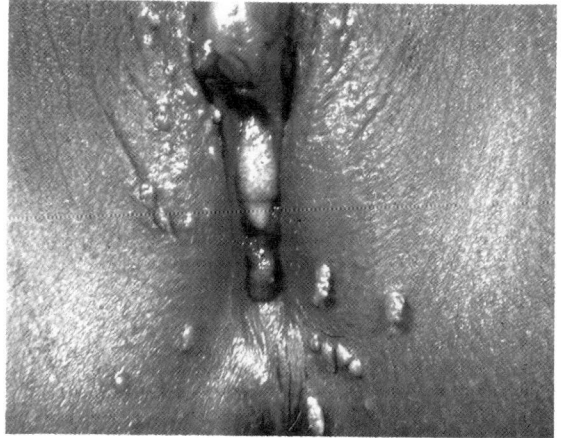

Fig. 10.4 Condylomata acuminata.

occur particularly in patients with spontaneous or iatrogenic immune impairment, in those with poor perineal hygiene, in pregnancy, when they may grow very rapidly, and in patients with diabetes mellitus. Whilst they are rare in children, their incidence appears to be increasing in prepubertal girls in whom the infection may have been acquired by close non-sexual contact (Stumpf 1980). Infection may also be transmitted by mothers to their offspring during parturition if there are extensive vulval or vaginal lesions, and as a consequence of this the child may develop laryngeal papillomata.

Clinical presentation. Condylomata form multiple, papillary or verrucous lesions or sessile rough-surfaced plaques on the skin and mucous membrane of the vulva, perineum and peri-anal region. They occur most frequently along the edges of the labia minora, in the interlabial sulcus or around the introitus (Fig. 10.4). They vary in colour, some being flesh coloured whilst others are pigmented and appear grey-brown or almost black. Flat and spiky condylomata also occur but are difficult or impossible to see without resource to colposcopic or histological examination. If they become secondarily infected condylomata may become painful and malodorous.

Histological appearance. The epithelial features are similar in all forms of the lesions. The epithelium, which is flat (Fig. 10.5) or covers fine fibrovascular cores (Fig. 10.6) is parakeratotic, or less commonly hyperkeratotic, and acanthotic; koilocytes, epithelial multinucleation and indi-

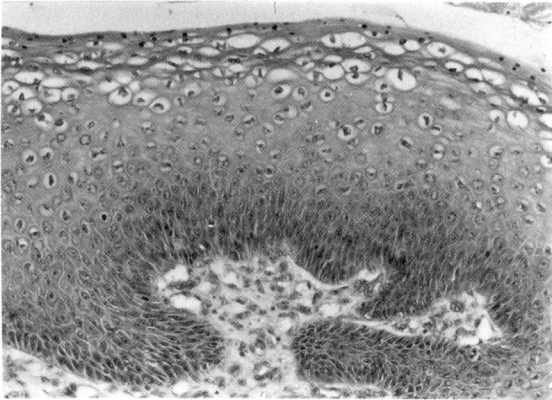

Fig. 10.5 Flat condyloma. The squamous epithelium is well stratified but the middle and upper layers contain large numbers of koilocytes, cells with clear cytoplasm and darkly staining, rather 'wrinkled' nuclei. There is no other evidence of cytological atypia. (H & E × 185)

vidual cell keratinisation may also be identified. The underlying stroma is usually chronically inflamed. Nuclear viral inclusions are not seen on light microscopic examination but electron-optic studies reveal viral inclusions in the nuclei of many cells, particularly those showing koilocytotic atypia (Kurman et al 1981). The inclusions are, however, sparse and relatively difficult to demonstrate even with electron microscopy, being found in only approximately 50% of condylomata (Dunn & Ogilvie 1968, Oriel & Almeida 1970, Oriel & Whimster 1971). They reach their greatest concentration after 6 to 12 months of growth and subsequently decline in number (Friedrich & Wilkinson 1982b). Immunohistochemistry demonstrates the viral antigen in tissue sections of 50% of vulval condylomata (Woodruff et al 1980, Kurman et al 1981, Toki et al 1986) and molecular hybridisation identifies the specific virus in up to 93% of condylomata; this is usually HPV6 (Gissmann et al 1982).

Interpretation of histological material from patients whose condylomata have recently been treated with podophyllin may be difficult as the preparation causes ballooning of the cells, vacuolation of the peripheral cytoplasm, nuclear enlargement and metaphase arrest. These appearances may be mistaken for intra-epithelial neoplasia, but can be distinguished by the absence of atypical mitoses and abnormality of chromatin dispersion (King & Sullivan 1947, Wade & Ackerman 1979).

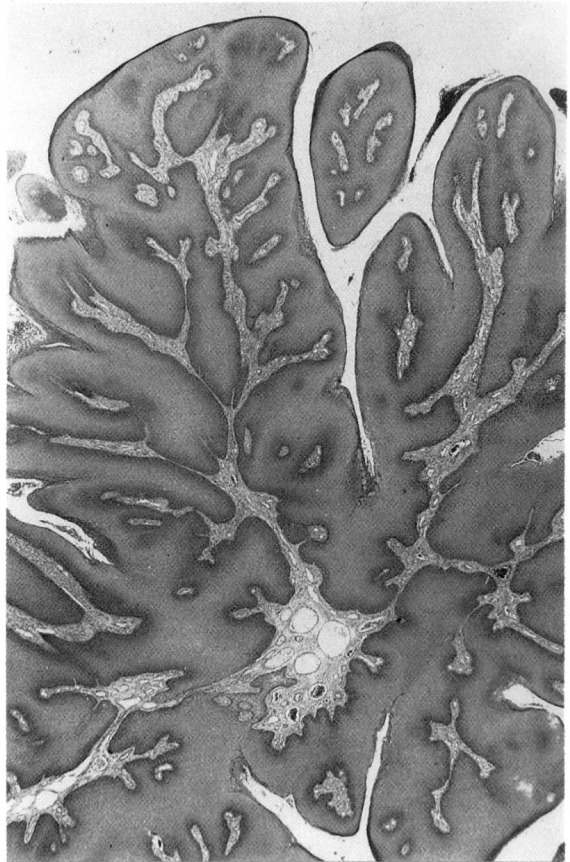

Fig. 10.6 Condyloma acuminatum. Fine fibro-vascular cores are covered by acanthotic squamous epithelium which is mildly hyperkeratotic. At this magnification, the cytological details are not apparent. (H & E × 17)

Treatment. Condylomata can be removed surgically, eradicated by cautery or laser or may be treated by the application of podophyllin (p. 115).

Prognosis. Spontaneous regression of condylomata can occur at any time, but is particularly common after pregnancy (Jablonska & Orth 1983). In contrast, recurrent disease is also common and there may be associated lesions in the vagina or on the cervix. Condylomata may therefore be difficult to eradicate. Such perpetuation of infection may be due to a partial impairment of immunity in some women (Seski et al 1978) who demonstrate abnormalities of lymphocyte transformation; such patients are also more likely to have repeated infection of other types and develop intra-epithelial neoplasia unduly frequently.

There is a history of condylomata in many patients who develop both VIN and squamous carcinoma of the vulva, but patients having only condylomata are infected with HPV6 whilst intraepithelial and invasive neoplasia are usually associated with HPV16 or 18. Many of the earlier reports identifying HPV within condylomata, squamous carcinomas and verrucous carcinomas were written at a time when identification of HPV type was not feasible and the reports should not therefore be regarded as indicating a common aetiology for all these lesions, although they are closely related. In determining the outcome in an individual patient, it is clear that in future virus type will be an important guide to prognosis.

Intra-epithelial neoplasia

The term dystrophy was introduced by Jeffcoate & Woodcock (1961) to describe a wide variety of disorders of squamous epithelial growth and maturation. It included both benign conditions and intraepithelial neoplasms of varying invasive potential but not specific dermatological disorders other than lichen sclerosus (see p. 172).

In 1976 the dystrophies were reclassified by the International Society for the Study of Vulvar Disease (ISSVD) into hyperplastic dystrophy, lichen sclerosus and mixed dystrophy, but this merely perpetuated the two main drawbacks to the classification. These are, firstly, that individual groups encompass benign and neoplastic conditions of quite different prognosis and, secondly, that it draws an artificial distinction between squamous eipthelium in which there are cytologically atypical cells showing some differentiation (dystrophy with atypia) and those in which the cells show little or no differentiation and which involve the full thickness of the epithelium and are termed carcinoma in situ. Recent recommendations by the International Society of Gynecological Pathologists seek to remedy this by distinguishing between, on the one hand, squamous epithelial abnormalities which are not premalignant and which show no cytological atypia, that is, squamous epithelial hyperplasia (Fig. 10.7) (hyperplastic dystrophy without cytological atypia) and lichen sclerosus and, on the other hand, those which are premalignant conditions or pre-invasive malignancies and which are characte-

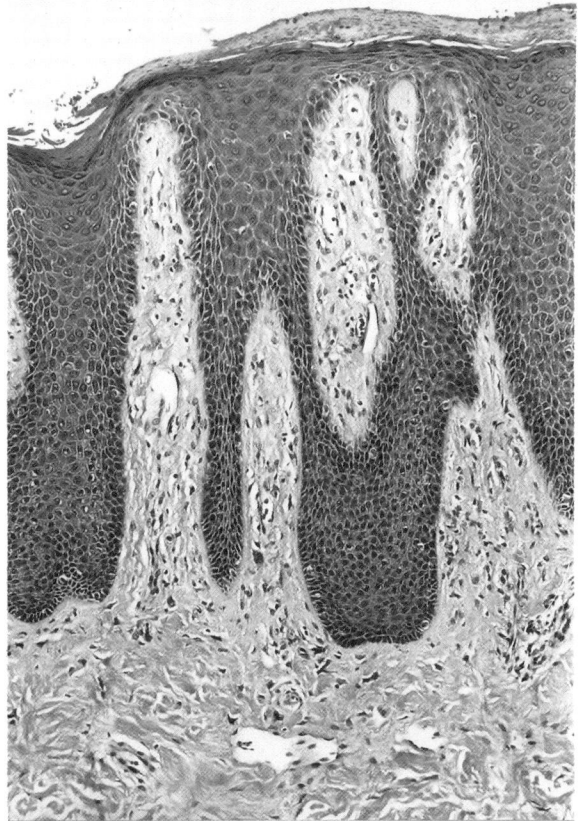

Fig. 10.7 Squamous epithelial hyperplasia. Although there is mild hyperkeratosis and marked elongation of the rete ridges, some of which are fused, there is normal stratification of the epithelium and a total absence of cellular atypia. (H & E × 115)

rised by cytological atypia, that is, the intra-epithelial neoplasias (see p. 192).

The term vulval intra-epithelial neoplasia (VIN) is considered by some authors to encompass all intra-epithelial malignant conditions affecting the vulval skin and mucosa. However, the clinical behaviour and prognostic significance of the non-squamous forms (Paget's disease and melanocytic lesions) are so different, both from each other and from the squamous forms, that they will be considered separately and the term vulval intra-eipthelial neoplasia will be used only for squamous cell abnormalities, encompassing those conditions known previously as Bowen's disease, erythroplasia of Queyrat, squamous carcinoma in situ of simplex type (Abell & Gosling 1961) and all forms of dystrophy showing squamous cell atypia (Buckley et al 1984).

Whilst the current proposals seek to distinguish between neoplastic and non-neoplastic intra-epithelial abnormalities, in approximately 10 to 15% of patients features of non-neoplastic and neo-plastic disorders co-exist. There are, however, no clinical features which permit identification of these mixed disorders prior to histological examination of the tissues, nor is there any reason to believe that the various components of the epithelial abnormality behave differently when they are in combination. It is recommended therefore that each pathological process should be separately identified in the histopathological report on such patients (Fig. 10.8).

Vulval intra-epithelial neoplasia (VIN)

The adoption of the VIN terminology is partly based on an analogy with cervical intra-epithelial neoplasia (Buckley et al 1982, Reid et al 1984) and allows for the discontinuation of such imprecise terms as 'mild dysplasia' and 'carcinoma in situ' (Crum 1982a). The single most important factor responsible for the introduction of the VIN terminology, however, has been the finding, using Feulgen microspectrophotometry (Fu et al 1981), that in most cases of mild or moderate atypia the abnormal cells are aneuploid (i.e. have a chromosome content which is not an exact multiple of 23—the normal haploid complement) (Crum et al 1982b); and there is no correlation between the degrees of abnormality within the squamous epithelium and the ploidy values. Most examples of vulval carcinoma in situ (92 to 100%) are also aneuploid (Friedrich et al 1980, Fu et al 1981) and there is no evidence that aneuploid atypia and carcinoma in situ differ biologically from each other in any way apart from the degree of maturation, or differentiation, of the intra-epithelial lesion.

VIN may arise in the setting of squamous hyperplasia or mixed epithelial disorders (mixed dystrophy, combining features of squamous hyperplasia and lichen sclerosus), may develop in condylomata or may occur in otherwise normal skin. It has been claimed that VIN may develop in skin showing features of lichen sclerosus (Lavery 1984); this has not been our experience, although the two conditions, LSA and VIN, may co-exist (Fig. 10.8).

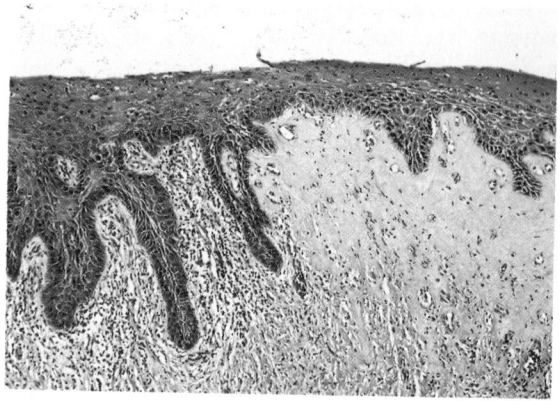

Fig. 10.8 Vulval intra-epithelial neoplasia with lichen sclerosus. On the left, there is acanthosis, elongation of the rete ridges and cytological atypia with disturbance of normal stratification, VIN; to the right, the epithelium is shallow and there is no cytological atypia, the underlying dermis is hyalinised and there is a mild chronic inflammatory cell infiltrate, lichen sclerosus. (H & E × 60)

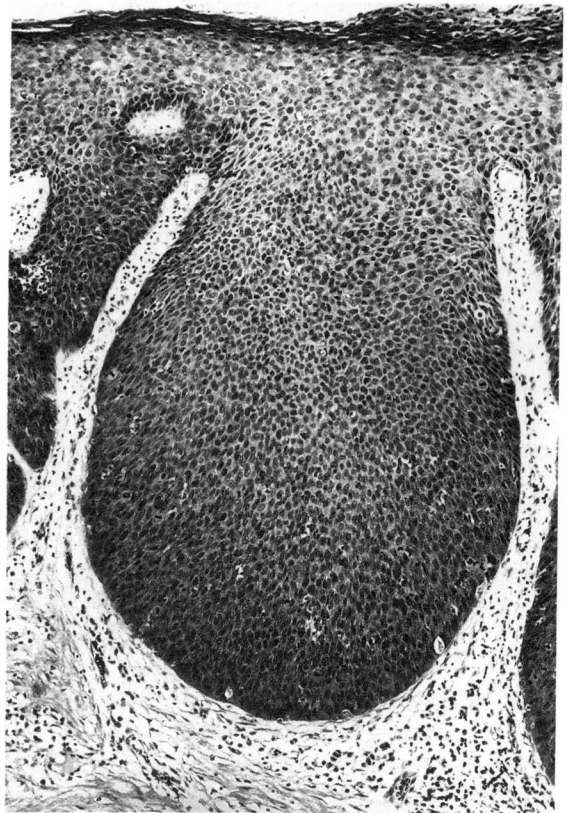

Fig. 10.9 Basaloid vulval intra-epithelial neoplasia. The epithelium is occupied throughout its depth by cells resembling those of the normal basal layer; there is parakeratosis. (H & E × 90)

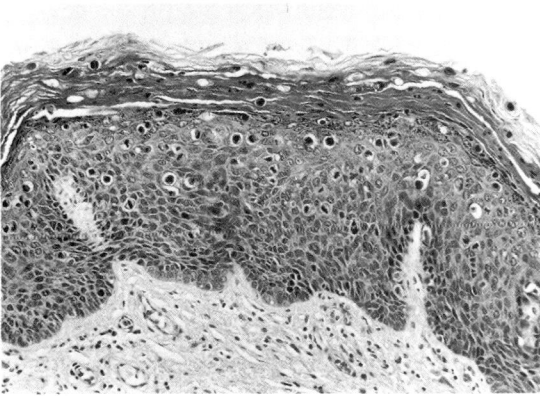

Fig. 10.10 Bowenoid vulval intra-epithelial neoplasia. The cellular atypia is characterised by the presence of koilocytes, corp ronds and frequent mitoses. (H & E × 120)

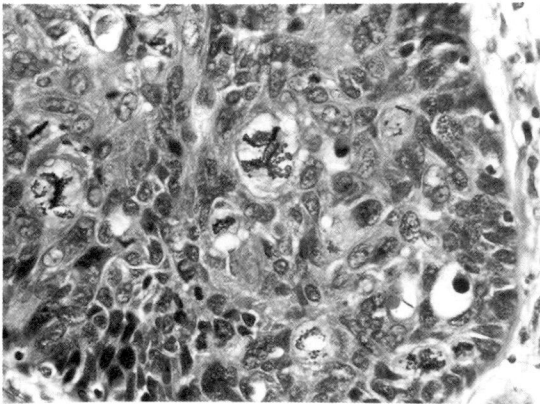

Fig. 10.11 Vulval intra-epithelial neoplasia. At the base of the rete ridge there are a number of bizarre, multipolar mitoses. (H & E × 310)

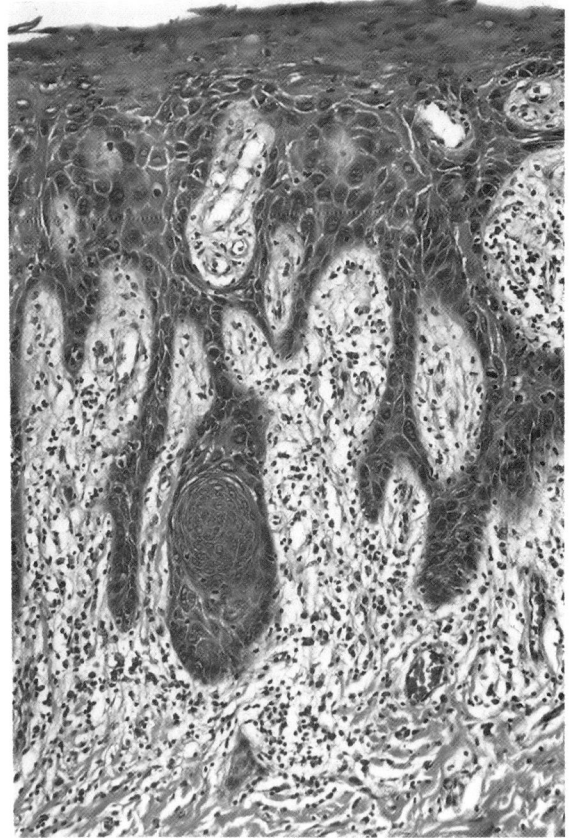

Fig. 10.12 Vulval intra-epithelial neoplasia. Within the elongated rete ridge in this example, there is a well-formed, squamous epithelial pearl. (H & E × 140)

Atypia within vulval squamous epithelium is manifested by disturbances of normal cellular stratification and abnormalities of maturation. Two basic patterns are seen (Buscema et al 1980b): one in which cells of basal or parabasal type extend into the upper layers of the epidermis (Abell 1965), basaloid VIN (Fig. 10.9), and the other in which premature cellular maturation occurs often in association with epithelial multinucleation, corps ronds and koilocytosis, which are the hallmark of papillomavirus infection (Abell & Gosling 1961), Bowenoid VIN (Fig. 10.10). Common to both forms of atypia (Fig. 10.11) are the presence of mitotic figures, sometimes of abnormal or bizarre form, above the basal layers of the epithelium, cellular and nuclear pleomorphism, a high nucleocytoplasmic ratio, irregular clumping of nuclear chromatin and, in many cases, either parakeratosis or hyperkeratosis. Bowenoid VIN is found typically in patients with current or previous evidence of papillomavirus infection having either flat or papillary condylomata in the lower genital tract. The two patterns of VIN may co-exist.

A further lesion, which is sometimes regarded as a variant of VIN III (International Society for the Study of Vulvar Disease, 1976, Friedrich 1976, Buscema & Woodruff 1980, Wilkinson et al 1986), is one in which there may be little evidence of cytological atypia, the principal abnormality being the presence of intra-epithelial pearls in the rete ridges (Fig. 10.12). Whether or not this abnormality truly merits inclusion within the VIN category remains a matter for further study.

Aetiology. There is a clear association between VIN III and both sexually transmitted diseases and neoplastic lesions elsewhere. Thus about 20 to 25% of patients with VIN III have concurrent, past or subsequent CIN (Buscema et al 1980b, Friedrich et al 1980, Benedet & Murphy 1982, Caglar et al 1982, DiPaola et al 1982, Andreasson & Bock 1985) whilst a substantial proportion, between 8 and 40%, have concurrent or subsequent invasive neoplasms, most commonly in the genital tract, but also elsewhere in the body (Abell 1965, Collins et al 1970, Boutselis 1972, Friedrich et al 1980, Caglar et al 1982, Bernstein et al 1983a). Friedrich et al (1980) noted that the overall incidence of sexually transmitted diseases in their series of 50 women with VIN III was 60%; this is a much higher incidence than those previously cited of 22% (Collins et al 1970) to 38% (Forney et al 1977). Whether this association between VIN III and sexually transmitted diseases is a true one or simply represents population bias remains to be resolved.

A history of herpes vulvitis is obtained in 10 to 12% of women with VIN III, whilst condylomata acuminata are present in between 15 and 30% (Abell 1965, Kovi et al 1974, Forney et al 1977, Buscema et al 1980b, Friedrich et al 1980, Caglar et al 1982, Bernstein et al 1983a, Daling et al 1984). This frequent association with condylomata does not, however, imply that patients with vulval condylomata run a very high risk of developing vulval carcinoma (Daling et al 1984).

A clear association between Bowenoid VIN and HPV infection has been demonstrated. Viral particles were identified in vulval condylomata (Dunn & Ogilvie 1968, Oriel & Almeida 1970); and in Bowenoid VIN (Olson et al 1968, Nordquist et al 1970) many years ago, and later immunohistochemistry and electron microscopic studies have confirmed that these were HPV (Jenson et al 1980, Jablonska & Orth 1983, Pilotti et al 1984, Rueda-Leverone et al 1987). More sophisticated molecular hybridisation studies have shown that whilst condylomata are caused by HPV 6 and 11 (Jablonska & Orth 1983, Gissman et al 1983), types 16 and 18 are more likely to be associated with intra-epithelial neoplasia and, possibly, invasive carcinoma (Pelisse et al 1985, Bergeron et al 1987, Gupta et al 1987, Reid et al 1987).

Evidence that Herpes simplex virus-2 (HSV2) may also play an aetiological role in the development of intra-epithelial neoplasia is provided by the finding of an early non-structural polypeptide of HSV2 in cases of severe vulval 'dysplasia' and 'carcinoma in situ' in the absence of productive viral infection (Cabral et al 1982), and an antigen induced by HSV2 has been found in patients with 'squamous carcinoma in situ' some of whom also had condylomata (Kaufman et al 1981). Only in the patients in whom the condylomata were associated with HSV2 did cytological atypia develop in this series, and other authors (Zur Hausen 1982) have also suggested that HPV and HSV2 may act synergistically in the development of intra-epithelial and invasive neoplasia of the vulva.

Other more general factors have been indicted in the formation of VIN, for example, arsenical insecticides (presumably by absorption) (Nordquist et al 1970, Friedrich 1972b), and ionising radiation (Figge & Gaudenz 1974, Choo & Morley 1980).

Clinical aspects. The clinical features of VIN I and II are poorly documented and the majority of the data refer only to cases of VIN III. The incidence of VIN III is low but it is being encountered more frequently than previously (Hilliard et al 1979, Buscema et al 1980b, Friedrich 1981, Benedet & Murphy 1982, Caglar et al 1982).

In general, Bowenoid VIN occurs in younger women than does the basaloid type and the age at which it occurs has become progressively younger (Jones & McLean 1986, Powell et al 1986). In the early 1960s Abell & Gosling (1961) and Abell (1965) reported that the average age for Bowenoid VIN was 42 years with a range of 23 to 65 years, whilst Wade et al (1979) in a rather small series reported a median age of 27 years with a range of 18 to 33 years. This latter figure is similar to that which many centres are recording.

The most common presenting complaint of women with VIN III is pruritus (Andreasson & Bock 1985), but about one-third have noticed some abnormality of the vulval skin and a substantial proportion ranging in different series from 18 to 46% (Buscema et al 1980b, Friedrich et al 1980, Caglar et al 1982, DiPaola et al 1982, Bernstein et al 1983a) are asymptomatic.

Macroscopically the lesions of VIN III are very variable, non-specific, and closely resemble the non-neoplastic epithelial abnormalities or shallow

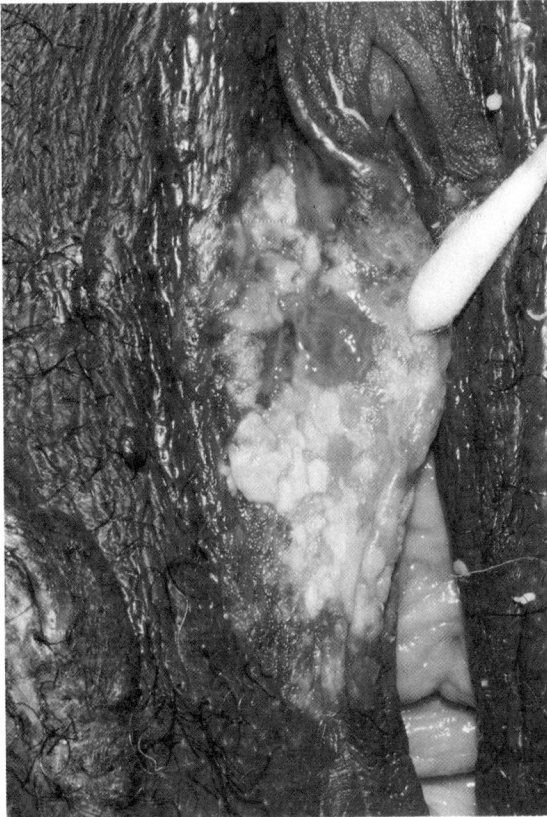 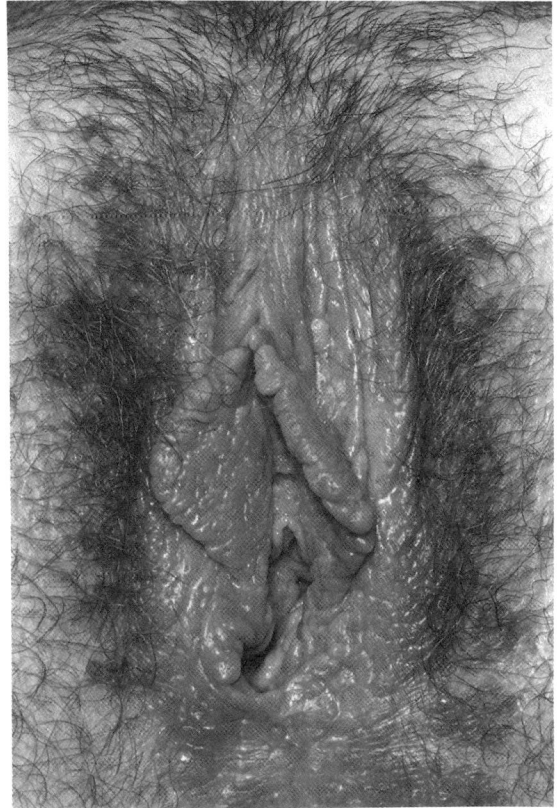

A   B

Fig. 10.13 (a and b) VIN III with warts (By Courtesy of Dr C M Ridley)

verrucosities. The diagnosis can be made only by biopsy, and the tendency towards a multicentric growth pattern makes multiple sampling mandatory (Buckley et al 1984). The lesions may be discrete and sharply localised to the labia and/or perineum or may affect the whole vulva: about 70 to 75% are multifocal, this being most common in the Bowenoid variety and in younger women (Hilliard et al 1979, Benedet & Murphy 1982, Pilotti et al 1984). Spread to involve the perineal skin, the peri-anal area and the anal canal occurs in between 14 and 35% of cases, particularly those in which the posterior part of the vulva is most severely affected (Schlaerth et al 1984). The lesions may be dull red and granular (Abell & Gosling 1961) or may present a variegated red and white pigmented appearance with interspersed warty areas in 20% of cases (Buscema et al 1980b) (Fig. 10.13 a). In many cases intra-epithelial or intradermal melanin, or both, is present and this may result in dark brown or black

lesions (Laohadtanaphorn et al 1979) (Fig. 10.13 b). Some of these pigmented cases of Bowenoid VIN present a specific clinical picture variously described as multiple, discoid, flat, grey brown lesions (Janovski & Barchet 1966, Kimura et al 1978, Kimura 1980), hyperpigmented raised lesions (Friedrich et al 1980), reddish-brown, violaceous papular or verrucous lesions (Wade et al 1979) or papillary or spiky condylomata (Lupulescu et al 1977, Hilliard et al 1979) and have been described as multicentric pigmented Bowen's disease (Kimura et al 1978, Bhawan 1980) or Bowenoid papulosis (Wade et al 1979). Histologically, aetiologically and in clinical behaviour, however, the lesions are similar to the non-pigmented forms of Bowenoid VIN III which are not overtly warty and the presence of pigment-laden macrophages is not even specific to VIN, for it merely indicates the presence of epidermal pigmentary incontinence.

Colposcopic examination reveals an abnormal

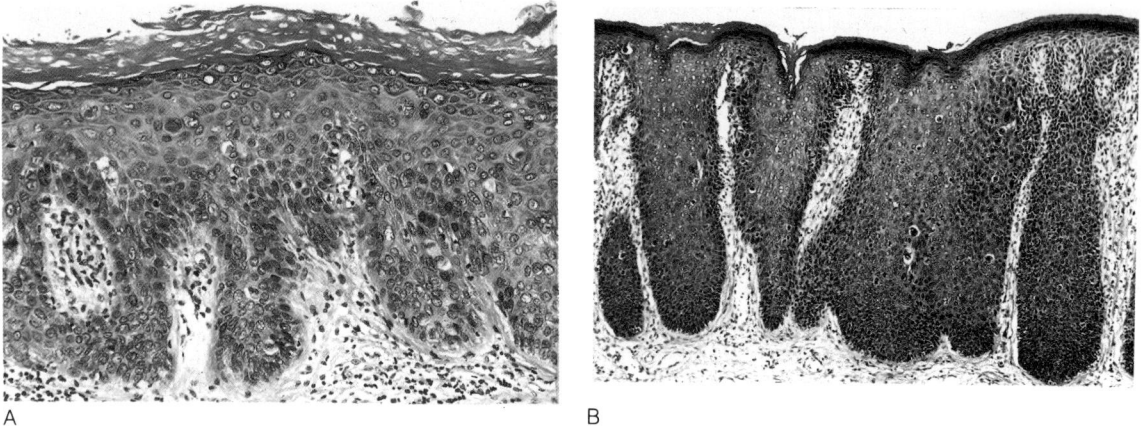

Fig. 10.14 (a) Bowenoid vulval intra-epithelial neoplasia. There is cellular stratification and cytoplasmic maturation but there is also cytological atypia characterised by multinucleation and mitoses, some of which are atypical, well above the basal layer. Grading of the degree of atypia in this example presents a problem but was regarded as representing VIN I. (H & E × 120) (b) Bowenoid vulval intra-epithelial neoplasia. A dense hyperkeratotic layer overlies an epithelium showing cytological atypia throughout its depth, notice the preservation of cytoplasmic maturation and individually keratinised cells. (H & E × 60)

vascular pattern with punctation, a mosaic pattern or vascular irregularities in up to 60% of patients (Buckley et al 1984, Andreasson and Bock 1985) with VIN III and this permits directed collection of cytological material or biopsy. However, in some cases, the epithelium is masked by the presence of a thick keratin layer, or the skin appears normal or there may be injection due to infection or scratching; in these cases colposcopy has nothing to offer and random biopsies are needed to establish a diagnosis.

Histopathology and cytology. When cellular abnormalities and lack of stratification are limited to the lower third of the squamous epithelium the lesion is classed as VIN I, which corresponds to 'mild atypia'; extension of the abnormal cells into the middle third of the epithelium puts the lesion into the category of VIN II, which is equivalent to 'moderate atypia'. Involvement of the upper third of the epithelium leads to a diagnosis of VIN III, a category encompassing both 'severe atypia' and carcinoma in situ. Grading of the form of VIN in which basal or parabasal cells extend into the upper epithelium is relatively easy, but grading of Bowenoid VIN is more difficult as it is characterised by a much greater degree of cytoplasmic maturation and cellular stratification than is seen in the basaloid form.

In basaloid VIN III a parakeratotic layer overlies an epithelium which is otherwise occupied throughout its thickness by closely packed, non-stratified cells which show nuclear crowding and a high nucleocytoplasmic ratio.

In the Bowenoid form (Fig. 10.14 a and b) there may be hyperkeratosis or parakeratosis; premature cellular maturation, variable retention of stratification, and pleomorphism, which may be extreme, and koilocytosis are key features. Koilocytes are most commonly, but not exclusively, found in the superficial layers of the epithelium. Often, however, in certain areas of such lesions the specific features are fewer and the epidermis is composed of large moderately pleomorphic cells with relatively scanty cytoplasm in which there are frequent mitoses (Fig. 10.15). It is not uncommon to find a mixture of basaloid and Bowenoid lesions in the same patient, demonstrating that the two forms are not mutually exclusive (Buscema et al 1980b). It is usual however, to distinguish between the basaloid and Bowenoid types because of various clinical, pathological and aetiological differences between the two conditions in their pure state.

Both basaloid VIN III and Bowenoid VIN III may extend into the pilosebaceous units (Abell & Gosling 1961, Abell 1965, Mene & Buckley 1985) and less commonly, into sweat gland ducts (Fig. 10.16).

Two main patterns of cytological abnormality are recognised in the smear preparations (Buckley et al 1984). In the first the smear is scanty and contains

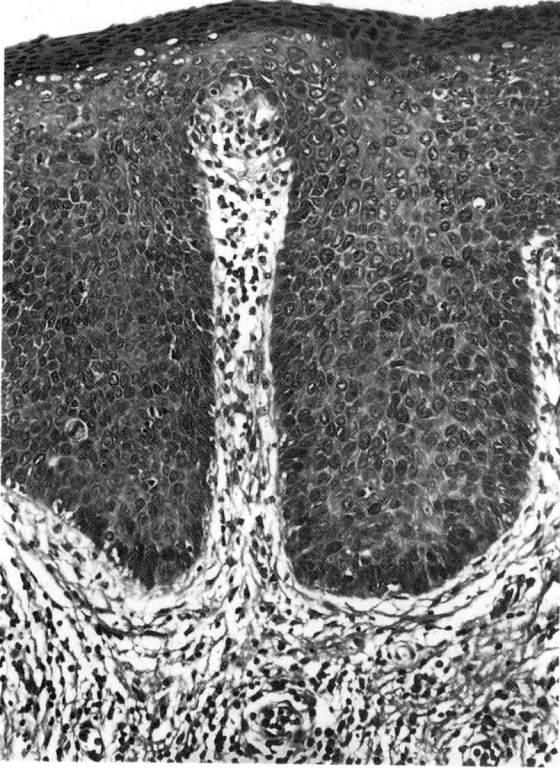

Fig. 10.15 Vulval intra-epithelial neoplasia. The epidermis is occupied by rather large cells which show little or no maturation: mitoses are frequent. Elsewhere in the vulva, the epithelium had the features of typical Bowenoid VIN, and even here, occasional koilocytes are present immediately below the surface parakeratosis. (H & E × 175)

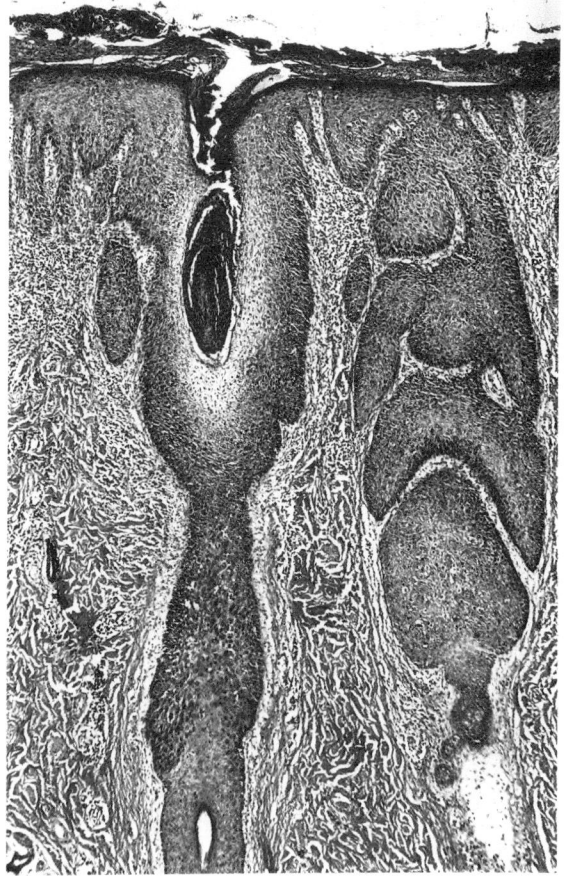

Fig. 10.16 Vulvar intra-epithelial neoplasia. Epithelium with atypical features extends into the hair follicle: note the abrupt transition to epithelium of normal appearance. (H & E × 45)

well-differentiated, often keratinised cells; nuclei may be large and degenerate with loss of recognisable chromatin pattern or hyperchromatic with a coarsely granular chromatin pattern similar to that seen in dyskaryotic cells in a cervical smear. The maturity of the dyskaryotic cells would point to a diagnosis of VIN I or II, but this is often an underestimate of the grade as the cells in the smear come from a thick layer of parakeratosis which may overlie the VIN. Careful examination may reveal occasional poorly differentiated dyskaryotic cells when vessels bring deeper epithelium near the surface. The second pattern is seen in the absence of pronounced hyperkeratosis or parakeratosis and is characterised by a more profuse exfoliation of cells. This pattern is more common in VIN III of basaloid type and the cells are immature with scanty cytoplasm. Chromatin patterns range from that typical of the dyskaryotic cell to nuclei of malignant type which suggest an invasive lesion. Cells of this type may certainly be seen in cases of early invasion, but more commonly biopsy of vulval lesions from which these cells have been shed shows only VIN III (Buckley et al 1984).

Prognosis. Very little is known about the natural history of VIN I and II and the risk of the lesions evolving into an invasive carcinoma has not been accurately determined; the risk is, however, almost certainly low (Friedrich 1981).

It is becoming clear that the behaviour of VIN III is not directly comparable to CIN III and that the incidence of progression to invasive neoplasia is low. In one series only 4 of 106 patients with VIN III developed an invasive tumour (Friedrich 1981), in a second only 1 in 37 did so (Friedrich et al 1980) and in a third 1 in 49 did so (Andreasson & Bock 1985). There is certainly no doubt that VIN III can progress to an invasive squamous cell carcinoma (Gardiner et al 1953, Collins et al 1970, Jones & Buntine 1978, Jones & McLean 1986) but it is clear that this is the exception rather than the rule. In most reported cases in which VIN has progressed to invasive carcinoma the patient has been either old or immunosuppressed (Buscema & Woodruff 1980, Buscema et al 1980b), and although well-documented cases of progression in younger immunologically normal patients are recorded they are less usual. By contrast, even untreated cases of aneuploid VIN III may undergo spontaneous regression (Friedrich 1972a, Skinner et al 1973, Friedrich et al 1980, Bernstein et al 1983a). This has been a particular feature in young women who are pregnant at the time of diagnosis and who have multicentric disease, although it is by no means limited to this group; Halasz et al (1986) reported a case in a child aged 3. Fu and colleagues (1981) demonstrated that Bowenoid VIN III, of which low invasive potential is a particular feature, had ploidy values frequently in excess of more than three times normal and that such lesions tend to recur or persist whilst those intra-epithelial lesions which progressed to carcinoma tended on the whole to be basaloid and have the same low ploidy values as invasive squamous carcinomas and the intra-epithelial neoplasm in the immediately adjacent epithelium.

Treatment. In view of the low rate of advance to invasive carcinoma there has been an increasing tendency to treat VIN III by more conservative means. Details of management are reviewed on page 334 et seq.

Micro-invasive squamous cell carcinoma

Attempts to define a micro-invasive carcinoma of the vulva comparable to that which has been described in the cervix, and for which conservative treatment proves an adequate and safe alternative to radical surgery or radiotherapy, have met with enormous difficulties. Some workers believe that such an entity can be recognised whilst others hold that any attempt to draw an analogy between cervical and vulval lesions is misguided and that a vulval carcinoma is either invasive or not (Douglas 1983). The inherent complexity of the problem has been confounded by a number of factors, which include differing concepts of micro-invasive carcinoma, the lack of an agreed definition, the use of imprecise pathological data and the accumulation of conflicting findings. The picture has not been made any clearer by the use of a variety of terms, thus 'superficial infiltrating carcinoma', 'superficially invasive carcinoma', 'occult carcinoma', 'early vulvar carcinoma', 'early invasive carcinoma', 'stage 1a carcinoma', and 'micro-invasive carcinoma', have often been used synonymously and interchangeably, and it is sometimes far from certain whether those using the terms are all referring to the same entity or not.

The most widely accepted definition of a micro-invasive carcinoma of the vulva (Kneale et al 1981), is: 'a squamous cell carcinoma 2 cm or less in diameter with no more than 5 mm stromal invasion where the depth of invasion is the maximum measured in any one high power field. The presence of confluence, vascular channel permeation or cellular anaplasia does not exclude the case from this category'. The maximum depth of 5 mm has been based on the report of Wharton et al (1974) that 25 patients with vulval carcinomas invading to a depth of 5 mm or less had no nodal metastases or recurrence of tumour and all survived, while, of 20 women whose neoplasms invaded beyond this level, 5 had lymph node spread and 3 died of vulval cancer. Wharton and his colleagues were, however, at pains to emphasise that the limit of 5 mm had been arbitrarily chosen and pointed out that further experience was required to determine whether or not this figure adequately characterised a micro-invasive stage. Their doubts on this point were fully justified for it has since become clear that about 12% of patients with tumour invasion to a depth of 5 mm or less have inguinal node metastases at the time of vulvectomy (Wilkinson et al 1982). The only truly valid concept of a micro-invasive carcinoma is of one which, though seen histologically to have broken out from the confines of the epithelium, is only invading the stroma to such an extent that it carries no risk of lymph node metastases. Therefore a definition employing 5 mm as a maximum depth of invasion is insufficient stringent and is associated with an unacceptably high incidence of nodal involvement. There has therefore been an increasing tendency for a cut-off point of 3 mm to be used for defining a micro-invasive lesion (Jafari & Cartnick 1976, Magrina et al 1979, Chu et al 1982, Hoffman et al 1983). Even this may be too lenient a figure, however, for there have been patients with tumours which though invading only to a depth of between 1 and 2 mm were associated with lymph node metastases either at the time of, or subsequent to, initial diagnosis (DiPaola et al 1975, Parker et al 1975, Yazigi et al 1978, Barnes et al 1980, Kolstad et al 1982) and some of these women eventually died of widespread disease. It has become apparent that it is only those tumours which invade to a depth of 1 mm or less which are not associated with any risk of lymph node involvement (Magrina et al 1979, Kolstad et al 1982, Hacker et al 1983), though the risk of spread is certainly low in carcinomas invading up to 1.5 mm (Wilkinson et al 1982). Some go further and suggest that any tumour invading to a depth greater than 0.8 mm carries a risk of metastases or recurrence (Buscema et al 1981, Woodruff 1982).

When considering these opinions, the fact must be taken into account that there has been no agreement as to the point from which the depth of invasion should be measured. The surface of the tumour, the surface of the intact adjacent epithelium, the lower margin of adjacent surface epithelium, the base of the adjacent most superficial dermal papilla, the tip of the deepest adjacent rete ridge and the superficial granular layer of the overlying epithelium have all been used as starting points for measuring tumour depth, and this makes comparison between different studies invidious. Wilkinson et al (1982), for example, used the base of the adjacent most superficial dermal papilla as their point from which tumour depth was measured and concluded that nodal metastasis was extremely unlikely if the depth of invasion was less than 1.5 mm. By contrast, Woodruff (1982) considered that tumour invasion to more than 0.8 mm was potentially dangerous but he was measuring this distance from the tip of the deepest rete ridge. It is obviously difficult to compare these two studies as they are based on different criteria, and it is even more difficult to interpret those far from uncommon studies in which no details are given about the point from which the depth of invasion was measured. There is probably no single site from which tumour invasion should be measured which has incontrovertible advantages over all other starting points, though the surface of the adjacent epithelium is least satisfactory because of variations in the keratin layer while the superficial granular layer appears an unsuitable starting point if only because it is sometimes absent in vulval skin. Until there is a measure of agreement as to the point from which depth of invasion is measured all comments about the importance of particular levels of invasion become almost meaningless.

Burghardt (1984) has argued that it is tumour volume rather than depth of tumour invasion which is most clearly and consistently related to the risk of nodal metastases and has pointed out that depth of invasion of a tumour is only of real importance when, in sites such as gastrointestinal tract, tissue boundaries are crossed and there is invasion from a lymphatic-free zone to an area which contains lymphatics. In the vulva, increasing depth of invasion does not involve the breaching of any anatomical barriers, and the available evidence suggests that lymphatic vessels must lie within 1–2 mm of the basement membrane of the surface epithelium. Very little is known about the volume of micro-invasive tumours of the vulva, though there is no clear correlation between depth of invasion and tumour mass. It is true that tumour volume remains below 1000 mm^3 when the depth of invasion is less than 1.5 mm but extension beyond that point is associated with a wide range of tumour volumes that do not relate in a linear manner to depth of invasion (Wilkinson et al 1982).

Even a tumour volume of 1000 mm^3 appears to be too large to fall within the category of a micro-invasive lesion (Pickel & Haas 1986), and this mass reflects, to a certain extent, the defining feature of a maximum diameter of 2 cm. It has been suggested that the maximum diameter of a micro-invasive carcinoma should be only 1 cm (DiSaia et al 1979), but Magrina et al (1979) noted that 10% of patients with tumours measuring 1 cm or less in diameter developed nodal metastases, while Kneale et al (1981) found a 4% incidence of lymph node involvement and a 16% incidence of local recurrence in association with neoplasms of 1 cm or less in

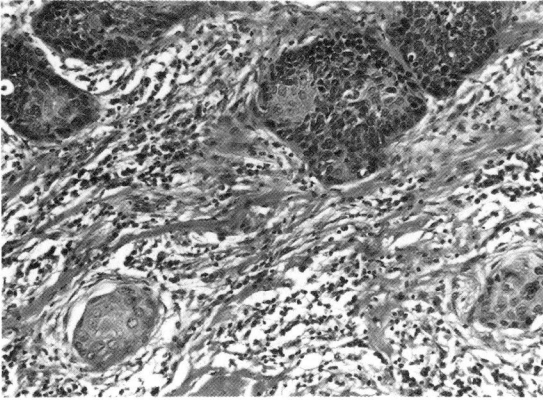

Fig. 10.17 Permeation, by tumour, of vascular-like spaces in the dermis beneath an epithelium with the features of VIN. (H & E × 120)

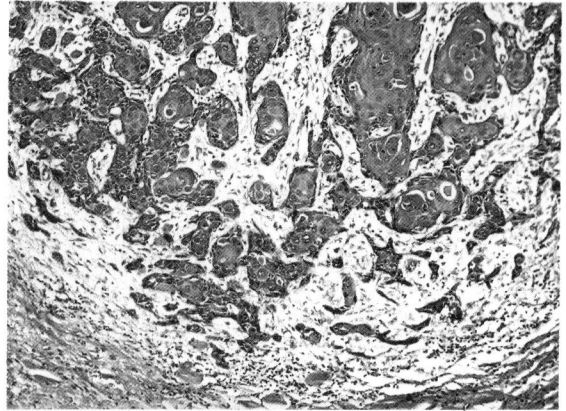

Fig. 10.18 A small, confluent invasive squamous carcinoma with a 'spray-like' pattern. (H & E × 60)

diameter. Hoffman et al (1983) have argued that tumour diameter correlates with the risk of nodal spread but only because the diameter of a neoplasm is closely related to its depth of invasion. They considered that variable depth was a better predictor of lymph node involvement than diameter and that a knowledge of tumour diameter did not add any further precision to the accuracy of prediction once tumour depth was known.

Other controversial aspects of the definition of a micro-invasive carcinoma of the vulva include the importance or otherwise of such features as vascular space involvement, confluence and degree of tumour differentiation and the significance of associated VIN.

In some studies, the invasion of vascular-like spaces (Fig. 10.17) has been significantly associated with an increased risk of nodal metastases (Parker et al 1975, Iversen et al 1981, Hoffman et al 1983, Husseinzadeh et al 1983) the most striking association being that of Kolstad et al (1982), in which 40% of patients in whom vascular-like spaces invasion was found had nodal metastases while only 3% of those without tumour involvement of these spaces showed evidence of lymph node spread. In contrast, others have failed to show any clearcut relationship between the presence of vascular space permeation and an increased risk of nodal metastases (Buscema et al 1981, Wilkinson et al 1982).

Two factors should be borne in mind when considering these conflicting reports: firstly, it may be

a difficult, subjective and arbitrary decision as to whether tumour cells are within a true vascular-like space or within a tissue cleft, and, secondly, the true incidence of vascular-like space involvement in vulval lesions of this type has not been assessed by serial sectioning—a technique, which, if findings in the cervix are relevant, could be expected to yield a much higher incidence of vascular-like involvement than is currently being reported.

Opinions differ as to the prognostic importance of tumour differentiation. While some authors have considered poor tumour differentiation as an important predictor of high risk of nodal metastases (Barnes et al 1980, Crissman & Azoury 1981, Husseinzadeh et al 1983) others (Magrina et al 1979, Iversen et al 1981, Chu et al 1982, Kolstad et al 1982, Woodruff 1982, Hoffman et al 1983) have shown no association between tumour differentiation and the risk of nodal metastases.

The importance of confluent tumour growth has also been a matter of debate. To some extent this is because an opinion as to whether a tumour is showing a confluent pattern or not is highly subjective. Attempts to define confluence have suggested either, 'a group of tumour cells filling an area of 2 mm or more' (Magrina et al 1979) or 'a mass of carcinoma filling a 1 mm or greater field' (Hoffman et al 1983). Clearly these differing definitions do little to solve the problem of how to assess confluence, but, within the limits imposed by this difficulty, Barnes et al (1980) and Hoffman et al (1983) considered that this pattern of growth (a 'spray-like' pattern) was clearly associated with an increased risk of nodal metastases (Fig. 10.18). Magrina et al (1979) showed that confluence was associated with a worse prognosis but not specifically with an increased risk of nodal spread, while Wilkinson et al (1982) found no correlation between a confluent growth pattern and lymph node involvement.

Some workers have reported that a microinvasive carcinoma which is arising from an epithelium having the features of VIN has an extremely good prognosis with little risk of nodal metastases (Magrina et al 1979, Barnes et al 1980), but Hacker et al (1983) demonstrated that the presence of VIN has no prognostic significance.

Conclusion. Faced with this array of conflicting opinion and the high incidence of nodal metastases in patients meeting the most widely accepted current definition of micro-invasive carcinoma, the International Society for the Study of Vulvar Disease recently agreed (Kneale 1984) that the term 'micro-invasive carcinoma of the vulva' is misleading and dangerous when taken with its current definition and recommended that its use be discontinued and that the designation stage 1a of the vulva be used to describe solitary lesions confined to a maximum of 2 cm diameter and 1 mm depth of invasion.

This recommendation is clearly justified but does not mean that attempts to delineate a minimally invasive lesion which can be treated conservatively should be abandoned. Barnes et al (1980) characterised a superficially invasive lesion which did not appear to be associated with any risk of lymph node metastases; this arose from an epithelium having the features of VIN as invading foci, single and multiple, formed of single cords or tongues of invading cells infiltrating the adjacent stroma to a distance of less than 2 mm from the limiting basement membrane of the epithelial site of origin (Fig. 10.19). If the foci were multiple, confluence or joining of these separate tongues of invading cells was not seen and vascular-like space permeation was not present. This is the pattern which corresponds to that in the cervix described as 'early stromal invasion' (Holzer et al 1982) and it is reasonable to suggest that this type of invasive lesion only should be treated conservatively. Any lesion exceeding this should be regarded as an invasive carcinoma of the vulva for treatment purposes.

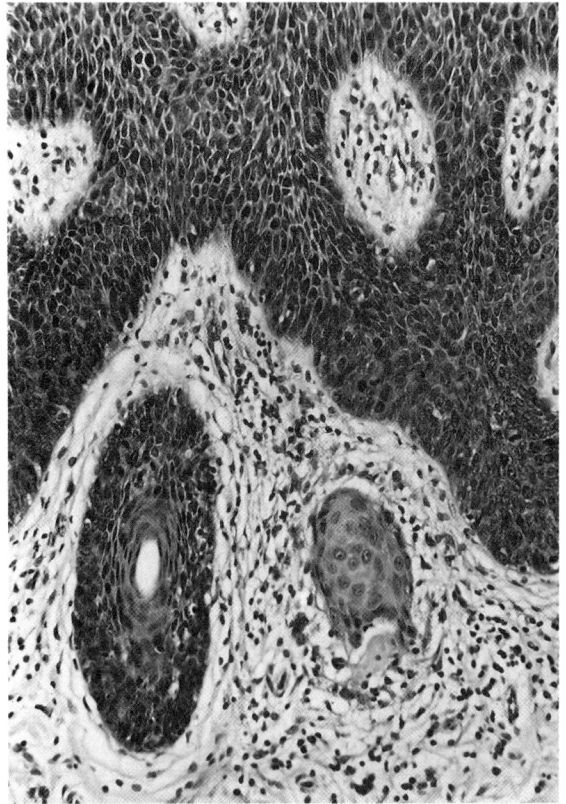

Fig. 10.19 Superficially invasive squamous carcinoma. A single cluster of invading cells lies immediately below an epithelium which has the features of VIN III. (H & E × 175)

Malignant epithelial neoplasms

Malignant tumours of the vulva comprise between 3 and 8% of all female genital tract malignancies and, of these, squamous carcinoma is by far the most common, accounting for almost 90% (Brunschwig & Brockunier 1967, Charles 1972, Kelly 1972, DiSaia & Creasman 1981) whilst adenocarcinoma of the vulva is distinctly rare (Ferenczy 1981). Just under 5% are malignant melanomas, 4% are described as undifferentiated carcinomas, 2.2% are sarcomas, 2–10% are basal cell carcinomas and 0.1–7% are primary carcinomas of Bartholin's gland (Crossen 1948, Barclay et al 1964, Kelly 1972, DiSaia & Creasman 1981, Merino et al 1982). Up to 10% of apparently primary vulval tumours are eventually found to be metastases (Japaze et al 1977).

Squamous carcinoma

Aetiology. The aetiology of squamous carcinoma is, in most cases, unknown but the tumour is associated generally with advanced age, the unmarried state, poverty, nulliparity (25 to 38% of patients are nulliparous), earlier than average menopause (Japaze et al 1977, DiSaia & Creasman 1981, Podratz et al 1983a), smoking (Chamberlain 1981), premature arteriosclerosis and immune deficiency (Lindeque et al 1987), and with local conditions such as poor hygiene, condylomata (Rutledge 1965) and granulomatous inflammation (Saltzstein et al 1956, Hay & Cole 1969, 1970) including syphilis, although the importance of the latter has declined in recent times. As the proportion of elderly women in the population has increased in recent years so too has the incidence of vulval carcinoma (Green 1978, Andreasson et al 1982b) and inevitably those associated general medical conditions which are also largely age related such as systemic hypertension, reported in 18 to 42% of patients, cardiac disease, 35%, arthritis, 18%, diabetes mellitus, 7 to 24%, hypothyroidism, 7% and obesity, 46% (Japaze et al 1977, Andreasson et al 1982b, Podratz et al 1983a).

In the past there was an established relationship between vulval carcinoma and industrial exposure to mineral oils in women working in the Lancashire cotton industry, the dyeing and bleaching industry in West Yorkshire and silver and cutlery buffers in Sheffield (Stacey 1939, Henry 1950).

An association with a second malignancy, which may be intra-epithelial or invasive, was noted by Taussig (1940) and this is most often in the cervix (Jimerson & Merrill 1970, Japaze et al 1977, Andreasson et al 1982b). Recent work has suggested that in a proportion of these cases a field change has occurred that is associated with papillomavirus infection and indeed an association between intra-epithelial and invasive squamous carcinoma and condylomata acuminata is well recognised (Charlewood & Shippell 1953, Woodruff & Rutledge 1965, Mickal et al 1966, Franklin & Rutledge 1971, Underwood & Hester 1971, Woodruff et al 1973, Kovi et al 1974, Josey et al 1976, Rhatigan & Saffos 1977, Shafeek et al 1979, Rastkar et al 1982, Stanbridge & Butler 1983, Daling et al 1984, Pilotti et al 1984) and may be

particularly important in the immunosuppressed patient. Patients in whom the intra-epithelial neoplasia has 'warty' features, that is, Bowenoid VIN, are, on the whole, younger and their lesions show less tendency to progress to invasion than do intra-epithelial neoplasms of more conventional form in the older women (Crum et al 1984). Herpes simplex virus type 2 (HSV2) has also been identified in the cells of an invasive carcinoma of the vulva (Josey et al 1976, Schwartz & Naftolin 1981, Cabral et al 1982). The role of radiation carcinogenicity in some of these patients is uncertain (Figge & Gaudenz 1974, Choo & Morley 1980). Certainly vulval malignancy may follow treatment of cervical carcinoma by radiotherapy, but whether the subsequent vulval malignancy is due to the radiation, or to potentiation of pre-existing carcinogens, or would have happened as a consequence of field change even in the absence of the radiotherapy, is open to question (Jimerson & Merrill 1970, Stanbridge & Butler 1983). The finding of an invasive squamous carcinoma of the vulva should, none the less, always arouse the suspicion of a simultaneous intra-epithelial or invasive carcinoma of the cervix. Conversely, in patients in whom cervical cancer has already been diagnosed, follow-up should include examination of the vulva (Choo & Morley 1980).

VIN is recognised by many authors as a precursor of squamous carcinoma and the concept is generally supported by the finding that women with intra-epithelial neoplasia of the vulva are younger than those with invasive lesions. VIN is present in the epithelium adjacent to the tumour in about 70% of patients (Zaino et al 1982, Hacker et al 1984); 'hyperplastic dystrophy' is present in about 50% of patients (Magrina et al 1979, Buscema et al 1980a, Zaino et al 1982, Podratz et al 1983a, Hacker et al 1984); 'mixed dystrophy' in about 10% (Zaino et al 1982, Hacker et al 1984) and lichen sclerosus in 6 to 25% (Zaino et al 1982, Hacker et al 1984) although a figure of 90% was reported by Hewitt (1984). Whilst there is some agreement that VIN is a precursor of invasive malignancy (McAdams & Kistner 1958), atypia is not usually seen in lichen sclerosus yet about 4% of cases are complicated by the development of invasive squamous carcinoma (Leighton & Langley 1975, Buscema et al 1980a). This may be a fortuitous association

Table 10.1 Clinical staging of vulval squamous carcinoma (after Friedrich and Wilkinson 1982)

Stage	Description
I	Tumour confined to the vulva and measures less than 2 cm in diameter. Regional lymph nodes are not clinically suspicious.
II	Tumour confined to the vulva but exceeds 2 cm in diameter. Regional lymph nodes are not clinically suspicious.
III	Tumour extends beyond the vulva and there are no suspicious lymph nodes or, a tumour of any size accompanied by clinically suspicious nodes.
IV	Grossly positive lymph nodes in the groins, regardless of the extent of the primary tumour or, evidence of metastatic disease anywhere.

Table 10.2 Errors in clinical staging (after Podratz et al 1983a)

Stage	Error (%)
I	18
II	22
III	31
IV	44

Table 10.3 Stage of disease: percentage of patients with nodal metastases

	Iversen et al 1980	Andreasson et al 1982b
I	10	11.5
II	30	13.3
III	45	27.4
IV	100	71.8

(Buscema et al 1980a, Fox & Buckley 1982, Zaino et al 1982). Some authors, however, believe that the condition does predispose to the development of carcinoma (Wallace 1971, Ridley 1983).

There is no evidence that vulval carcinoma, unlike many of the genital tract tumours, is in any way hormone dependent (Hoffman & Siiteri 1980, Ford et al 1983).

Clinical presentation. The age range is reported as 14 to 95 years (Benedet et al 1979, Cario et al 1984, Monaghan & Hammond 1984) and whilst more than three-quarters of patients are aged 60 years or more at the time of diagnosis (Green 1978), carcinoma of the vulva can, rarely, complicate pregnancy (Monaghan & Lindeque 1986).

Up to three-quarters of patients present with a lump, between 27 and 71% complain of pruritus, 6 to 41% have a discharge or bleeding and between 14.2 and 34.5% complain of pain (Brunschwig & Brockunier 1967, Kelly 1972, Benedet et al 1979, Podratz et al 1983a).

Clinical staging (Table 10.1) makes use of the size of the primary tumour and the clinical assessment of the regional lymph nodes. Many criticisms are made of this system: the choice of tumour diameter is somewhat arbitrary, no distinction is made between unilateral and bilateral inguinal nodal metastases and clinical detection of nodal metastases is notoriously unreliable; this is therefore an inaccurate method of staging. It is important to remember this when making use of epidemiological, prognostic and survival data based upon clinical staging. There is on average a 25% error in the clinical stage when compared with the pathological, histologically confirmed stage (Table 10.2) (Pod-

ratz et al 1983a) and the error reaches 44% for patients in stage IV, although this can be improved by fine needle aspiration biopsy of the suspicious nodes (James et al 1984). For the most part there is an underestimate, the occasional overestimate resulting from nodal enlargement in patients with an ulcerated and possibly infected neoplasm. The proportion of patients in each clinical stage with inguinal nodal metastases is shown in Table 10.3. An alternative clinical staging has been proposed by Krupp et al (1975) although Iversen et al (1980) and Boyce et al (1985) find the present system acceptable in their hands. A staging scheme based upon histopathological examination is clearly preferable and more accurate.

In a small, but well recognised, group of patients with squamous carcinoma of the vulva there is a significant degree of hypercalcaemia which returns to normal following the removal of the tumour (Schatten et al 1958, Nichols & Bonney 1973, Niebyl et al 1974, Shane & Naftolin 1975).

Gross pathology. The majority of squamous carcinomas, 70%, develop on the labia (Charles 1972, DiSaia & Creasman 1981), most commonly on the labia majora (40%, Janovski & Douglas 1972), but they also occur on the labia minora, clitoris (9 to 15%) and perineum (Benedet et al 1979). In about 10% of cases, the tumour is so large that its precise site of origin is uncertain (Benedet et al 1979). The neoplasms spread directly to the adjacent tissues, by lymphatics to the inguinal, femoral and pelvic lymph nodes and rarely, and late in the course of the disease, by the bloodstream (Stern & Kwon 1981) to the bones (Sharma & Isaacs 1985). Rutledge (1965) and

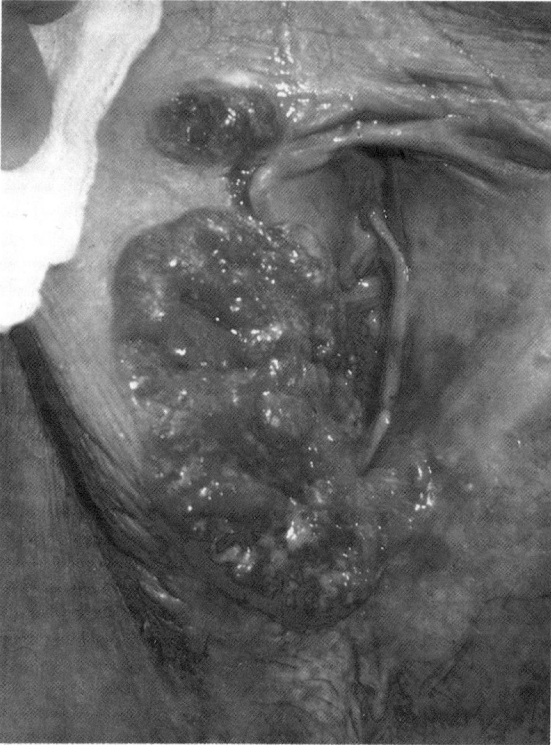

Fig. 10.20 Squamous cell carcinoma.

Charles (1972) reported that 10 to 20% of patients had multicentric disease, whilst Japaze et al (1977) and DiSaia & Creasman (1981) report that multifocal disease is uncommon with the exception of the rare 'kissing' tumours on the adjacent surfaces of the labia. Over half the tumours are ulcerated, 57.6% (Kelly 1972) to 62% (Andreasson et al 1982b), about one-third are papillary, 27% (Andreasson et al 1982b) to 40% (Kelly 1972), and 10 per cent are plaque-like (Fig. 10.20). Whatever the morphology of the tumour, nearly 30% already have inguinal nodal metastases at the time of diagnosis (Benedet et al 1979, Husseinzadeh et al 1983) and 16 to 22.5% have pelvic nodal metastases (Franklin & Rutledge 1971, Krupp & Bohm 1978). A small number of patients already have pelvic visceral spread at presentation (Stern & Kwon 1981, Monaghan & Hammond 1984), direct spread to the pelvic bones and occasionally distant metastases.

When the primary tumour is limited to one side of the vulva, more than 80% of inguinal nodal metastases occur to the ipsilateral nodes (Krupp & Bohm 1978), 5 to 15.3% only to the contralateral nodes and 14 to 30% are bilateral (Way, 1982). When the carcinoma is bilateral, 60% have bilateral inguinal node metastases (Krupp & Bohm 1978), which is probably a reflection of more advanced disease. Central and clitoral neoplasms show no greater tendency to spread to both inguinal regions than do unilateral tumours, 37.5% having bilateral metastases. This is not altogether surprising because not only do the clitoris and perineum have bilateral lymph flow but a small though significant quantity of contralateral lymph flow occurs from the anterior part of the labia minora (Eichner 1957, Iversen & Aas 1983). It is important to note that when the inguinal nodes are free from tumour the pelvic nodes are not usually affected (Curry et al 1980, Podratz et al 1983a, Shimm et al 1986). Krupp & Bohm (1978) have, however, reported one exception to this general rule.

Histopathology. Typical squamous carcinomas of the vulva differ morphologically in no way from those which occur in other parts of the body. The majority are well differentiated (53.6%), a similar number (40.5%) are moderately well differentiated; only 5 to 20% are poorly differentiated (Novak & Woodruff 1979, Hacker et al 1984) and these tend, according to some authors (Ferenczy 1981) to be more frequent in the vestibule and clitoral areas. A small number of specific, rather unusual histopathological variants are also described and, as noted above, attempts have been made to define a category of micro-invasive carcinomas comparable to those seen in the cervix.

Well-differentiated squamous carcinomas are composed of islands, anastamosing masses and infiltrating cords of squamous cells showing progressive nuclear and cytoplasmic maturation and keratinisation towards the centres of the masses where there are, in many areas, epithelial pearls (Fig. 10.21). The tumour surface is often ulcerated. Its margins are in continuity with the adjacent epithelium which may be normal, show evidence of a dystrophy or have the features of VIN. The underlying tissue is usually infiltrated by plasma cells and lymphocytes which vary in quantity. Nucleo-cytoplasmic ratios are low in these well-differentiated tumours, cytoplasmic maturation is present, nuclear pleomorphism and atypia are

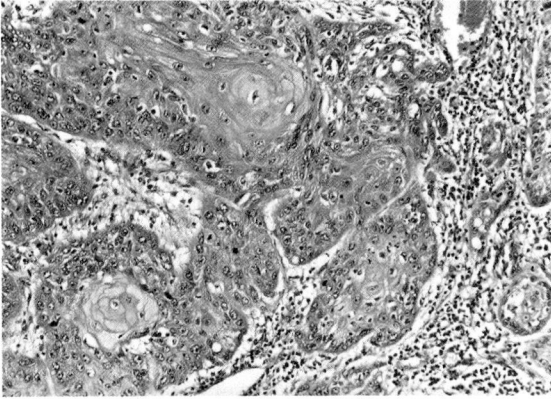

Fig. 10.21 Well-differentiated squamous carcinoma. The tumour is composed of nests of squamous cells showing cytoplasmic differentiation towards the centre of the nests with the formation of epithelial pearls. (H & E × 100)

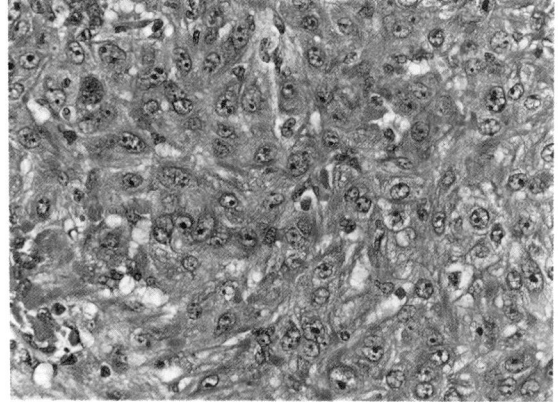

Fig. 10.22 Poorly differentiated squamous carcinoma. The tumour is composed of cells with copious cytoplasm and large nuclei in which there are prominent nucleoli. There are no specific squamous features in this field. (H & E × 240)

minimal and mitoses not conspicuous; intercellular bridges are prominent.

Dedifferentiation is characterised by the loss of cytoplasmic maturation, keratinisation and intercellular bridges and an increase in nuclear atypia, pleomorphism, nucleocytoplasmic ratios and mitoses. In the least differentiated forms the tumour consists of sheets and cords of cells which lack squamous features except in occasional individual cells (Fig. 10.22). Some exhibit marked pleomorphism whilst others are composed of small cells; frequent, often atypical, mitoses characterise the poorly differentiated neoplasm and intercellular bridges are not present. Unless cytoplasmic differentiation is present in some area, the term undifferentiated should be used. In such cases electron microscopy and immunocytochemistry may be useful in distinguishing the poorly differentiated carcinoma from other poorly differentiated neoplasms.

Variants of squamous carcinoma.

Verrucous carcinoma. Verrucous carcinoma of the vulva is extremely uncommon (Japaze et al 1982) and its distinction from other condyloma-like lesions of the vulva is somewhat confused for no definite criteria have been established which allow for a clear pathological distinction to be drawn between large squamous papilloma, large squamous papilloma with malignant change, giant condylo-

ma, giant condyloma with malignant change, well-differentiated squamous carcinoma and verrucous carcinoma. The confusion is greatest when attempting to distinguish between a giant condyloma and a verrucous carcinoma and indeed there is no agreement as to whether these are separate and distinct entities, arbitrarily defined morphological stages in a pathological continuum or identical lesions. In many reports, both of giant condyloma and of verrucous carcinoma of the vulva, these problems have been either ignored or evaded; in others the two lesions are considered as a single entity (Gallousis 1972) and in yet others a clear distinction is drawn between the two conditions (Partridge et al 1980a, b).

Faced with these uncertainties and ambiguities it is difficult to draw a clear picture of the pathology and clinical behaviour of verrucous carcinoma of the vulva; it is true that those cases which are unequivocally reported as verrucous carcinoma do appear to show a characteristic pattern of behaviour, but it is far from certain whether or not such reports tend to isolate one end of the pathological and clinical spectrum of this neoplasm. The same ambiguities must arise where HPV has been reported in verrucous carcinoma, for example the patients of Gissman et al (1982) and of Rando et al (1986) where an unusual type 6 HPV was found.

Verrucous carcinomas tend to occur at a generally older age than typical carcinomas, most patients

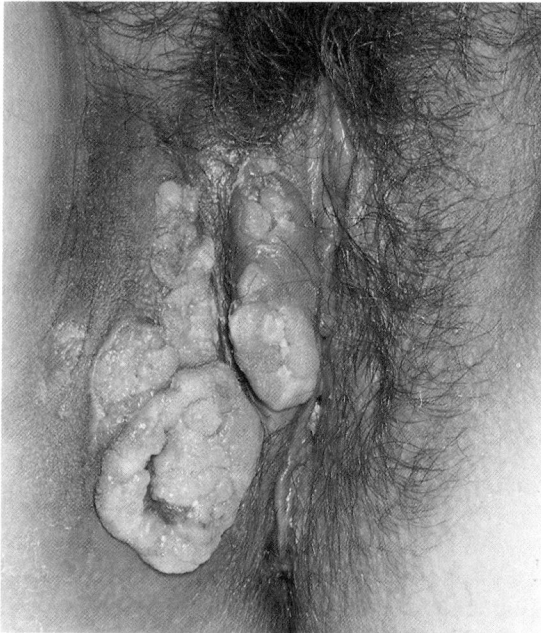

Fig. 10.23 Verrucous carcinoma (HPV 11 demonstrated) in a woman aged 25 years with myelodysplasia. (By courtesy of Dr C Howarth and Department of Medical Photography, Charing Cross Hospital)

being postmenopausal and a high proportion being in their eighth or ninth decade: the youngest reported case occurred in a woman of 21 years. In the series reported by Japaze et al (1982) there was serological evidence of syphilis in 12.5% of cases whilst 50% of the patients were known to have biopsy-proved vulval condylomas (Charlewood & Shippel 1953) during the 10 years prior to diagnosis; a further 25% were suffering from or later developed an invasive neoplasm either at other sites in the genital tract or elsewhere in the body.

The clinical presentation may be similar to that for typical squamous carcinoma but sometimes the lesion may grow very rapidly to reach, within say a 2-year period, a size sufficient to impede walking. The tumour classically appears as a warty or papillary, fungating, often ulcerated, mass to which the term 'cauliflower-like' is commonly applied. It may be grey, pink, yellow, white or pigmented like the adjacent skin. The most common site is the labia majora but not uncommonly the tumour involves both labia and, sometimes, the entire vulva (Fig. 10.23)

Histologically the tumour is composed of papillary fronds of mature stratified squamous epithelium with pushing, bulbous rete ridges. Hyperkeratosis is usually marked whilst acanthosis is often of a striking degree and sufficiently intricate as to make tangential sectioning difficult, or impossible, to avoid. The broad, bulbous rete ridges appear to be compressing and pushing against the underlying stroma rather than truly invading it and their basal margins are intact, smooth, regular and clearly defined. There is a striking lack of cellular atypia and of nuclear pleomorphism or hyperchromatism whilst a normal nucleo-cytoplasmic ratio is retained; delay in maturation is not a feature, with basal type cells being seen only in the two or three layers immediately abutting on the limiting basal membrane. There may be a scattering of mitotic figures but these are invariably confined to the basal layers and are always of normal form. There is commonly a well-defined granular layer and vacuolated cells and cells showing koilocytosis are a common, almost invariable feature (Gallousis 1972; Partridge et al 1980b, Fox 1986). There is always a well-marked, non-specific chronic inflammatory cell infiltrate adjacent to the base of the tumour.

In view of this bland histological appearance it is hardly surprising that the pathologist, especially one who is not fully aware of the clinical details, will usually report a biopsy from a verrucous carcinoma as being histologically benign, diagnoses of either a squamous papilloma or a condyloma usually being proffered. As a rule it is only when the tumour recurs or continues to show rapid growth and relentless invasive tendencies that the contrast between the aggressive nature of the neoplasm and its paradoxically innocuous histological appearance raises an awareness of the possibility of verrucous carcinoma.

The natural history of verrucous carcinoma is towards recurrence and local invasion (Lucas et al 1974). If primary removal is incomplete, and it can often be extremely difficult to ensure complete extirpation, recurrence is inevitable; about one-third of cases do so. The tumour invades the adjacent structures in a relentless manner, even to the extent of invading bone; perineural infiltration has been noted (Demian et al 1973) and tumour can sometimes encircle, without actually invading, lymph nodes. True lymphatic spread to nodes can occur from a vulval verrucous carcinoma (Vayrynen et al 1981) but is exceptional, as are distant metastases (Stehman et al 1980)

Spindle cell squamous cell carcinoma. Spindle cell carcinoma is an uncommon form of poorly differentiated squamous carcinoma (Brooks 1943, Sims & Kirsch, 1948) which occurs with extreme rarity on the vulva (Gosling et al 1961, Copas et al 1982).

There is sometimes a preceding history of radiotherapy (Brooks 1943, Sims & Kirsch 1948, Underwood et al 1951, Battifora 1976) and many of these tumours occur in areas of radiodermatitis. The neoplasm may be sessile, polypoidal or superficial, and is composed of bundles of spindle cells with basophilic cytoplasm and oval to round nuclei. Numerous mitoses are present and haemorrhage and necrosis are common (Copas et al 1982). The epidermis adjacent to one of the vulval tumours was described as having features of carcinoma in situ. Electron optic studies confirm the presence in these sarcoma-like tumours of features confirming their squamous nature, that is, keratohyalin, bundles of tonofilaments, premelanosomes and occasional well-developed desmosomes (Woyke et al 1974, Battifora 1976, Manglani et al 1980). Staining for keratin and intermediate filaments is also of value in distinguishing these tumours from sarcomas.

Most reports of tumours elsewhere in the body, especially on the head and neck, have indicated a variable prognosis with those tumours which are superficial and polypoidal apparently having a more favourable outcome than do the sessile forms (Manglani et al 1980). However, despite their polypoidal structure, the two fully described neoplasms occurring on the genitalia (the second being on the glans penis, Manglani et al 1980) had a rapidly fatal course and this generalisation may not apply to genital tumours. Merging of spindle cell and typical squamous cell carcinomatous elements in the tumour also correlates with a poor prognosis.

Adenoid squamous carcinoma. In some squamous carcinomas there is acantholysis in the centres of some or all of the infiltrating tumour cell nests and lobules as a consequence of which a pseudoglandular pattern develops (Lever 1947, Johnson & Helwig 1966). Cystic spaces are lined by a single layer of cubocolumnar neoplastic cells and contain somewhat pleomorphic isolated squamous cells. The term 'adenoid squamous cell carcinoma' is applied to these tumours, whether all or only part of the neoplasm has these features. Tests for mucin, however, are uniformly negative, refuting the argument that such tumours are a form of adenosquamous carcinoma. It is uncertain in what proportion of vulval neoplasms such a feature is present, but Lasser et al (1974) report it in 17 out of 50 patients with invasive squamous carcinoma of the vulva. Its development did not affect the prognosis to a statistically significant degree although 5 out of 17 patients with tumours showing this pattern (28%) died of their disease, compared with only 6 out of 33 patients with typical squamous carcinoma (18%), and 20% had a family history of skin cancer compared with 7% of patients with conventional squamous carcinoma (Johnson & Helwig 1966). The age of occurrence is similar to that for typical squamous carcinoma.

There is in the literature a tendency to confuse adenoid squamous carcinoma with adenosquamous carcinoma in which proved squamous and glandular elements are present. There is little doubt that both entities occur in the vulva, but whilst the former is probably simply a particular form of epidermal carcinoma the latter is more likely to be of Bartholin's gland, adnexal or cloacal origin.

Prognosis, prognostic factors and survival. A favourable outcome to the management of vulval carcinoma depends ultimately on the absence of metastases and this, in turn, depends upon early detection of the lesion, the size of the primary tumour and its depth of penetration, its histological differentiation and pattern of growth, the presence of lymphatic involvement adjacent to the primary tumour, and, according to some authors, the site of origin of the neoplasm and the bodily habitus of the patient. A combination of histopathological and clinical features affords a more accurate prediction of survival than does any one factor (Andreasson & Nyboe 1985).

Overall 5-year survival for patients with carcinoma of the vulva lies between 70% and 84.2% (corrected) (Iversen et al 1980, Andreasson et al 1982b, Podratz et al 1983a), which is not a great improvement on the 58.5% (uncorrected) reported by Taussig (1940). If the inguinal nodes contain metastatic tumour the 3-year survival for all stages of the disease is 46%, whilst if there is not metastatic disease survival at 3 years is 76.3% (Donaldson et al 1981). Curry et al (1980) attempted to refine the data somewhat and reported that if fewer than three ipsilateral inguinal nodes contained tumour the survival at 5 years was 69%, compared with 54% at 2 years when more than three unilateral nodes were affected and 52% at 2 years when bilateral inguinal nodal metastases were present—a statistically significant difference. Relating survival to clinical stage of the disease shows that for patients in stage I there is a 5-year survival of between 90 and 100%, for stage II between 81 and 83%, for stage III between 53 and 77% (Podratz et al 1983a, Boyce et al 1985, Malfetano et al 1986) and for stage IV up to 20% (Podratz et al 1983a, Malfetano et al 1986), although Kaplan & Kaufman (1975) reported a 50% 5-year survival for a small group of patients with stage IV disease treated by ultraradical procedures.

Generally speaking, the smaller the primary tumour and the less its depth of invasion, the fewer are the nodal metastases and the better the prognosis (Brunschwig & Brockunier 1967, Franklin & Rutledge 1971, Morley 1976, Krupp & Bohm 1978, Benedet et al 1979, Boyce et al 1985). When the tumour is less than 1 cm in diameter, inguinal nodal metastases are found in only up to 6.6% of cases (Franklin & Rutledge 1971, Wilkinson et al 1982, Boyce et al 1985). In small lesions of this type, depth of invasion may be a more accurate predictor of the presence of inguinal and pelvic lymph node metastases than is tumour diameter (Hoffman et al 1983, Husseinzadeh et al 1983) although Boyce et al (1985) showed that there is a statistically significant relationship between the diameter of the neoplasm and its depth of invasion, and measurement of diameter may be easier, particularly when the tumour is ulcerated or there is uncertainty about the plane of section. Patients with a tumour having a diameter between 1 and 2 cm have metastases in 15 to 21% of cases (Franklin & Rutledge 1971, Boyce et al 1985) and a 5-year survival of 90 to 100%, 35% of patients with tumour between 2 and 4 cm have metastases (Boyce et al 1985) and a 77% 5-year survival, whilst 30 to 55% of patients with tumours more than 4 cm in diameter have metastases and only 44 to 46% of patients survive for 5 years (Podratz et al 1983a, Boyce et al 1985). These figures suggest a direct relationship between

tumour size and the incidence of metastases but this is not a simple association. The figures are statistically significant only when the tumour size exceeds 4 cm (Andreasson et al 1982b) and the presence of metastases may depend to some extent upon poor histological differentiation of the tumour and a confluent, stellate or spray pattern of infiltration (Crissman & Azoury 1981, Hoffman et al 1983, Podratz et al 1983a, Hacker et al 1984, Boyce et al 1985). There are, for example, significantly fewer metastases from well-differentiated neoplasms measuring less than 4 cm in diameter, although Andreasson et al (1982a) found this to confer no prognostic advantage, possibly a consequence of the small sample. In the series of Boyce et al (1985), the histological grade of the tumour was, on the other hand, not related to the presence of nodal metastases or survival: histological grade I was considered an important factor, however, in the prediction of metastases by Way (1960), Husseinzadeh et al (1983) and Monaghan & Hammond (1984), all of whom found that poorly differentiated tumours were more likely than well-differentiated carcinomas to have metastasised even when there was no vascular space involvement around the primary poorly differentiated neoplasm, the risk being similar to that noted for well-differentiated tumours with vascular space involvement. The presence of vascular space infiltration adjacent to the tumour not only increases the risk of nodal metastases (Husseinzadeh et al 1983, Hacker et al 1984, Boyce et al 1985) but also increased the chance of local or vaginal recurrences and death from the disease (Iversen et al 1981).

Neither the gross morphology of the carcinoma nor the presence of an associated vulvar intraepithelial neoplasm has been shown to have any prognostic significance by Zaino et al (1982) and Hacker et al (1983), although an earlier report by Gosling et al (1961) suggested that patients in whom the carcinoma was associated with a 'leukoplakia' had a better chance of survival.

Recurrent disease, which may develop up to 12 years after initial treatment, occurs in 26.2 to 33% of patients (Andreasson et al 1982b, Monaghan & Hammond 1984) and is a serious problem. Generally, the earlier the recurrence, the worse the prognosis. Recurrence occurs most commonly at the vulva in about 18% of patients (Podratz et al 1982), which is three times more frequent than recurrence in the groins or in distant sites. Tumour histology does not seem to be related to the incidence of recurrences, but other factors which adversely affect survival do appear to be related to tumour recurrence, that is, a tumour size of more than 4 cm and inguinal nodal metastases, or both (Podratz et al 1982, Shimm et al 1986).

Treatment. Radical vulvectomy with dissection of the superficial and deep inguinal lymph nodes is the commonly accepted and preferred treatment for invasive squamous cell carcinoma of the vulva and gives the best results (Monaghan & Hammond 1984). Omission of inguinal lymphadenectomy cannot be justified and results, in a small proportion of patients, in the development of potentially preventable groin recurrences (Hacker et al 1984, Monaghan & Hammond 1984). Surgery can, if necessary, be extended for late stage disease, to include pelvic node dissection, anovulvectomy and exenteration (Podratz et al 1983, Monaghan & Hammond 1984). The latter provides, at present, the only hope of survival for patients with advanced disease and gives a 5-year survival of between 28 and 66% compared with an expected 20%, at best, with less aggressive therapy.

Treatment is considered further on page 342.

Surgery is the treatment of choice for verrucous carcinoma; it is usually limited to wide local excision (Lucas et al 1974, Isaacs 1976, Partridge et al 1980a, Stehman et al 1980, Japaze et al 1982) and recurrences are treated similarly. Lymphadenectomy has its advocates (Gallousis 1972, Selium & Lankeroni 1979) but in view of the extremely low incidence of lymph node metastases, even in advanced cases, this is an unnecessarily radical procedure (Isaacs 1976, Powell et al 1978). Recurrence of vulval verrucous carcinoma has been noted in about a third of cases, 30% having died as a direct result of their tumour. Seventy per cent of the patients have been treated solely by surgery, and amongst these 80% survived; by contrast only 46% of the patients treated with a combination of radiotherapy and surgery have survived. This striking discrepancy between the two modes of treatment could be explained in terms of radiotherapy being used only for those patients with far advanced tumours, but there is a general acceptance that not only are verrucous carcinomas radioresis-

tant (Demian et al 1973) but that in some cases irradiation may induce an anaplastic transformation of the neoplasm and an acceleration in the rate of tumour growth (Kraus & Perez-Mesa 1966).

Therapy for spindle cell carcinoma cannot be defined because of the paucity of cases. In view of the rapid course reported by Copas et al (1982) it would appear that radical vulvectomy with inguinal lymphadenectomy perhaps followed by chemotherapy may be advised and a similar approach is probably appropriate for adenoid squamous carcinoma.

Adenosquamous carcinoma

It is doubtful whether adenosquamous carcinoma ever arises directly from the epidermis of the vulva. When such neoplasms occur in the vulva they are usually said to be of cloacogenic origin (Rhatigan & Mojadidi 1973) (see p. 318), derived from skin appendages (Underwood et al 1978, Dissanayake & Salm 1980) (see p. 305), or carcinomas of Bartholin's gland (see p. 309). They are reputed to be aggressive tumours with a poor prognosis, and radical surgery with lymph node dissection is probably the appropriate treatment (Underwood et al 1979).

Adenocarcinoma

Adenocarcinoma is a rare primary neoplasm in the vulva and many such tumours are misdiagnosed initially as metastases. They may develop from the sweat glands (see p. 306), Bartholin's gland (see p. 310) or other similar, unnamed, mucus-secreting vestibular glands, mesonephric (Wolffian duct, Gärtner's duct) remnants, cloacal remnants (see below) or ectopic breast tissue (Hendrix & Behrman 1956) (see p. 229). It may be impossible to identify the precise tissue of origin, although the tumour morphology and cytological characteristics or residual non-neoplastic tissue may give a clue.

A mucus-secreting papillary, columnar cell adenocarcinoma has been described adjacent to the urethral meatus by Tiltman & Knutzen (1978) It was not thought to have developed from the paraurethral glands and the similarity of its epithelium to that found in large intestinal neoplasms and the presence of non-neoplastic intestinal-like epithelium containing Paneth cells immediately adjacent to it led to the suggestion that it had developed from a misplaced cloacal remnant. Indeed the morphology of the tumour, as illustrated, closely resembles that of large intestinal adenocarcinoma. It differs, however, from the usual cloacogenic carcinomas (see p. 320).

Treatment for vulval adenocarcinomas follows the pattern laid down for the treatment of vulval carcinomas in general.

Basal cell carcinoma

Basal cell carcinoma of the vulva is rare, accounting for only between 2 and 10% of all vulval malignancies (Siegler & Green 1951, Schueller 1965, Palladino et al 1969, Ambrosini et al 1980, Friedrich & Wilkinson 1982, Merino et al 1982, Dudzinski et al 1984).

Aetiology. These neoplasms occur most commonly on areas of the body exposed to solar radiation and this is most dramatically demonstrated in patients with xeroderma pigmentosum; such an aetiology is, however, unlikely in the development of vulval lesions. It has been suggested that chronic infection, environmental exposure to arsenic (Cabrera et al 1984), trauma, vaginal discharge, X-ray treatment and radiotherapy may be implicated (Breen et al 1975, Gordon & Kerr 1975, Dudzinski et al 1984) and in earlier days the use of medicinal arsenicals was associated with an increased risk of both basal cell and squamous carcinomas. These neoplasms also occur in patients with the basal cell naevus syndrome (Gorlin et al 1965) but apparently not on the vulva and have been described as a complication of a fibro-epitheliomatous polyp (Cruz-Jimenez & Abell 1975). There is evidence that immunocompromised patients are at increased risk of developing basal cell carcinomas (Murphy et al 1983) and this may be a factor in the development, not only of the basal cell carcinoma, but also of an associated second malignant neoplasm, which is present in 20% of these elderly patients (Palladino et al 1969). In some instances the second neoplasm may be a basal cell carcinoma elsewhere in the body (Cruz-Jimenez & Abell 1975, Deppisch 1978), or in very rare cases a second primary vulval basal cell carcinoma has been described (Deppisch 1978).

There is no evidence of a pre-invasive malignant phase although basal cell carcinoma has been associated with lichen sclerosus (McAdam & Kistner 1958, Meyrick-Thomas et al 1985) and in the majority of patients the aetiology remains unknown.

On the vulva, basal cell carcinomas occur most commonly in elderly white women, with a mean age of 58 to 73 years being quoted (Palladino et al 1969, Breen et al 1975, Cruz-Jimenez & Abell 1975, Zerner 1975) though occasional cases occur in younger women (Ambrosini et al 1980).

Clinical presentation. Basal cell carcinoma often presents with pruritus, serous or blood-stained discharge and bleeding; ulceration or a mass may be noted (Schueller 1965, Bean & Becker 1968, Palladino et al 1969, Breen et al 1975, Cruz-Jimenez & Abell 1975, Deppisch 1978). Frequently there is a delay in diagnosis due in some cases to the absence of symptoms (Merino et al 1982) but more commonly to patient neglect and perhaps to delay in performing a diagnostic biopsy (Palladino et al 1969, Dudzinski et al 1984). Symptoms may have been present for between 3 weeks and 34 years before diagnosis (Palladino et al 1969) and it is essential to carry out an adequate diagnostic biopsy to enable the correct histopathological interpretation to be made (Schueller 1965, Breen et al 1975, Cruz-Jimenez & Abell 1975, Goldstein & Kent 1975, Deppisch 1978, Merino et al 1982).

Gross pathology. Basal cell carcinoma is a locally aggressive, usually non-metastasising, carcinoma (Zerner 1975). Most lesions are confined to the labia majora (Zerner 1975, Friedrich & Wilkinson 1982c) and they are most common anteriorly although they may also develop around the clitoris, mons, urethra and fourchette (Schueller 1965, Palladino et al 1969, Deppisch 1978). They range in size from 1 to 7 cm (Breen et al 1975) and on rare occasions may reach 10 cm in their greatest axis (Dudzinski et al 1984). They may form a nodule with or without ulceration (Breen et al 1975), an exophytic lesion or an excoriated area; they may also be erythematous, polypoidal, papillomatous, cystic or plaque-like (Bean & Becker 1968, Breen et al 1975, Goldstein & Kent 1975, Deppisch 1978, Merino et al 1982) or resemble a dystrophic patch (Deppisch 1978) (Fig. 10.24). When the lesion contains melanin it may clinically resemble a malignant melanoma. The variable appearance of the basal cell carcinoma often leads to diagnostic problems,

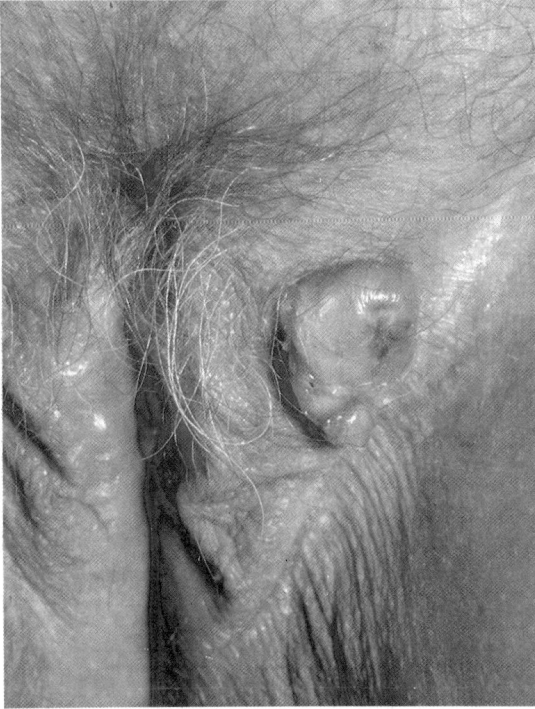

Fig. 10.24 Basal cell carcinoma. (Reproduced from Beilby and Ridley 1987 by courtesy of the authors and publisher)

particularly when the inguinal lymph nodes are enlarged secondary to local ulceration or infection.

Vulval basal cell carcinoma is not usually characterised by the development of nodal metastases but three cases have been described. Two patients (Jimenez et al 1975, Perrone et al 1987) had metastases in the inguinal nodes whilst the third (Sworn et al 1979) had involved nodes in the subcutaneous tissue beneath the tumour. These cases should, however, be regarded as exceptional.

Histopathology. Basal cell carcinomas of the vulva are similar histologically to those which occur in other parts of the body. The tumours, which develop from the epidermis, pilosebaceous units or sweat glands (Janovski & Douglas 1972), are composed of small, round, oval or slightly elongated cells with deeply basophilic nuclei and scanty cytoplasm. The constituent cells resemble morphologically those of the basal layer of the epidermis, but controversy existed for years (Zackheim 1963, Lever & Schaumburg-Lever 1975a, Gatter et al 1984) over the origin of these cells. Recent work, however (Gatter et al 1984), confirms the similarity of the immunohistochemical profile with that of the immature, pluripotential basal cells of the epidermis (Pollack et al 1982). Within the tumours and in the adjacent dermis and epidermis, it is usual to find an infiltrate of plasma cells, lymphocytes (largely T lymphocytes (Pollack et al 1982)) and histiocytes, and in some cases this may be very heavy. It is believed that this represents an active immunological response to the tumour (Murphy et al 1983).

Basal cell carcinomas grow in several distinct histological patterns, those which occur most commonly on the vulva being described as superficial, solid, sclerosing or morphea-like and keratotic (Siegler & Greene 1951, Ackles & Pratt 1956, Marcus 1960, Schueller 1965, Bean & Becker 1968, Cruz-Jimenez & Abell 1975, Goldstein & Kent 1975, Ferenczy 1981, Dudzinski et al 1984). A pure adenoid basal cell pattern is less common, although foci of adenoid pattern may occur in the more common solid varieties (Schueller 1965, Goldstein & Kent 1975, Sworn et al 1979, Merino et al 1982) and focal sebaceous differentiation may be seen (Rulon & Helwig 1974). Those rare vulval basal cell carcinomas which have metastasised are histologically unremarkable (Jimenez et al 1975, Sworn et al 1979), although atypical features have been described in metastasising tumours from other areas of the body (Farmer & Helwig 1980).

The histological patterns observed in basal cell carcinomas mimic, to some extent, those structures into which the pluripotential epidermal cells normally develop, i.e. hair follicles, sweat glands or sebaceous glands; hence the wide variety.

Superficial basal carcinoma appears in a histological section as a series of discrete, irregular proliferations of tumour cells budding downwards from the basal layer of the epidermis, the peripheral layer of cells forming a palisade (Fig. 10.25). The underlying dermis is often fibrotic. Opinions are divided as to whether each of the tumour structures is discrete (Sanderson 1961) or whether the nodules are interconnected and attached only at intervals to the epidermis (Madsen 1955).

The solid (undifferentiated) form is similar, but larger and more variably sized and shaped; cellular masses lie in the dermis although an origin from the epidermis, or occasionally a hair sheath, is usually apparent and each mass maintains the peripheral

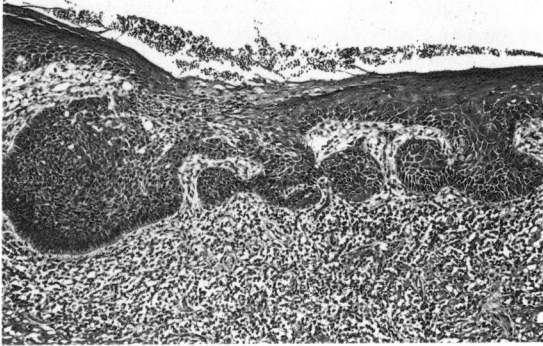

Fig. 10.25 Basal cell carcinoma, superficial pattern. Several irregularly sized tumour buds descend from the basal layer of the epidermis, into the dermis; the peripheral layer of cells forms a palisade. (H & E × 60)

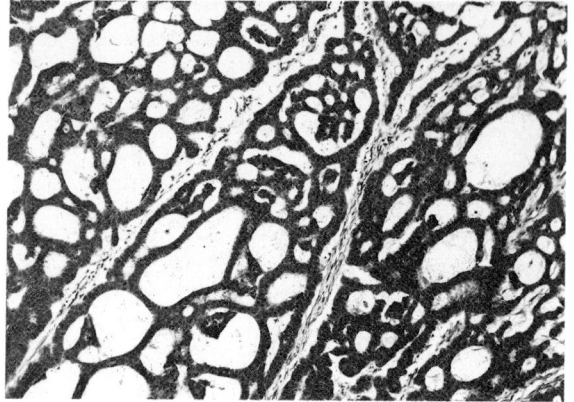

Fig. 10.27 Basal cell carcinoma, adenoid pattern. Fine cords and trabeculae of tumour cells form a cribriform pattern. (H & E × 60)

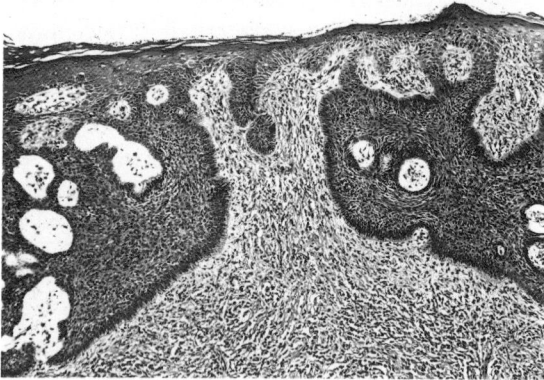

Fig. 10.26 Basal cell carcinoma, solid pattern. Irregular islands and buds of tumour, similar to those seen in the superficial pattern arise from the epidermis: small cystic spaces are seen in the cell masses. (H & E × 60)

layer of palisaded cells, those cells in the centres of the masses being arranged in a haphazard manner (Fig. 10.26). Sometimes cysts form in the centre of the masses (Dudzinski et al 1984) as a result of either degeneration or, occasionally, sebaceous differentiation.

The presence in the centres of the cellular masses of keratinising cells mimics pilar differentiation (Lever & Schaumburg-Lever 1975a). The keratinisation varies from a whorl of cells with slight cytoplasmic eosinophilia to complete keratinisation, without a granular layer, leading to the formation of a cyst lined by parakeratotic mature squamous epithelium. These squamous cells show

no atypia and in that respect differ from those seen in the metatypical or basosquamous carcinoma, in which both basal and squamous cells have the cytological features of malignancy (Borel 1973, Friedrich & Wilkinson 1982c).

The sclerosing, or morphea-like basal cell carcinoma consists of fine trabeculae and small clusters of tumour cells set in dense fibrous tissue (Ackles & Pratt 1956, Bean & Becker 1968).

In the adenoid pattern (Fig. 10.27), the cells form fine strands and trabeculae which enclose connective tissue islands to create a cribriform pattern (Merino et al 1982). True lumina containing amorphous or faintly granular material may form and an eccrine differentiation has been identified in some of these tumours (Freeman & Winkelman 1969).

About one-third of basal cell carcinomas are pigmented, the melanin lying between, rather than in, the tumour cells (Sanderson 1961).

Electron optic studies have shown (Pollack et al 1982), that desmosomes exist between the cells of basal cell carcinomas, and hemidesmosomes serve to anchor the tumour to the surrounding stroma— the latter are fewer in number, however, than in normal epidermis.

Treatment. In view of the rarity of metastatic disease, wide local excision is usually held to be the most appropriate form of treatment, radical vulvectomy and inguinal lymphadenectomy being reserved for those rare cases in which there are metastases, although Merino et al (1982) recommend dissection of the groin nodes for patients in whom the inguinal lymph nodes are enlarged and clinically 'suspicious'. Radiotherapy is usually reserved for those patients in poor general medical condition (Zerner 1975).

Prognosis. The outlook for patients with basal cell carcinoma of the vulva is excellent bearing in mind the age at which these tumours occur. There are, to the best of our knowledge, no recorded deaths from the disease but local recurrence occurs in about 20% of patients, probably due to inadequate primary excision (Palladino et al 1969). Recurrences are also treated surgically.

Merkel cell tumour (Trabecular carcinoma)

Merkel cell tumours are primary, small-cell, malignant neoplasms of the skin. Their constituent cells resemble the Merkel cells, which are slowly adapting, type I mechanoreceptors (Sinclair 1981, Camisa & Weissman 1982, Weissman & Camisa 1982). There is, however, no evidence at present that they develop from mature Merkel cells (Sibley et al 1985) nor that they are of neural crest origin, although they share several morphological and histochemical features with such cells (Tweedle 1978).

Aetiology. The tumours develop in older patients, the average age being about 70 years (Toker 1982). They are of unknown aetiology but an association with squamous carcinoma in situ and invasive squamous cell carcinoma suggests the possibility of either a common aetiological agent or a common histogenesis (Gomez et al 1981) (see below).

Pathology. The tumours occur most commonly on the head and neck and much less frequently on the extremities and trunk. Only three cases of vulval Merkel cell tumour have been reported to date (Tang et al 1982, Bottles et al 1984, Copeland et al 1985) and examination of extravulval lesions provides most of the pathological data.

Although it was recognised as a specific neoplasm in 1972 (Toker 1972), the Merkel cell tumour was originally believed to be of sweat gland origin and only more extensive electron optic and immunohistochemical studies have identified the cells as being similar to, and the neoplasms exhibiting similarities with, those of the diffuse endocrine system (van Dijk & Ten Seldam 1975, Mackay et al 1976, English 1977, Tang & Toker 1978, Abaci & Zak 1979, Tang & Toker 1979, De Wolf-Peeters et al 1980, Johannessen & Gould 1980, Sibley et al 1980, Sidhu et al 1980, Silva & Mackay 1980, Taxy et al 1980, Silva & Mackay 1981, Iwasaki et al 1981, Tang et al 1982, Frigerio et al 1983, Kirkham & Isaacson 1983, Rustin et al 1983, Sibley & Dahl 1985, Sibley et al 1985).

Gross pathology. The tumours present as small, sometimes painful, nodules or papules which may ulcerate and bleed on touch (Bottles et al 1984). They average just over 2 cm in diameter and are erythematous or violaceous (Frigerio et al 1983, Bottles et al 1984, Sibley et al 1985); occasionally they may be pale (Frigerio et al 1983). The neoplasms form a homogenous, grey-white to light brown, intradermal and subcutaneous mass (Toker 1972, Sibley et al 1985) which, to naked-eye examination, has apparently sharply demarcated margins (Wong et al 1981).

In the vulva, the lesions have been described on the labium minor (Tang et al 1982), the labium major (Bottles et al 1984) and in the region of Bartholin's gland (Copeland et al 1985). Inguinal nodal metastases and disseminated systemic disease occurred in all three cases.

Histopathology. The tumours are composed of fairly uniform cells with ill-defined cell margins and large, round, vesicular nuclei in which there are several small nucleoli (Bottles et al 1984, Sibley et al 1985); they have scanty amphophilic cytoplasm and are usually round, although spindled (oat-cell-like) hyperchromatic cells also occur (Bottles et al 1984, Sibley et al 1985) in morphologically less well-differentiated neoplasms (Tang et al 1982). Occasional groups of cells showing squamous differentiation and intermediate squamous/Merkel cell differentiation (Sidhu et al 1980, Tang et al 1982, Frigerio et al 1983) may be present. In about half the cases, the cells are Grimelius positive (Frigerio et al 1983) but negative to PAS, alcian blue and Masson Fontana stains.

Several histological patterns are recognised; the cells may form solid sheets, compact nests, cords or trabeculae. The cords and trabeculae tend to occur particularly at the margins of the more solid areas (Frigerio et al 1983, Bottles et al 1984, Sibley et al 1985). Occasional rosette arrangements may form (Tang & Toker 1979), and in the centres of these, amyloid may be identified (Abaci & Zak 1979); amyloid may also be found elsewhere in the stroma and cells. Loss of cellular cohesion in some tumours may produce a superficial resemblance to lymphomatous infiltration (Sibley et al 1985). The tumour margins are infiltrative and rarely 'pushing' (Frigerio et al 1983) and, whilst the neoplastic cells may enclose the skin appendages (Frigerio et al 1984), no continuity is seen between either the skin appendages or the covering epidermis (Sibley et al 1985). Small-vessel staining with DNA has been described, but appears to be a variable feature, as is tumour necrosis (Frigerio et al 1983, Sibley et al 1985).

A lymphoplasmacytic infiltrate is usually present at the tumour margins (Frigerio et al 1983, Sibley et al 1985), and metastases, when present, resemble closely the primary tumour.

Electron optic studies reveal peripheral, membrane-bound, dense-core cytoplasmic secretory granules and intermediate filaments which are like those found in APUD cells, and which are characteristic of the diffuse endocrine system (Hashimoto 1972, Carstens & Broghamer 1978, Tang & Toker 1979, Kirkham & Isaacson 1983, Sibley et al 1985). Macula (zonula) adherens junctions are seen (Frigerio et al 1983, Kirkham & Isaacson 1983), but desmosomes are rarely present except in areas of squamoid differentiation (Sidhu et al 1980, Frigerio et al 1983, Kirkham & Isaacson 1983, Sibley et al 1985) where the cells also have the typical cytoplasmic tonofibrils of squamous cells.

Immunohistochemical studies (Johannessen & Gould 1980, Iwasaki et al 1981, Gu et al 1983, Kirkham & Isaacson 1983, Silva et al 1984, Sibley & Dahl 1985) have demonstrated the presence in the cells of met-encephalin (Hartschuh & Grube 1979, Hartschuh et al 1980) and neurone-specific enolase (NSE), which act as markers for the diffuse endocrine system (Schmechel et al 1978, Gu et al 1981, Tapia et al 1981), cytokeratins of low molecular weight, vasoactive intestinal peptide (VIP), pancreatic polypeptide, calcitonin and other hormones. In some patients serum alphafetoprotein may be elevated (Rustin et al 1983).

In approximately one-third of patients described in some series (Gomez et al 1981) there has been an associated invasive or intra-epithelial squamous cell carcinoma. This finding and the squamous differentiation which has been described in some Merkel cell tumours (Tang et al 1982) suggest the possibility of a common histogenesis or a common carcinogen for squamous and Merkel cell tumours.

Two of the vulval tumours were associated with VIN III (Tang et al 1982, Bottles et al 1984) and in one there was squamous differentiation within the neoplasm (Tang et al 1982).

Prognosis. Tumour is present in the lymphatics around the primary neoplasm in many cases at the time of diagnosis (Sibley et al 1985) and occasionally in the arteries. Local recurrence occurs in 23 to 38% of patients (Tang & Toker 1979, Frigerio et al 1983, Sibley et al 1985), lymph node metastases in 60 to 70% (Tang & Toker 1979, Frigerio et al 1983, Sibley et al 1985), distant metastases in 25 to 40% (Sibley et al 1985) and about one-third of patients die of their disease (Tang et al 1982).

It has been suggested that the vulval Merkel cell tumour is particularly aggressive (Bottles et al 1984). This is based on the fact that all three reported patients had regional nodal metastases at the time of diagnosis and early systemic dissemination of the disease occurred in all cases. It may also be worth noting that the cases in which there is squamous differentiation are said to have a worse prognosis (Tang et al 1982, Frigerio et al 1983, Bottles et al 1984) and this was a feature of one of the vulval tumours (Tang et al 1982) although the metastases were of pure Merkel cell type. Tumours which appear less well differentiated and lack morphological differentiation into trabeculae, serpiginous or circular patterns are said to carry a particularly poor prognosis (Tang et al 1982).

Prognosis may also be adversely affected by the presence of a second neoplasm (Sibley et al 1985) but Gomez et al (1981) believe that co-existing VIN does not affect the behaviour of the tumour.

Treatment. Planned therapy for vulval Merkel cell tumour is difficult to formulate because of the small number of cases so far described; however, in view of the frequency of local recurrence and regional lymph node metastases, it is recommended that wide local excision with lymph node dissection should be carried out and that, when diagnosis has been made on a local excision biopsy, re-excision with nodal removal should follow.

It is also suggested (Copeland et al 1985), on the basis of experience with small-cell (oat-cell) carcinoma of the lung, that chemotherapy may be helpful.

Paget's disease

Paget's disease of the vulva, which was first described in 1901 by Dubreuilh, results from the presence in the vulval epidermis and skin appendages of secretory, glandular, adenocarcinoma cells (Roth et al 1977, Jones et al 1979).

Aetiology. The condition, which is uncommon and accounts for less than 0.2% of vulval carcinomas (Taylor et al 1975), affects patients ranging in age from 38 to 86 years (Koss et al 1968, Creasman et al 1975, Taylor et al 1975, Tsukada et al 1975, Lee et al 1977, Breen et al 1978, Jones et al 1979), with an average age of approximately 63 years (Breen et al 1978). In some patients, up to 50% in some series, there is a second neoplasm (Helwig & Graham 1963, Fenn et al 1971). The most common association is with a vulval adnexal carcinoma or other local tumour, for example, in Bartholin's gland (Tchang et al 1973), whilst of the more distant neoplasms carcinoma of the breast is the most common (Helwig & Graham 1963, Fetherston & Friedrich 1972, Friedrich et al 1975, Tsukada et al 1975, Hart & Millman 1977, Breen et al 1978); tumours in the urinary tract (Helwig & Graham 1963, Lee et al 1977, Tuck & Williams 1985, Degufu et al 1986), elsewhere in the female genital tract (Taylor et al 1975, Lee et al 1977, Breen et al 1978, Jones et al 1979, McKee & Hertogs 1980) in the anorectal area (Helwig & Graham 1963) and elsewhere on the body (Lee et al 1977) have also been reported in association with Paget's disease at this site.

In the 20 to 30% of women in whom there is an associated invasive neoplasm of the vulva or adjacent organ, the cells are believed to have migrated or metastasised from the tumour into the epidermis (Weiner 1937, Pinkus & Gould 1939, Dockerty & Pratt 1952, Kay & Hall 1954, Plachta & Speer 1954, Rosser & Hamlin 1957, Koss et al 1968, Boehm & Morris 1971, Demopoulos 1971, Tchang et al 1973, Creasman et al 1975, Friedrich et al 1975, Hart & Millman 1977, Lee et al 1977, Woodruff 1977). The possibility that the lesions are metastases from a more distant primary tumour has been considered (Helwig & Graham 1963) but has

been dismissed, because in most patients no such invasive tumour is identified.

In the vast majority of patients neither a locally invasive nor a distant invasive neoplasm is found and the neoplastic cells appear to have developed in situ (Woodruff 1955, Helwig & Graham 1963, Fetherston & Friedrich 1972, Neilson & Woodruff 1972, Friedrich et al 1975, Hart & Millman 1977, Gunn & Gallager 1980, Friedrich & Wilkinson 1982d), but whether the cells form in the epidermis and migrate into the adnexae (Woodruff 1955), develop in sweat gland ducts and migrate to the epidermis (Kariniemi et al 1984), or develop simultaneously in both the epidermis and the skin appendages (Helwig & Graham 1963, Fenn et al 1971, Medenica & Sahihi 1972) is a matter of debate.

Clinical presentation. Persistent pruritus and soreness are the most common problems (Tsukada et al 1975) and symptoms may have been present from a few months to 10 years (Jones et al 1979). In some patients there may be discharge and oozing from an ulcerated skin surface.

Gross pathology. Paget's disease appears as multiple (Gunn & Gallager 1980, Friedrich & Wilkinson 1982d), erythematous, apparently eczematous, moderately well-demarcated, scaly, map-like patches or plaques (Fig. 10.28). Sometimes the patches are hyperkeratotic and appear white (Helwig & Graham 1963, Tsukada et al 1975) whilst occasionally they are somewhat papillary (Helwig & Graham 1963). They occur most commonly on the labia majora (Breen et al 1978, Jones et al 1979) but they may also affect the perineum and peri-anal area. In some patients the lesions may extend to the inguinal folds, mons pubis (Koss et al 1968), the labia minora, vestibule and vagina (Jones et al 1979, DiSaia & Creasman 1981).

Histopathology. Paget's cells (Fig. 10.29) are large, round or oval and have copious, vacuolated cytoplasm and a large, vesicular, pale, oval or round nucleus which may be more hyperchromatic particularly when it lies peripherally and is indented, imparting a signet ring form to the cell. In some cells nucleoli are prominent and mitoses may be present (Jones et al 1979).

The cells form nests, sheets and aggregates with and without tubule formation (Fenn et al 1971). The larger nests (Fig. 10.30) lie more deeply in the

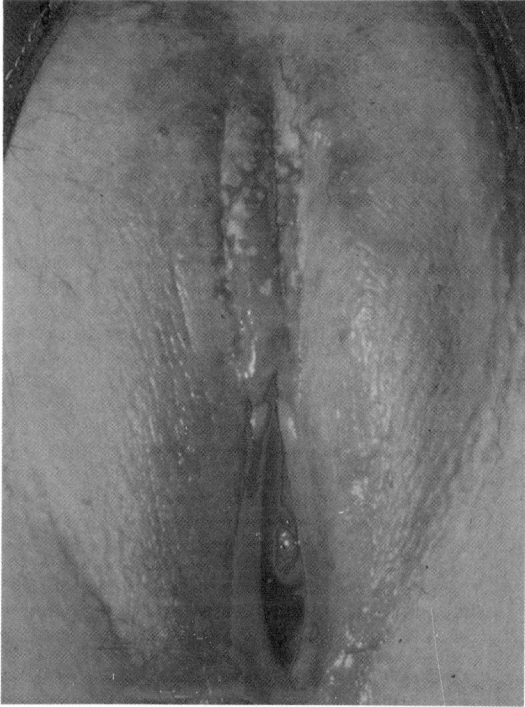

Fig. 10.28 Paget's disease (Reproduced from Beilby & Ridley (1987) by courtesy of the authors and publisher)

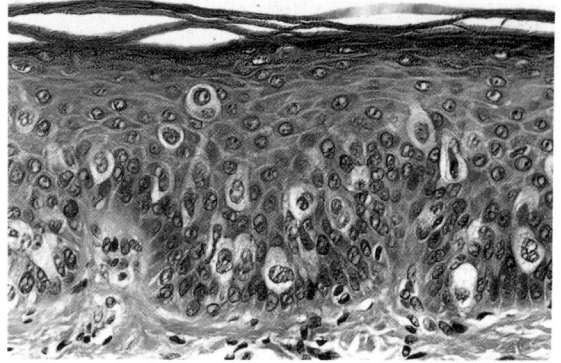

Fig. 10.29 Paget's disease. Large round cells with copious pale cytoplasm and rather irregular vesicular nuclei are scattered in the deeper layers of the epidermis. (H & E × 240)

epidermis whilst small nests of cells and single cells lie at the periphery of the lesion and in the more superficial layers of the epithelium where they may be identified in cytological scrape samples (Friedrich et al 1975, Masukawa & Friedrich 1978). Frequently the Paget cells extend histologically beyond the clinically apparent margins of the lesions (Taylor et al 1975, Jones et al 1979, Gunn & Gallager 1980). They may also be seen in the outer root sheath of the hair follicles (Tsukada et al 1975, Lee et al 1977), in eccrine sweat gland ducts (Jones et al 1979) and in sebaceous glands (Koss et al 1968) (Fig. 10.31). Reports of their presence in apocrine sweat gland ducts are conflicting; whilst Jones et al (1979) observed this rarely, Lee et al (1977) and Roth et al (1977) reported this in six of their 13 cases.

The affected epidermis can be normal, acanthotic, hyperkeratotic or parakeratotic and may contain atypical dyskeratotic cells (Taylor et al 1975, Tsukada et al 1975, Jones et al 1979). The underlying dermis is usually infiltrated by chronic inflammatory cells (Tsukada et al 1975).

Paget cells contain neutral and acid mucopolysaccharides (Tsukada et al 1975) and stain positively with mucicarmine, aldehyde fuchsin (Helwig & Graham 1963) and PAS/alcian blue even after diastase digestion (Belcher 1972). Sometimes, however, the staining is scanty and not seen in every cell. Melanin is usually absent from the cells (Helwig & Graham 1963, Salazar & Gonzalez-Angulo, 1984), but it has occasionally been identified in Paget cells from patients in whom the skin is heavily pigmented (Medenica & Sahihi 1972, Jones et al 1979) and this is believed to be due to phagocytosis of melanin from the adjacent cells and not to intracellular melanin production. None the less the finding of intracellular melanin in large cells with clear cytoplasm should raise the possibility of superficial spreading melanoma with which Paget's disease may be confused histologically (Stout 1938, Becker et al 1960, Jones et al 1979).

Carcinogenic embryonic antigen (CEA) has been identified in both mammary and extramammary Paget's disease and may be detectable in the serum if metastases are present (Kariniemi et al 1984, Oji et al 1984, Stapleton 1984, Nagle et al 1985, Anthony et al 1986).

Histogenesis. Histopathological, immunohistochemical and electron microscopic studies of the cells in patients with in situ lesions have led to different conclusions as to their histogenesis. Boehm & Morris (1971) identified them as being of apocrine type on the basis of their blue-staining reaction with colloidal iron and the electron microscopic studies of Demopoulos (1971), Neilson &

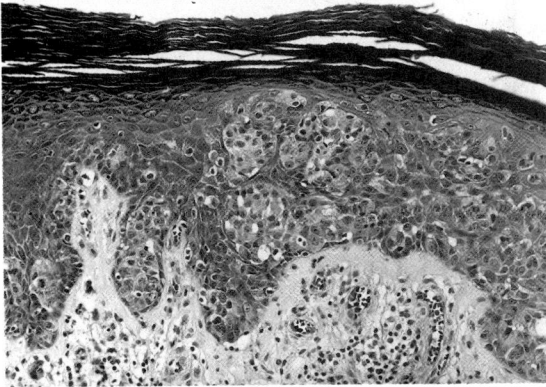

Fig. 10.30 Paget's disease. Large, pale-staining Paget cells form nests in the rete ridges and the Malpighian layer of the epidermis. (H & E × 130)

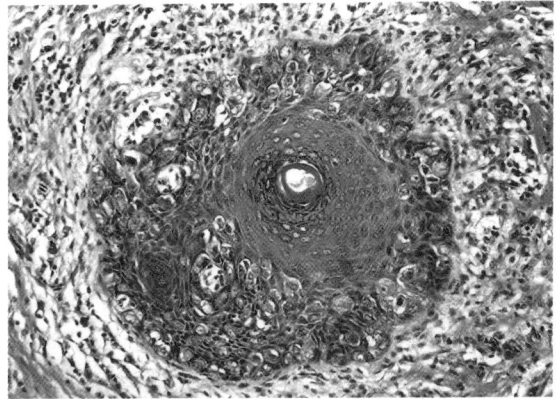

Fig. 10.31 Paget's disease. Paget cells are seen forming aggregates in the margin of this skin appendage. (H & E × 95)

Woodruff (1972) and Jones et al (1979), and the immunohistochemical identification of aprocrine epithelial antigen (Kariniemi et al 1984) and gross cystic disease fluid protein (GCDFP-15) (Mazoujian et al 1984) support this view. Tsukada et al (1975) found, however, no evidence of aprocrine differentiation and Koss & Brockunier (1969), Belcher (1972), Ferenczy & Richart (1972) and Webb & Beswick (1983) identified the cells as being of eccrine sweat gland type, whilst Moll & Moll (1985) and Nagle et al (1985) have demonstrated both eccrine- and apocrine-like features. Such diverse conclusions have led to the suggestion (Fetherston & Friedrich 1972, Roth et al 1977) that Paget's disease is actually a group of disorders which have similar appearances at the light microscopic level but with varying and distinct ultrastructural characteristics. This view is consistent with the more generally accepted concept that the in situ Paget's cell represents an aberrant differentiation from a multipotential basal layer cell derived from the embryonic germinative layer of the epidermis (Medenica & Sahihi 1972, Friedrich & Wilkinson 1982d, Salazar & Gonzalez-Angulo 1984). Further support for this latter concept lies in the finding that Paget's cells may be attached to other Paget cells and the adjacent squamous cells by desmosomes, an observation in keeping with a common origin for both the squamous cells of the eipdermis and the Paget cells (Demopoulos 1972, Medenica & Sahihi 1972, Roth et al 1977, Salazar & Gonzalez-Angulo 1984).

Prognosis. In those patients with an intraepithelial lesion recurrence following resection occurs in nearly 40% of cases (Helwig & Graham 1963, Koss et al 1968, Creasman et al 1975, Jones et al 1979, Gunn & Gallager 1980). This is thought to be due partly to the tendency of the lesion to extend microscopically beyond the clinically apparent limits thus making total excision difficult (Taylor et al 1975) and partly to the apparently multifocal nature of the disease. Recurrence may be delayed for many years and repeated resections are not uncommon. Recurrence in grafted skin has suggested the possibility that an unknown, possibly dermal, factor, may influence Pagetoid differentiation of the overlying epidermis (Beecham 1976). The condition is, however, not usually life endangering and the prognosis for survival is excellent (Lee et al 1977). However, whilst these in situ lesions show little tendency to invade the dermis (Fetherston & Friedrich 1972, Creasman et al 1975, Friedrich et al 1975, Parmley et al 1975) they can, albeit rarely, behave as an invasive malignant neoplasm which may give rise to lymph node metastases (Pierard & Kint 1968, Parmley et al 1975, Hart & Millman 1977, Breen et al 1978).

In those patients with an underlying invasive tumour, the prognosis is governed by the stage and spread of the neoplasm. The frequency with which local and more distant invasive tumour is present in patients with Paget's disease demands rigorous exclusion of such lesions (Fenn et al 1971, Fetherston & Friedrich 1972, Tsukada et al 1975, Lee et al 1977).

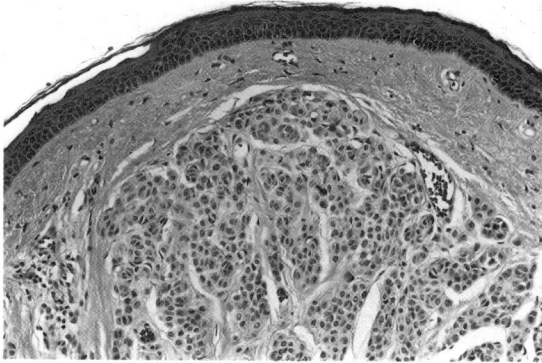

Fig. 10.32 Intradermal naevus. The dermis is occupied by nests of regular, focally pigmented cells which are distinct from the overlying epidermis. (H & E × 120)

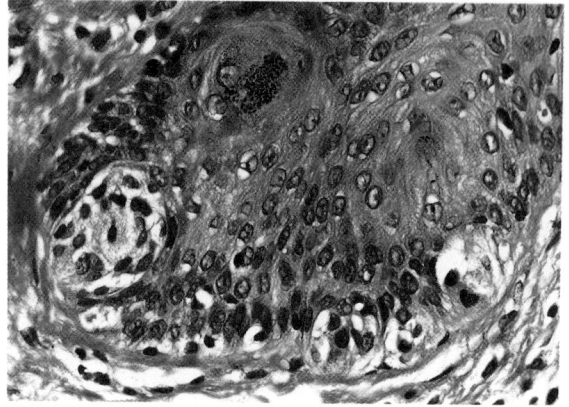

Fig. 10.34 Junctional naevus. Clusters of naevus cells are concentrated in the basal layer of the epidermis; there is no intradermal component. (H & E × 300)

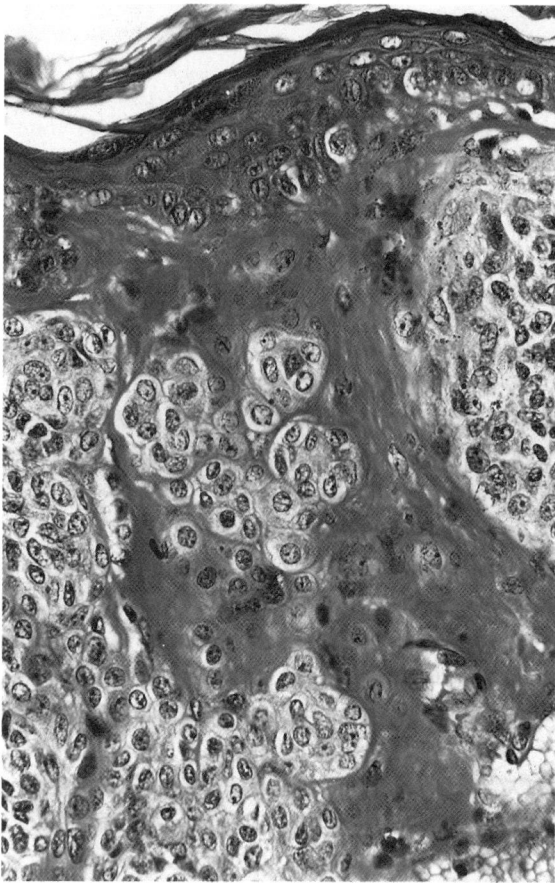

Fig. 10.33 Compound naevus. Pale-staining naevus cells form nests in the dermis and clusters are also seen in the covering epidermis. There is no evidence of mitotic activity and there is no migration of cells into the upper strata of the epidermis. (H & E × 350)

Treatment. Treatment for the intra-epithelial lesion is usually by wide local excision controlled by intra-operative frozen section examination of the resection margins (DiSaia & Creasman 1981, Stacy et al 1986). Recurrences are treated by further excision. Treatment is considered further on page 349. In the presence of a local carcinoma, however, radical vulvectomy and nodal dissection is the treatment of choice (Creasman et al 1975, Taylor et al 1975).

Melanocytic lesions

Naevi: Naevocellular Naevi, 'Moles'

These commonly acquired pigmented hamartomatous lesions occur in all areas of the body and show no particular predilection for the vulva. They consist of nests of well-defined aggregates of altered melanocytes (naevus cells) with regular oval or rounded nuclei lacking mitoses and nucleoli. All such naevi develop initially in the deeper layers of the epidermis as clusters of melanocytes which ultimately migrate into the dermis, where their nomenclature changes to that of naevus cell, to form an *intradermal naevus* (Fig. 10.32). The persistence of an intra-epidermal component identifies the lesion as a *compound naevus* (Fig. 10.33) whilst the term *junctional naevus* (Fig. 10.34) is used if there is no intradermal fraction.

Generally, intradermal and compound naevi are

elevated above the surrounding epithelium whilst junctional naevi are flat. Moles on the vulva may show junctional activity (Friedrich et al 1979) and such lesions are recognised as predisposing to the development of malignant melanoma; however, Christensen et al (1987) did not find junctional naevi to be significantly commoner on the vulva than on the trunk.

Naevus cells within the dermis show a variety of cellular maturation patterns. Cells in the superficial dermis most closely resemble melanocytes and tend to be large and heavily pigmented, whilst those in the deeper part of the lesion adopt a progressively more 'neural' appearance becoming smaller, more spindle shaped and less pigmented. Some naevi become more heavily pigmented in pregnancy (Janovski & Douglas 1972). As the cells become elongated they may resemble neural structures, particularly mimicking Meissner corpuscles; the cells may also be multinucleated, fusiform or ballooned. These changes in cell pattern are an important indicator of the maturation of the lesion.

Electron microscopy fails to reveal intercellular connections and there are no fibrils in the cytoplasm; the melanin content is variable.

Removal of all such lesions with an adequate margin of normal skin is required and careful histological examination obligatory.

Friedman & Ackerman (1981) noted that whereas vulval melanocytic naevi in older women are like those elsewhere on the body, some in premenopausal women can raise difficulties in the distinction from malignant melanoma. It has been alleged that most such lesions are junctional, but, in their series of seven, five were compound, and they all showed unusual features, for example nests of variably sized and shaped melanocytes in the epidermis. The general architecture of the lesion was most helpful in diagnosis. Christensen et al (1987) have further reviewed similar cases.

Figure 10.35 (a, b and c) shows a lesion of this compound type in a patient aged 26 years; the pigmentation was macular and quite widespread and further lesions developed after excision. The histology showed a dermal cellular component composed of small angulated cells as well as basal layer pigmentation and in some areas increased numbers of junctional melanocytes.

Biopsy will exclude malignancy but management in these cases with rather widespread lesions is difficult. Probably the wisest course is to advocate observation, with excision should the lesions give rise to symptoms or become thickened.

Lentigo (Lentigo simplex)

This is a benign pigmented proliferation of epidermal or mucous membrane melanocytes which forms smooth, non-infiltrating dark brown lesions on the mucosa of the labia minora and around the introitus. The lesion is of unknown aetiology and pathogenesis, and does not usually exceed 1.0 cm in diameter (Fig. 10.36 a). The histological features (Fig. 10.36 b) are those of mild elongation of the epidermal rete ridges with increased numbers of melanocytes and increased pigmentation of the basal layer of the skin or mucous membrane. Melanophages may be present in the squamous epithelium and in the underlying dermis. The lesions are not 'freckles', which in contrast contain fewer than normal or a normal number of melanocytes with hyperpigmentation of the basal layer of the epidermis. The lesions are sometimes removed for cosmetic reasons or because of their clinical resemblance to junctional naevi, but do not exhibit cytological atypia (Janovski & Douglas 1972). More widespread pigmentation probably of this type is noted on page 148.

Spitz naevus ('Juvenile melanoma')

The Spitz or spindle cell and epithelioid naevus may occasionally occur on the vulva (Janovski & Douglas 1972, Connors & Ackerman 1976). It appears as a pink-tan or light brown nodule or papule which may grow at an alarming rate; it is, however, entirely benign and melanocytes mature as they descend into the dermis (Connors & Ackerman, 1979). It is composed of spindle and epithelioid naevus cells, which are located in the dermis and at the dermo-epidermal junction and which infiltrate both the dermis and the epidermis. Nuclear atypia may be present, multinucleate giant cell forms are not uncommon and mitoses may be seen in the dermal component. However, in contrast to malignant melanoma, the naevus cells form well-demarcated, discrete groups in which the naevus cells appear to 'rain down' from the surface of the

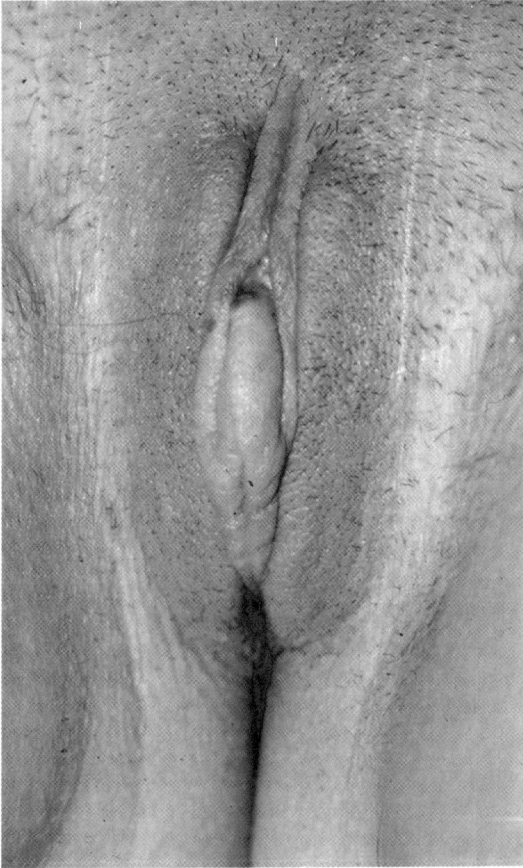 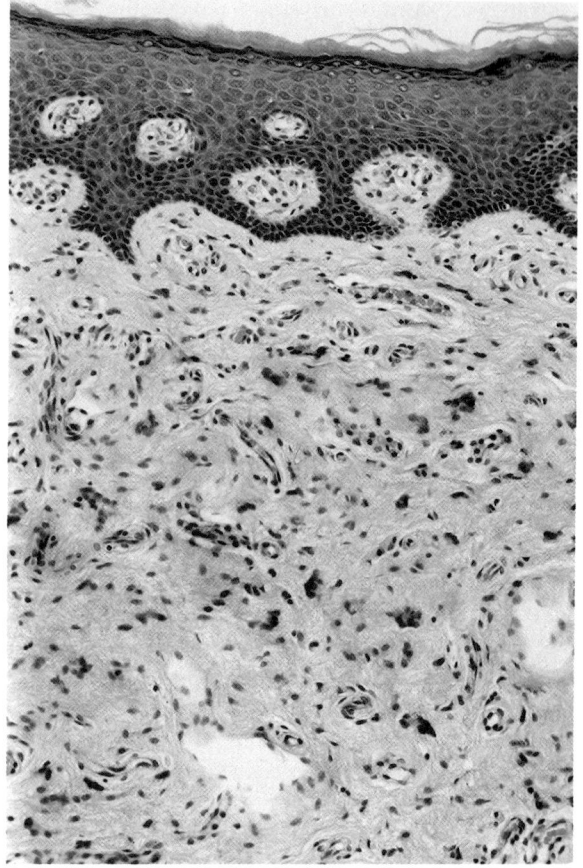

A   B

Fig. 10.35 (**a**) An unusual compound melanocytic naevus (Reproduced from Beilby and Ridley 1987 by courtesy of the authors and publisher) (**b** and **c**) Basal layer pigmentation, increased junctional melanocytes, angulated cells in dermis (H & E ×120, H & E ×300) (by courtesy of Dr Neil Smith and Dr E. Benjamin).

lesion and single-cell infiltration is not a feature. Simple excision with an adequate margin of visibly healthy tissue is sufficient treatment.

Halo naevus and inflammatory halo naevus

The halo naevus appears as a centrally pigmented 'mole' with a halo of depigmented or erythematous skin. Histologically it is composed of intradermal melanophages mixed with lymphocytes and histiocytes and residual naevus cells. Within the halo there is an absence of pigment. Despite the inflammatory infiltrate, which often raises the suspicion of a malignant lesion, the lateral margins of the halo naevus are sharply defined and there is no evidence of a malign nature (Connors & Ackerman 1976).

A similar appearance may occur following

trauma of a melanocytic naevus (Connors & Ackerman 1979).

Melanoma precursor lesions

Whilst junctional and compound naevi are known to progress to malignant melanoma, the proportion which do so is unknown but is probably small in view of the frequency of 'moles' and the rarity of melanomas. Histological examination of melanomas, however, reveals remnants of a benign melanocytic naevus in 35% of cases (Lever & Schaumburg-Lever 1983a).

The majority of atypical melanocytic proliferations, which are also recognised as leading to the development of melanomas, occur in sun-exposed areas of the body (Briggs 1985), but they are not limited to these areas and examination of the skin

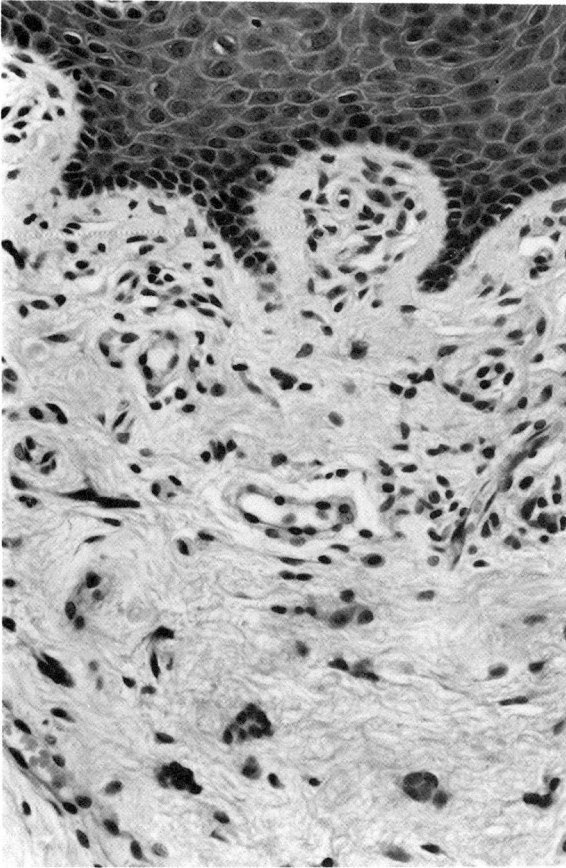

C

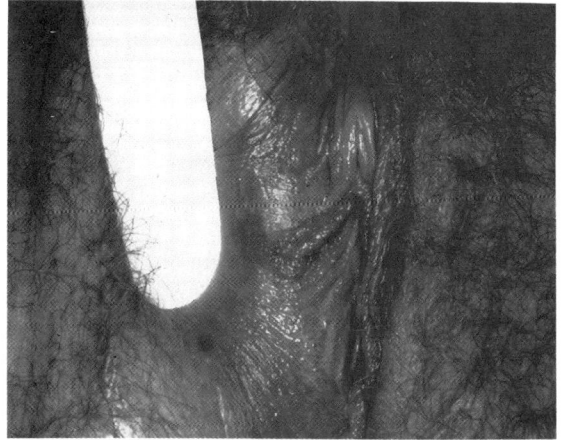

A

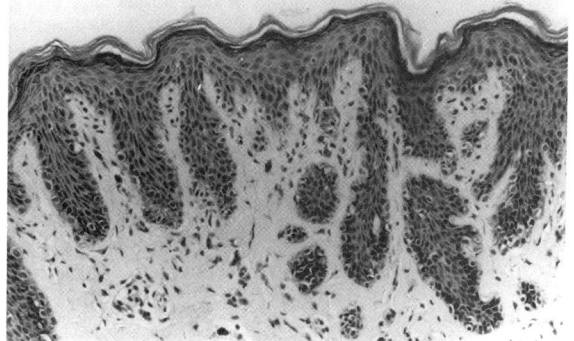

B

Fig. 10.36 (**a**) Lentigo. (**b**) increased number of melanocytes in the basal layer (H & E ×325) (by courtesy of Dr Neil Smith)

adjacent to vulval melanomas may reveal melanocytic atypia (Cook & Robertson 1985). Such abnormalities are identified, in general, in approximately

one-third of cases (Cook & Robertson 1985).

Three forms of atypical melanocytic proliferation are recognised (Cook & Robertson 1985); the dys-

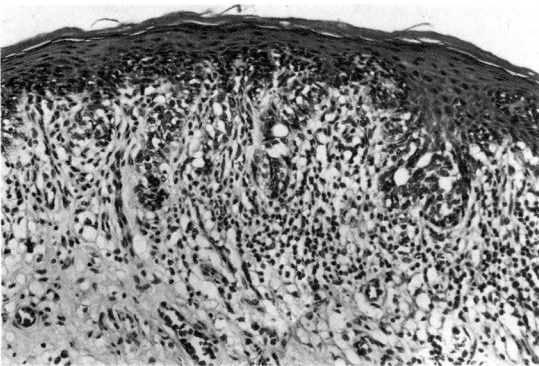

Fig. 10.37 Lentiginous melanocytic dysplasia. Atypical melanocytes lie along the basal layer of the elongated rete ridges. (H & E × 120)

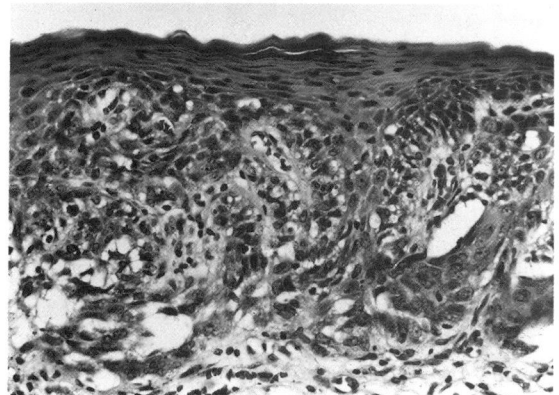

Fig. 10.38 Epithelioid melanocytic dysplasia. Atypical melanocytes, many of which are spindle shaped, form nests in the sides of the rete ridges. (H & E × 195)

plastic naevus or lentiginous melanocytic dysplasia, superficial spreading melanoma in situ or epithelioid melanocytic dysplasia, (spindle-celled melanocytic dysplasia: Pagetoid melanoma in situ: B-K mole) and atypical melanocytic hyperplasia (atypical melanocytic dysplasia).

Lentiginous melanocytic dysplasia (Fig. 10.37) is characterised by elongation of the rete ridges, with atypical melanocytes lying along the basal layer. The underlying dermis is usually infiltrated by lymphocytes and there is variable dermal fibrosis. In epithelioid melanocytic dysplasia (Fig. 10.38) atypical melanocytes, which may be spindle shaped (Cook & Robertson 1985) or spherical (Briggs 1985), form nests or clusters in the sides of the rete ridges. Atypical melanocytic hyperplasia is similar to lentiginous dysplasia but there is no elongation of the rete ridges. These atypical lesions are not mutually exclusive and different patterns may merge into one another. Should they be identified in a vulval biopsy, complete excision with an adequate margin of normal tissue is mandatory.

Malignant melanoma

A malignant melanoma of the vulva can, as elsewhere in the body, develop in a pre-existing junctional or compound naevus or can arise de novo from intra-epidermal melanocytes. Malignant melanomas at this site, rather surprisingly, occur more often than would be expected in terms of the proportion of the total skin surface accounted for by the vulva and represent approximately 4% of all malignant melanomas in females; they are probably the second commonest malignant neoplasm of the vulva and have been variously estimated as accounting for between 4 and 9% of vulval cancers. These figures should not, however, be allowed to conceal the fact that malignant melanomas of the vulva are, in absolute terms, very rare, to the extent that only a very few major centres have been able to accumulate and analyse more than a handful of cases.

Clinical features. Malignant melanoma of the vulva does not occur in prepubertal girls but thereafter its incidence rises steadily to reach a peak in the sixth and seventh decades: the mean age of women with this neoplasm is between 54 and 60 years.

Patients usually present with a relatively short history, varying from a few weeks to 8 months and it is unusual, though by no means unknown, for symptoms to have been present for longer than a year. The commonest initial complaint is of a lump or mass, whilst bleeding, itching or burning are also frequently noted; only a small proportion of women complain of changes in the physical appearance of a long-standing vulval 'mole' (Friedrich & Wilkinson 1982e) whilst a few patients present with an inguinal mass due to nodal metastases. The site of the tumour, a matter of some prognostic importance, has varied in different series: thus Morrow and Rutledge (1972) found that 75% of vulval malignant melanomas were centrally situated (i.e. involved the labia minora or the clitoris) whilst Podratz et al (1983b) noted a similar preponderance (77%) of centrally situated tumours; in other series, however, there has been an approximately equal distribution of central and lateral (i.e. involving labia majora) neoplasms (Phillips et al 1982, Jaramillo et al 1985). The melanoma may be flat, elevated nodular or polypoid and is often ulcerated. Characteristically a melanoma ranges in colour from brown to bluish-black (Fig. 10.39 a and b) but a small minority of lesions in this site are of the amelanotic variety and bear a close macroscopic resemblance to a squamous cell carcinoma. The melanoma is usually surrounded by a reddish flare, which indicates the cellular immune response to the neoplasm, and satellite skin metastases may be present.

Histological findings. In most series between 60 and 70% of vulval melanomas have been of the superficial spreading variety whilst the remainder were of the nodular type; the only notable exception to this general rule was in the series of Bouma et al (1982) in which 13 of 16 vulval malignant melanomas fell into the nodular category.

The superficial spreading melanoma evolves through a phase of radial growth (melanoma in situ) which precedes, often by several years, an invasive phase of vertical growth. The in situ lesion is characterised by the presence of atypical melanocytes, which form nests and Pagetoid patterns in the lower part of the epidermis with individual atypical cells in the upper layers of the epithelium. In the early invasive stage of a superficial spreading melanoma nests of atypical cells extend into the

A

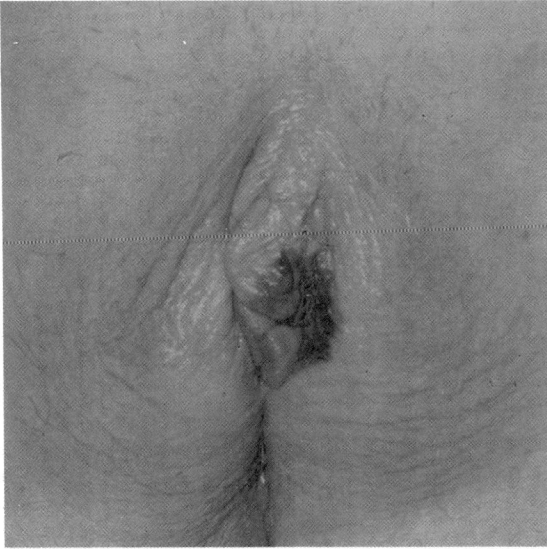

Fig. 10.39 (a) Superficial spreading malignant melanoma.
(b) Nodular melanoma. (By courtesy of C M Ridley 1975 The
Vulva. Major Problems in Dermatology 5. Lloyd Luke)

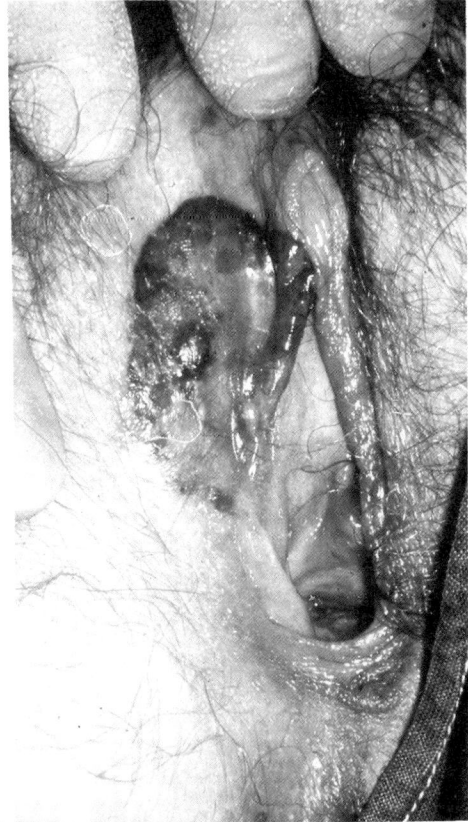

dermis; a proportion of superficial spreading melanomas will eventually enter into a vertical growth
phase and thus evolve into an apparently nodular
form of malignant melanoma.

The nodular malignant melanoma appears to
show only a vertical pattern of growth; it does not
have any preceding phase of radial growth and develops an invasive tendency at a very early stage in
its evolution. Histologically the lesion consists of

B

Fig. 10.40 Malignant melanoma. The tumour is composed of
epithelioid cells with large nuclei and very prominent, large
nucleoli. (H & E × 300)

discrete nodules or masses of invasive atypical
melanocytes extending both downwards into the
dermis and upwards into the epidermis. Two major
types of cell can be recognised, one having an
epithelioid appearance (Fig. 10.40) and the other
being spindle shaped; most tumours contain both
types of cell though as a rule one, usually the
epithelioid, predominates. A point of significance
in differentiating between a true nodular melanoma
and a superficial spreading melanoma which has
entered a vertical growth phase is that in the nodular form permeation of the epidermis by neoplastic
cells is limited to that part of the epithelium directly overlying the dermal tumour, whilst lateral intra-
epidermal extension of tumour cells beyond the
confines of the dermal lesion is characteristic of a
superficial spreading melanoma.

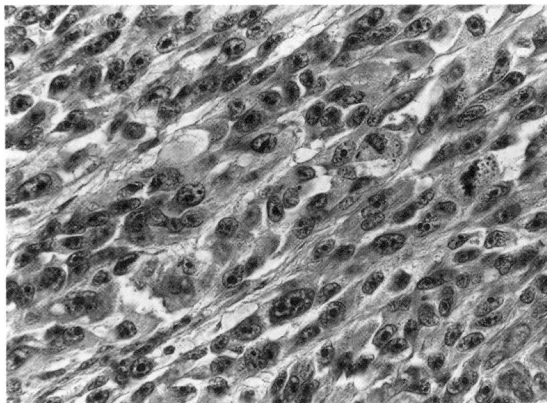

A rare variant of a malignant melanoma, only
one example of which has been reported as occurring in the vulva (Warner et al 1982), is the neuro-
trophic type, which has a particular affinity for

involving peripheral subcutaneous nerves. In the sole vulval case there was an intra-epithelial component, which appeared to be a lentigo malignant melanoma, and an invasive component, formed of spindle-shaped cells, which enveloped and invaded subcutaneous nerve fibres.

Staging and microstaging. The clinical staging system recommended by FIGO for squamous cell carcinoma of the vulva is also applied to vulval malignant melanomas; as with squamous tumours surgical and histological staging shows that clinical staging is incorrect in over 30% of cases (Podratz et al 1983b).

All melanomas which are clinically confined to the vulva should be subjected to histological microstaging. Two microstaging techniques are in current use—Clark's levels which define depth of tumour invasion in terms of dermal planes (Clark et al 1969) and Breslow's measurement of maximum tumour thickness (Breslow 1970).

Clark's levels are defined in the following terms:

level I: neoplastic cells are confined to the epidermis;
level II: tumour cells extend into the papillary dermis;
level III: invasive melanoma cells extend to the level of the subpapillary vessels but not into the reticular dermis;
level IV: neoplastic cells are invading the reticular dermis;
level V: tumour cells are invading the subcutaneous fat.

The Breslow technique measures the maximum tumour thickness either from the granular layer of the epidermis (if discernible) or from the surface of the epithelium to the deepest level of invasion and uses the following stages:

less than 0.76 mm;
0.76 to 1.50 mm;
1.51 to 2.25 mm;
2.26 to 3.00 mm;
more than 3 mm.

Chung et al (1975) maintained that Clark's levels could not be accurately measured in melanomas of the vulva because of lack of a clear distinction between the papillary and reticular dermis in this site and introduced their own microstaging system:

level 1:   tumour confined to the epithelium;
level 2:   penetration of tumour cells into the dermis or lamina propria to a depth of 1 mm from the granular layer of the epithelium;
level 3:   invasion of neoplastic cells to a depth of between 1 and 2 mm from the granular layer of the epithelium;
level 4:   invasion to a depth or of more than 2 mm from the granular layer into fibrous and fibrovascular tissue but not into subcutaneous fat;
level 5:   tumour invasion of the subcutaneous fat.

Prognosis and prognostic factors. The 5-year survival rate for patients suffering from a malignant melanoma of the vulva has ranged, in different series, from 24 to 54%, with a mean of about 35–40% (Symmonds et al 1960, Janovski et al 1962, Pack & Oropeza 1967, Yackel et al 1970, Morrow & Rutledge 1972, Fenn & Abell 1973, Bozzetti et al 1975, Chung et al 1975, Karlen et al 1975, Cleophax et al 1977, Ragni & Tobon 1979, Edington & Monaghan 1980, Bouma et al 1982, Phillips et al 1982, Podratz et al 1983b, Jaramillo et al 1985). It should be noted, however, that 5-year survival is not synonymous with cure; thus, Podratz et al (1983b) noted that four of their patients died of delayed recurrences, two at 7 years and two at 11 years after initial treatment, whilst four of the women in the series of Bouma et al (1982) developed either local recurrences or distant metastases between 6 and 13 years after primary therapy.

The prognostic value of the FIGO clinical staging system has been a matter for some debate. There is widespread agreement that the prognosis for stage II tumours is the same as is that for stage I neoplasms, both being associated with a 5-year survival rate of between 60 and 70%; there is also no doubt about the gloomy outlook for women with stage IV melanomas, very few of whom survive for more than 3 years. Conflicting views have, however, been expressed about the prognosis for women with stage III disease: Phillips et al (1982) noted that survival rates for such patients were the same as for those with stage I or II disease and Podratz et al (1983b) were also unable to prove that the prognosis for stage III tumours was significantly worse than that for tumours in earlier stages. By contrast, both Morrow (1981) and Jaramillo et al (1985) found that stage III melanomas were associated with an extremely poor prognosis and Johnson et al (1986) found that FIGO clinical staging was a useful prognostic indicator.

These disparate findings probably reflect both the small number of cases available for study and the equivocal nature of 'suspicious' nodes for it is clear that the presence of histologically proven nodal metastases is of grave import, 5-year survival rates of 55–60% for women without nodal lesions falling to between 0 and 30% for those with metastatic nodal tumour.

The diameter of a melanoma appears to be of little prognostic importance (at least up to 4 cm) but the site of the neoplasm is possibly more important, Podratz et al (1983b) reporting a 61% 10-year survival rate for women with lateral tumours and one of only 37% for those with centrally sited lesions; Morrow (1981) has, however, commented that central location of the tumour is only of prognostic significance if the urethra or vagina is involved.

The traditional belief that the prognosis for a superficial spreading melanoma is better than that for a nodular melanoma was upheld by Podratz et al (1983b) who noted a 10-year survival rate for patients with the former type of melanoma of 71% as contrasted to that for women with a nodular melanoma of only 38%, and by Johnson et al (1986); Chung et al (1975) found, however, a rather better survival rate for nodular melanomas (35%) than for superficial spreading melanomas. Other histological features, such as the degree of atypia, the number of mitotic figures, the content of pigment and the cell type (epithelioid or spindle shaped), appear to be of little prognostic import.

For melanomas confined to the vulva, histological microstaging has proved to be of considerable value. Podratz et al (1983b) found that tumours confined to Clark's levels I and II were associated with a 100% survival, those invading to levels III or IV with a survival rate of just over 80% and those extending to level V with a survival rate of only 28%. Phillips et al (1982) also found a survival rate of 100% for level II melanomas, of 50% for level III and 25% for levels IV and V.

Chung et al (1975), using their own microstaging system, found a 100% survival for tumours invading to their level II, a 40% survival for tumours reaching levels III or IV and a survival rate of only 20% for those melanomas extending to level V.

Using the Breslow technique of measuring tumour thickness, Podratz et al (1983b) found that neoplasms measuring less than 0.76 mm in thickness were associated with a 100% survival, tumours measuring between 0.76 and 3 mm in thickness were related to a 80% survival whilst those measuring more than 3 mm in thickness were accompanied by a survival rate of only 20%. Phillips et al (1982) and Jaramillo et al (1985) also found that all patients with melanomas less than 0.76 mm thick survived, and that survival rates plummeted with increasing thickness.

Management. The recommended standard treatment for a malignant melanoma of the vulva is radical vulvectomy with en bloc bilateral inguinal and femoral lymphadenectomy (Morrow 1981). It is recognised that the weakest points in this operation are the vaginal or urethral margins and Morrow (1981) has pointed out that partial resection of the involved terminal urethra or vagina seems to be inadequate; he recommends that superficial involvement of the vagina should be treated by total vaginectomy and hysterectomy and that extension to the urethra or bladder should be managed by exenteration.

This approach differs from that currently employed for cutaneous malignant melanomas elsewhere in the body where, increasingly, prophylactic lymphadenectomy is no longer being performed, this procedure only being undertaken if there is clinical evidence of nodal metastases. The arguments in favour of prophylactic lymphadenectomy have been that there is a relatively high incidence of clinically occult but histologically detectable lymph node metastases even in melanomas which appear to be at an early stage and that removal of the regional lymph nodes will prevent distant metastases. Whilst the former of these assertions may be true, two controlled trials have clearly shown that in cutaneous stage I malignant melanomas no benefit is conferred by routine prophylactic lymphadenectomy and that this procedure does not diminish the risk of distant metastases (Veronisi et al 1977, Sim et al 1978). Further positive arguments against routine prophylactic lymphadenopathy have been that the vast majority of patients will not have nodal metastases and will not therefore benefit from extended surgery, that some patients will develop chronic lymphoedema with the risk of stasis metastases from cells in transit (satellosis) and that the regional nodes play an important role in the patient's immunological defences against the tumour.

Despite these apparently compelling arguments for relatively conservative surgery in patients without clinically suspicious nodes there has been a marked reluctance to abandon routine groin node dissection for stage I and II melanomas of the vulva, it being maintained that a direct comparison between vulval melanomas and those elsewhere cannot be drawn in so far as at this site the primary lesion, the regional nodes and the intervening lymphatics can be removed en bloc, thus running no risk of stasis metastasis.

It has been questioned whether radical vulvectomy, let alone prophylactic lymphadenectomy, is necessary for all stage I and stage II vulval melanomas (Phillips et al 1982, Podratz et al 1983b, Jaramillo et al 1985). It is now widely recognised that cutaneous melanomas which extend only to Clark's level II and which are less than 0.76 mm thick as measured by the Breslow technique have a very low, virtually non-existent, risk of recurrence or metastasis if adequately excised; it seems highly probable that vulval melanomas of this type could be treated by partial vulvectomy without node dissection. It must be emphasised, however, that a 4–5 cm margin or margins approaching twice the diameter of the tumour should be aimed for and that whilst this margin of clearance may be readily attained in lateral melanomas this may well prove impossible for centrally sited neoplasms.

ADNEXAL NEOPLASMS

Benign adnexal (skin appendage) tumours

Tumours with eccrine differentiation

Syringoma. The syringoma is a benign organoid tumour which is regarded as an adenoma of the intra-epidermal eccrine sweat gland ducts (Hashimoto et al 1966, Hashimoto & Lever 1969). The lesions most commonly develop on the eyelids, cheeks, axillae, upper arms and abdomen and only rarely on the vulva (Brown & Freeman 1971, Carneiro et al 1971, Carneiro et al 1972, Isaacson & Turner 1979, Thomas et al 1979, Young et al 1980). Vulval lesions may occur in isolation (Carneiro et al 1971, 1972, Brown & Freeman 1971, Thomas et al 1979) or in association with lesions elsewhere on the body (Carneiro et al 1971, Young et al 1980).

They develop most commonly in adults, becoming apparent at puberty or shortly afterwards (Ridley 1975, Rook et al 1986). A family history is present in some cases (Woringer & Eichler 1951, Yesudian & Thambiah 1975, Young et al 1980) and the age range at presentation is from 9 to 43 years (Brown & Freeman 1971, Carneiro et al 1971, 1972).

The lesions are occasionally solitary but usually multiple, present in large numbers and are bilaterally symmetrical (Isaacson & Turner 1979) being concentrated on the labia majora but also occurring on the labia minora, suprapubic area and the inner aspects of the thighs where they may be asymptomatic or mildly pruritic (Hashimoto et al 1967a, Carneiro et al 1971, Young et al 1980). They are small, soft, firm to fleshy papules ranging from 1 to 4 mm in diameter; they vary from flesh colour to yellow.

Histologically, the lesion is ill-defined and appears as a series of small, comma-shaped ducts embedded in fibrous tissue in the dermis. The ducts are lined by two rows of epithelial cells that are often focally flattened due to pressure. The cells of the inner layer may be cuboidal or appear vacuolated: the lumina contain amorphous debris which is diastase resistant, PAS positive (Hashimoto et al 1966). In rare instances the cytoplasm of many of the tumour cells may appear clear due to the accumulation of glycogen (Headington et al 1972). There may also be solid strands and small islands of basaloid cells. Small epidermoid cysts may be present, particularly near the epidermis, these develop in cystic ductal lumina (Brownstein & Shapiro 1975, Lever & Schaumburg-Lever 1975b) and their rupture may lead to a foreign body response followed by calcification (Woringer & Eichler 1951, Hashimoto et al 1967a).

Mixed adnexoid tumours have been described in which syringomatous and pilosebaceous elements co-exist (Guindi et al 1974) or syringomatous elements may occur in a chondroid stroma (Headington 1961, Brownstein & Shapiro 1975).

Enzyme, histochemical and electron microscopic studies have established the syringoma as a tumour with differentiation towards intra-epidermal eccrine sweat gland ducts (Mustakallio 1959, Winkelman & Muller 1964, Hashimoto et al 1966, 1967a).

Treatment is unnecessary but the lesions may be treated by high frequency electrosurgical ablation or, rarely, by excision, if histological confirmation is required.

Clear-cell hidradenoma. The clear-cell hidradenoma is a rare eccrine sweat gland tumour which occurs most frequently on the face, scalp, thoracic wall and abdomen and only rarely on the vulva. It has in the past been referred to as nodular hidradenoma (Lund 1957), eccrine sweat gland adenoma of clear-cell type (O'Hara et al 1966, O'Hara & Bensch 1967), solid-cystic hidradenoma (Winkelman & Wolff 1967, 1968) and eccrine acrospiroma (Johnson & Helwig 1969).

The tumour may be painful on pressure but more commonly causes pruritus or burning (Johnson & Helwig 1969). The lesion forms a firm intradermal nodule which may extend into the subcutaneous tissue. The great majority range in size from 0.5 to 2 cm (Lever & Schaumburg-Lever 1975a) although they may be larger (Johnson & Helwig 1969). The skin covering the nodule is usually intact and of normal appearance but can be red to purple-blue (Johnson & Helwig 1969), and may ulcerate (Winkelman & Wolff 1968) and discharge serous fluid (Lever & Castleman 1952). The tumour is usually multilobular, well delineated but not encapsulated, varies in colour from grey to tan, is usually solid but may be partly cystic (Johnson & Helwig 1969) and may be haemorrhagic.

Histologically the tumour appears well circumscribed and is composed of lobular masses of cells separated by fine fibrous tissue bands. The lobules are concentrated in the upper and middle dermis but in some cases individual cells may extend into and replace the epidermis (Johnson & Helwig 1969) and, in the larger lesions, the lobules may extend into the deeper layers of the dermis and the subcutaneous tissue. The covering epidermis may be acanthotic, atrophic or ulcerated.

Within the cellular masses there are branching, tubular or ductal structures of various sizes lined by cuboidal ductal cells or secretory columnar cells and unlined cystic spaces containing pale, eosinophilic, homogenous material, which appear to develop as a result of degeneration (Winkelman & Wolff 1968, Johnson & Helwig 1969, Lever & Schaumburg-Lever 1975c). Two types of tumour cells are recognised (Lever & Castleman 1952, Kersting 1963, Hashimoto et al 1967b, Winkelman & Wolff 1968, Johnson & Helwig 1969); they vary in proportion from tumour to tumour and in different areas of the same neoplasm (Brownstein & Shapiro 1975). The first is epidermoid, fusiform and has an elongated nucleus and basophilic cytoplasm whilst the second is larger, has a round or oval nucleus with a regular or irregular outline and clear cytoplasm rich in glycogen (Kersting 1963), phosphorylase and esterolytic enzymes (Winkelman & Wolff 1968); the cell membranes are prominent. Cells occupying an intermediate position also occur; their cytoplasm is faintly eosinophilic (Lever & Schaumburg-Lever 1975c). At the margins of the cellular lobules, in occasional tumours, there are keratinised cells forming epithelial pearls (Lever & Castleman 1952, O'Hara et al 1966) and, when a slit-like lumen with an eosinophilic cuticle forms in the centre of the squamous cell clusters, there is a close resemblance to the intradermal portion of the eccrine sweat gland duct.

Electron microscopic studies reveal cells showing differentiation towards intra-epidermal and intradermal eccrine structures (Hashimoto et al 1976b).

Although the lesions are benign, 10% of those developing in the head, neck and trunk recur (Johnson & Helwig 1969). Recurrent lesions tend to be more fibrous and more deeply positioned than primary tumours and recurrence is believed to be the result of inadequate primary excision.

Tumours with apocrine differentiation

Papillary hidradenoma (hidradenoma papilliferum). The papillary hidradenoma is an almost invariably benign adenoma with apocrine sweat gland differentiation (Meeker et al 1962, Tappeiner & Wolff 1968, Hashimoto 1973, Brownstein & Shapiro 1975). The morphological similarity to an intraduct papilloma of the breast has led to suggestions that these neoplasms may develop from accessory breast tissue (Woodworth et al 1971) but this remains unproved. The tumours develop

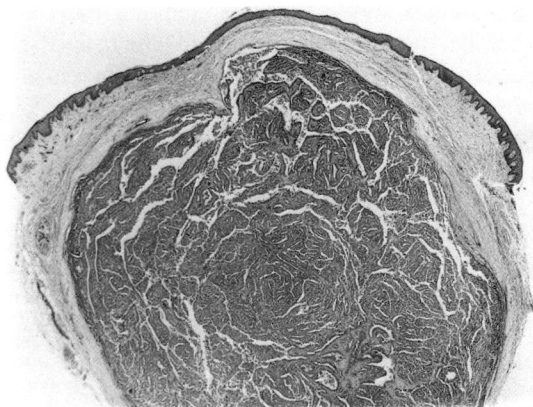

Fig. 10.41 Papillary hidradenoma. The complex, papillary pattern of this well-demarcated, intradermal lesion can be seen. (H & E × 12)

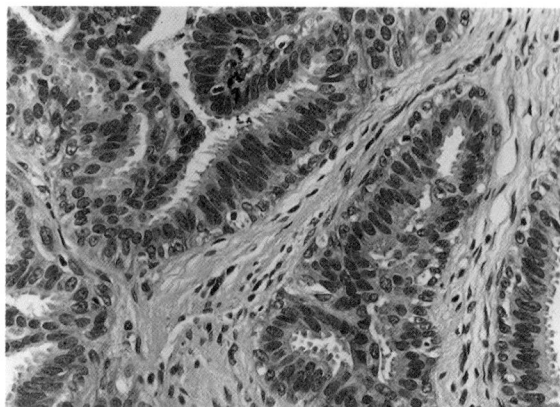

Fig. 10.42 Papillary hidradenoma. A group of tubules lined by an inner layer of tall columnar cells with an outer mantle of small, cuboidal, myo-epithelial cells. (H & E × 240)

after puberty, particularly in Caucasians, and almost exclusively in the anogenital region of middle-aged women (Meeker et al 1962, Donna et al 1978).

Hidradenomas are small, firm, often asymptomatic (Woodworth et al 1971), occasionally painful or irritating nodules usually less than 2 cm in diameter, and exceptionally, up to 8 cm in diameter (Kaufman et al 1987), which develop in the labia majora, interlabial sulcus, lateral surfaces of the labia minora (Friedrich & Wilkinson 1982f), perineal or peri-anal areas (Tappeiner & Wolff 1968, Lever & Schaumburg-Lever 1975d) and are occasionally multiple (Woodworth et al 1971). Curiously, when they are multiple Hobbs (1965) has observed that they may all develop on the same side of the vulva. In the majority of patients, the covering epidermis remains intact, but in a proportion of cases the elevated, overlying epithelium becomes ulcerated (Janovski & Douglas 1972, Donna et al 1978) and the red, fleshy, adenomatous tissue protrudes through the cutaneous defect. Such lesions may bleed on contact and can clinically mimic carcinoma; cytological smears may help to make the diagnosis in such cases (Hustin et al 1980).

The tumours lie deep in the dermis, have no connection with the epidermis (Brownstein & Shapiro 1975) and are often clearly delineated from the surrounding tissues by a layer of compressed connective tissue (Fig. 10.41). There is, however, no true capsule and the tumour acini may be seen microscopically to be infiltrating the connective tissue at

the margin of the lesion. Some of the tumours, however, have a peripheral epithelial wall which may show keratinisation (Hashimoto 1973). The neoplasm has a complex pattern of glandular acini, tubules and small cysts in which there are papillae. The epithelium lining the cysts, tubules and acini and covering the papillae is, for the most part, double layered (Fig. 10.42). One layer, the lining, is composed of cuboidal or columnar cells with oval, pale-staining, basal nuclei, faintly eosinophilic, PAS positive, diastase resistant cytoplasm which may show apocrine features as manifest by active, decapitation secretion (Lever & Schaumburg-Lever 1975d) and the other, the deeper layer, is formed by smaller, more darkly staining cuboidal or spindle-shaped myo-epithelial cells (Tappeiner & Wolff 1968, Hashimoto 1973). The luminal cells are positive for non-specific esterase and acid phosphatase (Lever & Schaumburg-Lever 1983b).

Exceptionally, concomitant focal tricho-epithelioma has been described (Donna et al 1978) and one case of metastasising squamous carcinoma developing in a peri-anal lesion has been recorded (Shenoy 1961). Treatment by local excision is, however, normally regarded as adequate (Woodworth et al 1971).

Tumours showing mixed sweat gland differentiation

Syringocystadenoma papilliferum (syringoadenoma papilliferum). These are rare tumours which may be present in childhood but usually develop de novo during adolescence and early adulthood. They appear usually as firm, rose-red papules varying in size from 1 to 3 mm, which may become papilliferous with exudation of fluid and formation of a crust.

One or more invaginations extend downwards from the epidermis, into the dermis. The superficial part of these may be lined by squamous epithelium, but in the deeper parts they are lined by two rows of cells. The luminal cells are tall, columnar and have faintly eosinophilic cytoplasm and oval nuclei; they may show decapitation secretion. The outer layer is composed of small cuboidal cells with round nuclei and scanty cytoplasm. The stroma of the tumour usually contains a plasma cell infiltrate.

There is no agreement about the differentiation of these lesions, the presented evidence being somewhat contradictory, some indicating eccrine differentiation whilst others suggest an apocrine pathway. It is probably true to say that both are correct and that differentiation may be either ductal or secretory (Lever & Schaumburg-Lever 1983b). Novak & Woodruff (1979) point out the difficulty that may occur in differentiating the lesion from one developing from vulval breast tissue.

Local excision of these lesions appears to be the correct treatment as there is no evidence that they ever behave in a malignant fashion (Domonkos et al 1982).

Tumours with hair structure differentiation

Pilar tumour. This neoplasm is thought to develop from the outer hair root sheath and is therefore distinct from the pilomatrixoma, which probably develops from the hair matrix cells. It usually occurs on the scalp of elderly women (Holmes 1968, Dabska 1971) but can very rarely occur on the vulva (Buchler et al 1978).

The tumour starts as a subcutaneous nodule which may become elevated, ulcerate and discharge serosanguineous fluid. It is composed of strands, and, more typically, lobules of squamous epithelium which undergo a rather abrupt change in their centres to eosinophilic, amorphous keratin which may be focally calcified. There may be a minor degree of cytological atypia and epithelial pearls may

develop. However, the tumour may be differentiated from squamous carcinoma by its sharp demarcation from the surrounding stroma and the abrupt, amorphous keratinisation without granular layer. The scalp tumours have been noted to develop cellular vacuolisation as the result of glycogen storage (Holmes 1968).

The tumour is usually regarded as benign, and is adequately treated by wide local excision, but in one case (Holmes 1968) metastases occurred. The tumour was, however, very extensive and it is possible that spread to the node occurred by direct infiltration rather than by true metastasis.

Tumours with sebaceous differentiation

Sebaceous adenoma. Sebaceous adenomas are rare, benign neoplasms rarely seen on the vulva. They appear as small, discrete, single or multiple nodules on the labia minora, and to a lesser extent on the labia majora. They are tan, pink-red or skin coloured and on section may appear yellow, or, less often, grey (Rulon & Helwig 1974). They are composed of well-demarcated, irregularly shaped, incompletely differentiated sebaceous lobules (Lever & Schaumburg-Lever 1983a). Cells similar to those at the periphery of the normal sebaceous glands, germinative cells, mature sebaceous cells and cells of intermediate differentiation all occur but the proportions of each cell type differ in different lobules.

They should be differentiated from sebaceous gland hyperplasia (Rocamora et al 1986) in which each of the constituent lobules drains into a dilated central sebaceous duct which may become plugged by keratin. Some authors believe that such a distinction is arbitrary (Rulon & Helwig 1974) but as up to 7% of those occurring elsewhere in the body recur, the differentiation is probably worthwhile. Adenomas do not show cytological atypia and are not known to dispose to the development of carcinoma (Janovski & Douglas 1972, Novak & Woodruff 1979).

Malignant adnexal (skin appendage) neoplasms

Introduction. Malignant sweat gland tumours of the vulva are rare and have, for the most part, been poorly documented. The tumours present a wide variety of histological appearances many of which may mimic the more common primary malignancies of the vulva and some of which may resemble metastatic adenocarcinoma from such common primary sites as breast or lung. Unless the surgeon and pathologist are alert to the possibility that a solid, intradermal malignant epithelial neoplasm may be of adnexal origin, such tumours will continue to go unrecognised.

The term adenocarcinoma or carcinoma of sweat gland origin is restricted in this account to infiltrating neoplasms and does not include Paget's disease of the intra-epithelial variety, although Paget's cells may be seen in the epidermis adjacent to an infiltrating carcinoma (Stout & Cooley 1951, Roth et al 1977, Rich et al 1981, Webb & Beswick 1983).

The reported frequency with which these tumours occur is complicated by the inclusion, in some of the older reports (McDonald 1941), of benign vulval tumours and the failure, in some of the reports of vulval Paget's disease, to distinguish between intra-epithelial and invasive sweat gland neoplasia. It is, however, reported that approximately 15% of malignant sweat gland tumours occur on the genitalia (Jacobson et al 1959).

Well-documented examples of invasive sweat gland neoplasms of the vulva are few; both eccrine and apocrine types are described although not infrequently, particularly in reports of vulval Paget's disease, whilst invasive sweat gland carcinomas are said to have been present they are either not described or so poorly differentiated that classification is impossible (Eichenberg 1934, Weiner 1937, Novak & Stevenson 1945, Dockerty & Pratt 1952, Plachta & Speer 1954, Rosser & Hamlin 1957, Miller 1967, Boehm & Morris 1971, El-Domeiri et al 1971, Tsukada et al 1975, Wilner et al 1976, Lee et al 1977, Roth et al 1977, Underwood et al 1978, Rich et al 1981, Webb & Beswick 1983, Wick et al 1985a, b).

Aetiology. The majority of malignant sweat gland tumours are of unknown aetiology but solar radiation may be a factor in those developing in exposed areas of the skin (Wick et al 1985b) and their development has been reported following radiotherapy (El-Domeiri et al 1972, Rich et al 1981, Webb & Beswick 1983) or exposure to ionizing radiation (Caccialanza et al 1979).

Clinical features. The usual age of occurrence lies between 50 and 70 years (Wick et al 1985b) although they can occur at any time from childhood to extreme old age (Dissanayake & Salm 1980, Wick et al 1985b) and may develop in pregnancy (Wick et al 1985b).

The tumours occur most frequently on the labia majora (Boehm & Morris 1971, Lee et al 1977, Underwood et al 1978, Wick et al 1985b), in the interlabial sulcus anteriorly adjacent to the clitoris (Rosser & Hamlin 1957, Webb & Beswick 1983) and, less commonly, on the posterior fourchette or perineum (Rich et al 1981, Wick et al 1985b). They most commonly form painless, or only mildly tender, firm, red-violet (Stout & Cooley 1951), nonulcerated dermal nodules which may or may not be fixed to the underlying tissues; mucinous tumours tend to be yellow-brown (Wright & Font 1979). Many tumours are small at the time of diagnosis, ranging in size from 0.5 to 10 cm and yet may have been present for several years.

Gross pathology. The tumours lie in the dermis and may extend into the subcutaneous tissue. Tumours of ductal origin tend to form homogenous grey white nodules, whilst those which secrete mucin are soft and mucoid (Wick et al 1985b). Recurrent tumours tend to resemble the original primary lesion.

Histological appearances. Malignant tumours of adnexal origin present a staggering variety of histological pictures varying from a very welldifferentiated small lesion which may, at first glance, appear to be benign, to a virtually undifferentiated infiltrating neoplasm (Fig. 10.43).

Guidelines have been established for the separation of benign adnexal tumours from those which can be expected to pursue a malignant course (Wick et al 1985b). Malignant tumours tend to have an infiltrating rather than a 'pushing' margin, nuclear pleomorphism, coarse clumping of the nuclear chromatin and hyperchromasia, an increased nucleo-cytoplasmic ratio, tumour necrosis and vascular space involvement.

The true nature of some of the less welldifferentiated neoplasms will probably be established only if appropriate stains, enzyme histochemistry and electron microscopy are carried out. However, whilst the detection of specific enzymes and CEA (Penneys et al 1982) may be useful in distinguishing sweat gland carcinomas from squamous

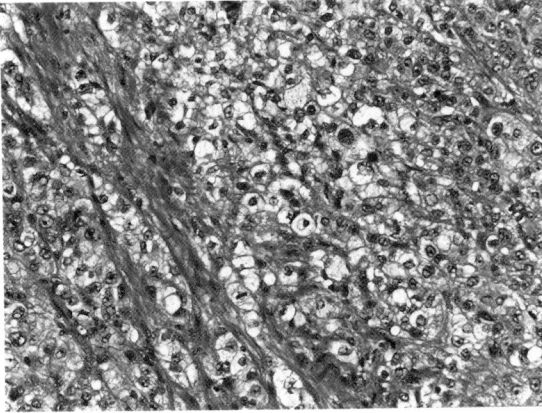

Fig. 10.43 Sweat gland carcinoma. In this example of poorly differentiated carcinoma, a focal, clear-celled pattern is reminiscent of clear-celled hidradenocarcinoma. (H & E × 150)

carcinomas and basal cell carcinomas, they are of no value in distinguishing adnexal adenocarcinomas from metastatic visceral adenocarcinoma and, with the least differentiated tumours, classification may be impossible (Roth et al 1977).

Tumours of eccrine gland origin

Ductal adenocarcinomas. The tumours are composed of polygonal or cuboidal cells with scanty eosinophilic cytoplasm and round vesicular nuclei containing amphophilic nucleoli; mitoses may be frequent. The cells form anastomosing cords and nests and in some tumours well-formed ducts with small lumina (Grant 1960) lined by an eosinophilic cuticle are a prominent feature; squamous metaplasia may be extensive (Teloh et al 1957). Indeed, some tumours have the features of muco-epidermoid carcinoma (adenosquamous carcinoma) being composed of squamous islands, within the margins of which there are acini. Some of the tumours described by Underwood and colleagues (1978) may come into this category.

Less commonly, spindle-celled areas are intermingled with the epithelial elements or the tumour may have a diffuse spindle-celled structure and the cells may assume striking concentric arrangements (Wick et al 1985b). Sometimes, long branching cords of spindle cells forming dilated, branching tubular structures are separated by a fibromyxoid stroma, syringoid eccrine carcinoma (Mehregan et

al 1983), malignant chondroid syringoma (Dissanayake & Salm 1980), or eccrine epithelioma (Freeman & Winkelmann 1969). The myxoid stroma stains positively with PAS (diastase resistant), alcian blue, sulphated alcian blue and colloidal iron. The tumour may also take the form of narrow epithelial cords growing in a serpiginous or lace-like pattern (Wick et al 1985b). Infiltration of the lymphatics adjacent to the primary tumour is often seen (Wick et al 1985b).

Electron optic examination reveals pericellular basal lamina, intercellular desmosomes, inter- and intra-microlumina containing microvillous projections (the latter being typical of eccrine ducts) and focal cytoplasmic tonofilaments. The features are similar in the epithelial and the spindle-celled forms.

The eccrine duct carcinomas can be distinguished from other vulval carcinomas which they resemble morphologically by the presence of phosphorylase, succinic dehydrogenase, indoxyl esterase and cytochrome oxidase, whilst stains for acid and alkaline phosphatase, ATPase, betaglucuronidase, acetate esterase, leucine aminopeptidase and monoamine oxidase are negative.

Wick et al (1985b) describe a ductal carcinoma with myxoid stroma and a lacy pattern reminiscent of adenoid basal cell carcinoma in a 22-year-old pregnant patient. The neoplasm had a rapid fatal course. Wilner et al (1976) also describe an eccrine ductal carcinoma in a 68-year-old woman; local extension had occurred to the vagina; and a third case was described by Fukuma et al (1986).

Mucinous adenocarcinoma (adenocystic eccrine adenocarcinoma). In this neoplasm, clusters and nests of small tumour cells are suspended in pools of mucin which are subdivided by fine fibrous tissue bands; cells are most numerous at the periphery of the lesion (Mendoza & Helwig 1971). The cells are small, relatively regular and the oval to round nuclei are moderately hyperchromatic and contain few mitoses. The cytoplasm is amphophilic, relatively scanty and rather vacuolated; a trace of mucin may be present (Webb & Beswick 1983). The cells form nests up to ten cells thick and duct-like structures which lack basement membrane material. At low magnification the lesions tend to appear well circumscribed but the margins are infiltrating and lymphatic invasion is often seen.

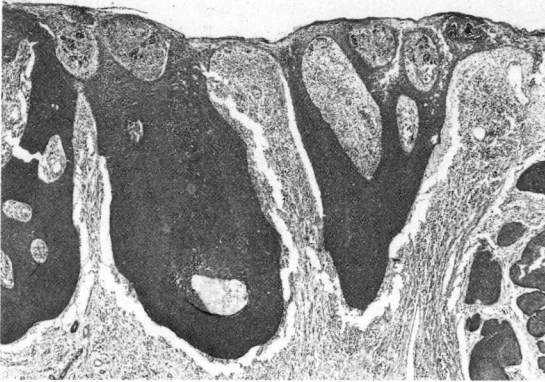

Fig. 10.44 Malignant eccrine poroma. The attachment of the cell nests to the covering epidermis is well shown. (H & E × 25)

The mucin is positive to PAS, mucicarmine, alcian blue, sulphated alcian blue and colloidal iron and is resistant to hyaluronidase and diastase digestion, the mucin continuing to stain positively with alcian blue at pH 2.5, even after hyaluronidase digestion (Grossman & Izuno 1974, Wright & Font 1979).

Vulval tumours of this type are described by Dockerty & Pratt (1952) and Webb & Beswick (1983).

Porocarcinoma (malignant eccrine poroma). A porocarcinoma is composed of rounded nests of either small basaloid cells with scanty cytoplasm and round to oval nuclei in which there is a central nucleolus or large cells with irregularly shaped hyperchromatic nuclei and abundant, glycogen-containing cytoplasm (Mehregan et al 1983). The cell nests are attached to the epidermis by cell cords and individual cells may extend up into the epidermis simulating an acrosyringium (Fig. 10.44). Typically the cells form a cribriform pattern or duct-like tumour and the centres of the cell nests may undergo necrosis and later calcify. The neoplasm shows a particular tendency to metastasise to the skin. A tumour of this type has been described in the vulva by Wick et al (1985a) and Wick et al (1985b), the patient being an 80-year-old woman.

Tumours of apocrine gland origin

Apocrine gland carcinoma. The tumours are composed of groups, sheets and cords of large globular polygonal cells with vesicular nuclei and vacuolated eosinophilic cytoplasm (Rosser & Hamlin 1957, Lee et al 1977, Roth et al 1977). Glandular lumina may form and decapitation secretion may be seen (Furtell et al 1971), although this is not a constant feature (Baes & Suurmond 1970, Lever & Schaumburg-Lever 1975e).

The cells stain positively with PAS, alcian blue and mucicarmine, staining is unaffected by diastase digestion and iron positive granules are present in the cytoplasm of some cells (Rosser & Hamlin 1957, Kipkie & Haust 1958). Best's stain for glycogen is negative, as is Sudan Black.

The cells also contain acid phosphatase and non-specific esterase but lack succinic dehydrogenase (Baes & Suurmond 1970).

Apocrine tumours may bear an acute resemblance to ductal carcinoma of the breast (Plachta & Speer 1954) and, in the vulva, distinction of apocrine carcinoma from carcinoma arising in heterotopic breast tissue may be impossible unless remains of the normal non-neoplastic tissue are intact (Rich et al 1981).

Vulval tumours of this type have been described by Plachta & Speer (1954), Rosser & Hamlin (1957), Boehm & Morris (1971), Lee et al (1977), Roth et al (1977) and perhaps by Weiner (1937).

Prognosis. Sweat gland tumours are said rarely to metastasise (Teloh et al 1957) yet, of those described in the vulva, many have done so (Eichenberg 1934, Weiner 1937, Dockerty & Pratt 1952, Rosser & Hamlin 1957, Boehm & Morris 1971, Wick et al 1985b).

The more usual course is for local recurrence (El-Domeiri et al 1971, Mehregan et al 1983, Wick et al 1985b) and a protracted course is not unusual (El-Domeiri et al 1972). In general the outcome depends upon the histological differentiation of the tumour (Berg & McDivitt 1968), its particular histological characteristics (Dissanayake & Salm 1980) and the extent of spread at the time of diagnosis. Generally speaking eccrine ductal carcinoma (syringocystadenocarcinomas), and mucinous carcinoma have a good prognosis though local recurrence may occur, whilst muco-epidermoid (adenosquamous) carcinoma and eccrine ductal carcinoma with myxoid stroma (chondroid syringoma) follow a more aggressive course (Dissanayake & Salm 1980, Wick et al 1985b).

Treatment. Well-differentiated tumours without clinically suspicious nodes may, it is said, be treated by wide local excision (El-Domeiri et al 1971), but palpable lymph nodes should be removed and poorly differentiated or undifferentiated tumours treated by local radical surgery and lymphadenectomy whether the nodes are clinically suspicious or not. Mucinous tumours rarely metastasise and lymphadenectomy may not be indicated in those cases (Mendoza & Helwig 1971, Grossman & Izuno 1974, Wright & Font 1979, Dissanayake & Salm 1980, Mehregan et al 1983).

The tumours are insensitive to radiotherapy (Grant 1960) but chemotherapy may be helpful in some advanced cases (El-Domeiri et al 1971) although the true value of this is not as yet established.

Sebaceous carcinoma

Sebaceous carcinomas are rare, only two cases having been reported to have developed on the vulva (Rulon & Helwig 1974, Jacobs et al 1986).

They form firm grey-white or yellow, indurated plaques or well-circumscribed intradermal nodules, and whilst the surface usually remains intact it may ulcerate, producing a lesion resembling a basal cell carcinoma.

The tumour forms irregularly shaped nests, masses or lobules which may vary in size. Many cells are undifferentiated but there is differentiation towards rather pleomorphic atypical sebaceous cells in the centres of the cell masses. Some of the larger lobules contain areas of atypical keratinizing cells (Lever & Schaumburg-Lever 1983b). The most differentiated cells are large, have oval or round nuclei in which eosinophilic nucleoli can be seen and have pale, eosinophilic cytoplasm which is finely foamy and within which vacuoles of varying sizes may form. In some areas the undifferentiated cells have eosinophilic cytoplasm which contains lipid; Oil-Red 0 gives a positive stain in the tumour cells, but stains for mucus are negative.

It is difficult to give an idea of the likely outcome in such rare conditions (Rulon & Helwig 1974). The tumour described by Rulon & Helwig (1974) did not, however, metastasise but tumours in other sites have done so, albeit rarely. It is important to differentiate sebaceous carcinoma from basal cell carcinoma showing sebaceous differentiation as basal cell carcinoma very rarely metastasises.

The current recommended therapy is to excise the lesion widely (Wick et al 1985c) with removal of the lymph nodes if they appear to be involved by metastatic disease. Too few cases have been described to evaluate the results of prophylactic lymph node dissection. Radiotherapy and chemotherapy have been employed, but as their use has tended to be in patients with extensive disseminated disease a failure of response may not be an accurate assessment of the radiosensitivity of the sebaceous carcinoma.

BARTHOLIN'S GLAND TUMOURS

Benign neoplasms and hamartomas

Benign neoplasms and hamartomas of Bartholin's gland are very rarely described (Smith Foushee et al 1968, Jeffcoate 1975, Honoré & O'Hara 1978) but one wonders whether this is a true reflection of their rarity or of the infrequency with which they are identified in patients suffering from a cyst or abscess of Bartholin's gland.

Adenoma

An adenoma presents as a permanent or intermittent swelling of the posterolateral part of the vulva which is clinically indistinguishable from a cyst, abscess or carcinoma of the gland; discharge and pain may be present. The tumours vary in size from 1 to 2 cm and appear as a homogenous, solid, grey-tan, ill-defined nodule associated with a ductal cyst which may or may not be inflamed (Smith Foushee et al 1968).

Histologically, the tumour margins are pushing and result in the formation of a fibrous pseudocapsule (Honoré & O'Hara 1978). The lesion is composed of closely packed secretory alveoli exhibiting a variable degree of branching and lined by a tall, pale, mucus-secreting epithelium with small basal nuclei which do not contain nucleoli or mitoses. There is some debate as to whether these lesions are really true benign neoplasms (Honoré & O'Hara 1978) or should, more correctly, be regarded as focal hyperplasias or hamartomas (Smith Foushee et al 1968). Similar lesions are also reported in the small, unnamed, minor vestibular glands (Axe et al 1986).

There is no evidence that adenomas, if so they be, are precursors of carcinomas, although adenoid cystic carcinoma has been observed to develop within a pleomorphic adenoma of mixed salivary type (Ordonez et al 1981). Other reports of pleomorphic adenoma (Hertig & Gore 1960, Janovski & Douglas 1972), papillary cystadenoma and leiomyoma have been published (Honoré & O'Hara 1978).

Malignant Bartholin's gland neoplasms

Carcinoma of Bartholin's gland

Carcinoma of Bartholin's gland constitutes between 0.1 and 7.25% of all vulval malignancies and 0.001% of female genital tract malignancies (Wharton & Everett 1951, Masterson & Goss 1954, Barclay et al 1964, Chamlian & Taylor 1972, Addison & Parker 1977, Wahlström et al 1978, Leuchter et al 1982, Webb et al 1984).

Clinical presentation. Bartholin's gland carcinoma most commonly presents as a vulval mass deep in the posterior part of the labium major, or with perineal pain (Barclay et al 1964, Leuchter et al 1982). There is often considerable delay between the onset of symptoms and the achievement of a correct diagnosis, in some cases amounting to several years (Trelford & Deos 1976, Wahlström et al 1978, Leuchter et al 1982). In about a quarter of patients the delay is due to the fact that the presenting complaint is an abscess in the gland and it is only when this lesion fails to respond to the usual antibiotics and drainage that the possibility of a more serious underlying disease is considered (Masterson & Goss 1954, Chamlian & Taylor 1972, Leuchter et al 1982). It is important therefore that the development of a Bartholin's gland abscess in the older patient, or persistent infection in the younger woman, should be thoroughly investigated by histological or cytological examination (Frable & Goplerud 1975, Schweppe & Schlake 1980).

The mean age at presentation varies from 50 to 62 years (Abell 1963, Barclay et al 1964, Leuchter et al 1982) and a substantial proportion of patients are postmenopausal. The condition has been des-cribed in a girl as young as 14 years (Addison 1977) and in pregnancy (Dennis et al 1955, Murphy et al 1962, Chamlian & Taylor 1972). Patients in whom investigation reveals the presence of a squamous carcinoma tend on the whole to be a little younger than those who develop adenocarcinoma (Leuchter et al 1982).

Gross pathology. The tumours form a firm nodule in the posterior part of the labium major and may extend superiorly into the vagina, posteriorly into the rectal sphincter and ischiorectal fossa and anteriorly along the labia (DiSaia & Creasman 1981, Leuchter et al 1982). They vary in size at presentation from 1 to 6 cm in their greatest axes (Leuchter et al 1982) and are usually solid, greywhite on section. It is unusual for the covering epidermis to ulcerate (Kuzuya et al 1981) but spontaneous or therapeutic drainage from an associated abscess may be present (Leuchter et al 1982) and the overlying epithelium and adjacent areas of the vulva may show the features of Paget's disease (Tchang et al 1973).

Metastases occur in the first instance to the inguinal and femoral lymph nodes and secondarily to the pelvic nodes. Metastases in the obturator nodes without detectable tumour in the iliac nodes, however, suggest the possibility of direct drainage from the deeper part of the gland directly to the pelvic nodes (Eichner 1957, Barclay et al 1964). At the time of diagnosis over one-third of the squamous and adenocarcinomas have already extended to the inguinal and femoral nodes whereas only 14.3% of adenoid cystic carcinomas have done so (Leuchter et al 1982).

Histopathology. It is usual for tumours of Bartholin's gland to be diagnosed only when the criteria as given by Honan (1897) or Chamlian & Taylor (1972) are fulfilled. In essence these state that there should be Bartholin's gland elements adjacent to the carcinoma, that areas of transiton from normal to neoplastic gland elements should be seen and that the tumour should be histologically compatible with an origin in the gland; no other concurrent primary tumour should be identified and the covering epithelium should be intact.

Reviews of the literature (Barclay et al 1964, Leuchter et al 1982) (Tables 10.4 and 10.5) show that the majority of the neoplasms are either squamous carcinomas, adenocarcinomas or adenoid

Table 10.4 Carcinoma of Bartholin's gland: histological patterns (Leuchter et al 1982)

Type	Number	Percentage
Squamous	34	37.8
Adenocarcinoma	29	32.2
Adenoid cystic	14	15.6
Mixed	4	5.6
Transitional	3	3.3
Anaplastic	4	4.4
Unknown	2	2.2
Total	90	100.0

Table 10.5 Carcinoma of Bartholin's gland: histological patterns (Barclay et al 1984, Leuchter et al 1982)

Type	Number	Percentage
Squamous	50	40.0
Adenocarcinoma	58	46.4
Total	108	86.4

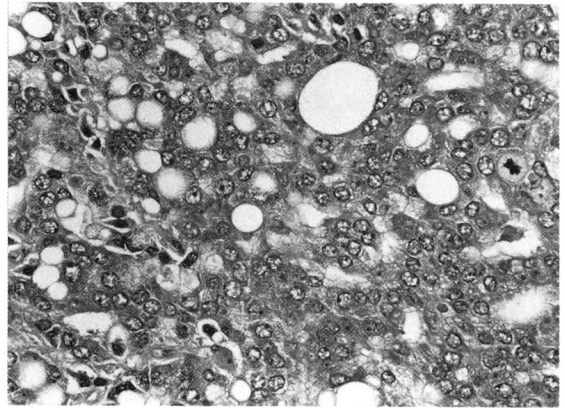

Fig. 10.45 Adenocarcinoma of Bartholin's gland. The tumour is composed of solid islands of small, rather poorly formed acini. (H & E × 240)

cystic carcinomas. Mixed tumours, which include both adenosquamous carcinoma and mixed transitional/squamous carcinoma, transitional carcinomas, adeno-acanthoma and anaplastic carcinoma together account for only just over 13% of the total. Instances of rare tumour combinations are also reported, for example, squamous carcinoma combined with adenoid cystic carcinoma (Webb et al 1984).

Squamous carcinoma. The histogenesis of squamous carcinoma is uncertain (Leuchter et al 1982) except in those cases in which antecedent inflammation is associated with glandular ductal squamous metaplasia (Boughton 1943), although overt (or clinical) inflammation is not a prerequisite for the development of metaplasia in Bartholin's gland. The majority are typical squamous carcinomas showing variable differentiation; rarely, spindle cell squamous carcinoma occurs and muco-epidermoid and adenosquamous forms are described (Ferenczy 1981).

Transitional cell carcinoma. Dodson et al (1970) and Wahlström et al (1978) reported what they believed to be the first Bartholin's gland transitional cell carcinoma. It is described as a non-papillary invasive transitional cell carcinoma reminiscent of the transitional cloacogenic carcinoma arising in the anal ducts. The atypical cells have a tendency to line cystic spaces of different sizes; small gland-like configurations and poorly developed squamous epithelial pearls may also occur. The cells are larger

than lymphocytes, have round, vesicular nuclei with prominent nucleoli and a moderate amount of homogenous cytoplasm. The tumour is considered to arise from the ductal epithelium, which is normally of transitional type.

Adenocarcinoma. Adenocarcinoma of Bartholin's gland may be well differentiated (Crossen 1948, Tchang et al 1973, Kuzuya et al 1981) or poorly differentiated (Advani et al 1978, Wahlström et al 1978) (Fig. 10.45) but unfortunately insufficient histopathological detail is provided in much of the literature to enable a complete picture of such tumours to be obtained.

In the well-differentiated mucus-secreting adenocarcinomas (Chamlian & Taylor 1972, Addison 1977, Ferenczy 1981, Kuzuya et al 1981) a papillary, tubular and cribriform pattern of growth is described. Three cell types are distinguished. The first, principal, columnar cells have abundant eosinophilic cytoplasm and resemble the Bartholin's gland ductal lining cells and the second have large mucous granules in their luminal cytoplasm and are goblet cell-like; they resemble the normal acinar cells. In both these types, the nuclei, which are basal, contain several nucleoli but mitoses are rarely seen. The third type is a stratified cuboidal cell with greater nucleo-cytoplasmic ratios and frequent mitoses. Mucus may be difficult to identify by light microscopy but electron microscopy reveals a similarity between these cells and those of eccrine sweat glands. It is suggested that these tumours develop from the cells of Bartholin's gland duct, which are capable of differentiating into both Bartholin's gland cells and eccrine sweat gland cells, the conclusions being based upon the electron optic studies (Kuzuya et al 1981). Ferenczy (1981) also mentions a papillary, clear-cell carcinoma of mesonephroid type similar to that seen elsewhere in the female genital tract.

Wahlström et al (1978) described three main types of poorly differentiated adenocarcinoma. They may be composed of fairly regular, cuboidal neoplastic cells with moderate amounts of cytoplasm and round, pale-staining nuclei with one nucleolus which form irregular glandular structures, cells with dark, pleomorphic nuclei with one or more conspicuous nucleoli and varying amounts of cytoplasm which form nests of gland-like structures and resemble the pattern of ductal carcinoma of the breast, or atypical epithelial cells with round dark nuclei and a moderate amount of cytoplasm which form strands and clumps without a regular growth pattern.

Advani et al (1978) described what appears to be yet a fourth form of poorly differentiated adenocarcinoma. It is composed of lobulated sheets of cells with well-defined cell membranes, clear or eosinophilic cytoplasm and round or oval nuclei. They do not form mucin, keratin, intercellular bridges or glandular structures and electron microscopy shows that the cells bear some resemblance to those of the upper zone of the main excretory duct of the Bartholin's gland.

Adenoid cystic carcinoma. In some series adenoid cystic carcinoma is included with adenocarcinomas of other types, but this is probably inappropriate as the tumour is distinctive in both its behaviour and histological appearance.

The tumour is composed of small, angular cells with hyperchromatic nuclei and scanty cytoplasm which resemble the luminal cells of the ductal epithelium, and modified myo-epithelial cells which have scanty cytoplasm and large angular nuclei without nucleoli. The cells form strands, trabeculae and well-circumscribed nests with a cribriform growth pattern within which there are lumina and pseudolumina containing basophilic fibrillar material (hyaline balls). The latter is a combination of reduplicated basal lamina material and proteoglycans (Orenstein et al 1985). The stroma

around the islands is dense fibrous tissue. The neoplasm characteristically invades the perineural space (Sayre 1949, Dennis et al 1955, Murphy et al 1962, Abell 1963, Dodson et al 1978), has a somewhat indolent course and tends to recur locally, sometimes many years after the removal of the initial lesion (Dodson et al 1978). Metastases may also occur, although less commonly than with other forms of adenocarcinoma (Sayre 1949, Abell 1963, Addison & Parker 1977, Dodson et al 1978, Wahlström et al 1978, Leuchter et al 1982, Bernstein et al 1983b, Chapman et al 1985, Abrao et al 1985). The histogenesis of these tumours is uncertain although Addison & Parker (1977) suggest a glandular or ductal epithelial origin, an origin from myo-epithelial elements of the vasculature or embryonic elements. Dodson et al (1978) reported an adenoid cystic carcinoma of the vulva which they believed had not developed in Bartholin's gland and it is not inconceivable that such tumours may arise from small unnamed vulval glands or ectopic breast tissue.

A combined adenoid cystic and squamous carcinoma has been recently reported (Webb et al 1984). Follow-up for 43 months at the time of reporting revealed no evidence of local recurrence or metastases.

Adenocarcinoma with benign squamous metaplasia (adeno-acanthoma). Van Nagell et al (1969) described a carcinoma in which the deeper invasive elements had a tubular and glandular pattern and in which the predominant epithelial cell was columnar with a round or oval nucleus set in clear cytoplasm. The superficial layers of the tumour were said to show squamous differentiation, with a transitional zone between the two components, although the photographic evidence which they present is far from convincing. A further example, described as a poorly differentiated adeno-acanthoma, was reported in 1980 by Dennefors and Bergman. Tumours with similar histopathological features may also develop from minor unnamed vestibular glands (Janovski & Douglas 1972).

Secondary neoplasms

Bartholin's gland may also, exceptionally rarely, be the site of metastatic carcinoma or become infiltrated by non-Hodgkin's lymphoma (Plouffe et al 1984, Leiman et al 1986).

Prognosis and survival. As with the majority of malignant tumours survival depends upon the extent to which the tumour has spread at the time of diagnosis and only partly upon the histological characteristics of the neoplasm. The main determinant is the status of the inguinal and femoral lymph nodes (Leuchter et al 1982) and unfortunately many patients present when the disease is already well advanced.

At the time of treatment, 37.3 to 55% of patients have inguinal/femoral lymph node metastases (Wheelock et al 1984) and of these 18% also have pelvic node involvement. It is unusual to find pelvic nodal metastases in the absence of inguinal node disease (Leuchter et al 1982), but direct communications are said to exist between the deep portion of the gland and the pelvic lymph nodes and occasionally metastatic disease is seen in the pelvic lymph nodes in the absence of inguinal/femoral disease (Eichner 1963).

Contralateral groin nodal metastases are found in 8.5% of patients (Sackett 1965, Van Nagell et al 1969, Chamlian & Taylor 1972, Leuchter et al 1982) and 5.1% have bilateral groin metastases (Leuchter et al 1982). Leuchter and colleagues (1982) also report one instance in which the contralateral inguinal nodes contained metastatic tumour in the absence of ipsilateral metastases. A general 5-year survival rate of 35.3% is quoted by Sackett (1965) and 84% by Copeland et al (1986).

In the absence of inguinal and femoral nodal metastases, the 3-year survival is 65% and the 5-year survival is 52%, whereas if there are nodal metastases the figures fall to 54% and 36% respectively (Leuchter et al 1982). If more than two nodes contain tumour then only 32% and 18% of patients survive the 3 years and 5 years respectively (Leuchter et al 1982).

Early reports suggested that adenoid cystic carcinomas do not metastasise to the regional lymph nodes (Abell 1963), but more recently it has been shown that whilst adenoid cystic carcinomas metastasise significantly less often than do other varieties they none the less do so (Dodson et al 1978, Wahlström et al 1978, Bernstein et al 1983b) in 14.3 to 25% of cases. This contrasts with figures of 44.4% for squamous carcinomas and 31.1% for adenocarcinomas. They also show a particular tendency to recur locally if inadequately excised and to have a prolonged course before metastases develop (Addison & Parker 1977). There is statistically no significance in the difference in metastatic rates between squamous carcinomas and adenocarcinomas (Leuchter et al 1982).

Treatment. There is agreement that adequate local excision of the primary neoplasm is mandatory and that this is usually best accomplished by radical vulvectomy (Leuchter et al 1982, Wheelock et al 1984) with, if necessary to ensure tumour-free tissue margins, excision of the lower part of the vagina, anal canal, rectum, levator ani and ischiorectal fossae (Addison & Parker 1977, DiSaia & Creasman 1981). There are differences of opinion, however, on the advisability of carrying out inguinal/femoral and pelvic node dissections and upon the necessity of using adjuvant radiotherapy (Wheelock et al 1984), largely because few authors have had sufficient experience with this rather rare condition.

Leuchter et al (1982) and Wheelock et al (1984) recommend routine femoral and inguinal lymphadenectomy for all types of tumour, despite the associated morbidity, leading on to pelvic node dissection only if multiple groin nodes contain tumour, whilst the finding of pelvic nodal metastases in the absence of inguinal disease makes pelvic nodal dissection the primary choice of other authors (Barclay et al 1964, Wahlström et al 1978) who, at that same time, state that such therapy may have no overall advantage in terms of survival compared with radical vulvectomy and inguinal lymphadenectomy with postoperative radiotherapy. Occasionally, prolonged survival has followed the use of radiotherapy only in patients with extensive disease in whom their general medical state rendered them unsuitable for extensive surgery (Leuchter et al 1982).

It has been suggested that local surgery alone (Addison & Parker 1977, Schweppe & Schlake 1980) may be adequate initial therapy for patients with adenoid cystic carcinomas and certainly radiotherapy does not seem to be appropriate (Dodson et al 1978). In those patients in whom there is already metastatic disease, however, the treatment is identical to that for any other form of neoplasm. The local recurrences which may occur are treated by wide local excision.

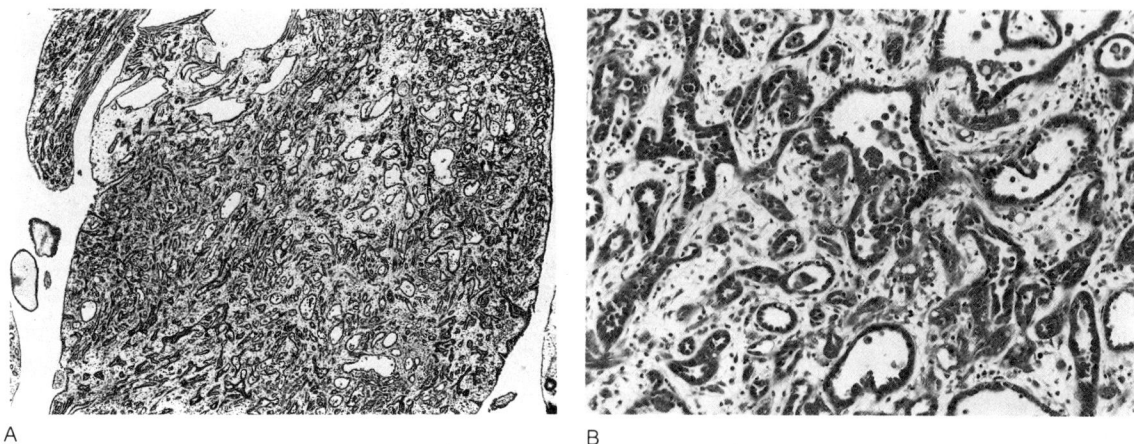

A   B

Fig. 10.46 Nephrogenic adenoma of the urethra. (**a**) A typical polypoidal lesion containing large numbers of glandular spaces of different sizes and shapes. (H & E × 25) (**b**) The glandular spaces are lined by cuboidal cells some of which have a 'hob-nailed' appearance. (H & E × 120)

URETHRAL TUMOURS

Benign neoplasms of the urethra

Benign neoplasms of the urethra are exceptionally rare. They may take the form of a so-called nephrogenic adenoma, an adenoma of Skene's glands, a transitional cell papilloma, a villous adenoma (Walker & Huffman 1947, Shield & Weiss 1973, Roberts & Melicow 1977, Peterson & Matsumoto 1978, Berger et al 1981, Howells et al 1985) or a leiomyoma (Shield & Weiss 1973).

Nephrogenic adenoma (adenomatoid tumour; mesonephroma)

A so-called adenomatoid tumour or nephrogenic adenoma is a polypoidal or papillary lesion composed of a series of small glandular spaces of varying sizes and shape, some of which are cystically dilated and contain pink amorphous material which may become focally calcified (Fig. 10.46). Some of the glands have a thick basement membrane and the lining cells, which may become rather flattened, are cuboidal and have faintly eosinophilic granular cytoplasm. The nuclei vary in size, are occasionally hyperchromatic and nucleoli may be present; mitoses are not usually seen. The lesions, which are usually found in the trigone of the male bladder, are believed to develop as a result of metaplasia in epithelium of mesonephric origin (Goldman 1972) and may form in either the urethral epithelium or in a urethral diverticulum (Goldman 1972, Sussman et al 1974, Gordon & Kerr 1975, Peterson & Matsumoto 1978). Indeed Goldman (1972) and Sussman et al (1974) prefer to regard the lesions simply as foci of metaplasia and not as neoplasms or hamartomas.

Transitional cell papilloma

Transitional cell papilloma of the urethra is described but it is doubtful whether any of these lesions should be considered as benign for they should, like similar lesions in the bladder, be regarded as of low grade malignancy and meticulous follow-up is required as recurrence or persistence may be a serious problem. They may also be associated with similar lesions elsewhere in the urinary tract (Roberts & Melicow 1977).

Villous adenoma

A papillary neoplasm resembling a villous adenoma of the large intestine may develop in the urethra (Howells et al 1985). It is composed of fine connective tissue cores covered by columnar epithelium, devoid of mucin, interspersed by mucus-containing goblet cells. Epithelial stratification and mitotic activity may be present but the lesion described by Howells et al (1985) had a benign course. It is suggested that the adenoma may develop as a consequence of metaplasia in urethral or paraurethral gland epithelium which have, in common with the rectum, a cloacogenic origin.

Leiomyoma

A small number of urethral leiomyomas presenting as a firm pink mass protruding from the urethral meatus have been described (Shield & Weiss 1973, Wani et al 1976). They usually develop in the posterior urethra but may become ulcerated as they protrude from the meatus. It has been suggested that they may develop due to the hormonal stimulus of pregnancy. Local removal proves satisfactory.

Malignant neoplasms of the urethra

Introduction

Primary carcinoma of the urethra is rare, and although more common in women than men, it still accounts for less than 1% of all malignancies developing in the female genital tract (Howe et al 1963, Grabstald et al 1966, Prempree et al 1978, 1984). The precise incidence varies, however, as it is customary, in some centres, to classify as vulval or vaginal those neoplasms which are large and develop at the urethral meatus or in the introitus respectively (Antoniades 1969).

Several types of carcinoma develop in the urethra and the site of origin within the urethra determines the histopathological pattern of the tumour, the clinical presentation and the ultimate outcome (Howe et al 1963). The extent to which the tumour has spread at the time of diagnosis, however, remains the most important prognostic factor.

Anatomy of the urethra

In its lower or distal two-thirds, the urethra is lined by stratified squamous epithelium which is in continuity below with the epithelium of the vulva. In its upper, or proximal, third the urethra is lined by transitional epithelium which is continuous at its upper end with that of the bladder. The submucosa contains the peri-urethral glands of Skene which are most frequent around the meatus but which may extend throughout its length (Walker & Huffman 1947, Levine 1980). The ducts of the glands of

Skene are lined by a pseudostratified and stratified columnar epithelium.

The lymphatic drainage of the distal urethra is, in common with that of the vulva, to the superficial and deep inguinal lymph nodes (Desai et al 1973). The proximal urethra drains to the deep pelvic chains (Desai et al 1973), that is, the external and internal liliac nodes, obturator nodes and occasionally a node over the promontory of the sacrum (Levine 1980).

Aetiology

Carcinoma of the urethra tends to occur in the older patient, the mean age at diagnosis being 63 years (Antoniades 1969, Roberts & Melicow 1977, Prempree et al 1984) though the age range is from 4 to 90 years. The tumour is more common in whites than in other ethnic groups (Levine 1980).

The cause is unknown but it has been suggested that it may be associated with chronic irritation from parturition, coitus or infection (Monaco et al 1958, Sullivan & Grabstald 1978). Although few authors have demonstrated any association between urethral carcinoma and such chronic inflammatory lesions as caruncles (Desai et al 1973). Adno (1957) noted the possibly coincidental development of a carcinoma in a caruncle and Janovski & Douglas (1972) and Roberts & Melicow (1977) describe a malignant change in the epithelium covering a caruncle. These are, however, the exception.

Transitional cell carcinoma may develop as part of a field change affecting the whole lower urinary tract in patients exposed to carcinogens (Riches & Cullen 1951, Gowing 1960, Richie & Skinner 1978) but industrial exposure such as this is less common in women than in men. On rare occasions, adenocarcinoma may develop in a urethral adenoma (Walker & Huffman 1947).

Clinical presentation

Tumours developing in the distal urethra are more common (Antoniades 1969, Roberts & Melicow 1977) and present clinically earlier than do those which arise in the proximal or upper urethra (Desai et al 1973, Levine 1980). Many of the symptoms are subtle or non-specific and only by maintaining a high level of suspicion, and adequately biopsying suspicious lesions (Desai et al 1973), can there be any real hope for a favourable clinical course which depends upon the early detection, identification and treatment of the disease.

The patient may have haematuria, urethral or vaginal bleeding, dysuria, frequency of micturition, itching, tenesmus, incontinence of urine, retention of urine, perineal pain, malodorous vaginal discharge, decreased urinary stream, difficulty in voiding urine, dyspareunia, urethrovaginal fistula, a palpable urethral mass, and on occasions, a protruding meatal mass (Ziegerman & Gordon 1970, Levine 1980). If the tumour becomes necrotic, ulcerated or infected, a malodorous discharge occurs (Walker & Huffman 1947) and in the advanced stages there may be a soft, fungating mass which bleeds easily on manipulation. Emaciation, weight loss and pelvic pain characterise the terminal stages (Knoblick 1960, Roberts & Melicow 1977).

Gross pathology

Tumours of the vulvo-urethral junction tend, as they grow, to resemble a caruncle and to form a sessile or polypoidal red nodule which may bleed on contact. Initially, as the tumour extends it grows circumferentially around the urethra which may, as a consequence, become fixed (Roberts & Melicow 1977). Later growth occurs along the urethra and down into the vulva.

Tumours arising from Skene's glands may form an indurated collar-like nodule around the meatus or protrude as a red fleshy mass from the meatus (Walker & Huffman 1947, Roberts & Melicow 1977).

Neoplasms developing in the middle and proximal thirds of the urethra may be sessile, polypoidal or papillary and may extend down to, and protrude through, the meatus (Roberts & Melicow 1977). Thus the finding of a meatal nodule does not necessarily indicate a tumour of meatal origin. Tumours of the middle third may also protrude into the vagina via a urethrovaginal fistula (Roberts & Melicow 1977) whilst neoplasms in the proximal or upper urethra tend to extend into the bladder.

Although the majority of tumours develop in the lower half of the urethra at the time of diagnosis

equal numbers affect the anterior and posterior or entire urethra (Sullivan & Grabstald 1978).

Rarely, and only in women, a carcinoma or carcinoma in situ (McLoughlin 1975) may develop in a urethral diverticulum, most often in the distal two-thirds of the urethra and only very occasionally in the proximal third (Hamilton & Leach 1951, Wishard & Nourse 1952, Hinman & Cohlan 1960, Melnick & Birdsall 1960, Wishard et al 1960, Nourse 1961, Wishard et al 1963, Grabstald et al 1966, Pathak & House 1970, Ney et al 1971, Torres & Quattlebaum 1972, Rhamy et al 1973, Marshall & Hirsch 1977, Gonzalez et al 1985). Tumours which develop in this site may protrude back into the vagina where they form a palpable lump, may be discovered as a papillary nodule within the diverticulum after surgery or may protrude from the mouth of the diverticulum into the urethral lumen (Cea et al 1977). Some tumours which are extensive at the time of diagnosis may also have originally developed in a diverticulum which has become obliterated by the growth of the neoplasm (Wishard et al 1960). The incidence of a neoplasm originating in this fashion may therefore be underestimated.

Carcinomas of the urethra spread locally to the labia, vagina (Roberts & Melicow 1977, Richie & Skinner 1978), bladder neck and peri-urethral tissue. Nodal metastases from the distal urethra occur in the superficial and deep inguinal lymph nodes (Gillenwater & Burros 1968, Desai et al 1973, Grabstald 1973), whilst those from the proximal urethra are found in the external and internal iliac nodes, obturator nodes and presacral node (Grabstald et al 1966, Desai et al 1973, Levine 1980). Distant metastases are usually a very late manifestation (Adler 1968). When they occur, their distribution corresponds to that which would be expected following haematogenous spread, that is, lungs, liver, bone and brain are most commonly affected, and Grabstald (1973) reports their presence more frequently with adenocarcinoma than with squamous carcinoma.

Lymph node metastases are more common in those patients in whom the tumour has extended to involve the whole distal half of the urethra, the proximal half of the urethra or the entire organ (Eisenstadt 1951, Antoniades 1969) than in patients in

Table 10.6 Staging of urethral carcinoma (Grabstald et al 1966, Levine 1980)

Stage 0	in situ carcinoma (limited to the urethra)	
Stage A	submucosal (limited to the mucosa and submucosa)	
Stage B	muscular (infiltrating the peri-urethral muscle)	
Stage C	peri-urethral	(i) infiltrating muscular wall of the vagina
		(ii) infiltrating the muscular wall of the vagina and the vaginal mucosa
		(iii) infiltrating other adjacent structures e.g. bladder, labia, clitoris
Stage D	metastases	(i) inguinal lymph nodes
		(ii) pelvic lymph nodes below the level of the aortic bifurcation
		(iii) lymph nodes above the aortic bifurcation
		(iv) distant

Table 10.7 Staging urethral carcinoma (Prempree et al 1984)

Stage I	disease limited to the distal half of the urethra	
Stage II	disease involves the whole urethra with extension to the peri-urethral tissues, but not involving the vulva or bladder	
Stage III	A involving urethra and vulva	
	B invading vaginal mucosa	
	C involving the urethra and bladder neck	
Stage IV	A invading parametrium or paracolpum	
	B metastases	(i) inguinal lymph nodes
		(ii) pelvic nodes
		(iii) para-aortic nodes
		(iv) distant

whom the primary tumour is limited to the meatus. They are also more frequent if the tumour has spread locally beyond the confines of the urethra. Up to 35% of patients already have nodal metastases at the time the tumour is diagnosed (Pointon & Poole-Wilson 1968).

Staging of the tumours

The carcinomas may be staged in a manner similar to that proposed for the staging of carcinoma of the male urethra (Levine 1980) (Table 10.6) or in a way which closely relates to the current methods of treatment and prognosis. The latter as described by Prempree et al (1978, 1984) is a modification of the staging outlined by Chau & Green (1965) and Taggart et al (1972) (Table 10.7).

Histopathology

Tumours at the vulvourethral junction are usually composed of a mixture of squamous and transitional epithelium whilst those that occur elsewhere in the urethra are more varied. The latter may be transitional or squamous cell carcinomas, adenocarcinomas of several types, mixed squamous/transitional cell carcinomas or undifferentiated carcinomas (Roberts & Melicow 1977).

Between 50 and 86% of the neoplasms developing in the distal half of the urethra are squamous carcinomas or contain a mixture of malignant squamous and transitional epithelium (Rogers &

Burns 1969, Skjaeraasen 1969, Desai et al 1973, Roberts & Melicow 1977, Sullivan & Grabstald 1978, Levine 1980). Adenocarcinomas are the second most common malignant neoplasms occurring in the urethra although the proportions vary in different series (Pointon & Poole-Wilson 1968, Grabstald 1973, Sullivan & Grabstald 1978); they are the predominant type in the proximal (upper) urethra (Knoblick 1960, Prempree et al 1984).

In urethral diverticula, the majority of invasive neoplasms are transitional carcinomas or adenocarcinomas and only a small proportion are squamous carcinomas (Wishard et al 1960, Nourse 1961, Spraitz & Welch 1965, Ney et al 1971, Torres & Quattlebaum 1972, Rhamy et al 1973, Cea et al 1977, Gonzalez et al 1985); transitional cell carcinoma in situ has also been described in a diverticulum (McLoughlin 1975).

A small number of urethral malignant melanomas have also been reported since the first report of such a neoplasm in 1896 (Levine 1980). Although rare, this is in fact the most common site of origin of malignant melanoma in the urinary tract (Katz & Grabstald 1976). The lesion may be pigmented or amelanotic (Monaco et al 1958). Most commonly it develops in the distal urethra or adjacent vulva and has a very poor prognosis (McBurney & Bale 1955, Monaco et al 1958, Gillenwater & Burros 1968, Pointon & Poole-Wilson 1968, Grabstald 1973, Miller & Raiman 1976, Robutti et al 1986).

Occasionally, sarcomas, lymphomas and undifferentiated carcinomas have been described (Ziegerman & Gordon 1970, Roberts & Melicow 1977) and metastatic tumours may, rarely, occur in the urethra. Roberts & Melicow (1977) describe a metastatic pulmonary carcinoma.

Transitional and squamous carcinoma. The transitional and squamous carcinomas may be papillary or solid. At one end of the spectrum, fine fibrovascular cores are covered by transitional or squamous epithelium showing varying degrees of cytological atypia, or by a mixture of squamous and transitional epithelium; at the other end of the spectrum, a solid, infiltrative carcinoma of mixed or pure cell type is found. Such tumours are often associated with, or are preceded by, an intra-epithelial neoplasm (Miller & Raiman 1976).

Adenocarcinomas. Approximately 10% of urethral adenocarcinomas are mucin secreting (Ney et al 1971, Rhamy et al 1973, Klotz 1974) and typically these develop from Skene's glands. Although an origin from urethritis cystica and glandularis has been observed in a male patient (Posso et al 1961) and a possible origin from ectopic cloacal cells of gut-like epithelium or from Gärtner's duct has been suggested (Hinman & Cohlan 1960, Marshall & Hirsch 1977). It is unlikely in fact that mucus-secreting tumours have an origin in Gärtner's duct but the clear-cell carcinoma described below may well have such a histogenesis.

Tumours developing from Skene's glands. These tumours consist of simple, often dilated, glands lined by cubocolumnar epithelium with mucin-containing cytoplasm; nuclear pleomorphism and mitoses are seen. The stroma is vascular connective tissue and smooth muscle (Nichol 1941, Walker & Huffman 1947, Knoblick 1960, Schnitzer 1964). The tumours are said to resemble those of the prostate of which Skene's glands are a homologue (Roberts & Melicow 1977, Svanholm et al 1987).

Signet-ring tumours. Exceptionally, signet-ringed (Menville & Counseller 1935, Klotz 1974) and mucoid forms are seen. The former is composed entirely of sheets of signet-ring cells or of pools of mucus-containing signet-ring cells and the latter of clusters of poorly differentiated adenocarcinoma cells, occasionally forming gland-like structures, lying in pools of mucus (Menville & Counseller 1935, Walker & Huffman 1947, De Haan & Johnson 1960, Helwig & Graham 1963).

Clear-cell 'mesonephroid' carcinoma. Tumours resembling those occurring in structures of Müllerian origin and ovary (Novak et al 1954) or Wolffian ducts, develop both in the urethral lumen (Adler 1968, Konnak 1973, Murayama et al 1978, Peven & Hidvegi 1985, Young & Scully 1985) and in urethral diverticula (Hinman & Cohlan 1960, Cea et al 1977, Tanabe et al 1982). Their histogenesis is unclear but the tumours are thought possibly to develop from mesonephric embryonal rests (Cea et al 1977, Peven & Hidvegi 1985), from mesonephric-associated intermediate mesoderm (Konnak 1973) or from some other congenital anomaly which also leads to the formation of the diverticulum (Hinman & Cohlan 1960, Spraitz & Welsh 1965). Electron optic studies (Tanabe et al 1982) have shown a similarity to the clear cells of the Müllerian carcinoma but the cells have long slender, closely packed microvilli on their luminal surfaces, unlike those of the Müllerian clear-cell carcinoma, which are short and blunt.

Typically the clear-cell carcinoma is composed of tubules, cysts or papillae with fine, vascular connective tissue cores covered by round or cuboidal, focally 'hob-nailed' cells with clear cytoplasm, distinct cell borders and moderately pleomorphic, large hyperchromatic nuclei with prominent nucleoli. The epithelium also forms clusters and buds into the interpapillary spaces; in some tumours the cells form sheets (Tanabe et al 1982). There may be intracellular glycogen or a trace of intracytoplasmic mucin (Cea et al 1977) whilst other tumours are PAS, alcian blue and mucicarmine negative demonstrating the absence of both glycogen and mucin (Cea et al 1977, Tanabe et al 1982). The mesonephric carcinoma described by Konnak (1973), whilst clearly illustrated as a clear-celled tumour, has none of the typical 'hob-nailed' cells characteristic of the mesonephroid carcinoma; indeed it is composed of tall, columnar cells with clear cytoplasm.

Prognosis

It is important to diagnose malignant disease of the urethra at an early stage when it is amenable to treatment because, overall, only 21.5% of patients with urethral carcinoma survive for 5 years (Ziegerman & Gordon 1970, Bracken et al 1976). A high level of suspicion and adequate biopsy are therefore essential if the early case is not to be missed (Desai et al 1973).

Patients in whom the disease is limited to the distal urethra may have a 100% 5-year survival when treated adequately (Prempree et al 1984), largely because distal lesions, by nature of their position of origin, are noticed earlier and inguinal node metastases are therefore unusual at the time of presentation. Involvement of the vulva or vagina does not adversely affect this favourable prognosis in some series (Prempree et al 1978) but in others it is highly detrimental (Chu 1973). If the tumour involves the whole urethra, however, or even the proximal urethra only, at the time of diagnosis, the outlook is grim, with only about 10% of patients surviving for 5 years (Ziegerman & Gordon 1970, Grabstald 1973). When the tumour is large (Rogers & Burns 1969), more than 3 cm in diameter, or has extended to the adjacent structures, stage III (Prempree et al 1984) or stage C (Levine 1980), there is an increased risk that nodal metastases will have already developed (Gradstald et al 1966, Bracken et al 1976, Prempree et al 1978, Turner & Hendry 1980).

Clinically, understaging is also a problem and may lead to inadequate therapy and therefore an unexpectedly poor result. This is a particular hazard when assessing the extent to which the tumour has infiltrated the neck of the bladder (Prempree et al 1984). It is recognised that if tumour involves the bladder, bladder neck, parametrium, or inguinal nodes, the prognosis is poor (Prempree et al 1978, 1984).

Opinions are divided as to the prognostic importance of histological types. There is a general belief that the histopathological type does not influence the outcome (Riches & Cullen 1951, Bracken et al 1976) when adjustments are made for the clinical stage and size of lesion at the time of diagnosis. Ziegerman & Gordon (1970), however, record that patients with adenocarcinoma do rather better than those with squamous carcinoma, as do Bracken et al (1972), but the latter are at pains to point out that the majority of adenocarcinomas in their series presented in early stage. The poor prognosis attributed by other authors to adenocarcinomas (Marshall & Hirsch 1977) may be related to their presence in the proximal urethra where prognosis is generally rather poor. Adenocarcinomas which develop in urethral diverticula may, however, be an exception in that patients with adenocarcinoma of a urethral diverticulum fare better than those with either transitional or squamous carcinomas arising in the

same site (Cea et al 1977) and well differentiated carcinomas in a diverticulum do better than poorly differentiated ones (Gonzalez et al 1985).

Treatment

Treatment is based upon the location and extent of the disease at the time of diagnosis and not upon the histological type.

Tumours which affect only the distal one-third of the urethra can be regarded as suitable for local treatment. Those affecting more than the distal one-third should, for the purposes of therapy, be regarded as involving the entire urethra (Grabstald et al 1966, Grabstald 1973).

Treatment of the distal lesions may be by definitive radiotherapy (Levine 1980, Prempree et al 1984) or by partial urethrectomy (Levine 1980). Results for these procedures are good in early stage disease and up to two-thirds of the urethra can be removed surgically without causing serious incontinence; however, it may also be necessary in these distal lesions to carry out a partial vulvectomy to clear the lower margins of the tumour (Levine 1980).

In patients with more advanced disease, surgery plus radiotherapy is usually indicated (Prempree et al 1984). Pre-operative radiation is given to reduce local recurrence, followed by exenterative surgery with or without vulvectomy and pelvic lymphadenectomy (Levine 1980). The role of chemotherapy has not yet been evaluated.

There are differences of opinion regarding the advisability of prophylactic lymphadenectomy in the treatment of urethral carcinoma, it being regarded as contra-indicated by Levine (1980). Removal of lymph nodes affected by metastatic disease is, however, recommended and it is useful when planning treatment to note that the presence of enlarged lymph nodes is almost always the consequence of metastatic disease rather than infection (Grabstald et al 1966, Grabstald 1973, Levine 1980) None the less, Desai et al (1973) recommends carrying out preliminary biopsy of the inguinal nodes prior to definitive treatment because of the morbidity associated with dissection of the groin nodes and their finding of metastases in only two of their six patients with palpable nodes.

Clear-cell carcinoma arising in the vagina and

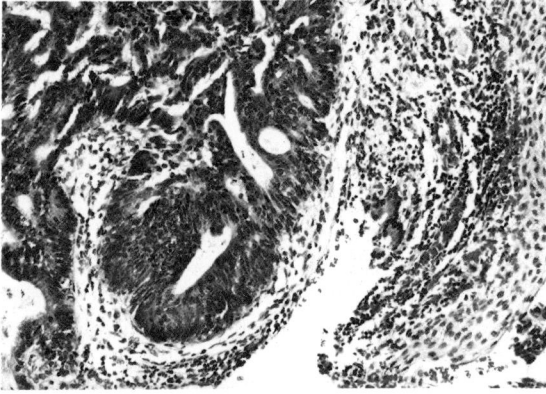

Fig. 10.47 Metastatic colonic adenocarcinoma of the vulva.
(H & E × 120)

cervix appears to be insensitive to radiotherapy
(Robboy et al 1974, Noller et al 1976) and very
limited experience with clear-cell adenocarcinoma
of the urethra suggests that this may also be true
for these tumours. Anterior exenteration or cysto-
urethrectomy appears to offer the best hope of a
cure (Tanabe et al 1982).

Malignant melanoma of the urethra is usually
treated by radiotherapy (Katz & Grabstald 1976,
Levine 1980) followed by radical surgery despite
the resistance of melanoma to radiotherapy.
Surgery may be followed by chemotherapy (Turner
& Hendry 1980) or local radiotherapy may be aug-
mented by cryosurgery (Grabstald 1973). Whatever the mode of treatment, the outlook is distinctly poor (Grabstald 1973, Turner & Hendry 1980).

MISCELLANEOUS MALIGNANT NEOPLASMS

Cloacogenic carcinoma (basaloid carcinoma)

This is a rare malignant neoplasm of the vulva
which forms a firm nodular tumour deep in the
labium major, rectovaginal septum or perineum
and which may cause pain on defaecation or dyspareunia. It is believed to develop in these sites
from epithelial rests or remnants of the urogenital
sinus or cloaca (Janovski & Douglas 1972, Ferenczy
1981). It may also develop from the transitional
epithelium of the anal canal or excretory duct of
Bartholin's gland.

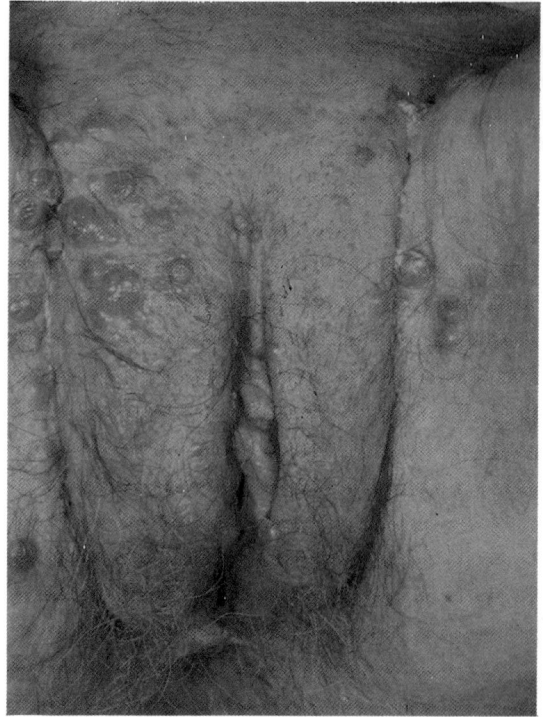

Fig. 10.48 Metastatic deposits (ovarian). (Reproduced from
Beilby and Ridley 1987 by courtesy of the authors and
publisher)

The tumour is composed of cells which on electron optic examination resemble the basal cells of
the squamous epithelium forming solid nests in
which foci of squamous and glandular differentiation may be seen. This latter finding has led some
to suggest that adenosquamous carcinoma of the
vulva may develop from this source (Rhatigan &
Mojadidi 1973) and, indeed, two of the adenosquamous carcinomas they described developed
deep in the labia majora in the region of Bartholin's
gland.

In general, cloacogenic carcinoma has a poor
prognosis and a tendency to metastasise early
(Ferenczy 1981).

Metastatic tumours of the vulva

Metastases occur to the vulva most frequently from
primary neoplasms of the cervix, endometrium,
vagina, ovary, urethra, kidney, breast, rectum
or lung (Fig. 10.47) (Dehner 1973; Mader &

Friedrich 1982) and, in addition to these predominantly adenocarcinomatous tumours, choriocarcinoma, melanoma and Burkitt's lymphoma may also metastasise to this site (Novak & Woodruff 1979, Egwuata et al 1980, Ferenczy 1981). It is not unusual for the metastatic lesion and the primary neoplasm to be diagnosed simultaneously; indeed, this happened in 27% of Dehner's (1973) cases.

Vulval metastases are found most commonly in the dermis or subcutaneous tissue of the labia majora or around the clitoris. They are composed of homogenous grey or reddish tissue and, whilst there is commonly only one nodule, it is not unusual to find several (Ferenczy 1981) (Fig. 10.48). Dehner (1973) noticed a tendency for metastatic

adenocarcinoma to invade the epidermis whilst metastatic squamous carcinoma remained within the dermis and subcutaneous tissue. An expansile growth pattern, multiple lesions and the absence of an intra-epithelial neoplastic component all argue in favour of a diagnosis of metastatic rather than primary tumour (Mader & Friedrich 1982). On rare occasions metastatic tumour in the vulva may present a clinical picture mimicking that of cellulitis, the skin becoming painful and red; this is the so-called inflammatory carcinoma (Hoogerland & Buchler 1979). The appearance of vulval metastases is associated with a very poor outlook indicating, as it does, disseminated malignancy.

REFERENCES

Abaci I F, Zak F G 1979 Multicentric amyloid containing cutaneous trabecular carcinoma. Case report with ultrastructural study. Journal of Cutaneous Pathology 6: 292–303

Abell M R 1963 Adenocystic (pseudoadenomatous) basal cell carcinoma of vestibular glands of vulva. American Journal of Obstetrics and Gynecology 86: 470–482

Abell M R 1965 Intraepithelial carcinomas of epidermis and squamous mucosa of vulva and perineum. Surgical Clinics of North America 45: 1179–1198

Abell M R, Gosling J R G 1961 Intraepithelial and infiltrative carcinoma of the vulva: Bowen's type. Cancer 14: 318–329

Abrao F S et al 1985 Adenoid cystic carcinoma of Bartholin's gland: review of the literature and report of two cases. Journal of Surgical Oncology 30: 132–137

Ackerman A B, Mihara I 1985 Dysplasia, dysplastic melanocytes, dysplastic nevi, the dysplastic nevus syndrome, and the relation between dysplastic nevi and malignant melanomas. Human Pathology 16: 87–91

Ackles R C, Pratt J P 1956 Basal cell carcinoma of the vulva. American Journal of Obstetrics and Gynecology 72: 1124–1126

Addison A 1977 Adenocarcinoma of Bartholin's gland in a 14 year-old girl. Report of a case. American Journal of Obstetrics and Gynecology 127: 214–215

Addison A, Parker R T 1977 Adenoid cystic carcinoma of Bartholin's gland: A review of the literature and report of a patient. Gynecologic Oncology 5: 196–201

Adler M 1968 Bericht über ein primäres Carcinoma urethrae als Beitrag zur Problematik der gynäkologisch-urologischen Grenzfälle. Zentralblatt für Gynäkologie 90: 123–124

Adno J 1957 Primary carcinoma of the female urethra with special reference to the urethral caruncle. British Journal of Urology 29: 52–57

Advani H, Waldo E D, Bigelow B 1978 Bartholin's gland carcinoma: an ultrastructural study. American Journal of Obstetrics and Gynecology 130: 362–364

Ambrosini L, Becagli L, Resta P 1980 Basal cell carcinoma of vulva. European Journal of Gynaecologic Oncology 1: 126–128

Andreasson B, Bock J E 1985 Intraepithelial neoplasia in the vulvar region. Gynecologic Oncology 21: 300–305

Andreasson B, Nyboe J 1985 Value of prognostic parameters in squamous cell carcinoma of the vulva. Gynecologic Oncology 22: 341–351

Andreasson B, Bock J E, Visfeldt J 1982 (a) Prognostic role of histology in squamous cell carcinoma in the vulvar region. Gynecologic Oncology 14: 373–381

Andreasson B, Bock J E, Weberg E 1982 (b) Invasive cancer in the vulvar region. Acta Obstetricia et Gynecologica Scandinavica 61: 113–119

Anthony P P, Freeman K, Warin A P 1986 Case reports: Extramammary Paget's disease. Clinical and Experimental Dermatology 11: 387–395

Antoniades J 1969 Radiation therapy in carcinoma of the female urethra. Cancer 24: 70–76

Axe S, Parmley T, Woodruff J D, Hlopak B 1986 Adenomas in minor vestibular glands. Obstetrics and Gynecology 68: 16–18

Baes H, Suurmond D 1970 Apocrine sweat gland carcinoma. British Journal of Dermatology 83: 483–486

Barclay D L, Collins C G, Macey H B Jr 1964 Cancer of the Bartholin's gland: A review and report of 8 cases. Obstetrics and Gynecology 24: 329–336

Barnes A E, Crissman J D, Schellhas H F, Azoury R S 1980 Microinvasive carcinoma of the vulva: a clinicopathologic evaluation. Obstetrics and Gynecology 56: 234–238

Battifora H 1976 Spindle cell carcinoma. Ultrastructural evidence of squamous origin and collagen production by the tumor cells. Cancer 37: 2275–2282

Bean S F, Becker F T 1968 Basal cell carcinoma of the vulva. A case report and review of the literature. Archives of Dermatology 98: 284–286

Becker S W, Brennan B, Weichselbaum P K 1960 Genital Paget's disease. Archives of Dermatology 82: 857–865

Beecham C T 1976 Paget's disease of the vulva. Obstetrics and Gynecology 47: 55S–58S

Beilby J O W, Ridley C M 1987 Pathology of the vulva. In: Fox H (ed) Haines' and Taylor's Obstetrical and Gynaecological pathology, 3rd edn. Churchill Livingstone, Edinburgh

Belcher R W 1972 Extramammary Paget's disease. Enzyme histochemical and electron microscopic study. Archives of Pathology 94: 59–64

Benedet J L, Murphy K J 1982 Squamous carcinoma *in situ* of the vulva. Gynecologic Oncology 14: 213–219

Benedet J L, Turko M, Fairey R N, Boyes D A 1979 Squamous carcinoma of the vulva: results of treatment 1938–1976. American Journal of Obstetrics and Gynecology 134: 201–207

Berg J W, McDivitt R W 1968 Pathology of sweat gland carcinoma. Pathology Annual 3: 123–144

Berger B W, Bhagavan S B S, Reiner W, Engel R, Lepor H 1981 Nephrogenic adenoma: clinical features and therapeutic considerations. Journal of Urology 126: 824–826

Bergeron C, Naghashfar Z, Canaan C, Shah K, Fu Y, Ferenczy A 1987 Human papillomavirus type 16 in intraepithelial neoplasia (Bowenoid papulosis) and coexistent invasive carcinoma of the vulva. International Journal of Gynecological Pathology 6: 1–11

Bernstein S G, Kovacs B R, Townsend D E, Morrow C P 1983a Vulvar carcinoma in situ. Obstetrics and Gynecology 61: 304–307

Bernstein S G, Voet R L, Lifshitz S, Buchsbaum, H J 1983b Adenoid cystic carcinoma of Bartholin's gland. Case report and review of the literature. American Journal of Obstetrics and Gynecology 147: 385–390

Bhawan J 1980 Multicentric pigmented Bowen's disease: a clinically benign squamous carcinoma *in situ*. Gynecologic Oncology 10: 201–205

Boehm B, Morris J McL 1971 Paget's disease and apocrine gland carcinoma of the vulva. Obstetrics and Gynecology 38: 185–192

Borel D M 1973 Cutaneous basosquamous carcinoma. Review of the literature and report of 35 cases. Archives of Pathology 95: 293–295

Bottles K, Lacey C G, Goldberg J, Lanner-Cusin K, Hom J, Miller T R 1984 Merkel cell carcinoma of the vulva. Obstetrics and Gynecology 63 (Supp 3): 61S–65S

Boughton T G 1943 Carcinoma of Bartholin's gland. American Journal of Surgery 59: 585–591

Bouma J, Weening J J, Elders A 1982 Malignant melanoma of the vulva: report of 18 cases. European Journal of Obstetrics and Gynaecology and Reproductive Biology 13: 237–251

Boutselis J G 1972 Intraepithelial carcinoma of the vulva. American Journal of Obstetrics and Gynecology 113: 733–738

Boyce J, Fruchter R G, Kasambilides E, Nicastri A D, Sedlis A, Remy J C 1985 Prognostic factors in carcinoma of the vulva. Gynecologic Oncology 20: 364–377

Bozzetti F, Cascinelli N, Cataldo I, Lupi G 1975 Prognosi del melanoma della vulva. Tumori 61: 393–399

Bracken R B, Johnson D E, Miller L S, Ayala A G, Gomez J J, Rutledge F 1976. Primary carcinoma of the female urethra. Journal of Urology 116: 188–192

Breen J L, Neubecker R D, Greenwald E, Gregori C A 1975 Basal cell carcinoma of the vulva. Obstetrics and Gynecology 46: 122–129

Breen J L, Smith C I, Gregori C A 1978 Extramammary Paget's disease. Clinical Obstetrics and Gynecology 21: 1107–1115

Breslow A 1970 Thickness, cross-sectional areas, and depth of invasion in the prognosis of cutaneous melanoma. Annals of Surgery 172: 902–908

Briggs J C 1985 Melanoma precursor lesions and borderline melanomas. Histopathology 9: 1251–1262

Brooks S M 1943 Carcinoma which simulates sarcoma. A study of 110 specimens from various sites. Archives of Pathology 36: 144–157

Brown S M, Freeman R G 1971 Syringoma limited to the vulva. Archives of Dermatology 104: 331

Brownstein M H, Shapiro L 1975 The sweat gland adenomas. International Journal of Dermatology 14: 397–411

Brunschwig A, Brockunier A Jr 1967 Surgical treatment of squamous-cell carcinoma of the vulva. Obstetrics and Gynecology 29: 362–368

Buchler D A, Sun F, Chuprevich T 1978 A pilar tumor of the vulva. Gynecologic Oncology 6: 479–486

Buckley C H, Butler E B, Fox H 1982 Cervical intraepithelial neoplasia. Journal of Clinical Pathology 35: 1–13

Buckley C H, Butler E B, Fox H 1984 Vulvar intraepithelial neoplasia and microinvasive carcinoma of the vulva. Journal of Clinical Pathology 37: 1201–1211

Burghardt E 1984 Microinvasive tumours of the female genital tract. Clinical Obstetrics and Gynecology 11: 239–257

Buscema J, Woodruff J D 1980 Progressive histobiologic alterations in the development of vulvar cancer. Report of five cases. American Journal of Obstetrics and Gynecology 138: 146–150

Buscema J, Stern J, Woodruff J D 1980a The significance of the histologic alteration adjacent to invasive vulvar carcinoma. American Journal of Obstetrics and Gynecology 137: 902–909

Buscema J, Woodruff J D, Parmley T H, Genadry R 1980b Carcinoma in situ of the vulva. Obstetrics and Gynecology 55: 225–230

Buscema J, Stern J L, Woodruff J D 1981 Early invasive carcinoma of the vulva. American Journal of Obstetrics and Gynecology 140: 563–569

Cabral G A, Marciano-Cabral F, Fry D, Lumpkin C K, Mercer L, Goplerud D 1982 Expression of herpes simplex virus type 2 antigens in premalignant and malignant human vulvar cells. American Journal of Obstetrics and Gynecology 143: 611–619

Cabrera H N, Cuda G, Lopez M, Costa J A 1984 Epitelioma basocelular de vulva en hacre. Medicina Cutanea Iber-Latino Americana 12: 81–85

Caccialanza M, Altomare G, Finzi A F 1979 Neoplasie cutanee multiple successive a ripetuti esami fluoroscopici. Radiological Medicine 65: 317–320

Caglar H, Tamer S, Hreshchysmn M M 1982 Vulvar intraepithelial neoplasia. Obstetrics and Gynecology 60: 346–349

Camisa C, Weissmann A 1982 Friedrich Sigmund Merkel. Part II. The cell. American Journal of Dermatopathology 4: 527–535

Cario G M, House M J, Paradinas F J 1984 Squamous cell carcinoma of the vulva in association with mixed vulvar dystrophy in an 18-year-old girl. Case report. British Journal of Obstetrics and Gynaecology 91: 87–90

Carneiro S J C, Gardner H L, Knox J M 1971 Syringoma of the vulva. Archives of Dermatology 103: 494–496

Carneiro S J C, Gardner H L, Knox J M 1972 Syringoma: Three cases with vulvar involvement. Obstetrics and Gynecology 39: 95–99

Carstens P H B Broghamer W L 1978 Duodenal carcinoid with cytoplasmic whorls of microfilaments. Journal of Pathology 124: 235–238

Cea P C, Ward J N, Lavengood R W, Gray G F 1977 Mesonephric adenocarcinomas in urethral diverticula. Urology 10: 58–61

Chamberlain G 1981 Aetiology of gynaecological cancer. Journal of the Royal Society of Medicine 74: 246–261

Chamlian D L, Taylor H B 1972 Primary carcinoma of Bartholin's gland: A report of 24 patients. Obstetrics and Gynecology 39: 489–494

Chapman G W Jr, Benda J B, Lifshitz S 1985 Adenoid cystic carcinoma of the vulva with lung metastases. A case report. Journal of Reproductive Medicine 30: 217–220

Charles A H 1972 Carcinoma of the vulva. British Medical Journal 1: 397–402

Charlewood G P, Shippel S 1953 Vulval condyloma acuminata as a premalignant lesion in the Bantu. South African Medical Journal 27: 149–151

Chau P M, Green A E 1965 Radiotherapeutic management of malignant tumors of the vagina. Progress in Clinical Cancer 1: 728–750

Choo Y C, Morley G W 1980 Double primary epidermoid carcinoma of the vulva and cervix. Gynecologic Oncology 9: 324–333

Christensen W N, Friedman K J, Woodruff J D, Hood A F 1987 Histologic characteristics of vulvar nevocellular nevi. Journal of Cutaneous Pathology 14: 87–91

Chu A M 1973 Female urethra carcinoma. Radiology 107: 627–630

Chu J, Tamimi H K, Ek M, Figge D C 1982 Stage I vulvar cancer: criteria for microinvasion. Obstetrics and Gynecology 59: 716–719

Chung A F, Woodruff J M, Lewis J L 1975 Malignant melanoma of the vulva: a report of 44 cases. Obstetrics and Gynecology 45: 638–646

Clark W H, From L, Bernardino E A, Mihm M C 1969 The histogenesis and biologic behaviour of primary human malignant melanomas of the skin. Cancer Research 29: 705–727

Cleophax J P, Pelleron J P, Durand J C, Lourant M 1977 Le mélanome de la vulve. Gynecologie 27: 333–339

Collins C G, Roman-Lopez J J, Lee F Y L 1970 Intraepithelial carcinoma of the vulva. American Journal of Obstetrics and Gynecology 108: 1187–1191

Connors R C, Ackerman A B 1976 Histologic pseudomalignancies of the skin. Archives of Dermatology 112: 1767–1780

Connors R C, Ackerman A B 1979 Pseudomalignancies. In: Helm F (ed) Cancer dermatology. Lea & Febiger, Philadelphia, p 285–310

Cook M G, Robertson I 1985 Melanocytic dysplasia and melanoma. Histopathology 9: 647–658

Copas P, Comas F V, Dyer M, Hall D J 1982 Spindle cell carcinoma of the vulva. Diagnostic Gynecology and Obstetrics 4: 235–241

Copeland L J, Cleary K, Sneige N, Edwards C L 1985 Neuroendocrine (Merkel cell) carcinoma of the vulva: a case report and review of the literature. Gynecologic Oncology 22: 367–378

Copeland L J, Sneige N, Gershenson D M, McGuffee V B, Abdul-Karim F, Rutledge F N 1986 Bartholin gland carcinoma. Obstetrics and Gynecology 67: 794–801

Creasman W T, Gallager H S, Rutledge F 1975 Paget's disease of the vulva. Gynecologic Oncology 3: 133–148

Crissman J D, Azoury R S 1981 Microinvasive carcinoma of the vulva. A report of two cases with regional lymph node metastasis. Diagnostic Gynecology and Obstetrics 3: 75–80

Crossen R J 1948 Primary carcinoma of Bartholin's gland. American Journal of Surgery 75: 597–600

Crum C P 1982 a Vulvar intraepithelial neoplasia: the concept and its application. Human Pathology 13: 187–189

Crum C P, Fu Y S, Levine R U, Richart R M, Townsend D E, Fenoglio C M 1982 b Intraepithelial squamous lesions of the vulva: biologic and histologic criteria for the distinction of condylomas from vulvar intraepithelial neoplasia. American Journal of Obstetrics and Gynecology 144: 77–83

Crum C P, Liskow A, Petras P, Keng W C, Frick H C 1984 Vulvar intraepithelial neoplasia (severe atypia and carcinoma in situ). Cancer 54: 1429–1434

Cruz-Jimenez P R, Abell M R 1975 Cutaneous basal cell carcinoma of the vulva. Cancer 36: 1860–1868

Curry S L, Wharton J T, Rutledge F 1980 Positive lymph nodes

in vulvar squamous carcinoma. Gynecologic Oncology 9: 63–67

Dabska M 1971 Giant hair matrix tumour. Cancer 28: 701–706

Daling J R, Chu J, Weiss N S, Emel L, Tamini H K 1984 The association of condylomata acuminata and squamous carcinoma of the vulva. British Journal of Cancer 50: 533–535

Degefu S, O'Quinn A G, Dhurandhar H N 1986 Paget's disease of the vulva and urogenital malignancies: a case report and review of the literature. Gynecologic Oncology 25: 347–354

De Haan Q C, Johnson C G 1960 Adenocarcinoma of paraurethral glands. American Journal of Obstetrics and Gynecology 80: 1108–1110

Dehner L P 1973 Metastatic and secondary tumors of the vulva. Obstetrics and Gynecology 42: 47–57

Demian S D E, Bushkin F L, Echevarria R A 1973 Perineural invasion and anaplastic transformation of verrucous carcinoma. Cancer. 32: 395–401

Demopoulos R I 1971 Fine structure of the extramammary Paget's cell. Cancer 27: 1202–1210

Dennefors B, Bergman B 1980 Primary carcinoma of the Bartholin gland. Acta Obstetricia et Gynecologica Scandinavica 59: 95–96

Dennis E J, Hester L L Jr, Wilson L A 1955 Primary carcinoma of Bartholin's glands. Review; report of a case. Obstetrics and Gynecology 6: 291–296

Deppisch L M 1978 Basal cell carcinoma of the vulva. Mt Sinai Journal of Medicine 45: 406–410

Desai S, Libertino J A, Zinman L 1973 Primary carcinoma of the female urethra. Journal of Urology 110: 693–695

De Wolf-Peeters C, Marien K, Mebis J, Desmet V 1980 A cutaneous APUDoma or Merkel cell tumor? A morphologically recognizable tumor with a biological and histological malignant aspect in contrast with its clinical behavior. Cancer 46: 1810–1816

DiPaola G R, Gomez-Rueda N, Arrighi L 1975 Relevance of microinvasion in carcinoma of the vulva. Obstetrics and Gynecology 45: 647–649

DiPaola G R, Rueda-Leverone N G, Belardi M G, Vighi S 1982 Vulvar carcinoma in situ: a report of 28 cases. Gynecologic Oncology 14: 236–242

DiSaia P J, Creasman W T 1981 Clinical gynecologic oncolgy. C V Mosby, St Louis, p 185–206

DiSaia P J, Creasman W T, Rich W M 1979 An alternate approach to early cancer of the vulva. American Journal of Obstetrics and Gynecology 133: 825–832

Dissanayake R V P, Salm R 1980 Sweat-gland carcinomas: prognosis related to histological type. Histopathology 4: 445–466

Dockerty M B, Pratt J H 1952 Extramammary Paget's disease. A report of four cases in which certain features of histogenesis were exhibited. Cancer 5: 1161–1169

Dodson M G, O'Leary J A, Averette H E 1970 Primary carcinoma of Bartholin's gland. Obstetrics and Gynecology 35: 578–584

Dodson M G, O'Leary J A, Orfei E 1978 Adenoid cystic carcinoma of the vulva. Malignant cylindroma. Obstetrics and Gynecology 51: 26S–29S

Domonkos A N, Arnold H L, Odom R B 1982 Epidermal nevi and tumors. In: Andrews' diseases of the skin. Clinical dermatology. W B Saunders, Philadelphia, p 792–858

Donaldson E S, Powell D E, Hanson M B, van Nagell J R 1981 Prognostic parameters in invasive vulvar cancer. Gynecologic Oncology 11: 184–190

Donna A, Torchio B, Lampertico P 1978 L'idroadenoma papillifero della vulva: contributo casistico e revisione della letteratura. Pathologica 70: 359–375

Douglas C P 1983 Vulvar dystrophies. In: Studd J (ed) Progress in obstetrics and gynaecology, Vol. 3. Churchill Livingstone, Edinburgh, p 166–212

Dubreuilh W 1901 Paget's disease of the vulva. British Journal of Dermatology 13: 407–413

Dudzinski M R, Askin F B, Fowler W C 1984 Giant basal cell carcinoma of the vulva. Obstetrics and Gynecology 63: 57S–60S

Dunn A E G, Ogilvie M M 1968 Intranuclear virus particles in human genital wart tissue: observations on the ultrastructure of the epidermal layer. Journal of Ultrastructure Research 22: 282–295

Edington P T, Monaghan J M 1980 Malignant melanoma of the vulva and vagina. British Journal of Obstetrics and Gynaecology 87: 422–424

Egwuata V E, Ejeckman G C, Okaro J M 1980 Burkitt's lymphoma of the vulva. Case report. British Journal of Obstetrics and Gynaecology 87: 827–830

Eichenberg 1934 Cited by Miller 1967

Eichner E 1957 In vivo studies on the pelvic lymphatics in women. Progress in Gynecology 3: 604–619

Eichner E 1963 Adenoid cystic carcinoma of the Bartholin gland. Obstetrics and Gynecology 21: 608–613

Eisenstadt J S 1951 Primary carcinoma of the female urethra. American Journal of Surgery 81: 612–617

El-Domeiri A A, Brasfield R D, Huvos A G, Strong E W 1971 Sweat gland carcinoma: A clinico-pathologic study of 83 patients. Annals of Surgery 173: 270–274

El-Domeiri A A, Huvos A G, Beattie E J Jr 1972 Sweat gland carcinoma arising in irradiated skin. American Journal of Roentgenology 114: 606–609

English K B 1977 Morphogenesis of Haarscheiben in rats. Journal of Investigative Dermatology 69: 58–67

Farmer E R, Helwig E B 1980 Metastatic basal cell carcinoma. Cancer 46: 748–757

Fenn M E, Abell M R 1973 Melanoma of vulva and vagina. Obstetrics and Gynecology 41: 902–911

Fenn M E, Morley G W, Abell M R 1971 Paget's disease of vulva. Obstetrics and Gynecology 38: 660–670

Ferenczy A 1981 Pathology of malignant tumors of the vulva and vagina. In: Coppleson M (ed) Gynecologic oncology. Churchill Livingstone, Edinburgh

Ferenczy A, Richart R M 1972 Ultrastructure of perineal Paget's disease. Cancer 29: 1141–1149

Fetherston W C, Friedrich E G Jr 1972 The origin and significance of vulvar Paget's disease. Obstetrics and Gynecology 39: 735–744

Figge D C, Gaudenz R 1974 Invasive carcinoma of the vulva. American Journal of Obstetrics and Gynecology 119: 382–394

Fisher E R, McCoy M M, Wechsler H L 1972 Analysis of histopathologic and electron microscopic determinants of keratoacanthoma and squamous cell carcinoma. Cancer 29: 1387–1397

Ford L C, Berek J S, Lagasse L D, Hacker N F, Heins Y L, Delange R J 1983 Estrogen and progesterone receptor sites in malignancies of the uterine cervix, vagina and vulva. Gynecologic Oncology 15: 27–31

Forney J P, Morrow C P, Townsend D E, DiSaia P J 1977 Management of carcinoma in situ of the vulva. American Journal of Obstetrics and Gynecology 127: 801–806

Fox H, Buckley C H 1982 Pathology for gynaecologists. Edward Arnold, London, p 104–105

Fox H 1986 Carcinoma verrugosa de la vulva. In: Gonzalez M J, Guiu J I, Burzaco I (eds) Advances en Obstetricia y Ginecologica. Salvatores Editores, Barcelona, p 127–134

Frable W J, Goplerud D R 1975 Adenoid cystic carcinoma of Bartholin's gland. Diagnosis by aspiration biopsy. Acta Cytologica 19: 152–153

Franklin E W III, Rutledge F D 1971 Prognostic factors in epidermoid carcinoma of the vulva. Obstetrics and Gynecology 37: 892–901

Freeman R G, Winkelmann R K 1969 Basal cell tumor with eccrine differentiation (Eccrine epithelioma). Archives of Dermatology 100: 234–242

Friedman R J, Ackerman A B 1981 Difficulties in the histologic diagnoses of melanocytic nevi on the vulvae of premenopausal women. In: Ackerman A B (ed) Pathology of Malignant Melanoma. Masson, New York 8: 119–127

Friedrich E G 1972a Reversible vulvar atypia: a case report. Obstetrics and Gynecology 39: 173–181

Friedrich E G 1972b Vulvar carcinoma in situ in identical twins. An occupational hazard. Obstetrics and Gynecology 39: 837–841

Friedrich E G 1976 New nomenclature for vulvar disease. Report of the committee on terminology. Obstetrics and Gynecology 47: 122–124

Friedrich E G 1981 Intraepithelial neoplasia of the vulva. In Coppleson M (ed) Gynecologic oncology. Churchill Livingstone, Edinburgh, p 303–319

Friedrich E G, Wilkinson E J 1982a The vulva. In: Blaustein A (ed) Pathology of the female genital tract, 2nd edn. Springer-Verlag, New York, p 33

Friedrich E G, Wilkinson E J 1982b The vulva. In: Blaustein A (ed) Pathology of the female genital tract, 2nd edn. Springer-Verlag, New York, p 16–18

Friedrich E G, Wilkinson E J 1982c The vulva. In: Blaustein A (ed) Pathology of the female genital tract, 2nd edn. Springer-Verlag, New York, p 49–50

Friedrich E G, Wilkinson E J 1982d The vulva. In: Blaustein A (ed) Pathology of the female genital tract, 2nd edn. Springer-Verlag, New York, p 42–45

Friedrich E G, Wilkinson E J 1982e The vulva. In: Blaustein A (ed) Pathology of the female genital tract, 2nd edn. Springer-Verlag, New York, p 48

Friedrich E G, Wilkinson E J 1982f The vulva. In: Blaustein A (ed) Pathology of the female genital tract, 2nd edn. Springer-Verlag, New York, p 30–32

Friedrich E G, Wilkinson E J Steingraeber P H, Lewis J D 1975 Paget's disease of the vulva and carcinoma of the breast. Obstetrics and Gynecology 46: 130–134

Friedrich E G, Burch K, Bahr J P 1979 The vulvar clinic: an eight year appraisal. American Journal of Obstetrics and Gynecology 135: 1036–1040

Friedrich E G, Wilkinson E J, Fu Y S 1980 Carcinoma in situ of the vulva: a continuing challenge. American Journal of Obstetrics and Gynecology 136: 830–843

Frigerio B, Capella C, Eusebi V, Tenti P, Azzopardi J G 1983 Merkel cell carcinoma of the skin: the structure and origin of normal Merkel cells. Histopathology 7: 229–249

Fu Y-S, Reagan J W, Townsend D E, Kaufman R H, Richart R M, Wentz W B 1981 Nuclear DNA study of vulvar intraepithelial and invasive squamous neoplasms. Obstetrics and Gynecology 57: 643–652

Fukuma K et al 1986 Eccrine adenocarcinoma of the vulva producing isolated alpha-subunit of glycoprotein hormones. Obstetrics and Gynecology 67: 293–296

Furtell J W, Krueger G, Chretien P B, Ketcham A S 1971 Multiple primary sweat gland carcinomas. Cancer 28: 686–691

Gallousis S 1972 Verrucous carcinoma: Report of three vulvar cases and review of the literature. Obstetrics and Gynecology 40: 502–507

Gardiner S H, Stout F E, Arbogast J L, Huber C P 1953 Intraepithelial carcinoma of the vulva. American Journal of Obstetrics and Gynecology 65: 539–549

Gatter K C, Pulford K A F, Vanstapel M J, Roach B, Mortimer P, Woolston R E, Taylor-Papadimitriou J, Lane E B, Mason D Y 1984 An immunohistological study of benign and malignant skin tumours: epithelial aspects. Histopathology 8: 209–227

Gillenwater J Y, Burros H M 1968 Unusual tumors of the female urethra. Obstetrics and Gynecology 31: 617–620

Gissmann L, DeVilliers E-M, zur Hausen H 1982 Analysis of human genital warts (condylomata acuminata) and other genital tumors for human papilloma-virus type 6 DNA. International Journal of Cancer 29: 143–146

Gissman L, Wolnik L, Ikenberg H et al 1983 Human papillomavirus types 6 & 11 sequences in genital and laryngeal papillomas and in some cervical cancers. Proceedings of the National Academy of Science USA 80: 560–563

Goldman R L 1972 Nephrogenic metaplasia (nephrogenic adenoma, adenomatoid tumor) of the bladder. Journal of Urology 108: 565–567

Goldstein A I, Kent D R 1975 All vulvar lesions should be biopsied. Basal cell carcinoma—an example of the futility of diagnosis by gross appearance. American Journal of Obstetrics and Gynecology 121: 173–174

Gomez L G, DiMaio S M, Silva E G, Mackay B 1981 The association between neuroendocrine (Merkel cell) carcinoma and squamous carcinoma of the skin. Laboratory Investigations 44: 24A

Gonzales M O, Harrison M L, Boileau M A 1985 Carcinoma in diverticulum of female urethra. Urology 26: 328–332

Gordon H L, Kerr S G 1975 Nephrogenic adenoma of the bladder in immunosuppressed renal transplantation. Urology 5: 275–277

Gorlin R J, Vickers R A, Kelln E, Williamson J J 1965 The multiple basal cell nevi syndrome. Cancer 18: 89–104

Gosling J R G, Abell M R, Drolette B M, Loughrin T D 1961 Infiltrative squamous cell carcinoma of the vulva. Cancer 14: 330–343

Gowing N F C 1960 Urethral carcinoma associated with cancer of the bladder. British Journal of Urology 32: 428–439

Grabstald H 1973 Tumors of the urethra in men and women. Cancer 32: 1236–1255

Grabstald H, Hilaris B, Henschke U, Whitmore W F 1966 Cancer of the female urethra. Journal of the American Medical Association 197: 835–842

Grant R A 1960 Sweat gland carcinoma with metastases. Journal of the American Medical Association 173: 490–492

Green T H 1978 Carcinoma of the vulva: a reassessment. Obstetrics and Gynecology 52: 462–469

Grossman J R, Izuno G T 1974 Primary mucinous (adenocystic) carcinoma of the skin. Archives of Dermatology 110: 274–276

Gu J, Polak J M, Tapia F J, Marangos P J, Pearse A G E 1981 Neuron-specific enolase in the Merkel cells of mammalian skin. American Journal of Pathology 104: 63–68

Gu J, Polak J M, van Noorden S, Pearse A G E, Marangos P J, Azzopardi J G 1983 Immunostaining of neuron-specific enolase as a diagnostic tool for Merkel cell tumors. Cancer 52: 1039–1043

Guindi S F, Silverberg B K, Evans T N 1974 Multifocal mixed adenoid tumors of the vulva. International Journal of Gynaecology and Obstetrics 12: 138–140

Gunn R A, Gallager H S 1980 Vulvar Paget's disease. A topographic study. Cancer 46: 590–594

Gupta J, Pilotti S, Shah K V, De Palo G, Rilke F 1987 Human papillomavirus-associated early vulvar neoplasia investigated by in situ hybridization. The American Journal of Surgical Pathology 11: 430–434

Hacker N F, Nieberg R K, Berek J S, Leuchter R S, Lucas W E, Tamimi H K, Nolan J F, Moore J G, Lagasse L D 1983 Superficially invasive vulvar cancer with nodal metastases. Gynecologic Oncology 15: 65–77

Hacker N F, Berek J S, Lagasse L D, Nieberg R K, Leuchter R S 1984 Individualization of the treatment for Stage I squamous cell vulvar carcinoma. Obstetrics and Gynecology 63: 155–162

Halasz C, Silvers D, Crum C P 1986 Bowenoid papulosis in a 3 year old girl. Journal of the American Academy of Dermatology 14: 326–330

Hamilton J D, Leach W B 1951 Adenocarcinoma arising in diverticulum of the female urethra. Archives of Pathology 51: 90–97

Hart W R, Millman J B 1977 Progression of intraepithelial Paget's disease of the vulva to invasive carcinoma. Cancer 40: 2333–2337

Hartschuh W, Grube D 1979 The Merkel cell—A member of the APUD cell system? Archives of Dermatological Research 265: 115–122

Hartschuh W, Weihe E, Büchler M 1980 Met-enkephalin-like immunoreactivity in Merkel cells of various species (Abstract). Journal of Investigative Dermatology 74: 453

Hashimoto K 1972 Fine structure of Merkel cell in human oral mucosa. Journal of Investigative Dermatology 58: 381–387

Hashimoto K 1973 Hidradenoma papilliferum. An electron microscopic study. Acta Dematovenerologica 53: 22–30

Hashimoto K, Lever W F 1969 Histogenesis of skin appendage tumors. Archives of Dermatology 100: 356–369

Hashimoto K, Gross B G, Lever W F 1966 Syringoma. Histochemical and electron microscopic studies. Archives of Investigative Dermatology 46: 150–166

Hashimoto K, DiBella R J, Borsuk G M, Lever W F 1967a Eruptive hidradenoma and syringoma. Histological, histochemical and electron microscopic studies. Archives of Dermatology 96: 500–519

Hashimoto K, DiBella R J, Lever W F 1967b Clear cell hidradenoma: Histological, histochemical and electron microscopic studies. Archives of Dermatology 96: 18–38

Hay D M, Cole F M 1969 Primary invasive carcinoma of the vulva in Jamaica. Journal of Obstetrics and Gynaecology of the British Commonwealth 76: 821–830

Hay D M, Cole F M 1970 Postgranulomatous epidermoid carcinoma of the vulva. American Journal of Obstetrics and Gynecology 108: 479–484

Headington J T 1961 Mixed tumors of skin: eccrine and apocrine types. Archives of Dermatology 84: 989–996

Headington J T, Koski J, Murphy P J 1972 Clear cell glycogenosis in multiple syringomas. Archives of Dermatology 106: 353–356

Helwig E B, Graham J H 1963 Anogenital (extramammary) Paget's disease. A clinicopathological study. Cancer 16: 387–403

Hendrix R C, Behrman S J 1956 Adenocarcinoma arising in a supernumerary mammary gland in the vulva. Obstetrics and Gynecology 8: 238–241

Henry S A 1950 Cutaneous cancer in relation to occupation. Annals of the Royal College of Surgeons of England 7: 425–454

Hertig A T, Gore H 1960 Tumors of the female sex organs.

Part 2. Armed Forces Institute of Pathology, Washington DC, p 68–85

Hewitt J 1984 Conditions étiologiques du carcinome invasif d'emblée de la vulve. Possibilité d'un traitement prophylactique? Journal of Gynaceology, Obstetrics and Reproductive Biology 13: 297–303

Hilliard G D, Massey F M, O'Toole R V 1979 Vulvar neoplasia in the young. American Journal of Obstetrics and Gynecology 135: 185–188

Iinman F Jr, Cohlan W R 1960 Gartner's duct carcinoma in a urethral diverticulum. Journal of Urology 83: 414–415

Hobbs J E 1965 Sweat gland tumours. Clinical Obstetrics and Gynecology 8: 946–951

Hoffman J S, Kumar N B, Morley G W 1983 Microinvasive squamous carcinoma of the vulva: search for a definition. Obstetrics and Gynecology 61: 615–618

Hoffman P G, Siiteri P K 1980 Sex steroid receptors in gynecologic cancer. Obstetrics and Gynecology 55: 648–652

Holmes E J 1968 Tumors of lower hair sheath. Common histogenesis of certain so-called 'sebaceous cysts', acanthomas and 'sebaceous carcinomas'. Cancer 21: 234–248

Holzer E 1982 Microinvasive carcinoma of the cervix—clinical aspects, treatment and follow-up. Clinics in Oncology 1: 315–322

Honan J H 1897 Über die Karzinome der Glandulae Bartholini (Inaugural dissertation). Berlin. E. Eberung

Honoré L H, O'Hara K E 1978 Adenoma of the Bartholin Gland: a report of three cases. European Journal of Obstetrics, Gynecology and Reproductive Biology 8: 335–340

Hoogerland D L, Buchler D A 1979 Inflammatory carcinoma of the vulva: case report. Gynecologic Oncology 8: 240–245

Howe G E, Prentiss R J, Mullenix R B, Fenny M J 1963 Carcinoma of the urethra, diagnosis and treatment. Journal of Urology 89: 232–235

Howells M R, Baylis M S, Howell S 1985 Benign urethral villous adenoma. Case report. British Journal of Obstetrics and Gynaecology 92: 1070–1071

Husseinzadeh N, Zaino R, Nahhas W A, Mortel R 1983 The significance of histologic findings in predicting nodal metastases in invasive squamous cell carcinoma of the vulva. Gynecologic Oncology 16: 105–111

Hustin J, Donnay M, Hamels J 1980 Identification of papillary hidradenoma of the vulva by imprint cytology. Acta Cytologica 24: 466–467

Isaacs J H 1976 Verrucous carcinoma of the female genital tract. Gynecologic Oncology 4: 259–269

Isaacson D, Turner M L 1979 Localized vulvar syringomas. Journal of the American Academy of Dermatology 1: 352–356

Iversen T 1981 Squamous cell carcinoma of the vulva. Localization of the primary tumor and lymph node metastases. Acta Obstetricia et Gynecologica Scandinavica 60: 211–214

Iversen T, Aas M 1983 Lymph drainage from the vulva. Gynecologic Oncology 16: 179–189

Iversen T, Aalders J G, Christensen A, Kolstad P 1980 Squamous cell carcinoma of the vulva: a review of 424 patients. Gynecologic Oncology 9: 271–279

Iversen T, Abeler V, Aalders J 1981 Individualised treatment of Stage I carcinoma of the vulva. Obstetrics and Gynecology 57: 85–89

Iwasaki H, Mitsui T, Kikuchi M, Imai T, Fukushima K 1981 Neuroendocrine carcinoma (trabecular carcinoma) of the skin with ectopic ACTH production. Cancer 48: 753–756

Jablonska S, Orth G 1983 Human papovaviruses. In: Rook A J, Maibach H I (eds) Recent advances in dermatology 6. Churchill Livingstone, Edinburgh, p 1–36

Jacobs D M, Sandles L G, Leboit P E 1986 Sebaceous carcinoma arising from Bowen's disease of the vulva. Archives of Dermatology 122: 1191–1193

Jacobson Y G, Rees T D, Grant R, Fitchett V H 1959 Metastasizing sweat-gland carcinoma. Notes on the surgical therapy. Archives of Surgery 78: 574–581

Jafari K, Cartnick F N 1976 Microinvasive squamous cell carcinoma of the vulva. Gynecologic Oncology 4: 158–166

James L P, Worsham G F, Hoskins W J, Belcik R 1984 Apocrine adenocarcinoma of the vulva with associated Paget's disease. Diagnosis of lymph node metastases by fine needle aspiration biopsy. Acta Cytologica 28: 178–184

Janovski N A, Barchet S 1966 Multicentric Bowen's disease of the vulva. Report of a case. Obstetrics and Gynecology 28: 170–174

Janovski N A, Douglas C P 1972 Diseases of the vulva, 1st American edn. Harper & Row, Maryland, p 92–95

Janovski N A, Marshall D, Taki I 1962 Malignant melanoma of the vulva. American Journal of Obstetrics and Gynecology 84: 523–536

Japaze H, Garcia-Bunuel R, Woodruff J D 1977 Primary vulvar neoplasia. A review of in situ and invasive carcinoma, 1935–1972. Obstetrics and Gynecology 49: 404–411

Japaze H, Dinh T V, Woodruff J D 1982 Verrucous carcinoma of the vulva: study of 24 cases. Obstetrics and Gynecology 60: 462–466

Jaramillo B A, Gansel P, Averette H E, Sevin B L, Lovecchio J L 1985 Malignant melanoma of the vulva. Obstetrics and Gynecology 66: 398–401

Jeffcoate, N. 1975 Principles of gynaecology, 4th edn. Butterworth, London, p 380

Jeffcoate T N A, Woodcock A S 1961 Premalignant conditions of the vulva, with particular reference to chronic epithelial dystrophies. British Medical Journal 2: 127–134

Jenson A B, Rosenthal J D, Olson C, Pass F, Lancaster W D, Shah K 1980 Immunological relatedness of papillomaviruses from different species. Journal of the National Cancer Institute 64: 495–500

Jimenez H T, Fenoglio C M, Richart R M 1975 Vulvar basal cell carcinoma with metastasis. A case report. American Journal of Obstetrics and Gynecology 121: 285–286

Jimerson G K, Merrill J A 1970 Multicentric squamous malignancy involving both cervix and vulva. Cancer 26: 150–153

Johannessen J V, Gould V E 1980 Neuroendocrine skin carcinoma associated with calcitonin production. A Merkel cell carcinoma? Human Pathology 11: 586–589

Johnson T L, Kumar N B, White C D, Morley G W 1986 Prognostic features of vulvar melanoma: A clinicopathologic analysis. International Journal of Gynecological Pathology 5: 110–118

Johnson W C, Helwig E B 1966 Adenoid squamous cell carcinoma adenoacanthoma: A clinicopathologic study of 155 patients. Cancer 18: 1639–1650

Johnson B L Jr, Helwig E B 1969 Eccrine acrospiroma. Cancer 23: 641–657

Jones I, Buntine D 1978 Progression of vulval carcinoma in situ. Australian and New Zealand Journal of Obstetrics and Gynaecology 18: 274–276

Jones R E Jr, Austin C, Ackerman A B 1979 Extramammary Paget's disease. A critical re-examination. American Journal of Dermatopathology 1: 101–132

Jones R W, McLean M R 1986 Carcinoma in situ of the vulva: a review of 31 treated cases and five untreated cases. Obstetrics and Gynecology 68: 499–503

Josey W E, Nahmias A J, Naib Z M 1976 Viruses and cancer of

the lower genital tract. Cancer 38: 526–533

Kaplan A L, Kaufman R H 1975 Management of advanced carcinoma of the vulva. Gynecologic Oncology 3: 220–232

Kariniemi A-L, Forsman L, Wahlström T, Vesterinen E, Andersson L 1984 Expression of differentiation antigens in mammary and extramammary Paget's disease. British Journal of Dermatology 110: 203–210

Karlen J R, Piver M S, Barlow J J 1975 Melanoma of the vulva. Obstetrics and Gynecology 45: 181–185

Katz J I, Grabstald H 1976 Primary malignant melanoma of the female urethra. Journal of Urology 116: 454–457

Kaufman R H, Dreesman G R, Burek J, Korhonen M O, Matson D O, Melnick J L, Powell K L, Purifoy D J M, Courtney R J, Adam E 1981 Herpesvirus-induced antigens in squamous cell carcinoma in situ of the vulva. New England Journal of Medicine 305: 483–488

Kaufmann T, Pawl N O, Soifer I, Greston W M, Kleiner G J 1987 Cystic papillary hidradenoma of the vulva: case report and review of the literature. Gynecologic Oncology 26: 240–245

Kay S, Hall W E B 1954 Sweat gland carcinoma with proved metastases. Report of a case. Cancer 7: 373–376

Kelly J 1972 Malignant disease of the vulva. Journal of Obstetrics and Gynaecology of the British Commonwealth 79: 265–272

Kersting D W 1963 Clear cell hidradenoma and hidradenocarcinoma. Archives of Dermatology 87: 323–333

Kimura S 1980 Condylomata acuminata with pigmented papular lesions. Dermatologica 160: 390–397

Kimura S, Hirai A, Harada R, Nagashima M 1978 So-called multicentric pigmented Bowen's disease. Dermatologica 157: 229–237

King L S, Sullivan M 1947 Effects of podophyllin and of colchicine on normal skin on condyloma acuminatum, and on verruca vulgaris. Archives of Pathology 43: 374–386

Kipkie G F, Haust M D 1958 Carcinoma of apocrine glands. Archives of Dermatology 78: 440–445

Kirkham N, Isaacson P 1983 Merkel cell carcinoma: a report of three cases with neurone-specific enolase activity. Histopathology 7: 251–259

Klotz P G 1974 Carcinoma of Skene's gland associated with urethral diverticulum. A case report. Journal of Urology 112: 487–488

Kneale B L 1984 Report of the ISSVD Task Force Journal of Reproductive Medicine 29: 454–456

Kneale B L G, Elliott P M, McDonald I A 1981 Microinvasive carcinoma of the vulva: clinical features and management. In: Coppleson M (ed) Gynecologic Oncology. Churchill Livingstone, Edinburgh, p 320–328

Knoblick R 1960 Primary adenocarcinoma of the female urethra. A review and report of 3 cases. American Journal of Obstetrics and Gynecology 80: 353–364

Kolstad P, Iversen T, Abeler V, Aalders J 1982 Microinvasive carcinoma of the vulva—definition and treatment problems. Clinical Oncology 1: 355–362

Konnak J W 1973 Mesonephric carcinoma involving the urethra. Journal of Urology 110: 76–78

Koss L G, Brockunier A Jr. 1969 Ultrastructural aspects of Paget's disease of the vulva. Archives of Pathology 87: 592–600

Koss L G, Ladinsky S, Brockunier A Jr 1968 Paget's disease of the vulva. Report of 10 cases. Obstetrics and Gynecology 31: 513–525

Kovi J, Tillman R L, Lee S M 1974 Malignant transformation of condyloma acuminatum. A light microscopic and ultra-structural study. American Journal of Clinical Pathology 61: 702–710

Kraus F T, Perez-Mesa C 1966 Verrucous carcinoma: clinical and pathologic study of 105 cases involving oral cavity, larynx and genitalia. Cancer 19: 26–38

Krupp P J, Bohm J W 1978 Lymph gland metastases in invasive squamous cell cancer of the vulva. American Journal of Obstetrics and Gynecology 130: 943–952

Krupp P J, Lee F Y L, Bohm J W, Batson H W, Diem J E, LeMire J E 1975 Prognostic parameters and clinical staging criteria in epidermoid carcinoma of the vulva. Obstetrics and Gynecology 46: 84–88

Kurman R J, Shah K H, Lancaster W D, Jenson A B 1981 Immunoperoxidase localization of papillomavirus antigens in cervical dysplasia and vulvar condylomas. American Journal of Obstetrics and Gynecology 140: 931–935

Kuzuya K, Matsuyama M, Nishi Y, Chihara T, Suchi T 1981 Ultrastructure of adenocarcinoma of Bartholin's gland. Cancer 48: 1392–1398

Laohadtanaphorn S, Hunter J C, Ansell I D 1979 Multicentric, pigmented carcinoma in situ of the vulva in association with vulval condyloma acuminata. Australian and New Zealand Journal of Obstetrics and Gynaecology 19: 249–252

Lasser A, Cornog J L, Morris J McL 1974 Adenoid squamous cell carcinoma of the vulva. Cancer 33: 224–227

Lavery H A, Pinkerton J H M, Middleton D 1984 HLA tissue typing and chronic vulval dystrophy. British Journal of Obstetrics and Gynaecology 91: 694–696

Lee S C, Roth L M, Ehrlich C, Hall J A 1977 Extramammary Paget's disease of the vulva. A clinicopathologic study of 13 cases. Cancer 39: 2540–2549

Leighton P C, Langley F A 1975 A clinico-pathological study of vulval dermatoses. Journal of Clinical Pathology 28: 394–402

Leiman G, Markowitz S, Veiga-Ferreira M M, Margolius K A 1986 Renal adenocarcinoma presenting with bilateral metastases to Bartholin's glands: primary diagnosis by aspiration cytology. Diagnostic Cytopathology 2: 252–255

Leuchter R S, Hacker N F, Voet R L, Berek J S, Townsend D E, Lagasse L D 1982 Primary carcinoma of the Bartholin Gland: A report of 14 cases and review of the literature. Obstetrics and Gynecology 60: 361–367

Lever W F 1947 Adenoacanthoma of sweat glands. Carcinoma of sweat glands with glandular and epidermal elements. Report of four cases. Archives of Dermatology and Syphilology 56: 157–171

Lever W F, Castleman B 1952 Clear cell myo-epithelioma of the skin. Report of ten cases. American Journal of Pathology 28: 691–699

Lever W F, Schaumburg-Lever G 1975a Tumours of the epidermal appendages. In: Histopathology of the skin, 5th edn. J B Lippincott, Philadephia, p 537–551

Lever W F, Schaumburg-Lever G 1975b In: Histopathology of the skin, 5th edn. J B Lippincott, Philadelphia, p 513–514

Lever W F, Schaumburg-Lever G 1975c Clear cell hidradenoma. In: Histopathology of the skin, 5th edn. J B Lippincott, Philadelphia. p 527–530

Lever W F, Schaumburg-Lever G 1975d Histopathology of the skin, 5th edn. J B Lippincott, Philadelphia, p 507–509

Lever W F, Schaumburg-Lever G 1975e Histopathology of the skin, 5th edn. J B Lippincott, Philadelphia, p 553–554

Lever W F, Schaumburg-Lever G 1983a Histopathology of the skin, 6th edn. J B Lippincott, Philadelphia, p 706–717

Lever W F, Schaumburg-Lever G 1983b Histopathology of the skin, 6th edn. J B Lippincott, Philadelphia, p 536–580

Levine R L 1980 Urethral cancer. Cancer 45: 1965–1972 supplement

Lindeque B G, Nel A E, Du Toit J P 1987 Immune deficiency and invasive carcinoma of the vulva in a young woman: a case report. Gynecologic Oncology 26: 112–118

Lucas W E, Benirschke K, Lebherz T B 1974 Verrucous carcinoma of the female genital tract. American Journal of Obstetrics and Gynecology 119: 435–440

Lupulescu A, Mehregan A H, Rahbari H, Pinkus H, Birmingham D J 1977 Venereal warts vs Bowen's disease. A histologic and ultrastructural study of five cases. Journal of the American Medical Association 237: 2520–2522

Lund H Z 1957 Tumors of the skin. In: Atlas of tumor pathology, Section I. Fascicle 2. Armed Forces Institute of Pathology, Washington D C

McAdams A, Kistner R 1958 The relationship of chronic vulvar disease, leukoplakia, and carcinoma in situ to carcinoma of the vulva. Cancer 11: 740–757

McBurney R P, Bale G F 1955 Primary melanoma of the female urethra. Surgery 37: 973–978

McDonald J R 1941 Apocrine sweat gland carcinoma of the vulva. American Journal of Clinical Pathology 11: 890–897

Mackay B, Luna M A, Butler J J 1976 Adult neuroblastoma. Electron microscopic observations in nine cases. Cancer 37: 1334–1351

McKee P H, Hertogs K T 1980 Endocervical adenocarcinoma and vulval Paget's disease: a significant association. British Journal of Dermatology 103: 443–448

McLoughlin M G 1975 Carcinoma in situ in urethral diverticulum: pitfalls of marsupialization alone. Urology 6: 343

Mader M H, Friedrich E G Jr 1982 Vulvar metastasis of breast carcinoma. A case report. Journal of Reproductive Medicine 27: 169–171

Madsen A 1955 The histogenesis of superficial basal-cell epithelioma. Unicentric or multicentric origin. Archives of Dermatology 72: 29–30

Magrina J F, Webb M J, Gaffey T A, Symmonds R E 1979 Stage I squamous cell cancer of the vulva. American Journal of Obstetrics and Gynecology 134: 453–459

Malfetano J, Piver M S, Tsukada Y 1986 Stage III and IV squamous cell carcinoma of the vulva. Gynecologic Oncology 23: 192–198

Manglani K S, Manaligod J R, Ray B 1980 Spindle cell carcinoma of the glans penis: a light and electron microscopic study. Cancer 46: 2266–2272

Marcus S L 1960 Basal cell and basal-squamous cell carcinoma of the vulva. American Journal of Obstetrics and Gynecology 79: 461–469

Marshall S, Hirsch K 1977 Carcinoma within urethral diverticula. Urology 10: 161–163

Masterson J G, Goss A S 1954 Carcinoma of Bartholin Gland. Review of the literature and report of a new case in an elderly patient treated by radical operation. American Journal of Obstetrics and Gynecology 69: 1323–1332

Masukawa T, Friedrich E G Jr 1978 Cytopathology of Paget's disease of the vulva: diagnostic abrasive cytology. Acta Cytologica (Balt.) 22: 476–478

Mazoujian G, Pinkus G S, Haagensen D E Jr 1984 Extramammary Paget's disease—Evidence for an apocrine origin. An immunoperoxidase study of gross cystic disease fluid protein-15, carcino-embryonic antigen, and keratin proteins. American Journal of Surgical Pathology 8: 43–50

Medenica M, Sahihi T 1972 Ultrastructural study of a case of extramammary Paget's disease of the vulva. Archives of Dermatology 105: 236–243

Meeker J H, Neubecker R D, Helwig E B 1962 Hidradenoma papilliferum. American Journal of Clinical Pathology 37: 182–195

Mehregan A H, Hashimoto K, Rahbari H 1983 Eccrine adenocarcinoma. A clinicopathologic study of 35 cases. Archives of Dermatology 119: 104–114

Melnick J L, Birdsall T M 1960 Carcinoma of a diverticulum of the female urethra. American Journal of Obstetrics and Gynecology 80: 347–352

Mendoza S, Helwig E B 1971 Mucinous (adenocystic) carcinoma of the skin. Archives of Dermatology 103: 68–78

Mene A, Buckley C H 1985 Involvement of the vulval skin appendages by intraepithelial neoplasia. British Journal of Obstetrics and Gynaecology 92: 634–638

Menville J G, Counseller V S 1935 Mucoid carcinoma of the female urethra. Journal of Urology 33: 76–81

Merino M J, LiVolsi V A, Schwartz P E, Rudnicki J 1982 Adenoid basal cell carcinoma of the vulva. International Journal of Gynecological Pathology 1: 299–306

Meyrick Thomas R H, McGibbon D H, Munro D D 1985 Basal cell carcinoma of the vulva in association with lichen sclerosus et atrophicus. Journal of the Royal Society of Medicine 78 (Supplement 11): 16–18

Mickal A, Andonie J A, Dougherty C M 1966 Squamous cell carcinoma of the vulva. Obstetrics and Gynecology 28: 670–674

Miller J D, Raiman R J 1976 Carcinoma of the female urethra. International Surgery 61: 431–432

Miller W L 1967 Sweat gland carcinoma—a clinicopathologic problem. American Journal of Clinical Pathology 47: 767–780

Moll I, Moll R 1985 Cells of extramammary Paget's disease express cytokeratins different from those of epidermal cells. Journal of Investigative Dermatology 84: 3–8

Monaco A P, Murphy G B, Dowling W 1958 Primary cancer of the female urethra. Cancer 11: 1215–1221

Monaghan J M, Hammond I G 1984 Pelvic node dissection in the treatment of vulval carcinoma—is it necessary? British Journal of Obstetrics and Gynaecology 91: 270–274

Monaghan J M, Lindeque G 1986 Vulvar carcinoma in pregnancy (Commentary). British Journal of Obstetrics and Gynaecology 93: 785–786

Morley G W 1976 Infiltrative carcinoma of the vulva: results of surgical treatment. American Journal of Obstetrics and Gynecology 124: 874–888

Morrow C P 1981 Melanoma of female genital tract. In: Coppleson M (ed) Gynecologic oncology. Churchill Livingstone, Edinburgh, ch 59, p 784

Morrow C P, Rutledge F N 1972 Melanoma of the vulva. Obstetrics and Gynecology 39: 745–752

Murayama T, Komatsu H, Asano M, Tahara M, Nakamura T 1978 Mesonephric adenocarcinoma of the urethra in a woman: report of a case. Journal of Urology 120: 500–501

Murphy G F, Krusinski P A, Myzak L A, Ershler W B 1983 Local immune response in basal cell carcinoma: characterization by transmission electron microscopy and monoclonal anti-T6 antibody. Journal of the American Academy of Dermatology 8: 477–485

Murphy G F, Kwan T H, Mihm M C Jr 1984a The skin. In: Robbins S L, Cotran R S, Kumar V (eds) Pathologic basis of disease, 3rd edition. W B Saunders, Philadelphia, p 1262–1263

Murphy G F, Kwan T H, Mihm M C 1984b The skin. In: Robbins S L, Cotran R S, Kumar V (eds) Pathologic basis of disease, 3rd edn. W B Saunders, Philadelphia, p 1265–1266

Murphy J, Wilson J M, Bickel D A 1962 Adenoid cystic

carcinoma of the Bartholin gland and pregnancy. American Journal of Obstetrics and Gynecology 83: 612–614

Mustakallio K K 1959 Succinic dehydrogenase activity of syringomas. Acta Dermatoven 39: 318–323

Nagle R B, Lucas D O, McDaniel K M, Clark V A. Schmalzel G M 1985 New evidence linking mammary and extramammary cells to a common cell phenotype. American Journal of Clinical Pathology 83: 431–438

Neilson D, Woodruff J D 1972 Electron microscopy in in situ and invasive vulvar Paget's disease. American Journal of Obstetrics and Gynecology 113: 719–732

Ney C, Miller H L, Ochs D 1971 Adenocarcinoma in a diverticulum of the female urethra: a case report of mucous adenocarcinoma with a summary of the literature. Journal of Urology 106: 874–877

Nichol J E 1941 Two cases of carcinoma of the urethra. Canadian Medical Association Journal 45: 155–156

Nichols C E, Bonney W A Jr 1973 Carcinoma of the vulva producing hypercalcemia. Obstetrics and Gynecology 42: 58–61

Niebyl J R, Genadry R, Friedrich E G Jr, Wilkinson E J, Woodruff J D 1974 Vulvar carcinoma with hypercalcemia. Obstetrics and Gynecology 45: 343–348

Noller K L, Decker D G, Symmonds R E, Dockerty M B, Kurland L T 1976 Clear cell adenocarcinoma of the vagina and cervix. Survival data. American Journal of Obstetrics and Gynecology 124: 285–288

Nordquist R E, Olson R L, Everett M A, Condit P T 1970 Virus-like particles in Bowen's disease. Cancer Research 30: 288–293

Nourse M H 1961 Diverticulum of the female urethra. West Journal of Surgery Obstetrics and Gynecology 69: 286–287

Novak E, Stevenson R R 1945 Sweat gland tumors of the vulva. Benign (hidradenoma) and malignant (adenocarcinoma). American Journal of Obstetrics and Gynecology 50: 641–659

Novak E R, Woodruff J D 1979 Gynecologic and obstetric pathology, 8th edition. W B Saunders, Philadelphia, ch 1, p 1–58

Novak E, Woodruff J D, Novak E R 1954 Probable mesonephric origin of certain female genital tract tumors. American Journal of Obstetrics and Gynecology 68: 1222–1242

O'Hara J M, Bensch K G 1967 Fine structure of eccrine sweat gland adenoma, clear cell type. Journal of Investigative Dermatology 49: 261–272

O'Hara J M, Bensch K, Ioannides G, Klaus S N 1966 Eccrine sweat gland adenoma, clear cell type. Cancer 19: 1438–1450

Oji M, Furue M, Tamaki K 1984 Serum carcinoembryonic antigen level in Paget's disease. British Journal of Dermatology 110: 211–213

Olson R L, Nordquist R E, Everett M A 1968 An electron microscopic study of Bowen's disease. Cancer Research 28: 2078–2085

Ordonez N G, Manning J T, Luna M A 1981 Mixed tumor of the vulva: a report of two cases probably arising in Bartholin's gland. Cancer 48: 181–186

Orenstein J M, Dardick I, Van Nostrand A W P 1985 Ultrastructural similarities of adenoid cystic carcinoma and pleomorphic adenoma. Histopathology 9: 623–638

Oriel J D, Almeida J D 1970 Demonstration of virus particles in human genital warts. British Journal of Venereal Diseases 46: 37–42

Oriel J D, Whimster I W 1971 Carcinoma in situ associated with virus containing anal warts. British Journal of Dermatology 84: 71–73

Pack G T, Oropeza R A 1967 A comparative study of melano-

mas and epidermoid carcinomas of the vulva: a review of 44 melanomas and 58 epidermoid carcinomas (1930–1965). Reviews in Surgery 24: 305–324

Palladino V S, Duffy J L, Bures G J 1969 Basal cell carcinoma of the vulva. Cancer 24: 460–470

Parker R T, Duncan I, Rampone J, Creasman W 1975 Operating management of early invasive epidermoid carcinoma of the vulva. American Journal of Obstetrics and Gynecology 123: 349–354

Parmley T H, Woodruff J D, Julian C G 1975 Invasive vulvar Paget's disease. Obstetrics and Gynecology 46: 341–346

Partridge E E, Murad T, Shingleton H M, Austin J M, Hatch K D 1980a Verrucous lesions of the female genitalia. I. Giant condylomata. American Journal of Obstetrics and Gynecology 137: 412–418

Partridge E E, Murad T, Shingleton H M, Austin J M, Hatch K D 1980b Verrucous lesions of the female genitalia. II. Verrucous carcinoma. American Journal of Obstetrics and Gynecology 137: 419–424

Pathak U N, House M J 1970 Diverticulum of the female urethra. Obstetrics and Gynecology 36: 789–794

Pelisse M, Orth G, Croissant O et al 1985 Données anatomo—cliniques et virologiques dans vingt cas de maladie de Bowen Vulvaire. Annales de Dermatologie et de Vénérologie 112: 749–750

Penneys N S, Nadji M, Ziegels-Weissman J, Ketabchi M, Morales A R 1982 Carcinoembryonic antigen in sweat-gland carcinomas. Cancer 50: 1608–1611

Perrone T, Twiggs L B, Adcock L L, Dehner L P 1987 Vulvar basal cell carcinoma: an infrequently metastasizing neoplasm. International Journal of Gynecological Pathology 6: 152–165

Peterson L J, Matsumoto L M 1978 Nephrogenic adenoma in urethral diverticulum. Urology 11: 193–195

Peven D R, Hidvegi D F 1985 Clear-cell adenocarcinoma of the female urethra. Acta Cytologica 29: 142–146

Phillips G L, Twiggs L B, Okagaki T 1982 Vulvar melanoma: a microstaging study. Gynecologic Oncology 14: 80–88

Pickel H, Haas J 1986 Microcarcinoma of the vulva. Journal of Reproductive Medicine 31: 831–835

Pierard J, Kint A 1968 Maladie de Paget extramammaire. Étude d'un cas en microscopie electronique. Archives Belges de Dermatologie et de Syphiligraphie 24: 335–347

Pilotti S, Rilke F, Shah K V, Torre G D, De Palo G 1984 Immunohistochemical and ultrastructural evidence of papilloma virus infection association with in situ and microinvasive squamous cell carcinoma of the vulva. American Journal of Surgical Pathology 8: 751–761

Pinkus H, Gould S E 1939 Extramammary Paget's disease and intraepidermal carcinoma. Archives of Dermatology and Syphilology 39: 479–502

Plachta A, Speer F D 1954 Apocrine gland adenocarcinoma and extramammary Paget's disease of the vulva. Review of the literature and report of a case. Cancer 7: 910–919

Plouffe L, Tulandi T, Rosenberg A, Ferenczy A 1984 Non-Hodgkin's lymphoma in Bartholin's gland. Case report and review of the literature. American Journal of Obstetrics and Gynecology 148: 608–609

Podratz K C, Symmonds R E, Taylor W F 1982 Carcinoma of the vulva: analysis of treatment failures. American Journal of Obstetrics and Gynecology 143: 340–347

Podratz K C, Symmonds R E, Taylor W F, Williams T J 1983a Carcinoma of the vulva: analysis of treatment and survival. Obstetrics and Gynecology 61: 63–74

Podratz K C, Gaffey T A, Symmonds R E, Johansen K L, O'Brien P C 1983b Melanoma of the vulva: an update. Gynecologic Oncology 16: 153–168

Pointon R C S, Poole-Wilson D S 1968 Primary carcinoma of the urethra. British Journal of Urology 40: 682–693

Pollack S V, Goslen J B, Sherertz E F, Jegasothy B V 1982 The biology of basal cell carcinoma: a review. Journal of the American Academy of Dermatology 7: 569–577

Posso M A, Berg G A, Murphy A I, Totten R S 1961 Mucinous adenocarcinoma of the urethra. Report of a case associated with urethritis glandularis. Journal of Urology 85: 944–948

Powell J L, Franklin E W III, Nickerson J F, Burrell M O 1978 Verrucous carcinoma of the female genital tract. Gynecologic Oncology 6: 565–573

Powell L C, Dinh T V, Rajaraman S, Hannigan E V, Dillard E A Jr, Yandell R B, To T 1986 Carcinoma in situ of the vulva. A clinicopathologic study of 50 cases. Journal of Reproductive Medicine 31: 808–814

Prempree T, Wizenberg M J, Scott R M 1978 Radiation treatment of primary carcinoma of the female urethra. Cancer 42: 1177–1184

Prempree T, Amornmarn R, Patanaphan V 1984 Radiation therapy in primary carcinoma of the female urethra. II. An update on results. Cancer 54: 729–733

Ragni M V, Tobon H 1974 Primary malignant melanoma of the vagina and vulva. Obstetrics and Gynecology 43: 658–664

Rando R F, Sedlacek T V, Hunt J, Jenson A B, Kurman R J, Lancaster W D 1986 Verrucous Carcinoma of the Vulva associated with an unusual Type 6 Human Papilloma virus. Obstetrics and Gynecology 67 (Supplement): 70S–75S

Rastkar G, Okagaki T, Twiggs L B, Clark B A 1982 Early invasive and in situ warty carcinoma of the vulva: clinical histologic and electron microscopic study with particular reference to viral association. American Journal of Obstetrics and Gynecology 143: 814–820

Reid R, Fu Y S, Herschman B R, Crum C P, Braun L, Shah K V, Agronow S J, Stanhope C R 1984 Genital warts and cervical cancer. VI. The relationship between aneuploid and polyploid cervical lesions. American Journal of Obstetrics and Gynecology 150: 189–199

Reid R, Greenberg M, Jenson A B, Hussain M, Willett J, Daoud Y, Temple G, Stanhope C R, Sherman A I, Phibbs G D, Lorincz A T 1987 Sexually transmitted papillomaviral infections. I The anatomic distribution and pathologic grade of neoplastic lesions associated with different viral types. American Journal of Obstetrics and Gynecology 156: 212–222

Rhamy R K, Boldus R A, Allison R C, Tapper R I 1973 Therapeutic modalities in adenocarcinoma of the female urethra. Journal of Urology 109: 638–640

Rhatigan R M, Mojadidi O 1973 Adenosquamous carcinomas of the vulva and vagina. American Journal of Clinical Pathology 59: 208–217

Rhatigan R M, Nuss R C 1985 Keratoacanthoma of the vulva. Gynecologic Oncology 21: 118–123

Rhatigan R M, Saffos R O 1977 Condyloma acuminatum and squamous carcinoma of the vulva. Southern Medical Journal 70: 591–594

Rich P M, Okagaki T, Clark B, Prem K A 1981 Adenocarcinoma of the sweat gland of the vulva. Light and electron microscopic study. Cancer 47: 1352–1357

Riches E W, Cullen T H 1951 Carcinoma of the urethra. British Journal of Urology 23: 209–221

Richie J P, Skinner D G 1978 Carcinoma in situ of the urethra associated with bladder carcinoma: the role of urethrectomy. Journal of Urology 119: 80–81

Ridley C M 1975 The vulva. Major problems in dermatology. W B Saunders, London, p 224–225

Ridley C M 1983 Vulval 'dysplasia'. British Journal of Hospital Medicine 30: 158–166

Robboy S J, Herbst A L, Scully R E 1974 Clear cell adenocarcinoma of the vagina and cervix. Cancer 34: 606–614

Roberts T W, Melicow M M 1977 Pathology and natural history of urethral tumors in females. Review of 65 cases. Urology 10: 583–589

Robutti F et al 1986 Primary malignant melanoma of the female urethra. European Urology 12: 62–63

Rocamora A, Santonja C, Vives R, Varona C 1986 Sebaceous gland hyperplasia of the vulva. A case report. Obstetrics and Gynecology 68 (3 Supplement): 63S–65S

Rogers R E, Burns B 1969 Carcinoma of the female urethra. Obstetrics and Gynecology 33: 54–57

Rosser E ap I, Hamlin I M E 1957 Paget's disease of the vulva. Journal of Obstetrics and Gynaecology of the British Empire 64: 127–130

Roth L M, Lee S C, Ehrlich C E 1977 Paget's disease of the vulva. A histogenetic study of five cases including ultrastructural observations and review of the literature. American Journal of Surgical Pathology 1: 193–206

Rueda-Leverone N G, Di Paola G R, Meiss R P, Vighi S G, Llamosas F 1987 Association of human papillomavirus infection and vulvar intraepithelial neoplasia: a morphological and imunohistochemical study of 30 cases. Gynecologic Oncology 26: 331–339

Rulon D B, Helwig E B 1974 Cutaneous sebaceous neoplasms. Cancer 33: 82–102

Rustin M H A, Chambers T J, Levison D A, Munro D D 1983 Merkel cell tumour: report of a case. British Journal of Dermatology 108: 711–715

Rutledge F N 1965 Cancer of the vulva and vagina. Clinical Obstetrics and Gynecology 8: 1051–1079

Sackett N B 1965 Carcinoma primary in Bartholin's gland—5 year survivals after radical surgery. American Journal of Obstetrics and Gynecology 91: 1149–1150

Salazar H, Gonzalez-Angulo A 1984 Ultrastructural diagnosis in gynaecological pathology. Clinics in Obstetrics and Gynaecology 11: 25–77

Saltzstein S L, Woodruff J D, Novak E R 1956 Postgranulomatous carcinoma of the vulva. Obstetrics and Gynecology 7: 80–90

Sanderson K V 1961 The architecture of basal-cell carcinoma. British Journal of Dermatology 73: 455–474

Sanderson K V, MacKie R M 1986 In: Rook A, Wilkinson D S, Ebling T J G (eds) Textbook of dermatology, 4th edn. Blackwell Scientific, Oxford, p 2162

Sayre G P 1949 Cylindroma of the vulva: Adenocarcinoma, cylindroma type, of the vulva. Report of a case of twenty-seven years' duration. Proceedings of Staff Meeting Mayo Clinic 24: 224–233

Schatten W E, Ship A G, Pieper W J, Bartter F C 1958 Syndrome resembling hyperparathyroidism associated with squamous cell carcinoma. Annals of Surgery 148: 890–894

Schlaerth J B, Morrow C P, Nalick R H, Gaddis O 1984 Anal involvement by carcinoma in situ of the perineum in women. Obstetrics and Gynecology 64: 406–411

Schmechel D, Marangos P J, Brightman M 1978 Neurone-specific enolase as a molecular marker for peripheral and central neuroendocrine cells. Nature 276: 834–836

Schnitzer B 1964 Primary adenocarcinoma of female urethra. A review and report of two cases. Journal of Urology 92: 135–139

Schueller E F 1965 Basal cell cancer of the vulva. American Journal of Obstetrics and Gynecology 93: 199–208

Schwartz P E, Naftolin F 1981 Type 2 herpes simplex virus and vulvar carcinoma in situ. New England Journal of Medicine 305: 517–518

Schweppe K W, Schlake W 1980 Adenocarcinoma of Bartholin's gland. Geburtshilfe Frauenheilkunde 40: 437–443

Selium M A, Lankeroni M R 1979 Verrucous carcinoma of the vulva. Journal of Reproductive Medicine 22: 92–96

Seski J C, Reinhalter E R, Silva J Jr 1978 Abnormalities of lymphocyte transformations in women with condylomata acuminata. Obstetrics and Gynecology 51: 188–192

Shafeek M A, Osman M I, Hussein M A 1979 Carcinoma of the vulva arising in condylomata acuminata. Obstetrics and Gynecology 54: 120–122

Shane J M, Naftolin F 1975 Aberrant hormone activity by tumors of gynecologic importance. American Journal of Obstetrics and Gynecology 121: 133–147

Sharma S K, Isaacs J H 1985 Bone metastasis in vulvar carcinoma. Gynecologic Oncology 20: 156–161

Shenoy Y M V 1961 Malignant perianal papillary hidradenoma. Archives of Dermatology 83: 965–967

Shield D E, Weiss R M 1973 Leiomyoma of the female urethra. Journal of Urology 109: 430–431

Shimm D S, Fuller A F, Orlow E L, Dosoretz D E, Aristizabal S A 1986 Prognostic variables in the treatment of squamous cell carcinoma of the vulva. Gynecologic Oncology 24: 343–358

Sibley R K, Dahl D 1985 Primary neuroendocrine (Merkel cell?) carcinoma of the skin. II. An immunocytochemical study of 21 cases. American Journal of Surgical Pathology 9: 109–116

Sibley R K, Rosai J, Foucar E, Dehner L P, Bosl G 1980 Neuroendocrine (Merkel cell) carcinoma of the skin. A histologic and ultrastructural study of two cases. American Journal of Surgical Pathology 4: 211–221

Sibley R K, Dehner L P, Rosai J 1985 Primary neuroendocrine (Merkel cell?) carcinoma of the skin. I. A clinicopathologic and ultrastructural study of 43 cases. American Journal of Surgical Pathology 9: 95–108

Sidhu G S, Mullins J D, Feiner H, Schaefler K, Flotte T J, Schultenover S J 1980 Merkel cell neoplasms. Histology, electron microscopy, biology and histogenesis. American Journal of Dermatopathology 2: 101–119

Siegler A M, Greene H J 1951 Basal-cell carcinoma of the vulva. A report of 5 cases and review of the literature. American Journal of Obstetrics and Gynecology 62: 1219–1224

Silva E G, Mackay B 1980 Small cell neuroepithelial tumor of the skin. Laboratory Investigations 42: 151

Silva E G, Mackay B 1981 Neuroendocrine (Merkel cell) carcinomas of the skin: An ultrastructural study of nine cases. Ultrastructural Pathology 2: 1–9

Silva E G, Ordóñez N G, Lechago J 1984 Immunohistochemical studies in endocrine carcinoma of the skin. American Journal of Clinical Pathology 81: 558–562

Sim F H, Taylor W F, Ivins J C, Pritchard D J, Soule E H 1978 A prospective randomized study of the efficacy of routine elective lymphadenectomy in management of malignant melanoma: preliminary results. Cancer 41: 948–956

Sims C F, Kirsch N 1948 Spindle cell epidermoid epithelioma simulating sarcoma in chronic radiodermatitis. Archives of Dermatology and Syphilology 57: 63–68

Sinclair D 1981 Mechanisms of cutaneous sensation, 2nd edn. Oxford University Press, p 53–80

Skinner M S, Sternberg W H, Ichinose H, Collins J 1973 Spontaneous regression of Bowenoid atypia of the vulva. Obstetrics and Gynecology 42: 40–46

Skjaeraasen E 1969 Cancer of the female urethra: a clinical study of 25 cases. Acta Obstetricia et and Gynecologica Scandinavica 48: 589–597

Smith Foushee J H, Reeves W J, McCool J A 1968 Benign masses of Bartholin's gland. Solid adenomas, adenomas with cyst and Bartholin's gland with varices and thrombosis or cavernous hemangioma. Obstetrics and Gynecology 31: 695–701

Spraitz A F, Welch J S 1965 Diverticulum of the female urethra. American Journal of Obstetrics and Gynecology 91: 1013–1016

Stacey J E 1939 Epithelioma of the vulva. Proceedings of the Royal Society of Medicine 32: 304–308

Stacy D, Burrell M O, Franklin E W 1986 Extramammary Paget's disease of the vulva and anus: use of intraoperative frozen-section margins. American Journal of Obstetrics and Gynecology 155: 519–523

Stanbridge C M, Butler E B 1983 Human papillomavirus infection of the lower female genital tract: association with multicentric neoplasia. International Journal of Gynecological Pathology 2: 264–274

Stapleton J J 1984 Extramammary Paget's disease of the vulva in a young black woman. A case report with histogenic confirmation by immunostaining. Journal of Reproductive Medicine 29: 444–446

Stehman F B, Castaloo T W, Charles E H, Lagasse L 1980 Verrucous carcinoma of the vulva. International Journal of Obstetrics and Gynecology 17: 523–525

Stern J B, Kwon T H 1981 Vulvar carcinoma with metastases to the uterus. Gynecologic Oncology 11: 246–251

Stout A P 1938 The relationship of malignant amelanotic melanoma (naevocarcinoma) to extramammary Paget's disease. American Journal of Cancer 33: 196–204

Stout A P, Cooley S G E 1951 Carcinoma of sweat glands. Cancer 4: 521–536

Stumpf P G 1980 Increasing occurrence of condylomata acuminata in premenstrual children. Obstetrics and Gynecology 56: 262–264

Sullivan J, Grabstald H 1978 Management of carcinoma of the urethra. In: Skinner D G, de Kernion J B (eds) Genitourinary cancer. W B Saunders, Philadelphia, p 419–429

Sussman E B, Brice M II, Gray G F 1974 Nephrogenic metaplasia of the bladder. Journal of Urology 111: 34–35

Svanholm H, Andersen O P, Røhl H 1987 Tumour of female paraurethral duct. Immunohistochemical similarity with prostatic carcinoma. Virchows Archiv A 411: 395–398

Sworn M J, Hammond G T, Buchanan R 1979 Metastatic basal cell carcinoma of the vulva case report. British Journal of Obstetrics and Gynecology 86: 332–334

Symmonds R E, Pratt J H, Dockerty M D 1960 Melanoma of the vulva. Obstetrics and Gynecology 15: 543–553

Taggart C G, Castro J R, Rutledge F N 1972 Carcinoma of the female urethra. American Journal of Roentgenology 114: 145–151

Tanabe E T, Mazur M T, Schaeffer A J 1982 Clear cell adenocarcinoma of the female urethra. Cancer 49: 372–378

Tang C-K, Toker R C 1978 Trabecular carcinoma of the skin. An ultrastructural study. Cancer 42: 2311–2321

Tang C-K, Toker R C 1979 Trabecular carcinoma of the skin: Further clinicopathologic and ultrastructural study. Mt Sinai Journal of Medicine 46: 516–523

Tang C-K, Nedwich A, Toker C, Zaman A N F 1982 Unusual cutaneous carcinoma with features of small cell (oat cell-like) and squamous cell carcinomas. A variant of malignant Merkel cell neoplasm. American Journal of Dermatopathology 4:

537–548

Tapia F J, Polak J M, Barbosa A J A, Bloom S R, Marangos P J, Dermody C, Pearse A G E 1981 Neuron-specific enolase is produced by neuroendocrine tumours. Lancet i: 808–810

Tappeiner J, Wolff K 1968 Hidradenoma papilliferum. Eine enzymhistochemische und electronenmikroskopische Studie. Hautarzt 19: 101–109

Taussig F J 1940 Cancer of the vulva: an analysis of 155 cases (1911–1940). American Journal of Obstetrics and Gynecology 40: 764–779

Taxy J B, Ettinger D S, Wharam M D 1980 Primary small cell carcinoma of the skin. Cancer 46: 2308–2311

Taylor P T, Stenwig J T, Klausen H 1975 Paget's disease of the vulva: A report of 18 cases. Gynecologic Oncology, 46–60

Tchang F, Okagaki T, Richart R M 1973 Adenocarcinoma of Bartholin's gland associated with Paget's disease of vulvar area. Cancer 31: 221–225

Teloh H A, Balkin R B, Grier J P 1957 Metastasizing sweat-gland carcinoma. Archives of Dermatology 76: 80–86

Thomas J, Majmudar B, Gorelkin L 1979 Syringoma localized to the vulva. Archives of Dermatology 115: 95–96

Tiltman A J, Knutzen V K 1978 Primary adenocarcinoma of the vulva originating in misplaced cloacal tissue. Obstetrics and Gynecology 51: 30S–33S

Toker C 1972 Trabecular carcinoma of the skin. Archives of Dermatology 105: 107–110

Toker C 1982 Trabecular carcinoma of the skin. A question of title. American Journal of Dermatopathology 4: 497–500

Toki T, Oikawa N, Tase T, Satoh S, Wada Y, Yajima A 1986 Immunohistochemical demonstration of papillomavirus antigen in cervical dysplasia and vulvar condyloma. Gynecological and Obstetric Investigation 22: 97–101

Torres S A, Quattlebaum R B 1972 Carcinoma in a urethral diverticulum. Southern Medical Journal 65: 1374–1376

Trelford J D, Deos P H 1976 Bartholin's gland carcinomas: Five cases. Gynecologic Oncology 4: 212–221

Tsukada Y, Lopez R G, Pickren J W, Piver M S, Barlow J J 1975 Paget's disease of the vulva. A clinocopathologic study of eight cases. Obstetrics and Gynecology 45: 73–78

Tuck S M, Williams A 1985 Paget's disease of the vulva complicated by bladder carcinoma. Case report. British Journal of Obstetrics and Gynecology 92: 416–418

Turner A G, Hendry W F 1980 Primary carcinoma of the female urethra. British Journal of Urology 52: 549–554

Tweedle C D 1978 Ultrastructure of Merkel cell development in aneurogenic and control amphibian larvae (Ambystoma). Neuroscience 3: 481–486

Underwood J W, Adcock L L, Okagaki T 1978 Adeno-squamous carcinoma of skin appendages (Adenoid squamous cell carcinoma, pseudoglandular squamous cell carcinoma, adenoacanthoma of sweat gland of Lever) of the vulva. Cancer 42: 1851–1855

Underwood L J, Montgomery H, Broders A C 1951 Squamous-cell epithelioma that simulates sarcoma. Archives of Dermatology and Syphilology 64: 149–158

Underwood P B, Hester L L 1971 Diagnosis and treatment of premalignant lesions of the vulva: a review. American Journal of Obstetrics and Gynecology 110: 849–857

Van Dijk C, Ten Seldam R E J 1975 A possible primary cutaneous carcinoid. Cancer 36: 1016–1020

Van Nagell J R Jr, Tweeddale D N, Roddick J W Jr 1969 Primary adenoacanthoma of the Bartholin gland. Report of a case. Obstetrics and Gynecology 34: 87–90

Vayrynen M, Romppanen T, Koskela E, Castren A O, Syrjänen K 1981 Verrucous squamous cell carcinoma of the female genital tract: report of three cases and survey of the literature. International Journal of Gynaecology and Obstetrics 19: 351–356

Veronisi U, Adamus J, Bandiera D C, Brennhond I O, Caceres E, Cascinelli N, Claudio F, Ikonopisov R L, Javorskj V V, Kirov S, Kulakowski A, Lacour J, Lejeune F, Mechl Z, Marabito A, Rodé J, Sergeev S, van Slooten E, Szczygiel K, Trapeznikov N N, Wagner R I 1977 Inefficacy of immediate node dissection in Stage I melanoma of the limbs. New England Journal of Medicine 297: 627–630

Wade T R, Ackerman A B 1979 The effects of podophyllum resin on condylomata acuminata. Archives of Dermatology 115: 1349

Wade T R, Kopf A W, Ackerman A B 1979 Bowenoid papulosis of the genitalia. Archives of Dermatology 115: 306–308

Wahlström T, Vesterinen E, Saksela E 1978 Primary carcinoma of Bartholin's Glands: A morphological and clinical study of six cases including a transitional cell carcinoma. Gynecologic Oncology 6: 354–362

Walker L M, Huffman J W 1947 Adenocarcinoma of the female urethra. A review. Quarterly Bulletin of the Northwestern University 21: 115–125

Wallace H J 1971 Lichen sclerosus et atrophicus. Transactions of St John's Hospital Dermatological Society 57: 9–30

Wani N A, Bhan B L, Guru A A, Garyali R K 1976 Leiomyoma of the female urethra: a case report. Journal of Urology 116: 120–121

Warner F C S, Hafez G R, Buchler D A 1982 Neurotropic melanoma of the vulva. Cancer 49: 999–1004

Way S 1960 Carcinoma of the vulva. American Journal of Obstetrics and Gynecology 79: 692–697

Way S 1982 Malignant disease of the vulva. Churchill Livingstone, Edinburgh

Webb J B, Beswick I P 1983 Eccrine hidradenocarcinoma of the vulva with Paget's disease. Case report with a review of the literature. British Journal of Obstetrics and Gynecology 90: 90–95

Webb J B, Lott M, O'Sullivan J C, Azzopardi J G 1984 Combined adenoid cystic and squamous carcinoma of Bartholin's gland. Case report. British Journal of Obstetrics and Gynaecology 91: 291–295

Weiner H A 1937 Paget's disease of the skin and its relation to carcinoma of the apocrine sweat glands. American Journal of Cancer 31: 373–403

Weissmann A, Camisa C 1982 Friedrich Sigmund Merkel Part I. The man. American Journal of Dermatopathology 4: 521–526

Wharton J T, Gallager S, Rutledge F N 1974 Microinvasive carcinoma of the vulva. American Journal of Obstetrics and Gynecology 118: 159–162

Wharton L R, Everett H S 1951 Primary malignant Bartholin's gland tumors. Obstetrics and Gynecology Surveys 6: 1–8

Wheelock J B, Gopelrud D R, Dunn L T, Oates J F 1984 Primary carcinoma of the Bartholin gland: a report of ten cases. Obstetrics and Gynecology 63: 820–824

Wick M R, Goellner J R, Wolfe J T III, Su W P D 1985a Vulvar sweat gland carcinomas. Archives of Pathology and Laboratory Medicine 109: 43–47

Wick M R, Goellner J R, Wolfe J T III, Su W P D 1985b Adnexal carcinomas of the skin. I. Eccrine carcinomas. Cancer 56: 1147–1162

Wick M R, Goellner J R, Wolfe J T III, Su W P D 1985c Adnexal carcinomas of the skin II. Extraocular sebaceous carcinomas. Cancer 56: 1163–1172

Wilkinson E J, Rico M J, Pierson K K 1982 Microinvasive

carcinoma of the vulva. International Journal of Gynecological Pathology 1: 29–39

Wilkinson E J, Kneale B, Lynch P J 1986 Report of the ISSVD terminology committee. In: Journal of Reproductive Medicine 31: 973–974

Wilner R B, Greenwald M, Wendelken H 1976 Eccrine carcinoma of the vulva: report of a case. Journal of the American Osteopathic Association 76: 282–285

Winkelmann R K, Muller S A 1964 Sweat gland tumors. Archives of Dermatology 89: 827–831

Winkelmann R K, Wolff K 1967 Solid-cystic hidradenoma of the skin. Archives of Dermatology 97: 651–661

Winkelmann R K, Wolff K 1968 Histochemistry of hidradenoma and eccrine spiradenoma. Journal of Investigative Dermatology 49: 173–180

Wishard W N Jr, Nourse M H 1952 Carcinoma in diverticulum of female urethra. Journal of Urology 68: 320–323

Wishard W N Jr, Nourse M H, Mertz J H O 1960 Carcinoma in diverticulum of female urethra. Journal of Urology 83: 409–413

Wishard W N Jr, Nourse M H, Mertz J H O 1963 Carcinoma in a diverticulum of the female urethra. Journal of Urology 89: 431–432

Wong S W, Dao A H, Glick A D 1981 Trabecular carcinoma of the skin: a case report. Human Pathology 12: 838–840

Woodruff J D 1955 Paget's disease of the vulva. Obstetrics and Gynecology 5: 175–185

Woodruff J D 1977 Paget's disease. Obstetrics and Gynecology 49: 511–512

Woodruff J D 1982 Early invasive carcinoma of the vulva. Clinical Oncology 1: 349–354

Woodruff J D, Novak E R 1962 Premalignant lesions of the vulva. A pathological and clinical survey. Clinical Obstetrics and Gynecology 5: 1102–1118

Woodruff J D, Julian C, Puray T, Mermut S, Katayama P 1973 The contemporary challenge of carcinoma in situ of the vulva. American Journal of Obstetrics and Gynecology 115: 667–686

Woodruff J D, Braun L, Cavalieri R, Gupta P, Pass F, Shah K V 1980 Immunologic identification of papillomavirus antigen in condyloma tissues from the female genital tract. Obstetrics and Gynecology 56: 727–732

Woodworth H, Dockerty M B, Wilson R B, Pratt J H 1971

Papillary hidradenoma of the vulva. A clinicopathologic study of 69 cases. American Journal of Obstetrics and Gynecology 110: 501–508

Woringer Fr, Eichler A 1951 Constatations et réflexions au sujet d'un cas d'hidradénomes éruptifs. Annales de Dermatologie et Syphiligraphie (Paris) 78: 152–164

Woyke S, Domagala W, Olszewski W, Korabiec M 1974 Pseudosarcoma of the skin. An electron microscopic study and comparison with the fine structure of the spindle-cell variant of squamous carcinoma. Cancer 33: 970–980

Wright J D, Font R L 1979 Mucinous sweat gland adenocarcinoma of the eyelid. A clinicopathologic study of 21 cases with histochemical and electron microscopic observations. Cancer 44: 1757–1768

Yackel D B, Symmonds R E, Kempers R D 1970 Melanoma of the vulva. Obstetrics and Gynecology 35: 625–631

Yazigi R, Piver M S, Tsukada Y 1978 Microinvasive carcinoma of the vulva. Obstetrics and Gynecology 51: 368–370

Yesudian P, Thambiah A 1975 Familial syringoma. Dermatologica 150: 32–35

Young A W Jr, Herman E W, Tovell H M M 1980 Syringoma of the vulva: incidence, diagnosis and cause of pruritus. Obstetrics and Gynecology 55: 515–518

Young R H, Scully R E 1985 Clear cell adenocarcinoma of the bladder and urethra. A report of three cases and review of the literature. The American Journal of Surgical Pathology 9: 816–826

Zackheim H S 1963 Origin of the human basal cell epithelioma. Journal of Investigative Dermatology 40: 283–297

Zaino R J, Husseinzadeh N, Nahhas W, Mortel R 1982 Epithelial alterations in proximity to invasive squamous carcinoma of the vulva. International Journal of Gynecological Pathology 1: 173–184

Zerner J 1975 Basal cell carcinoma of the vulva. A report of six cases and review of the literature. Journal of the Maine Medical Association 65: 127–129

Ziegerman J H, Gordon S F 1970 Cancer of the female urethra—a curable disease. Obstetrics and Gynecology 36: 785–789

Zur Hausen H 1982 Human genital cancer: synergism between two virus infections or synergism between a virus infection and initiating events? Lancet ii 1370–1372

11

Some surgical modalities of treatment in vulval conditions
M J Campion and A Singer

MANAGEMENT OF VULVAL NEOPLASIA

Vulval intra-epithelial neoplasia (squamous type)

Compelling changes in the clinical profile of vulval intra-epithelial neoplasia (VIN) in recent years have necessitated change in the philosophy of management. The disease now affects younger women in greater frequency, with the modal age of diagnosis of VIN III (Fig. 11.1) falling to 30 years or less in recent studies (Friedrich et al 1980, Bernstein et al 1983, Campion & Singer 1987). Up to 30% of women with VIN are nulligravid and thus attention must be focused on maintenance of sexual fuction

and reproductive capacity as well as on psychological effects of treatment (Campion et al 1985).

The pathophysiology and natural history of VIN have not been fully elucidated and thus recommendations regarding therapy must remain cautions. However, progression of VIN to malignancy has been reported, particularly in the immunosuppressed or elderly woman (Gardiner et al 1953, Buscema et al 1980, Friedrich et al 1980, Jones & McLean 1986). Small, early invasive vulval cancers are now more frequently diagnosed in younger women. Many women with VIN are symptomatic and at risk of neoplasia elsewhere in the genital

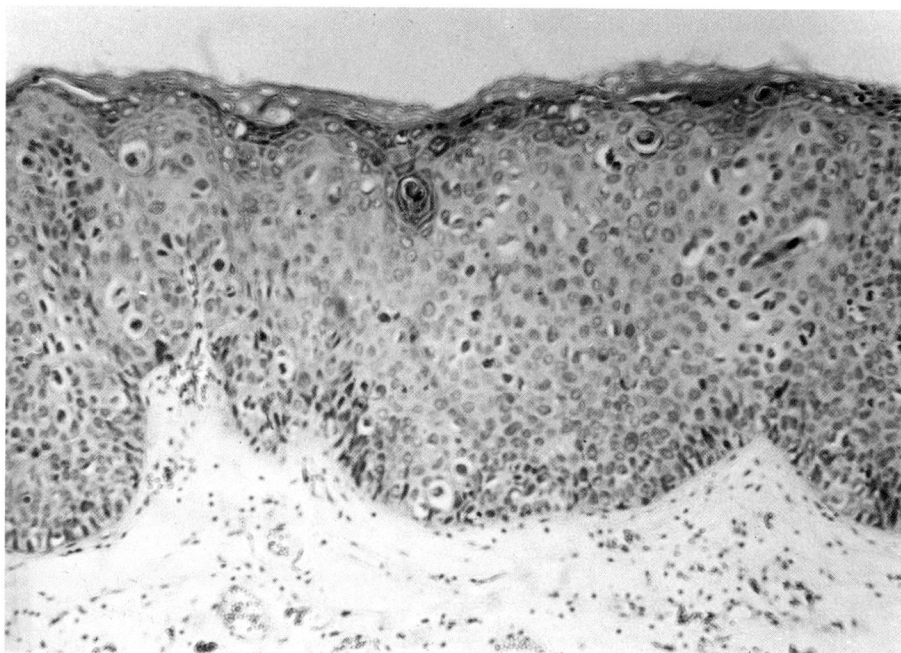

Fig. 11.1 VIN III: epithelial atypia with pleomorphic pyknotic nuclei and disordered maturation involving the full thickness of the vulval epithelium

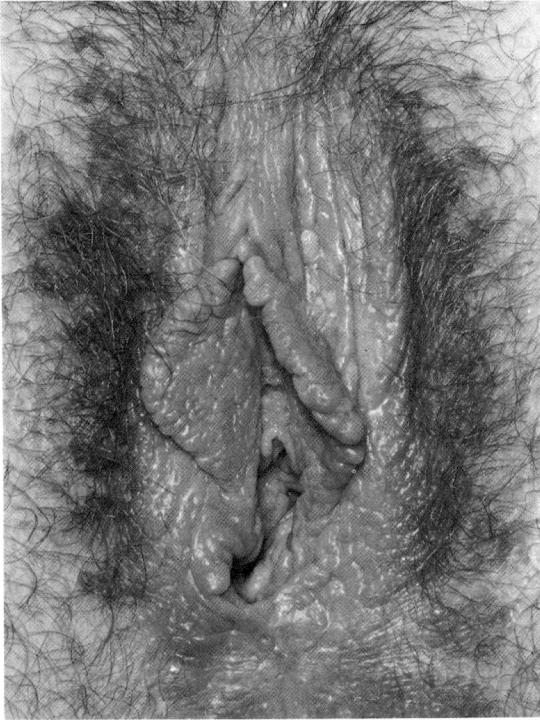

Fig. 11.2 VIN III: extensive warty lesions, pigmented at periphery

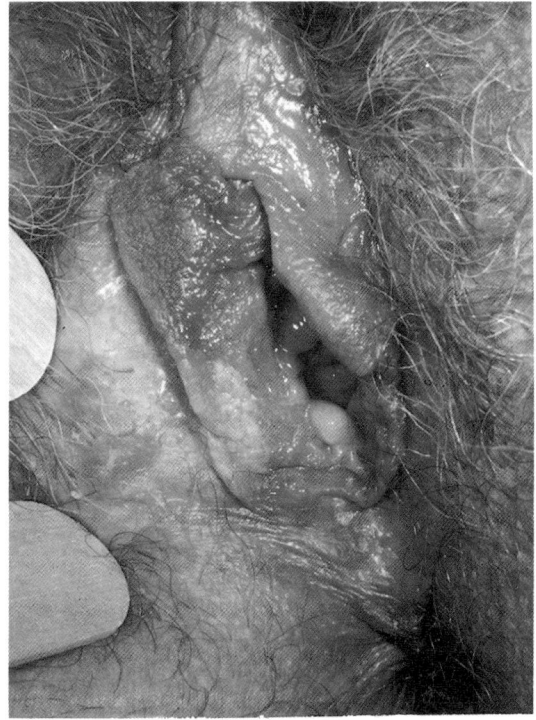

Fig. 11.3 VIN III: macular lesions. (Reproduced from Beilby & Ridley 1987 by courtesy of the authors and publisher)

tract (Campion & Singer 1987). Thus the changes in this clinical profile of VIN demand care and accuracy in diagnosis and formulation of a conservative but effective and individualised approach to therapy.

Diagnosis

In the absence of a sensitive screening test for detection of pre-invasive vulval disease, the diagnosis of VIN depends on awareness of symptomatology, familiarity with clinical appearance, a high index of suspicion on the part of the examiner and readiness to perform a confirmatory biopsy. The value of careful inspection of the vulva during routine gynaecological examination cannot be overstated and remains a most productive diagnostic technique. The magnified illumination of the colposcope improves accuracy of diagnosis and is particularly effective in detecting multifocal lesions within the vulva. The proclivity to multicentricity of squamous neoplasia in the lower genital tract (Campion et al 1985, McCance et al 1985, Bergeron et al 1987) demands that the cervix, vagina and peri-anal regions be examined carefully by colposcopy also.

The clinical appearance of VIN III is variable (Figs. 11.2, 11.3). The lesions may be papular or macular, coalescent or discrete, single or multiple. Lesions on the cutaneous surface of the vulva usually appear as white or pigmented, thickened and hyperkeratotic plaques. By contrast, lesions of the mucosal surface are usually macular and pink or red in colour. The milder forms of VIN present clinically as pale areas varying in optical density. The addition of 5% acetic acid to the vulval skin produces prominent blanching of the lesion after 3 to 5 minutes. Such areas of white epithelium are clearly visible through the colposcope and there is no associated patient discomfort. Vulval pre-invasive lesions are hyperpigmented in 10 to 15% of patients. These lesions range in colour from mahogany to dark brown and stand out sharply when observed with the naked eye.

Parakeratosis is a common feature. This is defined as retention of nuclear chromatin material in the usually acellular keratin layer of the epithelium and as such is a manifestation of abnormal maturation. It is identifiable using the Collins et al (1966) toluidine blue test. A 1% aqueous solution of the dye is applied to the external genital area. Toluidine blue is a nuclear stain and will become fixed to superficial nuclei (ulcers, fissures, parakeratosis). After drying for 2 to 3 minutes, the area is decolourised with a solution of 1% acetic acid. Areas of parakeratosis and suspicious foci of increased nuclear atypia retain the dye and acquire a deep blue tinge while normal skin accepts little or none of the dye. Unfortunately, hyperkeratotic lesions, although often neoplastic, are poorly stained, whereas benign excoriations are often brilliant; that is, there are high false positive and false negative rates (Lancet 1982). Thus colposcopic examination has emerged as a more accurate diagnostic technique and toluidine blue must not be applied until a thorough colposcopy has been performed.

Colposcopic examination may itself at times be compromised by vulval inflammation or other disease processes such as hyperkeratosis. Colposcopically suspicious epithelium may occur in association with herpetic infections, trauma, healing and scar formation. Therefore, following identification of suspicious lesions, vulval biopsy must be used liberally to obtain definitive diagnosis. Extensive disease may demand examination and biopsy under general anaesthetic. However, biopsies may often be taken under local anaesthetic, producing minimal patient discomfort. Adequate biopsies are obtainable using an 'alligator joints' instrument such as the Patterson rectal biopsy forceps which allow adequate skin traction and sampling of deeper layers of epithelium. Similarly a Keyes dermatological punch (4 mm or 6 mm size) allows removal of an adequate tissue sample and permits ready orientation for future sectioning. After obtaining the biopsy specimen a small piece of gel foam cut with the Keyes punch or biopsy forceps may be positioned in the skin defect with a small dressing for 24 hours. Invasive carcinoma can virtually al-

ways be excluded by expert colposcopy and multiple biopsies (Campion 1987). These conservative and cosmetically acceptable diagnostic modalities have become the mainstay of diagnosis of vulval premalignancy.

Contiguous structures which may also be involved with intra-epithelial neoplasia are the perianal and anal region, the glans of the clitoris, the lower vagina and urethral meatus. These areas are readily assessed using the colposcope and biopsies must be taken of suspicious lesions.

The high incidence of associated and sometimes silent sexually transmitted disease in women with VIN calls for a thorough search for evidence of HPV and HSV infection, *Chlamydia trachomatis*, *Trichomonas vaginalis* and *Gardnerella vaginalis*. An endocervical culture for gonorrhoea and a serological screening test for syphilis should be performed in all cases.

Modes of treatment

The different therapeutic modalities employed in the treatment of the more severe degrees of VIN, in particular VIN III (severe dysplasia, carcinoma in situ), will now be critically reviewed.

Surgical techniques.

Vulvectomy. Although the original treatment advocated by Knight (1943) for carcinoma in situ of the vulva was wide local excision, in the 1960s simple vulvectomy became standard management (Collins et al 1970, Boutselis 1972). There were several reasons for the more aggressive surgical approach:

1. Vulval carcinoma in situ was considered a pre-invasive lesion with a high risk of malignant progression.
2. The disease was frequently multifocal and complete removal therefore required more extensive surgery.
3. Complete histological evaluation of the vulvectomy specimen permitted exclusion of occult invasion.
4. Vulval epithelium at risk of future neoplasia could be removed.

Certainly, the recurrence rate of carcinoma in situ after vulvectomy in most series is low, Boutselis (1972) reporting an incidence of less than 10%.

However, recurrence of disease after an adequate lesser procedure, such as wide local excision, is not significantly greater. Indeed, in the series of Buscema et al (1980) the recurrence rate of VIN after vulvectomy was 32%; after local excision it was 30%. Further, the area at risk of recurrence includes the entire lower genital tract, perineum and anal skin and thus even a total vulvectomy is not adequate to remove all the epithelium at risk.

Recently the trend has been to more conservative therapeutic modalities in managing pre-invasive vulval disease. The risk of progress of VIN to invasive cancer is considered lower and slower to take effect than was previously thought. Spontaneous regressions have been reported (Bernstein et al 1983), particularly in pregnancy (Friedrich et al 1980). As vulval carcinoma in situ is presenting with increasing frequency in younger women the sequelae of vulvectomy are particularly undesirable, for example loss of peri-anal padding and protection, introital stenosis and dyspareunia, loss of secretions from vulval glands, loss of sensation (particularly with clitoral amputation), loss of elasticity for vaginal delivery, urinary stream problems and a castration-like self image.

Major postoperative complications such as pulmonary embolism do occur. Wound breakdown following primary closure is uncommon but scarring may impair sexual function and reproductive capacity. Perhaps the greatest cost is in emotional terms as, despite the relief following treatment for a potentially malignant lesion, the patients regret the loss of the vulva and regard themselves as 'disfigured'.

Experience in diagnosis of vulva-epithelial neoplasia and thorough mapping of lesions using the colposcope, after application of acetic acid, obviate the need for vulvectomy to exclude invasive disease. Less radical treatment can then be offered. Many series have now demonstrated the accuracy of colposcopic diagnosis with liberal use of biopsy, DiSaia & Rich (1981) finding no invasion in 39 patients diagnosed as having carcinoma in situ. In this unit, occult invasion was diagnosed on biopsy in a single patient in 50 initially diagnosed as VIN by colposcopy. The invasive lesion occurred in association with recurrence of severe vulval condylomata acuminata. Friedrich et al (1980) described superficial invasion in three of 50 patients diagnosed

initially as having carcinoma in situ but none of the three patients had more than 1 mm of invasion. Accurate clinical assessment and colposcopy of the vulva permits less radical management, thus avoiding complications and improving the cosmetic result.

Skinning vulvectomy with split thickness skin graft: Rutledge & Sinclair (1968) introduced the skinning (cutaneous) vulvectomy and skin graft procedure. The technique has been modified and promoted by DiSaia (DiSaia et al 1984, Rettenmaier et al 1987) (Fig. 11.4). A shallow 'skinning' excision of the vulval skin is performed following careful mapping of lesions to determine extent of disease. The skin at risk in the vulval site is replaced with epidermis from a donor site on the thigh or buttock. The clitoris is always preserved, any lesions on the glans being superficially excised, and the epithelium regenerates without loss of sensation. The skinning vulvectomy and skin graft procedure is indicated particularly for extensive, multifocal VIN (Rettenmaier et al 1987). The subcutaneous tissue of the vulva is preserved, giving optimal cosmetic and functional results, but the method has the disadvantage of producing an additional scar at the donor site.

Using this technique, a low recurrence rate is achieved. Forney et al (1977) describe one recurrence in eight patients so treated. Recent reports have suggested that donated skin might be susceptible to a similar disease process, and that disease might recur within the skin graft. However, DiSaia et al (1984) describe recurrence outside the grafted area (in preserved vulval skin) but never in the graft itself. They suggest that the neoplastic potential is inherent in the original vulval skin and does not translate to skin from other parts of the body placed at the vulval site.

Following skinning vulvectomy and skin graft, prolonged bed rest for 1 week is required whilst the split thickness graft adheres to the graft bed. Such immobilisation increases the potential for morbidity. Thus care must be taken to encourage circulation to avoid thrombo-embolic phenomena and to assess respiratory status, particularly in the elderly.

Wide local excision: recent series report increasing use of wide local excision for VIN (Friedrich et al 1980). Certainly, most localised lesions are managed very effectively by wide local excision, allow-

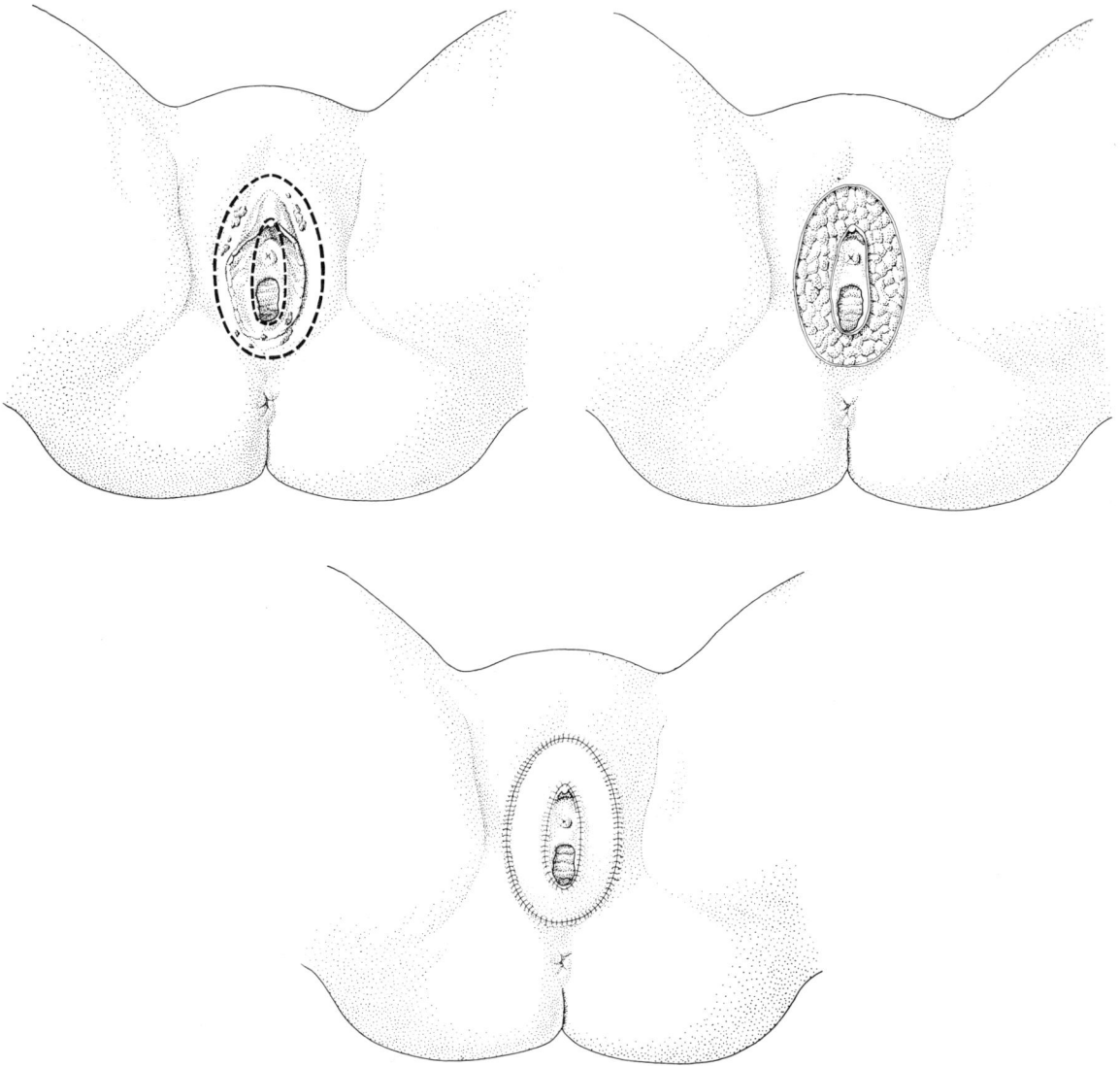

Fig. 11.4 Schematic representation of skinning vulvectomy with split thickness skin graft (after DiSaia et al 1984)

ing a disease-free border of at least 5 to 10 mm, with primary approximation of the defect. Healing is usually uncomplicated with good cosmetic and functional outcome. The vulval skin and mucous membrane have a great deal of elasticity; thus sexual and reproductive functions are preserved, which is of importance particularly in the young patient.

The important advantage of surgical excision is that complete histological assessment of the biopsy is possible. Lesions with foci of micro-invasive disease will be diagnosed. Histological evaluation of

the margins of excised tissue is essential. Of 37 patients treated surgically by Friedrich et al (1980), 31 had disease-free margins. Three (10%) of these developed a recurrence. Three of six (50%) with positive margins developed a recurrence. Thus the probability of recurrence of vulval carcinoma in situ depends more on the histological quality of the surgical margins than on the magnitude of the operative procedure.

The preferred surgical approach to more severe degrees of VIN, particularly vulval carcinoma in situ, is therefore wide excision, encompassing all lesions with a wide margin and sparing areas of vulval skin not involved with disease. Wide local excision will usually achieve this, but with extensive, widespread disease skinning vulvectomy with split thickness skin graft to the vulva from a donor site may be indicated. The clitoris should be preserved even if overlying skin requires excision due to involvement with VIN. The patient must be carefully reassessed at regular intervals for life with attention being paid to the cervix and entire lower genital tract extending into the peri-anal and anal regions. Recurrence of intra-epithelial disease does not carry the ominous implications of an invasive recurrence and can be managed with further wide excision.

Local destruction. Laser vaporisation: the carbon dioxide laser has become more widely used in the management of VIN over the past decade, providing an effective but non-mutilating treatment (Reid 1985, Campion & Singer 1987, Wright & Davies 1987). This has been important in view of the increased prevalence of VIN in younger women, the disease being commonly multifocal and associated with more widespread clinical and subclinical sexually transmitted papillomavirus infection. The carbon dioxide laser allows destruction of the entire area of abnormal epithelium to a shallow depth permitting rapid healing from keratinocytes in underlying pilosebaecous glands. A cosmetically pleasing end result will be obtained, irrespective of the area ablated, provided destruction does not extend beyond the mid-dermis.

The success of any destructive surgical modality depends on accurate appraisal of the extent and nature of disease to be eradicated. This is achieved by performing a very thorough pre-operative and intra-operative colposcopy of vulva, vagina, cervix, urethra and anus to delineate all areas of VIN or HPV infection. Any areas of prominent induration or ulceration, large or solitary nodules, and lesions characterised colposcopically by bizarre dilated capillaries or friable yellowish epithelium must be evaluated by wide local excision to exclude occult invasion. Lesions superimposed on long-standing condylomata acuminata or on chronic dermatological conditions, especially in elderly or immunosuppressed patients, must also be managed with extreme caution.

After exclusion of occult invasion and delineation of the extent of disease by careful mapping of lesions, the carbon dioxide laser permits precise but minimal tissue destruction to optimise cure potential and minimise sequelae. The laser is employed with as high a power density as the surgeon can control, although experience has shown that power densities over 600 W/cm^2 are very difficult to control on the vulva (Reid et al 1985). Choice of appropriate laser beam geometry is the key to safe vulval laser therapy. The vulval mucosa, in particular, is fragile tissue and extreme care must be taken to control depth of vaporisation. The area of disease is outlined to include a 3 to 5 mm outer peripheral margin of normal tissue. Large areas can be subdivided and vaporised in turn.

After the initial impact of the laser, the wound is immediately covered by a layer of char that precludes depth orientation. The surface char is wiped away uncovering the plump keratinocytes of the prickle and basal layers. This next layer is destroyed by rapid oscillation of the laser beam over the tissue and without overlapping of beam paths. The area is then wiped with moistened cotton wool, exposing the smooth surface of the basement membrane, beneath which can be seen the anatomically intact papillary dermis. The area is then vaporised to the level of the reticular dermis, the coarse collagen and elastic bundles becoming visible through the operating microscope as grey-white fibres. This is the deepest level from which optimum healing will result and large areas can be ablated to this depth without scarring or loss of function. Thus laser vaporisation in the treatment of VIN is usually performed to a mid-dermal level, or second surgical plane, that is, a depth of about 3 mm (Figs. 11.5–11.9)

However, most of the hair follicles and apocrine glands are located within the lower half of the reticular dermis. Mene & Buckley (1985) recently have reported disease involving skin appendages in 28 of 50 patients with VIN and the maximum depth of involvement reached 4.6 mm from the surface of the epidermis. Thus the surgeon must be aware of the depth of involvement of skin appendages with disease on histology. If disease penetrates beyond the mid-dermal level wide local excision, or laser vaporisation followed by split skin grafting, may be indicated to avoid scarring or keloid formation, or residual disease due to in-

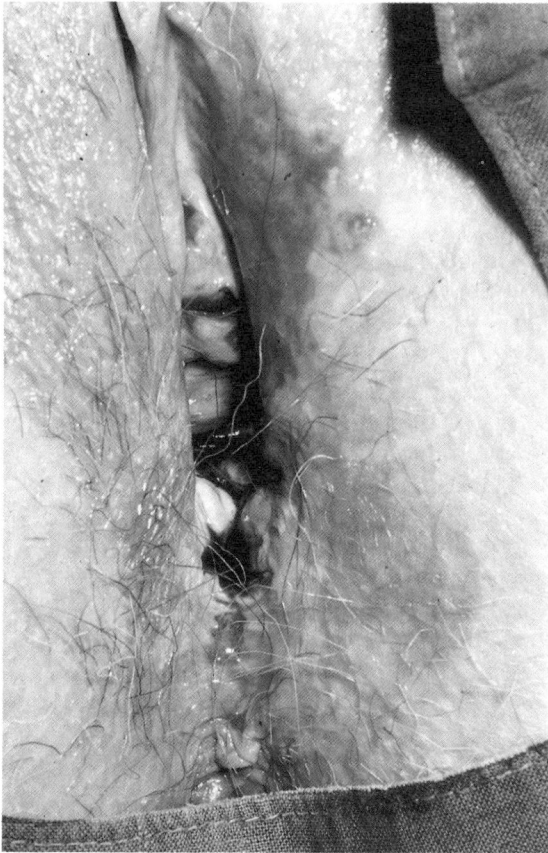

Fig. 11.5 Lesion of VIN.

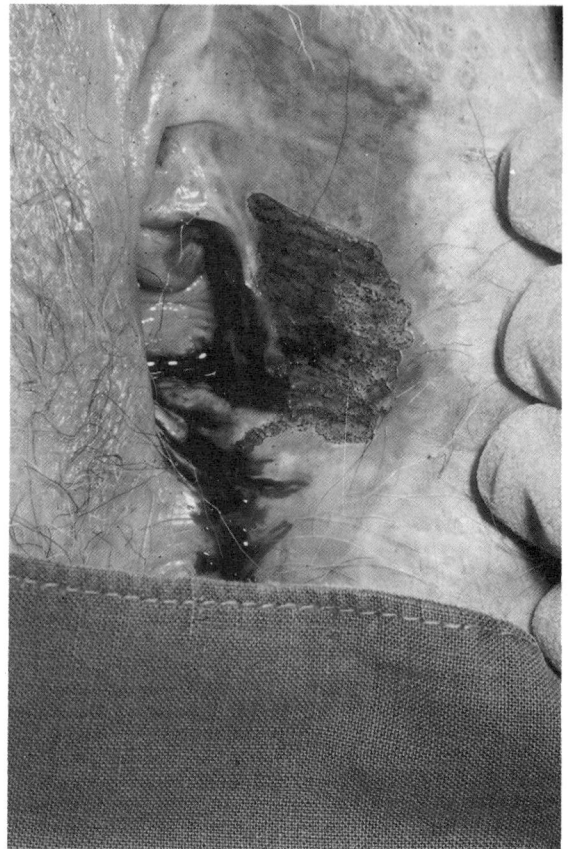

Fig. 11.6 Initial laser process.

adequate depth of destruction. Disease involving both hair-bearing areas of the vulva and mucous membrane may be best treated by combining wide local excision of the lateral lesion with laser vaporisation of the inner lesions. Destruction of the skin appendages produces an effective third-degree burn. Such wounds heal by granulation from the base and epithelial ingrowth from the sides yielding atrophic scars devoid of physiological skin functions and too weak to withstand vigorous coital function.

After vulval laser surgery, charred desiccated tissue remains. Within 12–24 hours induration, exudation and oedema are noted followed by formation of a thin, grey, necrotic membrane over the defect. At this time, 48 to 60 hours after surgery, the discomfort is maximal (Jordan 1981). It can be relieved by saline or sea-water sitz baths several times a day. The perineum should be dried with a

blow dryer after bathing. Following urination, perineal irrigation and air cooling are advised. Micturition may be very painful and hence a catheter may be required in cases of extensive laser treatment to avoid retention of urine. Oedema, induration and pain subside towards the end of the second week. Healing is rapid with complete re-epithelialisation occurring over 4 to 6 weeks. The cosmetic results are excellent.

Bleeding is unusual but if it occurs it will be about 4 to 7 days after surgery. Infection is uncommon with adherence to the postoperative regimes. Coaptation of the labia is a potential sequel of extensive laser therapy of opposing surfaces but this is rare with good surgical technique and meticulous postoperative care.

The carbon dioxide laser therefore provides an increasingly popular therapeutic option in the management of VIN. However, the patient must be

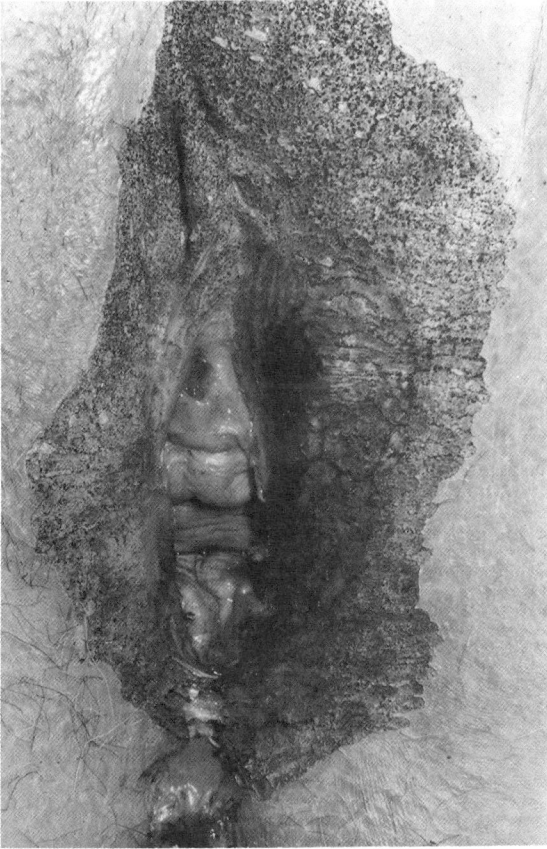

Fig. 11.7 Later stage of laser process.

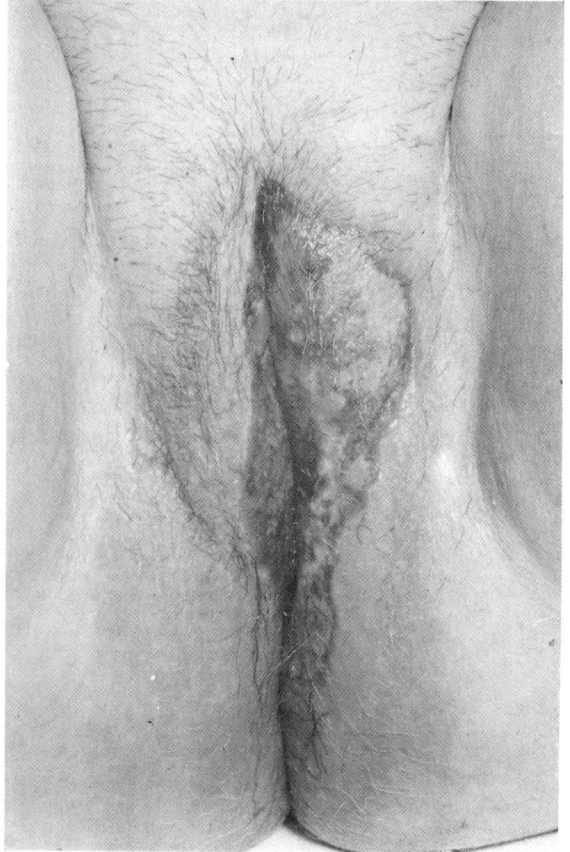

Fig. 11.8 End of laser treatment.

carefully assessed postoperati ely to exclude invasive disease and the surgeon must have a detailed knowledge of vulval anatomy and be trained in the use of the laser in order to achieve cure without unnecessary morbidity. Multiple treatments will frequently be necessary. Patient follow-up must be meticulous, particularly in the first 5 years after treatment, and should continue for life. Recurrent disease may be further managed with the laser after exclusion of occult invasion. In our experience most recurrences occur outside previously treated areas. In this unit, 44 of 50 (88%) of women with VIN III have been cured using the carbon dioxide laser (with a minimum of 12 months follow-up) (Campion & Singer 1987). Similar results are obtained by others; Townsend et al (1982) successfully treated 31 of 33 patients (94%) with VIN III. Baggish & Dorsey (1981) reported that 31 of 35 patients were cured of their disease.

Management of peri-anal and anal extension of

VIN. Vulval intra-epithelial neoplasia may involve a large area of skin extending at times into the peri-anal region and may involve the anal mucosa. Management of such extensive disease requires individualisation and may involve a combination of therapeutic modalities often spread over a period of time.

Intra-epithelial neoplasia of peri-anal skin extending to the anal mucosa may be managed by total excision of the involved epithelium followed by split skin grafts, which may be applied to the anal canal and sutured circumferentially to the rectal mucosa (Schlauth et al 1984). Sphincter function is preserved (Reynolds et al 1984). The carbon dioxide laser may also be used for peri-anal and anal disease with or without subsequent skin grafting. We have treated five women with extensive peri-anal disease involving the anal mucosa using the carbon dioxide laser with satisfactory results.

Other local destructive techniques. Cryosurgery has

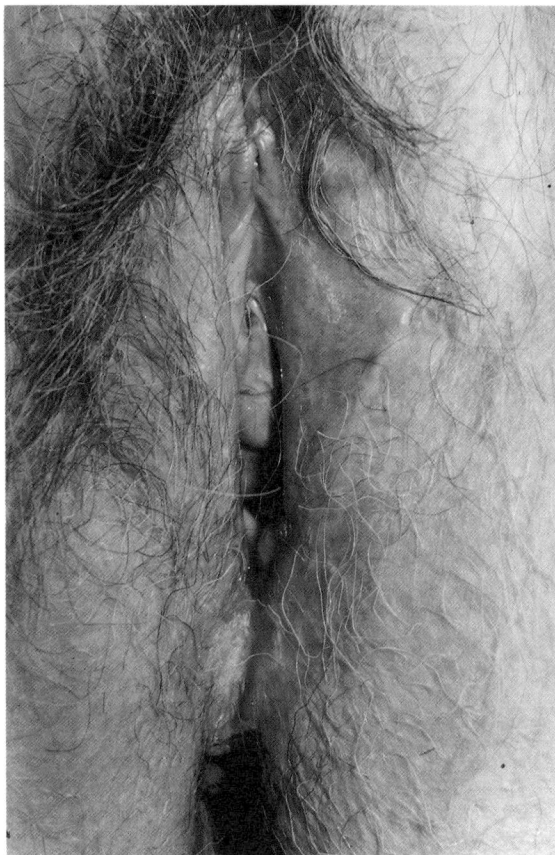

Fig. 11.9 Postoperative result following laser treatment.

been used with some success for small unifocal lesions (Forney et al 1977). Similarly, electrocoagulation diathermy has been used in the treatment of VIN. However, particularly with more extensive disease, the injury produces an ulcerated area, the healing of which is protracted and painful. Disease frequently persists after complete tissue repair. These techniques are thus rarely used.

Non-surgical techniques.

Topical 5-fluorouracil (5-FU). The first reports of using 5-FU cream for VIN were by Jansen et al in 1967 and were followed by those of Woodruff et al in 1973. Review of the literature since that time (Silman et al 1985) indicates the remission rate of VIN following treatment with topical 5-FU to be 30% with a further 10% showing improvement. The 60% failure rate for 5-FU contrasts with the 10% failure rate of laser destruction or wide local excision with clear excision margins.

Most authors agree that a 6-week course is required to achieve remission (Friedrich et al 1980). Ulceration occurs after about 2 weeks and this is associated with burning and pain. Large, confluent lesions develop into painful ulcerations and the associated discomfort leads to poor patient compliance. The keratinised skin of the lateral labia majora is particularly unfavourable for 5-FU. However, the poor results of treatment are largely due to the severe discomfort from chemo-inflammation, which inhibits the patient's ability to use enough 5-FU to achieve an adequate therapeutic effect.

2,4-dinitrochlorobenzene. Several authors have reported the use of topical dinitrochlorobenzene (Weintraub & Lagasse 1973) or dinitrofluorobenzene (DiSaia et al 1984) applied topically 2 weeks after systemic sensitisation of the patient with the same mitogen. Treatment again results in production of a necrotic, slowly healing ulcer associated with considerable discomfort. Such techniques are not widely used.

Invasive vulval neoplasia (squamous carcinoma)

Over the past two decades, the incidence of vulval cancer, which accounts for 5% of gynaecological malignancies, has increased (Green 1978, DiSaia et al 1984).

Delay in diagnosis and treatment of vulval cancer, due either to patients' reluctance to seek medical attention or to protracted medical treatment without definitive diagnosis or referral, remains an important clinical problem. Such delays were noted over 40 years ago by Taussig (1940) but Monaghan (1985) still reports delay in diagnosis of more than 24 months in 14% of a large personal series. Hacker et al (1981) reported a mean delay of 10 months with a range of 1–36 months.

Histological diagnosis of an adequate and representative biopsy is the basic component of assessment but thorough evaluation of the patient followed by accurate evaluation of the lesion are required for decision on management.

Evaluation of the patient

As carcinoma of the vulva most commonly affects elderly women, many patients have significant medical problems such as diabetes mellitus, hypertension, obesity, cardiovascular and respiratory disorders, blood dyscrasias and malignancy elsewhere. Thus, a careful general history of previous disease and treatment thereof, followed by thorough general examination, is essential to determine the patient's ability to withstand the rigors of radical surgery. The nutritional status of the elderly patient is also important and assessment by physician, anaesthetist and surgeon is required prior to therapeutic decisions being taken. However, in centres experienced in management of vulval cancer, such a team approach permits high operability rates in the order of 90 to 95%. This has been achieved with increased use of spinal and epidural anaesthesia.

Evaluation of the lesion

Frankly invasive vulval cancer usually presents little difficulty in diagnosis and may be readily confirmed by an adequate biopsy. However, early invasive disease, as with in situ carcinoma, is not easily distinguished from other vulval lesions. Suspicious areas appear as ulcers, tumours and pigmented or white epithelium.

Ulcerated lesions require investigation to exclude syphilis including dark-ground examination and serology. Neoplasia is confirmed by biopsy of the advancing edge of the ulcer. Vulval tumours are assessed by biopsy or excision. Areas of epithelial abnormality are best assessed using the magnified illumination of the colposcope after application of 5% acetic acid. This reveals abnormalities of blood vessel patterns, skin colour and skin contour, the common associates of early invasive disease. Colposcopically directed biopsy again permits more accurate diagnosis, having regard to the often large area of vulval skin to be screened. Careful assessment of the entire lower genital tract comprising cervix, vagina, vulva, perianal and anal region is necessary if vulval malignancy is suspected and several biopsies may be required with multifocal disease. Thus examination under anaesthesia is frequently preferred for pre-operative assessment if the patient is considered to be fit for anaesthesia.

Choice of treatment

After Taussig (1940) and Way (1948) reported very much improved survival rates for carcinoma of the vulva by using the en bloc dissection of radical vulvectomy with bilateral groin and deep pelvic lymphadenectomy, this operation became the mainstay of treatment in vulval malignancy. A corrected 5-year survival rate of over 90% for stage I and II disease is achieved using this operation. Hence deep pelvic lymphadenectomy was performed routinely for many years with radical vulvectomy and inguinal lymphadenectomy, irrespective of presence or absence of disease in the inguinal lymph nodes or the size of the vulval tumour. The deep pelvic node dissection, however, is associated with increased operative mortality and morbidity, delayed healing and prolonged hospitalisation, particularly in the elderly woman. Thus, in recent years, attempts have been made to individualise the treatment of vulval cancer, modifying the surgical approach to perform a less radical operation without decreasing survival.

It is now more common practice to limit the initial operation to radical vulvectomy with bilateral inguinal lymphadenectomy. Deep pelvic node dissection is performed only in those patients considered at high risk of pelvic node involvement and who are considered fit for more aggressive surgery. In certain specific circumstances, vulvectomy alone or wide local excision may be adequate and appropriate treatment. Further to decrease morbidity associated with groin lymphadenectomy, the dissection is occasionally performed through separate groin incisions (Hacker et al 1981), although the efficacy of this approach awaits appraisal.

The efforts to individualise the surgical approach to vulval cancer has required rationalisation of indications for bilateral inguinal node dissection and deep pelvic node dissection in addition to removal of the tumour. This has been based on consideration of four factors:

1. Stage of tumour.
2. Size of tumour.
3. Site of tumour and pattern of spread.
4. Depth of invasion.

(A further factor, histological differentiation, is considered on p. 284.)

The system of staging carcinoma of the vulva adopted by FIGO in 1970 is a non-operative method based on clinical assessment of tumour size, regional lymph node status and the presence of distant metastases (TNM system). However, this system is associated with unacceptably high errors in staging of disease, reaching 25%, largely due to inaccuracy in clinical detection of involved regional lymph nodes. Palpation of groin nodes is an unreliable method of assessment. In Monaghan's (1985) large series of 212 cases of vulval cancer, over 50% of patients with palpable groin lymph nodes had no histological evidence of disease in these nodes; conversely in over 50% of cases with involved groin nodes, these nodes were not clinically palpable prior to surgery.

The early promise of lymphangiography in diagnosis of involved groin nodes has not been fulfilled. Access to the groin lymphatic vessels and nodes is readily achieved; but small impalpable nodes filled with cancer do not permit entry of contrast, producing false negative results, and local fat deposits cause filling defects in nodes, producing false positive results. Fine-needle aspiration of suspicious nodes is of limited value, particularly with early metastatic disease. Groin node biopsy is fraught with risk due to the large number of nodes present over a wide area.

Thus, whilst involvement of groin lymph nodes is an important prognostic factor, reliable pre-operative assessment is often not possible. It is therefore unwise to decide upon operative approach to vulval cancer based on the clinical assessment of regional lymph node status unless there is extensive, apparent nodal involvement.

In 1980, Curry et al reported that in 191 patients, only nine (47%) had positive deep pelvic nodes and all nine patients had metastatic disease in the groin nodes, suggesting that deep pelvic nodes are not involved with metastatic disease when the inguinal nodes are clear of cancer. It is accepted that deep pelvic nodes will be positive in approximately 25% of cases with proved inguinal node metastases. Curry et al (1980) therefore recommended that if four or more groin nodes are involved at the time of operation, deep pelvic node dissection should be performed.

Whilst the FIGO classification defines tumours greater than 2 cm in diameter as representing a higher stage of disease, of greater value to the surgeon in determining appropriate therapy is the realisation that the larger the primary tumour, the greater is the risk of inguinal and pelvic node in-

volvement (Podratz et al 1982). Indeed, Monaghan & Hammond (1984), in a large series of over 150 groin and/or groin and pelvic node dissections, observed that only lesions greater than 4 cm in diameter were associated with deep pelvic node metastases. The authors recommend that deep pelvic node dissection be therefore reserved for vulval cancers greater than 4 cm in diameter, a clinical assessment readily made in the pre-operative examination.

In an endeavour to rationalise indications for radical surgery for vulval malignancy, it has been suggested that labial malignancies not involving midline structures such as clitoris, urethra, vagina, fourchette or peri-anal regions are at low risk of involvement of contralateral groin nodes. Hacker et al (1984) considered bilateral spread and contralateral spread alone from laterally placed tumours to be rare. They recommend that if the ipsilateral nodes are negative, contralateral node dissection is unnecessary. Thus in some centres labial cancers, particularly if small tumours, are managed by vulvectomy or even wide local excision with ipsilateral node dissection but preservation of contralateral nodes.

However, Monaghan (1985) describes a small but significant number of patients with small lateral tumours and bilateral lymph node involvement or contralateral spread alone. Thus, until more accurate means of assessment of groin node involvement are available and demonstrated to be reliable, radical vulvectomy with bilateral inguinal node dissection is the appropriate treatment of squamous vulval cancers less than 4 cm in diameter, regardless of position, providing the patient is fit for radical surgery. Techniques such as monoclonal radionucleotide labelling are currently being investigated as means of identifying involved nodes. There is no convincing evidence that deep pelvic node dissection should be routinely performed for vulval cancer arising from or involving the clitoris, unless there is clear evidence of groin node involvement or the tumour is greater than 4 cm in diameter.

Wide local excision is considered adequate treatment for stage 1A vulval carcinoma (Kneale 1984) without groin node dissection. Careful follow-up is mandatory and local recurrence must be anticipated, particularly in the patient at risk. All other cases of invasion greater than 1 mm depth should be managed by radical vulvectomy with bilateral groin node dissection if the patient is fit for surgery. No attempt should be made to distinguish between superficial and deep inguinal node systems (Zucker & Berkowitz 1985).

Conclusion

It is now generally accepted that the optimum basic management for vulval carcinoma is to perform a radical vulvectomy and bilateral groin node dissection. The bilateral groin node dissection should be dispensed with only if the depth of invasion of the carcinoma is less than 1 mm or if the patient is considered to be unfit for radical surgery. In these situations wide local excision of the tumour or vulvectomy alone may be performed with close and long term follow-up of the patient.

Unilateral cancers may be associated with contralateral groin node spread even if ipsilateral nodes are clear. Thus a bilateral en bloc inguinal node dissection is routinely performed with no attempt to distinguish between different anatomical levels of nodes.

Dissection of deep pelvic nodes is performed routinely only when the carcinoma is greater than 4 cm in diameter. If however the groin nodes are clearly extensively involved with disease on clinical examination, deep pelvic node dissection should be performed regardless of size of primary tumour, although, in this case, the vulval cancer is usually large. The deep pelvic nodes are not involved without groin node involvement but there is currently no reliable clinical assessment of groin node status as an indication to proceed to pelvic node dissection.

Surgical treatment

Invasive squamous cell carcinoma of the vulva, stage I, II and III, responds to correct surgical therapy so that the poor survival prior to 1950 is now replaced by an improved prognosis. The patient should be admitted to hospital at least 2 days prior to surgery for routine pre-operative preparation and assessment, management of incidental disease and intensive cleaning of the vulval region by antiseptic bathing.

Operative technique: lymphadenectomy.

The traditional skin incision for radical vulvectomy and bilateral groin node dissection, described by Way (1948), involved removal of a wide area of skin resulting in failure to achieve primary skin closure of the wound or skin apposition under considerable tension. This was associated with immobilisation, wound breakdown, increased morbidity and mortality. Monaghan's (1985) modification to the original 'butterfly incision' permits removal of the tumour with an adequate tumour-free margin but with minimal skin removal from the groin (Fig. 11.10). Primary closure is regularly achieved without tension. The patient is nursed prone with full movement in the postoperative period.

The skin incisions in the groin are undercut down to the aponeurosis of the external oblique muscle above the groin and to the fascia over the sartorius muscle which forms the lateral boundary of the femoral canal. The fascia is incised from the anterior superior iliac spine to the apex of the femoral triangle. This will now permit removal of the entire groin nodes en bloc. Haemostasis is meticulously secured in the extensive raw area beneath the skin flaps with particular attention to larger vessels to diminish the risk of secondary haemorrhage.

If a deep pelvic node dissection is indicated, the external and common iliac, hypogastric and obturator nodes are removed bilaterally using a retroperitoneal approach.

The abdomen is closed, reconstituting the fascial layers carefully to prevent hernia formation and without pressure on the femoral vessels. Groin skin closure is performed using interrupted sutures or skin staples. Continuous drainage using large diameter drains is mandatory, up to 250–300 ml of serosanguinous fluid collecting on each side per day.

Operative technique: vulvectomy.

The vulvectomy involves excising the carcinoma with a wide margin of normal skin, all dystrophic skin being removed with the specimen. If the tumour extends close to the urethra, it may be necessary to remove the distal 1 cm but this will not affect continence. Care is taken not to remove the sphincter ani or to enter the rectum. Occasionally, however, it is necessary to excise part of the vagina and the anus to achieve a tumour-free margin. The levator muscles may, if deficient, require plication to prevent a

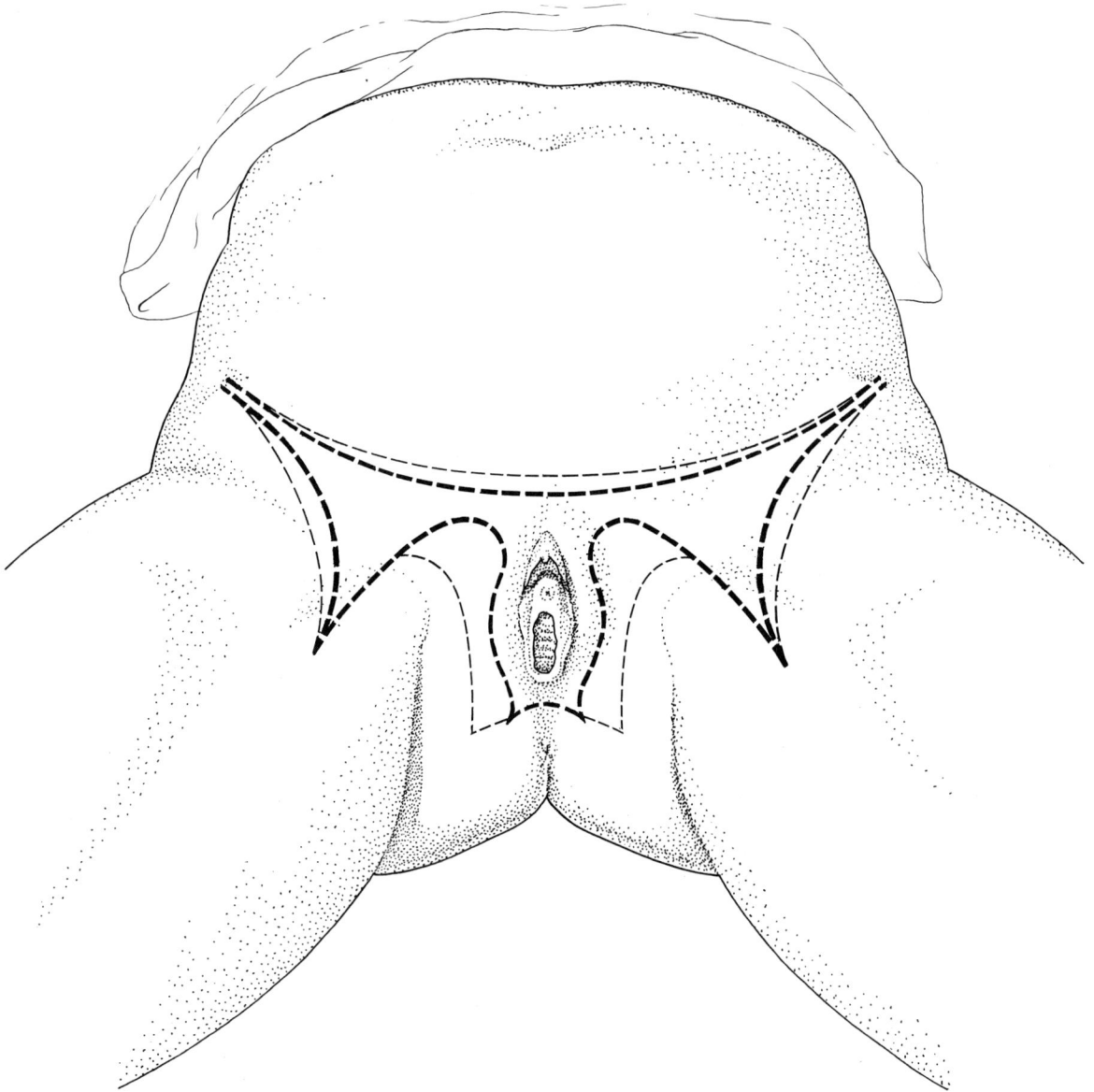

Fig. 11.10 Monaghan modification of the 'butterfly' skin incision for radical vulvectomy with bilateral groin node dissection.

rectocoele. Primary closure of the wounds is usually achieved. A soft drain may be placed in the base of the wound for 72 hours.

Postoperative care. Meticulous postoperative care is important. After removal of the epidural catheter (if inserted) at the end of the operation, the patient is started on subcutaneous heparin 5000 units b.d. for 10 days. The patient is not immobilised; thus leg exercises are taught and begun immediate-

ly. The patient is made to walk as soon as possible. Anti-embolic stockings are helpful until the patient is adequately mobile. This regime contributes to a very low incidence of thrombo-embolic disease in the postoperative period. Monaghan reports a 4% incidence of significant thrombo-embolic disease postoperatively but with no associated death.

The patient is given metronidazole, 1 g as a suppository, pre-operatively but prophylactic antibiotics are not used in the postoperative period as a routine. However, the patient is closely monitored for signs of systemic infection and appropriate antibiotics prescribed rapidly if such develop. Blood volume should be ascertained and corrected with the first 24 hours. Optimum nutrition must be maintained. An indwelling urethral or suprapubic catheter is maintained in situ on continuous drainage for at least 10 postoperative days to keep the vulva as dry as possible.

Complications. In the early series of Way (1978), the operative mortality approached 20%. However, with modification of surgical technique, closer attention to pre-operative assessment and postoperative monitoring and the development of centres experienced in the management of vulval cancer, the operative mortality has been reduced to 1% (Monaghan 1985). This has occurred although surgery is frequently performed on patients in the ninth and tenth decades of life, clearly with surprising safety.

The commonest complication of surgical treatment is wound breakdown and infection, encountered in about 50% of patients. However, by removing lesser amounts of skin and minimising the undermining of skin flaps, primary wound healing is achieved in the remaining 50% of patients. Infection and wound breakdown are decreased by suction drainage of wounds.

Lymphoedema of the lower extremities is another important complication, especially following both inguinal and deep pelvic node dissection. The incidence of this distressing complication is reported at between 13 and 65% of patients (Monaghan & Hammond 1984) but it can be reduced by routine use of custom-made elastic support stockings for 3 months to 1 year postoperatively while collateral lymph channels develop. Rutledge et al (1970) have advised low dose prophylactic antibiotic therapy in postlymphadenectomy patients to prevent streptococcal infection in the lower extremities, which may be associated with an acute toxic illness as well as dramatically increasing the incidence of significant chronic lymphoedema.

Lymphocysts may occur in the inguinal region following inguinal lymphadenectomy or more frequently in the pelvis following pelvic lymphadenectomy. These collections may at times be symptomatic and require drainage.

Urinary tract infection is a common postoperative complication, probably secondary to catheterisation. A suprapubic catheter may decrease this risk. Misdirection of urinary stream due to hooding or scarring of the urethral orifice, stress incontinence and development of cystocoele or rectocoele due to loss of support of the lower vagina are long term complications.

Removal of the vulva, particularly the clitoris, and the associated introital scarring and decreased mobility of perineal tissue can result in diminished sexual function, satisfaction and pleasure as well as causing significant dyspareunia at times. Alteration of body image associated with radical genital surgery is variable but patients must be adequately counselled pre-operatively and following surgery regarding possible psychosexual sequelae of treatment (p. 225). This is clearly of particular importance in the young patient. Satisfactory sexual function and response, pregnancy and vaginal delivery have been reported following radical surgery for vulval cancer.

Surgical treatment of metastatic vulval cancer

Patients presenting with stage IV squamous cell cancer of the vulva may still be treated surgically. Whilst cure of the disease is only occasionally achieved, more frequently the patient's quality of life may be improved, allowing her to live the remainder of her life without problems associated with an often large, fungating or ulcerated vulval tumour and associated nodal disease. Radical vulvectomy and groin node dissection, if the patient is fit for surgery, removes all local disease and, although the patient may die of the cancer, the mode of death will be improved. Fungating groin nodes should be removed en bloc with the vulva and pelvic node dissection performed. Negative pelvic nodes significantly improve prognosis.

If the vulval cancer has spread to pelvic organs, particularly bladder and rectum, removal at this stage requires an exenterative approach together with bilateral inguinal and pelvic lymphadenectomy. Krupp & Bohm (1978) report an increased operative mortality without improved 5-year survival for women in the eighth and later decades and thus exenteration vulvectomy is indicated in this group only if the patient is considered fit enough for and wishes such aggressive treatment. Extra-pelvic extension and distant metastases to bone, liver, kidney and skin are uncommon with vulval carcinoma and are considered contra-indications to pelvic exenteration. However, Way (1971) and Monaghan (1985) both report management of pubic arch metastases by resection of a segment of bone with the surgical specimen without impairing later ambulation.

Recurrent vulval carcinoma

Local or distant recurrence of vulval carcinoma occurs in up to 26% of treated cases (Podratz et al 1982), over 80% occurring in the first 2 years after surgery. Most recurrences are local and near the site of the primary lesion, occurring particularly if the primary tumour was large or if the lymph nodes were involved with metastatic disease. This high incidence of local recurrence demands close atten-tion to adequate surgical margins in resection of the primary tumour, although local recurrences occur even when margins are declared clear of disease. In many cases, local recurrence is successfully treated by wide local excision with adequate tumour-free margins. Radiotherapy may be indicated if adequate resection is not achieved but morbidity is then significantly increased. Recurrent local disease in groin nodes is difficult to treat; it usually requires radiotherapy but the prognosis is poor.

Prognosis with surgical treatment

Survival with carcinoma of the vulva is directly related to the extent of disease, that is, tumour size and presence or absence of nodal and other metastases, at the time of diagnosis and treatment. Whilst many elderly women treated for vulval cancer will succumb to intercurrent disease while tumour free, the corrected 5-year survival rate for carcinoma of the vulva when groin nodes are negative is over 90%. Many series report an overall corrected 5-year survival rate of 75% for all stages of vulval carcinoma (Monaghan 1985). If groin nodes are involved with disease, the corrected 5-year survival is between 30 and 50%, but if deep pelvic nodes are involved, 5-year survival falls to less than 20%. These figures emphasise the importance of prompt diagnosis and adequate therapy.

Non-surgical techniques

Radiotherapy

Despite recent improvements in methods of delivering irradiation such as cobalt-60 and linear accelerators, the role of radiotherapy in treatment of vulval cancer remains limited. The results have been poor, with as low as 10% 3-year survival (Lifshitz et al 1982). The tumour itself is relatively insensitive to radiotherapy and the tumour bed is extremely radiosensitive. The collateral circulation of the vulval skin is poor and thus serious complications, such as severe vulvitis, radiation necrosis, fistula, urethral obstruction and death, range in incidence from 8 to 50%. The frequent presence of vulval dermatoses (especially atrophic lesions) in association with malignant disease makes the lesion even less suitable for irradiation.

Modern radiation techniques produce less damage to a radiosensitive skin; thus aggressive radiotherapy may enhance survival if the patient is unsuitable for surgery or if appropriate surgical expertise is not available. If radiotherapy is used as the sole therapeutic modality, irradiation of regional lymph nodes is mandatory. Radiotherapy is also used in some centres in lesser dosage to reduce the size of a larger tumour mass to facilitate a definitive surgical procedure. It is also used for recurrent disease and as palliative treatment of inoperable node involvement.

Verrucous carcinoma of the vulva should never be irradiated. This locally invasive and indolent cancer is insensitive to radiotherapy and can be stimulated to rapid dissemination by irradiation et (Kraus & Perez-Mesa 1966).

Chemotherapy

Five-year survival following surgical treatment of vulval cancer falls significantly with nodal metastases. Postoperative radiotherapy in these patients is of limited value. Thus, chemotherapy has been used experimentally to improve the poor prognosis for more advanced disease. Deppe et al (1979) described significant tumour responses in regimens with both bleomycin and methotrexate but the treatment was not curative. Advanced vulval carcinomas including tumours involving the anus initially considered inoperable have been successfully treated with 5-fluorouracil plus mitomycin C, achieving remission and subsequent operability (Bruchner et al 1979, Kalva et al 1981). However, at present, there is no single agent or combination chemotherapeutic regime to treat vulval cancer adequately and its use remains essentially experimental.

Conclusion. The improved prognosis for carcinoma of the vulva over the past 3 decades has been the result of improved surgical skills, modified surgical technique, thorough pre-operative assessment and meticulous postoperative care. These factors have evolved against the background of emergence of specialised units with facilities and skills for radical treatment of malignant disease in high risk patients. The poorer prognosis associated with advanced disease, particularly with lymph node involvement, underlies the need for a high index of suspicion in the at-risk patient to enable early diagnosis and prompt, effective therapy.

Management of some other forms of vulval neoplasia

Verrucous carcinoma

Radiotherapy is contra-indicated and excision is the treatment of choice (p. 285); if the tumour is large, wide local excision may in fact entail complete excision of the vulva (simple vulvectomy).

Rare variants of epithelial tumours (pp. 283, 285, 289)

Treatment for adenosquamous carcinoma and adenocarcinoma is on similar lines to that of squamous carcinoma. Chemotherapy in addition to surgery may be indicated in spindle-cell carcinoma, adenoid squamous carcinoma and Merkel cell tumour.

Basal cell carcinoma

Except for the rare metastasising lesions (p. 288) the tumour is invasive only locally and then slowly; and the preferred treatment is wide local excision.

Paget's disease of the vulva

Paget's disease of the vulva usually remains as an intraepithelial disease but is associated with an underlying carcinoma of the vulva or adjacent organ in up to 30 per cent of cases. Wide local excision is usually the recommended treatment with careful histological examination of the surgical specimen. Particular attention should be paid to the resection margins as Paget's disease can extend laterally beyond the clinical margin and is often multicentric (Gunn & Gallager 1980). Frozen sections from the surgical margins may indicate whether excision is complete (Stacy et al 1986). The Mohs technique of micrographic surgery may be valuable (Mohs & Blanchaid 1979). Recurrence is managed usually by further wide local excision, Woodruff et al (1977) reporting up to 10 excisions on one patient with recurrent Paget's disease over a 23 year period. Extensive disease is seen as an indication for vulvectomy as the treatment of choice, particularly if early invasive disease is confirmed or suspected. Topical bleomycin has also been recommended as effective therapy for Paget's disease particularly for recurrent disease (Watring 1978). However excision with careful histological examination of the surgical specimen is the recommended approach.

Occasionally Paget's disease may present as a frank invasive cancer in which case radical vulvectomy, usually with bilateral groin dissection, is indicated.

Melanoma

The only hope of cure is early diagnosis and sufficiently radical surgery. Depth of invasion and metastatic disease in lymph nodes or distant organs are important factors influencing management. The management is under continuous review (p. 301) but radical vulvectomy with bilateral groin dissection is the usual approach. Chemotherapy has been used to treat metastatic disease but does not significantly improve outcome.

Adnexal tumours, tumours of the urethra

Details of appropriate treatments are discussed on the relevant pages of Chapter 10.

Metastases from other sites

Treatment is that appropriate for metastatic spread of the primary cancer.

Sarcoma and other non-epithelial and mixed tumours

Treatment must be individualised but radical vulvectomy with bilateral node dissection is the usual surgical approach. The problem is discussed in the light of available knowledge for each type in Chapter 9.

SURGERY IN NON-NEOPLASTIC CONDITIONS OF THE VULVA

Surgery for congenital vulval abnormalities

Hypertrophy of the labia minora—Labioplasty

One labium minus or both may be hypertrophied. The diagnosis of this congenital abnormality is usually made after puberty when the patient presents complaining of a vulval protrusion. Occasionally, hypertrophy of the labia minora may be associated with local irritation, discomfort in walking or sitting and problems with personal hygiene. Chafing, oedema and ulceration may occur particularly with exercise. Sexual intercourse may at times be impaired.

No treatment other than reassurance and attention to hygiene is usually necessary. However, if symptoms persist despite conservative measures, reduction labioplasty is a simple technique producing excellent results, and is described in full by Hodgkinson & Hait (1984).

Surgical management of the absent vagina

Congenital absence of the vagina is a rare abnormality. The diagnosis is usually made in adolescence when the commonest presenting symptom is primary amenorrhoea; there is a commonly associated congenital absence of the uterus. The ovaries are usually present and the patient is of normal female build and secondary sexual characteristics. The vulva looks normal though the vagina is absent or short (Fig. 11.11). Rectal examination fails to reveal either an upper vaginal compartment distended with menstruum or, in most cases, a uterus.

Before surgical construction of an artifical vagina is contemplated, karyotyping of the patient should be performed. If an XY complement of chromosomes is detected, then a diagnosis of intersex is made and the management is more complex. In an

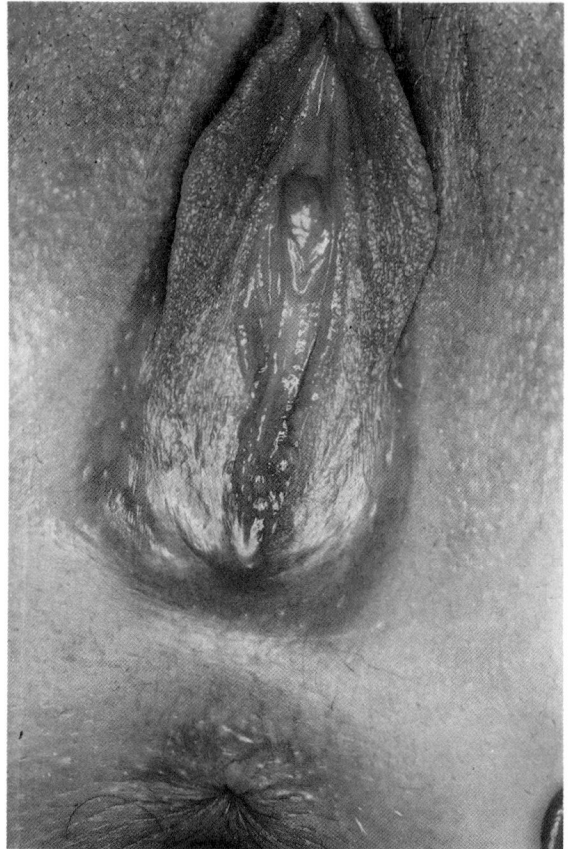

Fig. 11.11 Vulva in patient with absent vagina

XX patient, an intravenous pyelogram is desirable to exclude associated sexual anomalies such as duplication and congenital absence of a kidney. Laparoscopic examination to assess pelvic organs is a useful investigation which may convert clinical suspicion into diagnostic certainty in relation to other congenital abnormalities. The psychological status and needs of the patient must also be sympathetically assessed.

Construction of an artificial vagina in such cases may then be desirable. A short blind vagina may be of sufficient capacity to permit coital penetration and regular intercourse may establish an adequate, functional vagina. Dewhurst (1980) has recommended the use of vaginal dilators to increase the length of this lower pouch in well-motivated women.

An earlier surgical approach to construction of an artificial vagina (McIndoe & Bannister 1938)

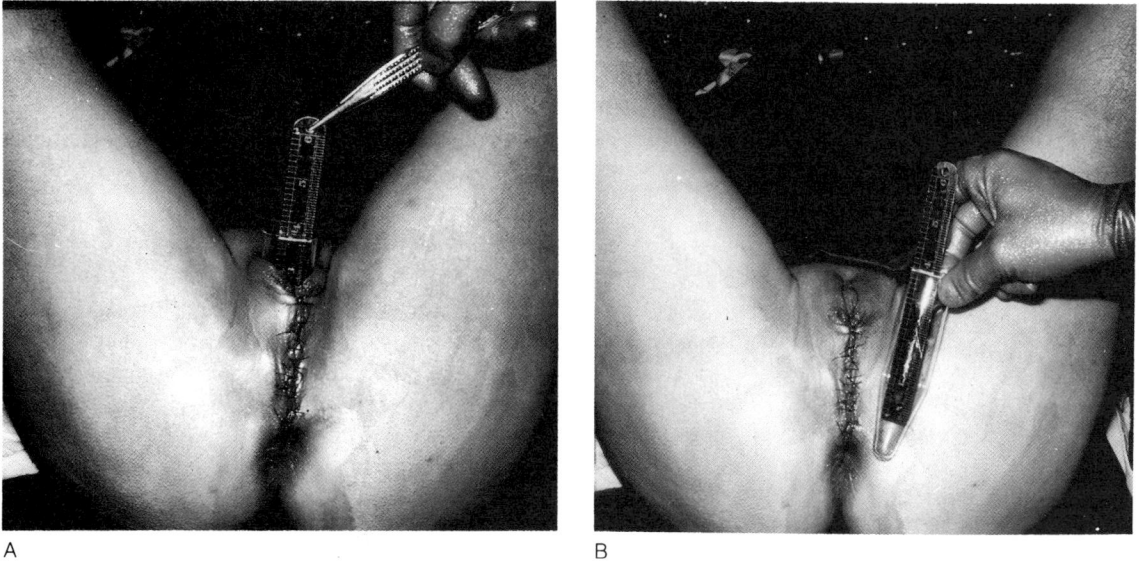

A   B

Fig. 11.12 (a and b) Creation of artificial vagina (vulvovaginoplasty).

was to create a cavity between the bladder and bowel at the site which the natural vagina would occupy. The cavity was lined with a split graft from the thigh, applied on a plastic mould. This technique was commonly used but was associated with considerable postoperative discomfort as well as with a high risk of graft breakdown and stenosis. This technique has since been improved by using amnion to cover the new vaginal wall (Ashworth et al 1986) and results of this procedure are encouraging.

The operation of vulvovaginoplasty was introduced by Williams (1964) and has been modified and improved. An artificial vagina is produced by surgically apposing the labia majora to produce an enclosed cavity. A skin graft is not necessary (Figs. 11.12 a and b). Prominent labia minora may require removal prior to forming the pouch as the artificial vagina may otherwise be occupied by the enfolded nymphae. The operation is simple and quick. It can be performed on younger, teenage unmarried girls preparing them physically and psychologically for normal coital relationships. The functional result is good (Fig. 11.13) and disuse does not result in contraction. Regular use of vaginal dilators is not necessary and the development of granulation tissue is not a problem. The first two approaches were reviewed by Feroze et al (1975) and vulvovaginoplasty was considered the prefer-

able surgical approach in construction of an artificial vagina, by reason of its surgical simplicity and fewer complications.

Surgical procedures for the whole range of congenital abnormalities are considered in detail by Dewhurst (1980).

Management of injuries to the vulva

Severe laceration injuries

Ice packs are useful to reduce oedema and the pelvis should be elevated as far as possible; an indwelling Foley catheter should be in situ.

Management also includes the treatment of shock, and fluid replacement as necessary. Examination under general anaesthetic may be required; blood clot is cleared from the area and the extent of the damage is ascertained. Haemostasis should be meticulously secured. It is unwise to insert tight stitches to control venous oozing as they will only result in postoperative pain and eventual infection and sloughing of tissue. If oozing of blood continues some degree of infection must be anticipated and antibiotics are given for 7 days.

Haemorrhage from the hymen

This is the commonest coital accident, the tear usually resulting from a first attempt at coitus.

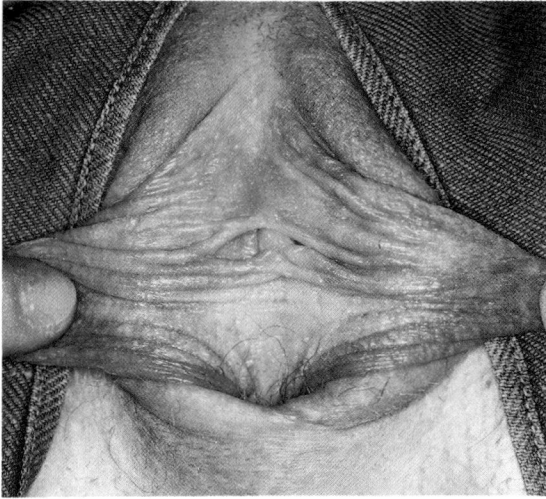

Fig. 11.13 Postoperative result of vulvovaginoplasty.

Under a general anaesthetic obvious small arterial bleeding is readily stopped with a haemostatic suture. Where necessary radial incision and dilatation of the hymen can be carried out.

Surgery for contraction of vaginal introitus

There are two types of permanent contraction of the vaginal introitus. One follows badly performed colpoperineorrhaphy operations which may also have become infected postoperatively. The perineal closure has generally been carried too far forward and forms a narrow shelf of fibrous tissue which obstructs penetration. The superficial perineal muscles may also have been built up into an obstructive barrier. Inside the narrowed introitus the vagina is of adequate capacity thanks to the abundance of loosely applied vaginal mucosa at that level. In most cases there is no actual shortage of skin and treatment is directed towards correcting the artificially produced defect by a simple operation of the Fenton type.

The second type of introital narrowing is consequent upon long-standing atrophic changes in the vulval skin and is usually seen in older women. The skin is thin, chronically inflamed and inelastic; the underlying muscle is of poor tone so that the introitus is narrow and non-distensible. Since the skin of the vaginal wall and particularly the posterior wall is poorly oestrogenised and atrophic, the narrowing is continued into the lower vagina. There is an absolute shortage of skin, and enlargement of the introitus can only be achieved by bringing in a flap of normal thickness healthy skin by a vaginoplasty type of procedure.

Fenton's operation

The term Fenton's operation tends to be applied to any operation where the introital opening is increased by making a vertical incision in the perineum and suturing it horizontally. Fenton's operation, however, was designed to deal with more than superficial contraction, and necessitates division of the overtight superficial perineal muscles in the perineal body so that they fall laterally. This is the step which increases the introital opening. The operation is completed by tailoring the skin to the new perineal surface and suturing it transversely.

Vaginoplasty

When there is not only a shortage of skin but it is thin and atrophic with poor blood supply and loss of subcutaneous areolar tissue, healthy unaffected full thickness skin is required to enlarge the contracted introitus and lower vagina and is obtained from the lateral aspect of the labium majus and adjacent thigh. The principle of the operation is to split the posterior vaginal wall longitudinally in its lower half, to undermine and free the skin edges until the introitus and lumen are of adequate size and then to 'swing in' or rotate the graft to make up the defect posteriorly. The graft is triangular in shape and is not detached distally at its base so that there is little fear of necrosis. It is carefully sutured in position and lightly supported in its new site by a vaginal pack which is retained for 24 hours postoperatively. A more detailed description has been given by Lees & Singer (1982). Paniel et al 1984, 1986 have devised a procedure which utilises vaginal mucosa rather than skin. A somewhat similar operation has been advocated to remove minor vestibular glands. Ashworth et al (1986) have achieved satisfactory functional results using amnion as a graft.

Surgery of Bartholin's gland and duct

Cysts

Cysts of Bartholin's gland and of its duct may be infective or non-infective in origin. The ducts of Bartholin's gland are situated in a position where they are vulnerable to infection and to trauma. Chronic inflammation, particularly due to recurrent infection, may result in obstruction of the duct and cyst formation. Similarly trauma, particularly associated with parturition, for example with a lateral episiotomy not originating in the midline, may cause scarring and distortion of the duct, leading to cyst formation. The clinical appearance is of an enlargement in the lateral part of the posterior fourchette. The edge of the labium minus may be raised over the swelling, appearing to bisect it. The cyst is tender, liable to trauma in walking and even sitting and frequently flares up to form an abscess.

Abscesses

Acute Bartholin's abscess is usually due to infection of both gland and duct by gram negative coliform bacteria but *Neisseria gonorrhoeae* and *Staphylococcus aureus* may also be responsible. There is frequently a pre-existing Bartholin's cyst which becomes secondarily infected. The patient develops an acutely painful and injected Bartholin's abscess involving both gland and duct. The natural history of the abscess is spontaneous discharge with relief from pain and swelling. However, the condition may recur several months later, running an identical course, and this may be repeated several times. Antibiotic therapy has a minimal effect on the natural history of the Bartholin's abscess.

Surgical treatment

Incision and drainage of an acute Bartholin's abscess, or an abscess supervening on a cyst, will, as with spontaneous discharge, often result in recurrence. Such lesions should be incised and marsupialised. In marsupialisation, the edges of the vestibular incision over the swelling are sutured to an underlying incision in the cyst wall. The operation is simple and takes only a few minutes. It may be performed under local or general anaesthetic and

there should be minimal bleeding. Haematomata should not occur. The procedure can be undertaken during the acute inflammatory stage and gland function with production of secretion often returns to normal. Recurrence remains a problem but, if the roof of the cyst or abscess is largely excised to leave what is in effect a basal hemisphere, it must be uncommon. The secret of success is in making an adequate incision of the cyst wall. Kaufman (1981) reviewed this subject.

An alternative to surgical marsupialisation is the formation of a fistula by insertion of a spinal catheter with an inflatable bulb at the distal end into the Bartholin's duct. The catheter is retained in situ over a period of a few weeks and a fistulous track forms around it. This procedure was described by Word in 1968. However, it has not gained widespread popularity as a therapeutic approach.

Non-infected Bartholin's cysts are also usually managed by marsupialisation. However, failure of a previous marsupialisation operation or chronic Bartholinitis with formation of a smaller, discrete cyst may be treated by excision of the Bartholin's duct and gland. This operation has no application in the presence of acute infection. To avoid significant bleeding, the plane of cleavage in dissection should be obtained and maintained by directing the scalpel against the gland itself. The enucleated cavity must be carefully obliterated in layers by fine sutures with fastidious attention to haemostasis. The patient should remain in hospital largely at rest for a few days. Hurried or careless surgery or premature return to activity will bring certain retribution in the form of bleeding, haematomata and infection.

Neoplasia

In determining the surgical approach to a Bartholin's gland tumour, the unlikely possibility of neoplasm rather than inflammation should not be forgotten. Such an occurrence should be suspected in an elderly patient or in a younger woman if she has repeated problems. The tumour presents as a hard, indurated swelling in the region of Bartholin's gland. Ulceration frequently occurs. Treatment is as for carcinoma of the vulva, with radical vulvectomy and bilateral inguinal lymphadenectomy the mainstay of treatment.

354   THE VULVA

REFERENCES

Andreasson, B, Bock J E, Visfeldt J 1982 Prognostic role of histology in squamous cell carcinoma in the vulvar region. Gynecologic Oncology 14: 373–381

Ashworth M F, Morton R E, Dewhurst J, Lilford R J, Bates R G 1986 Vaginoplasty using amnion. Obstetrics and Gynecology 67: 443–446

Baggish M S, Dorsey J H 1981 CO_2 laser for treatment of vulvar carcinoma-in-situ. Obstetrics and Gynecology 57: 371

Bergeron C, Ferenczy A, Shah K V, Naghashfar Z 1987 Multicentric human papillomavirus infections of the female genital tract: correlation of viral types with abnormal mitotic figures, colposcopic presentation and location. Obstetrics and Gynecology 69: 736–742

Bernstein S G, Kovacs B R, Townsend D E, Morrow C P 1983 Vulvar intraepithelial neoplasia. Journal of Clinical Pathology 37: 1201–1211

Boutselis I G 1972 Intraepithelial carcinoma of the vulva. Am Journal of Obstetrics and Gynecology 113: 433

Bruchner H W, Spigelman M K et al 1979 Carcinoma of the anus treated with a combination of radiotherapy and chemotherapy. Cancer Treatment Reports 63: 395–398

Buscema J, Woodruff J D, Parmley T H, Genadry R 1980 Carcinoma in situ of the vulva. Obstetrics and Gynecology 55: 225–230

Campion M J, 1987 Néoplasie intraépithéliales de la vulve (VIN). Médicine et Hygiene 45: 1325–1329

Campion M J, Clarkson P K, McCance D J 1985 Squamous neoplasia of the cervix in relation to other genital tract neoplasia. In: Clinics in Obstetrics and Gynaecology, Vol. 12, no. 1 W B Saunders, London, p 265

Campion M J, Singer A 1987 Vulval intraepithelial neoplasia: a clinical review. Genito-urinary Medicine 63: 147–152

Campion M J, Clarkson P K, McCance D J 1985 Squamous neoplasia of the cervix in relation to other genital tract neoplasia. In: Clinics in Obstetrics and Gynaecology, Vol. 12, no. 1 W B Saunders, London, p 265

Collins C G, Hansen L H, Theriot E 1966 A Clinical stain for use in selecting biopsy sites in patients with vulvar disease. Obstetrics and Gynecology 28: 158

Collins C G, Roman-Lopez J J, Lee, F Y L 1970 Intraepithelial carcinoma of the vulva. American Journal of Obstetrics and Gynecology 108: 1187

Curry S L, Wharton J T, Rutledge F N 1980 Positive lymph nodes in vulvar squamous carcinoma. Gynecologic Oncology 9: 63–67

Deppe G, Cohen C J, Burchner H W 1979 Chemotherapy of squamous cell carcinoma of the vulva; a review. Gynecologic Oncology 7: 345–348

Dewhurst C D 1980 Practical pediatric and adolescent gynecology. Marcel Dekker, New York

DiSaia P J, Rich W M 1981 Surgical Approach to multifocal carcinoma in situ of the vulva. American Journal of Obstetrics and Gynecology 140: 136

DiSaia P J, Morrow G P, Townsend D E 1984 Synopsis of Gynecologic Oncology. New York, Wiley

Feroze R M, Dewhurst C J, Wepley G A C 1975 Vaginoplasty at The Chelsea Hospital for Women: a comparison of two techniques. British Journal of Obstetrics and Gynaecology 82: 536

Forney J P, Morrow C P, Townsend D E, DiSaia P J 1977 Management of carcinoma in situ of the vulva. American Journal of Obstetrics and Gynecology 127: 801

Franklin E W, Rutledge F D 1972 Epidemiology of epidermoid carcinoma of the vulva. Obstetrics and Gynecology 39: 165–72

Friedrich E G, Wilkinson E J, Fu Y S 1980 Carcinoma in situ of the vulva: a continuing challenge. American Journal of Obstetrics and Gynecology 136: 880

Jones R W, McLean M R 1986 Carcinoma in situ of the vulva: a review of thirty one treated and five untreated cases. Obstetrics and Gynecology 68: 499–503

Gardiner S H, Stout F G, Arbogast J L, Huber C P 1953 Intraepithelial carcinoma of the vulva. American Journal of Obstetrics and Gynecology 65: 539

Green T H 1978 Carcinoma of the vulva, a reassessment. Obstetrics and Gynecology 52: 426

Hacker N F, Leuchter R S, Berek J S, Castaldo T W, Lagasse L D 1981 Radical vulvectomy and bilateral inguinal lymphadenectomy through separate groin incisions. Obstetrics and Gynecology 58: 574–9

Lees D H, Singer A 1980 Colour Atlas of Gynaecological Surgery. Wolfe Medical, London, Vol 4, p 22

Lees D H, Singer A 1982 Vaginal surgery for Congenital Acquired Abnormalities. Clinical Obstetrics and Gynaecology 25, 4: 883

Lifshitz F, Savage J E, Yates S J, Buchsbaum H J 1982 Primary epidermoid carcinoma of the vulva. Surgery in Gynecology and Obstetrics 155: 59–61

McCance D J, Clarkson P K, Walker P J, Singer a 1985 Human papillomavirus DNA sequences in multicentric lower genital tract neoplasia. British Journal of Obstetrics and Gynaecology

McIndoe A H, Bannister J B 1938 Operation for cure of congenital absence of the vagina. Journal of Obstetrics and Gynaecology of the British Empire 45: 490–494

Mene A, Buckley H C 1985 Involvement of the vulval skin appendages by intraepithelial neoplasia. British Journal of Obstetrics and Gynaecology 92: 634–638

Monaghan J M 1985 The management of carcinoma of the vulva. In: Shepherd J H, Monaghan J M (eds) Clinical Gynaecological Oncology. Blackwell, Oxford

Monaghan J M, Hammond I G 1984 Pelvic node dissection in treatment of vulval carcinoma—is it necessary? British Journal of Obstetrics and Gynaecology 91: 270–4

Podratz K C, Symonds R E, Taylor W F 1982 Carcinoma of the vulva: analysis of treatment failures. American Journal of Obstetrics and Gynecology 143: 340–351

Reid R 1985 Superficial laser vulvectomy. III. A new surgical technique for appendage conserving ablation of refractory condylomas and vulvar intraepithelial neoplasia. American Journal of Obstetrics and Gynecology 152: 504–509

Reid R, Elfont E A, Zirkin R M, Fuller T A 1985 Superficial laser vulvectomy. II. The anatomic and biophysical principles permitting accurate control over the depth of dermal destruction with the carbon dioxide laser. American Journal of Obstetrics and Gynecology

Rettenmaier M A, Berman M C, DiSaia P J 1987 Skinning vulvectomy for the treatment of multifocal vulval intraepithelial neoplasia. Obstetrics and Gynecology 69: 247–250

Reynolds, V H, Madden J J, Franlin J D 1984 Preservation of anal function after fetal excision of the anal mucosa for Bowen's disease. Annals of Surgery 119/563–568

Rutledge F, Sinclair M 1968 Treatment of intraepithelial carcinoma of the vulva by skin excision and graft. American Journal of Obstetrics and Gynecology 102: 806

Rutledge F, Smith J P, Franklin E K 1970 Carcinoma of the

vulva. American Journal of Obstetrics and Gynecology 106: 1117

Schlaerth J B, Marrow C P, Nalick R H, Gaddis O 1984 Anal involvement by carcinoma-in-situ of the Perineum in women. Obstetrics and Gynecology 64: 406–411

Silman F H, Sedlis A, Boyce J G 1985 A review of lower genital intraepithelial neoplasia and the use of topical 5-Fluorouracil. Obstetric and Gynecologic Survey 40(4): 190–220

Stacy D, Burrell M O, Franklin E W 1986 Extramammary Paget's disease of the vulva and anus: use of intraoperative frozen-section margins. American Journal of Obstetrics and Gynecology 155: 519–523

Taussig F J 1940 Cancer of the vulva: an analysis of 155 cases (1911–1940). American Journal of Obstetrics and Gynecology 40: 764–79

Townsend D E, Levine R V, Richart R M, Crum C P, Petrilli E S 1982 Management of vulvar intraepithelial neoplasia by carbon dioxide laser. Obstetrics and Gynecology 60: 49–52

Watring W G 1978 Treatment of concurrent Pagets' disease of the vulva with topical bleomycin. Cancer 41: 10–14

Way S 1948 The anatomy of the lymphatic drainage of the vulva and its influence on radical operation for carcinoma. Annals of The Royal College of Surgeons of England

Way S 1971 Carcinoma of the vulva. In: Deeley T J (ed) Modern Radiotherapy: Gynaecological Cancer. Butterworths, London. pp 203–213

Way S 1978 The surgery of vulvar carcinoma: an appraisal. Clinical Obstetrics and Gynecology 5(3): 623

Way S 1984 Results of a planned attack on carcinoma of the vulva. British Medical Journal 2: 780

Weintraub I, Lagasse L D 1973 Reversibility of vulvar atypia by DNCB-induced delayed hypersensitivity. Obstetrics and Gynecology 41: 195

Williams E A 1964 Congenital absence of the vagina: a simple operation for its relief. Journal of Obstetrics and Gynaecology of the British Commonwealth 71: 511–516

Williams E A 1976 Utero-vaginal aginesir. Annals of the Royal College of Surgeons of England 58: 266–277

Woodruff J D, Julian C, Pinay T, Mermut S, Katayama P 1973 The contemporary challenge of carcinoma-in-situ fo the vulva. American Journal of Obstetrics and Gynecology 115: 677

Word B 1968 Office treatment of cyst and abscess of Bartholin's gland duct. Southern Medical Journal 61: 514–518

Wright V C, Davies E 1987 Laser surgery for vulvar intraepithelial neoplasia: principles and results. American Journal of Obstetrics and Gynecology, 152: 374–378

Zucker P K, Berkowitz R S 1985 The issue of microinvasive squamous cell carcinoma of the vulva: an evaluation of criteria of diagnosis and methods of therapy. Obstetrics and Gynecologic Survey 40(3): 136–143

Index

The Vulva

Professor. W. Thompson
Dept O + G.